Quality of Life in Asia

Volume 17

This series, the first of its kind, examines both the objective and subjective dimensions of life quality in Asia, especially East Asia. It unravels and compares the contours, dynamics and patterns of building nations by offering innovative works that discuss basic and applied research and emphasizing inter- and multi-disciplinary approaches to the various domains of life quality. The series appeals to a variety of fields in humanities, social sciences and other professional disciplines. Asia is the largest, most populous continent on Earth, and it is home to the world's most dynamic region, East Asia. In the past three decades, East Asia has been the most successful region in the world in expanding its economies and integrating them into the global economy, offering lessons on how poor countries, even with limited natural resources, can achieve rapid economic development. Yet while scholars and policymakers have focused on why East Asia has prospered, little has been written on how its economic expansion has affected the quality of life of its citizens. This series publish several volumes a year, either single or multiple-authored monographs or collections of essays.

Daniel T. L. Shek

Promoting Holistic Development in University Students

Springer

Daniel T. L. Shek
Department of Applied Social Sciences
The Hong Kong Polytechnic University
Hung Hom, Kowloon, Hong Kong

ISSN 2211-0550 ISSN 2211-0569 (electronic)
Quality of Life in Asia
ISBN 978-981-96-0250-6 ISBN 978-981-96-0251-3 (eBook)
https://doi.org/10.1007/978-981-96-0251-3

This Springer imprint is published by the registered company Springer Nature Singapore Pte Ltd.
The registered company address is: 152 Beach Road, #21-01/04 Gateway East, Singapore 189721, Singapore

This book is dedicated to:

God who has abided, provided and guided my life;
My mother and Ruth who are the anchors of my family of origin;
Jannifer who has supported me and the children in a loving and gentle manner;
Moses and Esther who have taught me about adolescence and emerging adulthood.

Foreword

The Hong Kong Polytechnic University (PolyU) aspires to be an innovative world-class university with a strong sense of social responsibility. We are committed to pursuing excellence in education, research and knowledge transfer for the benefit of Hong Kong, the Nation and the world. By doing so, we live up to our motto, *"To learn and to apply, for the benefit of mankind"*.

Our educational philosophy is that students should embody both competence and virtue, with an emphasis on virtue. Indeed, we strive to nurture future professionals and leaders committed to the betterment of society. To cultivate a sense of social responsibility among students, one of our key initiatives is that undergraduate students have to pass one Service-Learning subject as a graduation requirement, which provides them with real-world experience in meeting societal needs. To promote holistic education and whole-person development, our General Education curriculum also requires undergraduate students to take a leadership subject which covers transversal skills, learn to learn competences, academic integrity, and law-abiding leadership. Different departments are working hard to achieve these institutional learning outcomes. The Leadership Education and Development (LEAD) programme of the Department of Applied Social Sciences under the leadership of Professor Daniel Shek is a very good exemplification of this concerted effort.

Hence, it is with great pleasure that I present this book about four innovative LEAD subjects developed at PolyU. These include two leadership subjects and two Service-Learning subjects. For the leadership subjects, "Tomorrow's Leaders" is offered to all PolyU students (except students of the Faculty of Business) and focuses on twenty-first century skills and holistic youth development. For the subject entitled "Service Leadership", it is a timely and relevant subject responding to the growing global service economy and nurtures the competence, character and care (3Cs) of students. It is also an outcome of the collaboration between Professor Shek and the late Dr Po Chung, Co-founder of DHL International. Professor Shek has also facilitated, co-developed and supervised two Service-Learning subjects, including one on the promotion of children and adolescent development and another one on the application of Service Leadership theory and concepts to Service-Learning contexts.

These subjects have many innovative and unique features. First, they embrace the philosophy that "every student can shine and thrive". Second, they cover soft skills that are much needed in our VUCA (volatile, uncertain, complex and ambiguous) world. Third, they adopt experiential, collaborative and reflective learning strategies. Fourth, they utilize different strategies to evaluate the impact of the subjects on student outcomes. Fifth, they promote a scholarship of teaching and learning, with wide dissemination of teaching experiences and student outcomes. Sixth, the subjects are making a real impact in Mainland China and Hong Kong. Finally, these subjects have received many prestigious teaching awards, which is impressive in the higher education sector in Hong Kong. These include five QS Reimagine Education Awards (two Gold Awards, one Silver Award and two Bronze Awards) and a University Grants Committee Teaching Award.

The publication of this book during the 2024/25 academic year is particularly meaningful since the year 2024 marked the 30th anniversary of PolyU achieving full university status, a major milestone in our institution's history. On behalf of the PolyU community, I would like to commend Professor Shek for his significant contribution via this book to the promotion of holistic development in the higher education sector both within and beyond Hong Kong.

President, The Hong Kong Polytechnic University — Jin-Guang Teng

Preface

Writing an authored book is a herculean task. Besides, compared with articles in Q1 or Q2 journals, books may not be formally and seriously counted as reputable publications. As such, many colleagues are not interested in writing an authored book. Instead, they may concentrate their effort on writing ten papers in Q1 journals. Hence, why did I decide to write this authored book, which has taken us more than two years?

There are several reasons why I decided to write this book. First, there are growing developmental issues among university students, such as mental health problems and moral issues (e.g., plagiarism, egocentrism, and materialism). Hence, many stakeholders, including educators, policymakers, parents, and university students, have asked one crucial question, "How can we promote the well-being and holistic development of university students?" In particular, with the growing emphasis on technology (such as artificial intelligence) as well as entrepreneurship in undergraduate education, there is a strong need to rethink the nature of holistic development in university students as well as the way to nurture students to have a better quality of life as well as holistic development.

The second reason for writing this book is to provide an opportunity for colleagues to reflect on the institutional learning outcomes and desired graduate attributes that should be cherished in university education. Typically, university education focuses on the cultivation of cognitive or intellectual skills (such as computational and analytical skills), which cannot be regarded as unreasonable. However, with the growing complexity of the contemporary world, there is a call to cultivate "non-cognitive" skills in university students, such as dealing with adversity, properly handling negative emotions, and learning how to communicate and resolve interpersonal conflicts. Essentially, these are "soft" skills that university students should acquire in contrast to "hard skills" that are typically assessed via examinations.

Thirdly, educators should realize that there are changing conceptions of "optimal" student development. While the traditional conception of desirable youth development is operated in terms of cognitive intelligence (intelligence quotient), there is an alternative conception focusing on the importance of "multiple intelligences," highlighting the importance of non-cognitive skills. With reference to the positive youth development (PYD) approach, the Search Institute focuses on youth developmental assets such as internal assets (e.g., psychosocial competence) and external assets (e.g., support from significant others). Richard Lerner's 5Cs (connection, competence, confidence, character, and compassion) highlight the importance of psychosocial competence and character, which are commonly ignored in the formal curriculum. These models prompt us to reflect on what should be nurtured in university students.

Additionally, there is dissatisfaction with the quality of higher education. Concerning the qualities of graduates, many studies show that employers are not satisfied with the qualities of university graduates, particularly in the areas of interpersonal communication, resilience, emotional competence, and work attitudes. In other words, there is a mismatch between graduate qualities and the perceptions of the expected graduate qualities. Besides, there is the criticism that contemporary universities fail to cultivate "better people." In fact, contemporary universities are obsessive about rankings and "overt" achievements without much reflection on the importance of the inner qualities and psychosocial competencies of university graduates.

The reason for writing this book is simple. University students are leaders and pillars of society for the future, and we have to assure them of holistic development and a good quality of life. Historically, university students have been regarded as "intellectuals" who shoulder the responsibility of shaping a better society. However, the focus is on the outcome of intellectual performance (e.g., examination results) rather than the essence of intellectuals, such as promoting social justice and civic engagement. With reference to holistic development (physical, psychological, social, and spiritual domains), university education focuses primarily on cognitive development. Besides, in a system focusing on the "survival of the fittest," examination results and achievements, instead of inner personal development, have become the focus of many universities.

Therefore, I decided to write this book to document the effectiveness and possible application of the PYD approach in the university context. PYD highlights the importance of young people's strengths and potential, and it also upholds the importance of providing opportunities for young people to thrive. I have been working on the P.A.T.H.S. Project (2005–2018) and the Tin Ka Ping P.A.T.H.S. Project (2011–2018) to promote the quality of life of high school students. To expand the impact of the PYD approach, I developed a subject entitled "Tomorrow's Leaders," which can be regarded as a university version of the P.A.T.H.S. Project. In this subject, we focus on PYD attributes, such as resilience, self-efficacy, and spirituality, as the foundation of successful leaders. Apart from "Tomorrow's Leaders," I have also collaborated with other colleagues (particularly Dr. Po Chung, who proposed the Service Leadership Theory) to develop subjects of "Service Leadership" (focusing on competencies, character, and care) and "Service Leadership through Serving Children and Families with Special Needs." Throughout the years, different evaluation studies have clearly documented the positive impact of these subjects. Hence, it is exhilarating to share these subjects with colleagues in the field.

Finally, I am going to retire soon. This book represents a snapshot of my work done to promote leadership and Service-Learning (SL) using the PYD approach under the new 4-year undergraduate program. Hence, I am pleased to share the two award-winning leadership subjects and two SL subjects with readers who are passionate about the holistic development of university students. I also look forward to having an intellectual discussion on the related issues and the possible future directions on using leadership and SL subjects as vehicles to promote the quality of life of university students.

This book will not exist without the enthusiastic support of The Hong Kong Polytechnic University (PolyU). In particular, I wish to thank the University for providing financial support to write this book. Besides, the financial support of the Li and Fung Endowed Professorship in supporting the research on Service Leadership and this book project is much appreciated. I am also indebted to several important persons who have provided unfailing support for the development of the four subjects covered in this book. First, I must thank Prof. Walter Yuen, the architect of the new 4-year undergraduate program, for implementing the leadership and Service-Learning subjects. My memory of the Senate meeting on approving the curriculum framework of the new 4-year undergraduate program is still fresh. The initiative was only approved by three-quarters of the Senate members. In other words, one-fourth of the Senate members were skeptical about these new elements in the undergraduate curriculum. Also, I wish to thank Prof. Timothy Tong and Prof. Philip Chan for their support in consolidating the Leadership and Service-Learning subjects in the new 4-year undergraduate program. Last but not least, I must thank Prof. J. G. Teng, President of PolyU, for his strong beliefs on the importance of nurturing leadership and social responsibility in university students, as well as his staunch support for the development of leadership and SL subjects in the University. His vision about holistic development of students is truly exemplary for university presidents.

When I wrote this book, I continually reflected on the Chinese saying, "Throwing a brick to attract a jade" (pao zhuan yin yu). It is my earnest hope that this book is a "brick" that will attract "jades" so that we can have fruitful dialogues and debates on how we can nurture the holistic development of university students, mainly through credit-bearing leadership and SL subjects in the formal curriculum. Besides, I also constantly think about "ideal" youth development in the traditional Chinese culture (e.g., Confucianism) and contemporary scientific literature on desired youth developmental outcomes.

Finally, although I am the lead author of this book, I would like to give credit to those colleagues who have helped to teach and evaluate leadership and Service-Learning subjects in the past decade as well as to contribute to the materials in this book. Without them, it would not be possible to tell good stories about these subjects. Hence, it is my pleasure to invite them to be chapter co-authors. They are Lu Yu, Xiang Li, Ginger C. C. Chau, Xiaoqin Zhu, and Diya Dou. It is my humble wish that this book will be a milestone in the use of leadership and Service-Learning education to enhance the holistic development of university students.

Hung Hom, Hong Kong Daniel T. L. Shek

Acknowledgments The preparation of chapters in this book and related research is financially supported by The Hong Kong Polytechnic University (Grants 97G1 and ZZUE), Li and Fung Endowed Professorship in Service Leadership Education, Wofoo Foundation, and Matching Fund of Research Grants Council (ZECL and ZH4Q).

Contents

Chapter 1
Developmental Issues of University Students

Daniel T. L. Shek

Abstract University students are the pillars of society's future, and the cultivation of holistic development of university students through university education is essential. Unfortunately, there is worrying evidence of the developmental issues faced by university students in both international and local contexts. These issues include psychological well-being problems (e.g., depression, anxiety, suicide, and non-suicidal self-injury), psychosocial stressors (e.g., academic burden, interpersonal stress, and financial pressure), addictive behaviors (e.g., substance abuse and Internet addiction), interpersonal problems (e.g., interpersonal conflicts and violence), conflict and communication issues with parents, lifestyle issues (e.g., sleep problems, nutrition issues, or lack of exercise), and character, value, or law abidance problems (e.g., plagiarism, over-materialistic, growing egocentrism, and sexual harassment). This chapter examines international and local news on these developmental issues among university students, highlights the urgent need to nurture holistic development in university students, suggests ways to improve the well-being of university students, and briefly outlines the organization of the fourteen chapters in this book.

Keywords University students · Holistic development · Developmental issues · Psychological well-being · International and local news

1.1 Introduction

In many societies, university students are usually regarded as "leaders of tomorrow." Besides, a university education is also a vehicle for climbing up the social ladder. Hence, cultivating the holistic development of university students, including their cognitive and non-cognitive skills, is essential. Meanwhile, as Prince et al. (2007) pointed out, if there is no mental health, there is no health. Therefore, it is also necessary to enhance the well-being of university students (Shek, 2010; Shek & Wong, 2011). Unfortunately, there is worrying evidence of the developmental issues faced by university students in both international and local contexts (Shek, 2010; Shek & Cheung, 2013; Shek & Wong, 2011). There are several categories of problems nowadays. First, psychological well-being issues, such as depression, anxiety,

D. T. L. Shek, *Promoting Holistic Development in University Students*, Quality of Life in Asia 17, https://doi.org/10.1007/978-981-96-0251-3_1

suicide, and non-suicidal self-injury, are common among university students. Second, university students are faced with many psychosocial stressors, such as academic burden, interpersonal stress, and financial pressure. Third, addictive behaviors, such as substance abuse, are common among university students in the West. Moreover, with the growing popularity of Internet users, Internet addiction has become another challenge. Fourth, interpersonal problems such as interpersonal conflicts and interpersonal violence are present in university students. Fifth, entering the university may create parent-adolescent conflict and family communication problems. Sixth, there are lifestyle issues (e.g., sleep problems, nutrition issues, or lack of exercise) in university students. Finally, character problems (e.g., plagiarism, cheating in examinations, or discipline problems); value confusion (e.g., over-materialistic, growing egocentrism, or lack of life meaning); or law abidance issues (e.g., stealing in hostels, sexual harassment, or vandalism) are also emerging concerns for university students.

1.2 News Reflecting Developmental Issues in University Students

In the following sections, we will investigate some international and local news that can reflect the developmental issues in university students to set the stage for our reflection. We focus on the news because it gives real-life examples of developmental issues in university students. Of course, we have to bear in mind the limitations of news because they may not be generalizable. However, it can be argued that news can be regarded as "layman cases" that are food for thought.

1.2.1 International News

Besides empirical studies on the prevalence of mental problems, there are many news that can give us some ideas about the developmental issues and challenges faced by university students. In the following section, we will focus on some international news reflecting such concerns.

First, there are many news reports on the mental health issues that concern university students, especially under the influence of COVID-19. In a report covering the increasing rate of depression and anxiety disorders among university students in America, Joseph (2019) highlighted that mental problems (anxiety and severe depression) and low flourishing have more than doubled in the past years. The rate of moderate-to-severe anxiety was 17.9% in 2013, which rose to 34.4% in 2018. In terms of moderate-to-severe depression rate, it was 23.2% in 2007, and this figure rose to 41.1% in 2018. One of the possible factors contributing to these problems is the increasing popularity of smartphones since 2012, which negatively influenced the quality of sleep and reduced real-time interpersonal communications among phone users. The report also highlighted the inadequacies of campus and community mental health services. In another report, Hall (2022b) reported that university students in the United Kingdom who became the "COVID generation" experienced a mental health crisis. The National Union of Students highlighted an increase in mental problems such as anxiety disorders, eating disorders, loneliness, and self-harming among students, with around 47% of students being negatively affected by mental health issues, leading to higher dropout rates. Besides, in the news headline, Fawcett (2022) reported that it is challenging for the "COVID-19 generation" to attend universities as they are suffering from increased rates of anxiety, depression, and suicide. At the same time, many US college students might exhibit reservedness, apathy, and lack of motivation in online teaching and learning. For example, the University of Oregon reported that the students were apathetic toward college. They have a desire to connect but are not sure about the strategies.

Crucially, suicide among university students is also another concern. The Guardian reported that university students in the UK are still affected by the great pandemic. There was an increase in calls to Nightline, a peer-run helpline for UK university students who are facing mental health challenges amid the pandemic, with 7.4% of calls from students attempting suicide in 2022 (Hall, 2022a). There were many factors leading to this problem, including uncertainty, loneliness, economic recession, increased cost of living triggered by the pandemic, and stress of readjusting to the pandemic and post-pandemic challenges. Additionally, the mental health issue is also prevalent in non-Western contexts. In a BBC News report, Limaye (2023) highlighted that the suicidal mental health crisis is the worst ever in Afghanistan. The headline reads, "Afghan women in mental health crisis over bleak future," showing that the crisis was intensive among female university students who have lost the right to access to education and enjoy freedom under Taliban rule. One psychiatrist said that the hotline received 170 distress calls from women within two days when they got the news that they could no longer receive a university education. Sadly, six families whose daughters committed suicide surveyed accused the closure of universities because it created hopelessness for their children. While the United Nations warned about rising mental health problems and suicides, the Taliban has no practical answers. Besides, suicides remain overlooked due to the stigma surrounding mental health issues in Afghanistan, in conjunction with the problems of hunger and economic crisis in the country.

Besides mental health problems, the international news also revealed addiction issues among university students. In the news entitled "'I just can't stop': Online porn addiction becoming a serious issue in Japan," Kawakami (2023) reported the issue of Internet pornography addiction among Japanese university students as well as its negative consequences on their mental health and daily living. In 2019, Japan ranked second globally in terms of traffic to adult websites, with 5.7% of Japanese college students in 2021 admitted to having such viewing habits. The news illustrated the experience of a student on how excessive pornography consumption led to academic failures and mental health issues like depression, anxiety, and insomnia—the unrestricted availability of unlimited content and the heightened stimulation it provides contributed to this addiction problem significantly.

Furthermore, there was also news on substance abuse. According to Paúl's (2021) report in the Washington Post, the COVID-19 pandemic intensified cannabis consumption among US college students. Although alcohol addiction rates dropped to a record low of 24% in 2021 (a figure which is still very high), marijuana use increased from 38% in 2015 to 44% in 2020. Moreover, in 2015, only 5% of students consumed marijuana daily, while this rate rose to 8% over five years, and the use of psychedelic drugs reached 9% in 2020. It seems that the students used marijuana to cope with social isolation and monotony. While researchers had concerns about the link between marijuana use and psychiatric disorders such as anxiety and suicide, students generally had perceptions of the low risks involved. Moreover, students were pushing for further relaxation of marijuana rules on campuses with its legalization in many states.

Additionally, interpersonal issues and feelings of loneliness were intensifying among university students. Firstly, loneliness was regarded as a common problem among the youngsters. In the news titled "No one would even know if I had died in my room: Coronavirus leaves international students in dire straits," Morris et al. (2020) reported their research findings in The Conversation that there was heightened loneliness experienced by international university students residing in private rental housing in Australia during the COVID-19 pandemic. Before the outbreak, only a third of the participants reported feelings of loneliness, while that number increased to 63% since the outbreak because of job losses and struggles in paying rent and tuition fees. One student expressed the common feeling among the international student group that nobody would even know if they had died in their room if not for the owner coming to ask for rent. This issue highlighted the urgent need for the government to consider providing financial support and resources to assist international students during the pandemic. In Belgium, Tielemans (2021) reported in Brussels Times that three-quarters of students at the KU Leuven in Belgium said the coronavirus made them feel lonely, citing a survey finding by the student union of the KU Leuven. The university's mental health policy officer also noted that the situation had worsened and that some students shared their feelings of exclusion. While KU Leuven provided resources such as chat lines and sensitization campaigns to support students, psychologists argued that these measures were inadequate. Additionally, many students were reluctant to seek help.

Besides, family issues contribute to another stressor for university students. For example, in a report by ABC Australia, Russian students in Australia were negatively affected by Russia's invasion of Ukraine in the forms of discrimination and family conflicts. The headline revealed that Moscow's invasion of Ukraine has affected Russian students in Australia in negative ways. The news article covered stories and experiences of several Russian students who had experienced various difficulties, including obstacles in accessing financial resources, feelings of isolation and fear due to their nationality, and even rejection from universities. Additionally, the students had conflicts and tensions within their own families because they held different perspectives on the war (ABC Australia, 2023).

In addition to the above concerns, there is also much news coverage on character issues in university students. Sun (2020) reported with the headline, "Coronavirus:

NUS students allegedly abuse COVID-19 measures to cheat on exam." The National University of Singapore was investigating a case involving students who allegedly shared and plagiarized answers in a practical exam for a programming module, taking advantage of the opportunity to take the practice exams at home as a precautionary measure against contracting COVID-19. While the National University of Singapore (NUS) had received confessions of cheating from some students, others have resorted to social media to appeal for leniency or justify their actions, and some students even blamed the university for this problem. This incident has raised serious concerns about academic integrity and the impact of the pandemic on the education system. As reported by Foxe (2022), at least 1500 Irish university students were reported for cheating, plagiarism, or utilizing "essay mills" between 2019 and 2022. While universities remain dedicated to upholding academic standards and integrity, with varying disciplinary measures being given, universities generally adopted a relatively lenient stance toward students involved in academic dishonesty, particularly for those considered "first offense," resulting in fewer instances of expulsion reported as severe disciplinary measures.

With the headline entitled "COVID-19 at college: Shaming and blaming students can make it worse, experts say," Syal (2022) in NBC News reported that college students in the United States have faced accusations of selfishness and a lack of responsibility in several universities in the US regarding students' violations of group activities during the pandemic, leading to universities implementing penalties for students who have broken the law by violating coronavirus policies. However, some experts argued that zero-tolerance policies may make the situation worse and that universities should adopt a harm-reduction approach rather than strictly enforcing abstinence-based policies. Besides, Mafolo (2019) reported on the growing trend of low turnout and political apathy among South African university students. The headline reads, "SRC elections: Students see little value in campus politics." Data obtained from several universities showed that less than one-quarter of students participated in Student Representative Council (SRC) elections over three years until 2019. Students cited a lack of trust in politicians, feeling unrepresented, and a perceived absence of tangible changes resulting from previous elections as reasons for non-participation. This lack of engagement and interest in campus politics may mirror the broader trend of political apathy among young people, as evidenced by the fact that 6 million young individuals were not registered to vote in the 2019 national elections.

Tragically, university students also show law-abiding issues. McShane et al. (2023) reported on three stabbings in five days at the University of California, Davis, raising concerns about campus crime in the US. The headline reads, "Ex-UC Davis student arrested in fatal stabbings near campus, police say." The suspect in these attacks was identified as a former UC Davis student who was separated from the university due to academic reasons, and no evidence showed that the suspect had any personal connection or prior knowledge of the victims involved. UC Davis decided to convert evening classes to distance learning and increase security after the incident, but fears and anxieties about campus safety persist among students and staff. Similarly, The Toronto Star reported on the incidents of sexual violence and student death that occurred at Western University in Canada during Orientation Week (Teotonio & Yousif, 2021). The headline was entitled "Arrests made as Western University tightens campus security after reports of sexual violence, student death." Four formal complaints of sexual assault had been received by the university, leading to arrests and removal of some students from residence. In addition, a first-year student was tragically killed after being violently assaulted near the campus in the same week. Students have expressed feeling unsafe and criticized the university for lacking immediate action to address the toxic culture that seems to permeate the campus community.

1.2.2 Local News

Apart from the news worrying about the psychological well-being of university students in the international context, there is also much news on this topic in Hong Kong. Similar to other places, mental health issues are covered in the media. The Hong Kong Federation of Youth Groups (Wong et al., 2017) revealed in their report that, from 2015 to 2016, the counseling hotline received over 16,400 calls from young people who were suffering from mental disorders. Among those cases, more than 2100 university students made the call, which was 60% higher than the same period one year ago. Additionally, Am730 (2023) covered a local survey in 2018 that 27% of university students suffered from moderate or above levels of depression, while 20% of them experienced anxiety disorders. These prevalence rates were higher than the rate for the general rate of mental illness in Hong Kong in 2015, which was 13.3%. A specialist in psychiatry stated that the identity change of college students from students to adults has invisibly added much pressure on them.

Although many universities and organizations are implementing mental health programs or school counseling services for students, the impact is limited. Wu (2020) reported the launch of an online tutoring program for Hong Kong university students called "Rest Online." This online tutoring program taught university students how to understand their own negative emotions and behaviors, thereby alleviating the pressure related to study and personal growth. A professor revealed figures from recent studies that about 30–50% of Hong Kong college students were faced with mental stress, which was likely to be related to the 2019 social unrest and the COVID-19 pandemic. However, she pointed out that the average ratio of university counselors to students in Hong Kong was 1:1342, while the related ratio in the US was about three times that of Hong Kong, reflecting that Hong Kong had insufficient university counselors. In another report, Auyeung (2018) reported that a fourth-year college student in Hong Kong suffered from emotional problems due to her inability to adapt to college and heavy academic pressure. However, the attitude of the campus counselor made her depression worse. She felt that the university's counseling team could not help her get out of her emotional predicament.

Crucially, there is much news on the psychosocial stress encountered by university students. Lun et al. (2018) surveyed 1119 undergraduates from eight public universities in 2018 and found that 68.5% of students showed mild to severe depression, and around 9% had moderately severe to severe depression. Besides, 54.4% of students were experiencing mild to severe anxiety, and 5.8% had severe anxiety. Compared with the findings a decade ago, the prevalence rate of depression increased slightly, while the prevalence rate of anxiety was similar. The study also showed several reasons for high stress, including examination pressure, coursework burden, difficulty in adapting to the university learning model, and worrying about graduation and future employment. Similarly, a news article reported the pressure faced by Hong Kong university students in 2016 (HKET, 2016). Past research findings showed that around 10–15% of students suffer from anxiety and adjustment problems every year. Many students reported that they were nervous before exams and suffered from psychological and physical problems, such as insomnia, loss of appetite, and difficulty swallowing. Some students also had hand tremors after entering the examination room, poor concentration, and were unable to take the exam. Those who were too stressed even needed to suspend school or delay graduation.

Besides, news on student suicide and self-injury situations is concerning. Lau (2016) reported that a student committed suicide in March 2016, which was the 20th student suicide case since the start of the academic year in September 2015. Among over 20 student suicide cases, 13 were primary or secondary school students, and 11 were college students. Most of the people suspected that the cause of the suicide was related to academic stress. Unfortunately, perceived difficulty in upward social mobility was one of the causes of suicide among Hong Kong youth. Noteworthy, most of the suicide cases came from single-parent families with insufficient social support. In another report, Wenweipo (2017) revealed that the "Blue Whale" game was suspected of having been circulating among Hong Kong university students. A self-proclaimed student from The University of Hong Kong (HKU) posted on Facebook that three friends had coincidentally written the words "I AM A WHALE" on the Internet. They also noticed that their left hands were injured and bandaged. This game took advantage of the curiosity of teenagers, lured their personal information or nude photos, and then coerced the victim to carry out a "mission" of a series of self-injury and, finally, suicide.

Likewise, the local news also revealed addiction issues among university students. In 2014, the management of a student dormitory at The Hong Kong University of Science and Technology (HKUST) noticed the smell of marijuana smoke coming from the back of the dormitory (Auyeung, 2014). In 2007, a female student from Hong Kong Baptist University drank and celebrated in the dormitory with her classmates. The next day, her roommate found her unconscious with red "alcohol blisters" on her body. She died after being sent to the hospital (Lee, 2007). In another news, On.cc (2017) reported illegal behaviors of students in the dormitories of various universities in Hong Kong involving drugs and alcohol abuse and marijuana cultivation.

Interpersonal issues were also observed in college students. Oriental Daily (2013) reported the findings of the HKU's Students' Union's magazine *Undergrad*. The report showed that around 6% of The University of Hong Kong (HKU) students surveyed revealed that they had had sex on campus, and another 9% had had sex in the dormitory. Based on the results of this survey, the editor of *Undergrad* recommended that the university should reflect on the need to provide more related courses and workshops. Besides, there is news on the interpersonal problems of university students in the political domain. Gou (2022) reported that a Mainland Chinese student had been harassed by other students in a dormitory. According to the recording, a group of dormitory students kept knocking on the door of two non-local dormitory students and joking in Mandarin, "Let us come out to play" and "Hong Kong welcomes you." One of the non-local students repeatedly begged the resident outside the door to "go away" but was ignored. The university had punished the three dormitory students—two were permanently banned from dormitories, and one was banned from dormitories for one semester. The school also issued warnings to two other dormitory students.

University students are also facing stress and trauma due to socio-political issues. Lam (2019) reported that the 2019 social unrest had torn society apart, and this kind of conflict and division had also affected many families in Hong Kong. The article reported that Radio Television Hong Kong found at least 50 young people quarreled with their families during the demonstrations and were kicked out of their homes in mid-August 2019. BBC News Chinese (Lam, 2019) interviewed a 55-year-old mother and her son, a college student. The son and his father quarreled over political opinions in mid-July 2019 and never returned home. The student once lived temporarily with a classmate and then lived in a university dormitory after school started.

Lack of personal space and family issues contribute to significant stress for young people in Hong Kong. For example, HKET (2023b) reported the conflict between a female college student and her family because of the lack of private space in the small residential units in Hong Kong. The female college student was in a family of four living in public housing, and she had to share the same room with her younger brother since childhood. However, her outbursts of dissatisfaction started when she entered university. She said that in middle school, her classmates had similar backgrounds, so she would not feel the gap in family circumstances. However, after entering university, she found that many of her classmates had their own rooms even if they were not living in private housing. So, she became dissatisfied with her living environment. She lamented that in the past, her mother had always criticized her for poor grades, and her father had often played loud videos at home, so they often argued with each other.

In addition, some news outlets have highlighted the lifestyle problems of university students. Mingpao-Health (2018) reported an interview with a psychiatrist who revealed that gaming disorder is becoming more severe among young people. He received 30 to 40 cases, most of whom were male students aged 10 to 30 years. The phenomenon was rarely seen in 5 years ago. Kwok et al. (2021) conducted a study to show how video games on the Internet and social media overuse are problematic and can create addictive symptoms. Fifteen university students joined the research. The findings revealed that internet and social media addiction had negative impacts on physical activity, well-being, sleep quality, and academic performance of university students.

University students also showed signs of moral confusion. Chau (2015) reported that the Lingnan University Student Union held a concert and allowed the musical band to use vulgar lyrics to insult the police and incite hatred, raising public concern about the university's standards for students' moral conduct. The Chairman of the Education Policy Concern Organization pointed out that in the early years, obscene games appeared in university orientation camps. Therefore, he believed that the Lingnan University Student Union incident was a reminder for the eight major universities that activity guidelines and student codes needed to be more specific. Students cannot be allowed to use so-called artistic freedom and "freedom of speech" as a shield, and relevant penalties should be strictly enforced. In another news (Singtao, 2020), the Chairman of the Board of Trustees of the Education University of Hong Kong criticized some college students for not respecting teachers. He reiterated that during the social unrest in 2019, some college students abused the principal with vulgar language and threw "ghost banknotes" at the principal, showing that students did not know how to respect teachers. He revealed that an official once expressed to him that some teachers took an extreme approach when teaching liberal studies. In 2023, HKET (2023a) reported that in response to the indent games played in the orientation camps, the Chairperson of the Legislative Council's Education Affairs Committee said she was shocked to hear the suspected cases involving sexual assault, sexual harassment, and rape in orientation camps. She stressed that sexual bullying scandals had been occurring in the orientation camps in various universities in Hong Kong for a long time. The phenomenon was caused by the school management problem and students' weak moral awareness.

There are also media reports on value confusion among university students. In a study, Kwok Lai (2019) found that 82.1% and 70.3% of the students had moderate or above levels of meaning needs (e.g., consciously needing the meaning of life) and meaning exploration (e.g., consciously needing to explore the meaning of life), respectively. Besides, 67.9% of the students had a low sense of life meaning (e.g., feeling that life is meaningful), and 64.3% of the students had above medium levels of meaning confusion (e.g., being confused about whether life is meaningful).

There is some news on the law abidance issues in university students. Yeung and Chiu (2021) reported that the police had smashed a drug warehouse in an industrial building and arrested a 22-year-old male college student for trafficking dangerous drugs. They also seized approximately HK$195 million in methamphetamine and heroin. The police found that the operation of the group was sophisticated and systematic. The second news article is a commentary by the HKET (2023a). The article pointed out that the orientation camp scandals had reached the level of illegality, which was caused by the young people's weak moral concepts and law-abiding awareness. They also misunderstood freedom and thought that they would be free after entering universities. It was pointed out that university orientation is not unique to Hong Kong. In fact, many universities in the US have relevant regulations on orientation activities.

These developmental issues highlight the questions of how we can promote the healthy or optimal development of university students and through what means. We argue that in view of such problems, there is an urgent need to promote the well-being of university students, cultivate "healthy," "optimal," "balanced," and "holistic" development of young people, and value the role of psychosocial competence plays in the process. Regarding the question of how to achieve the above tasks, our second argument is that credit-bearing Leadership and Service-Learning (SL) subjects are promising tools to promote the holistic development of students. Our third argument is that there are successful credit-bearing subjects that can help promote the holistic development of university students. We will share our experience in Hong Kong to illustrate the possibility of achieving the above objectives. Our fourth argument is that evaluation is an essential component of understanding the usefulness of credit-bearing Leadership and SL subjects to promote the holistic development of students. In other words, we have to apply scientific research methods and convincing evidence to examine this topic, particularly in connection with the scholarship of teaching and learning. Our final argument is that we have to rethink whether universities fulfill their role of nurturing university students to be "better people" and reflecting on the related issues.

1.3 Holistic Development in University Students: Definitions and Conceptual Frameworks

Before we proceed further, there is a need to clarify several terms that are commonly used to understand holistic development in university students. The first term is "institutional learning outcomes," which refers to the qualities that graduates are expected to gain through university education. These outcomes are commonly achieved by achieving "program outcomes" and "subject outcomes." The second term is "desired graduate attributes," which are qualities of graduates that the university desires with reference to the expectations and needs of society, such as problem-solving skills, cognitive competence, and interpersonal communication skills. Typically, university administrators and teachers develop institutional learning outcomes with reference to desired graduate attributes. Additionally, the third term is "holistic student development," which means that students should have good development in different domains of their development. With reference to the usage of the term in the health fields, holistic development includes physical, psychological, social, and spiritual domains. Another related term is "balanced student development," which refers to the emphasis on both academic and non-academic development in the students. As far as related skills are concerned, academic outcome requires "cognitive" skills, whereas non-academic outcome requires "non-cognitive" skills, such as resilience, emotional competence, self-efficacy, and communication skills. Researchers have referred to "non-cognitive" skills as "psychosocial competence" or "social-emotional learning" skills. In short, it is helpful to examine whether psychosocial competencies or non-cognitive skills are emphasized to promote the holistic development of university students in the institutional learning outcomes or desired graduate attributes of university students. Obviously, one promising way is to strengthen the psychosocial competence of the students.

Conceptually speaking, the cultivation of psychosocial competence can also improve the well-being of the students. Felce and Perry (1995) proposed different domains of quality of life, including physical well-being (e.g., health), material well-being (e.g., financial stability), social well-being (e.g., interpersonal relationship), development (e.g., competence), and emotional well-being (e.g., self-esteem). Based on this conception, the promotion of psychosocial competence of university students can promote their social and emotional well-being. Another concept is the construct of well-being. As far as the concept of well-being is concerned, a common way is to differentiate between hedonic and eudaimonic well-being. Hedonic well-being refers to the presence of positive effects, such as life satisfaction, and the absence of negative effects (Deci & Ryan, 2008). In contrast, eudaimonic well-being, always operationalized as psychological well-being, represents human flourishing and living to one's self-actualization. It goes beyond pleasure-driven happiness to work toward personal growth and a sense of fulfillment (Tatarkiewicz, 1976). Deci and Ryan (2008) further defined the concepts of eudaimonic motives (exploring development, growth, and purpose), hedonic enjoyment drives (pursuing happiness and joy), and hedonic comfort impulse (chasing pleasure). Braaten et al. (2019) revealed that pursuing eudaimonic and hedonic enjoyment can improve university students' quality of life, while chasing hedonic comfort does not have such a positive effect. Moreover, eudaimonic motives have positive influences on life satisfaction, meaning in life, and self-connection. At the same time, motives for hedonic enjoyment do not reveal such an impact. Therefore, it is necessary to distinguish between eudaimonic and hedonic enjoyment and hedonic comfort motives in cultivating the holistic development of university students.

The purpose of this book is to highlight the importance of looking at the holistic developmental needs of university students and examine the ways through which their needs could be met. The basic conceptual framework is that besides the intellectual development of university students, universities should also nurture the non-cognitive skills (or transversal skills or soft skills) of university students. While many models cover holistic development in students, we highlight 21st-century skills and the positive youth development approach in our discussion. In particular, we focus on the scope of 21st-century skills and the OECD Learning Compass 2030, which highlights the importance of non-cognitive skills, psychosocial competence, and positive values underlying learning. We further reinforce the importance of this conceptual framework in Chap. 5, which outlines the positive youth development approach and focuses on the importance of developmental assets in young people, such as adversity quotient, emotional quotient, and spiritual quotient (Shek et al., 2019). Essentially, these two areas form the conceptual framework for holistic student development. In fact, there are many studies showing that PYD attributes are related to the developmental outcomes of university students, particularly during the social event (Shek, 2020) and the COVID-19 pandemic (Shek, 2021; Shek et al., 2023a, 2023b, 2023c).

Regarding the question of how we can nurture holistic student development, we argue that leadership education and SL are two important vehicles that can be used to build up psychosocial competencies in university students. With reference to the role of General Education, we describe the General University Requirements at The Hong Kong Polytechnic University under the education reform where the university system was changed from a 3-year system to a 4-year system, in which we have developed new credit-bearing subjects on leadership and SL.

1.4 Layout of This Book

There are fourteen chapters in this book. In this introductory chapter, we highlight the need to nurture holistic development in university students based on a cursory examination of the news on the developmental issues of university students in the local and international contexts. We also highlight our arguments on ways to improve the well-being of university students. In Chap. 2, based on universities ranked in the first 100 places in Times Higher Education, we examine the institutional learning outcomes and desired graduate attributes, particularly on whether they cover holistic student development. In Chap. 3, we focus on the institutional learning outcomes and desired graduate attributes in universities in Hong Kong and identify the gaps in this topic. When we move on to Chap. 4, we present the development of 21st-century skills and make a comprehensive analysis based on the OECD Learning Compass 2030. In Chap. 5, we discuss that both positive youth development attributes and non-cognitive attributes are essential in promoting holistic development in university students. We then discuss leadership training in Chap. 6 and SL as vehicles to nurture holistic student development in Chap. 7. In Chap. 8, we outline the General University Requirements at The Hong Kong Polytechnic University, which include Leadership and SL as graduation requirements.

Additionally, in Chap. 9, we introduce the subject entitled "Tomorrow's Leaders," which emphasizes leadership qualities based on the positive youth development approach. It can also be regarded as a "university version" of the Project P.A.T.H.S. (Shek & Sun, 2013). In the next chapter, we outline the features of the subject entitled "Service Leadership," which emphasizes the importance of leadership qualities in the service economy, including competence, character, and care. Chapter 11 presents an SL subject entitled "Promotion of Children and Adolescent Development," which also highlights the importance of positive youth development attributes. When it comes to Chap. 12, we present another SL subject entitled "Service Leadership through Serving Children and Adolescents with Special Needs." In the next chapter, we discuss how we can promote law abidance in university students, which is of utmost importance to the well-being of themselves and the community. In Chap. 14, we consider the way forward and highlight some recommendations.

Acknowledgements The preparation of this chapter is financially supported by The Hong Kong Polytechnic University (ZZ4U and ZZUE), Li and Fung Endowed Professorship in Service Leadership Education, Wofoo Foundation, and the Matching Fund of Research Grants Council (ZECL and ZH4Q).

References

ABC Australia. (2023, April 14). What Mosco's invasion of Ukraine has meant for Russian students studying in Australia. *ABC Australia.* https://www.abc.net.au/news/2023-04-14/russian-students-in-australia-ukraine-war/102172504

Am730. (2023, June 06). Cing seoi beng daai hok saang jik wat bei lai gou, sei tip si jyu zi gei wo gaai [Emotional disorders. The high percentage of depression in college students, four tips to reconcile with yourself]. *Am730.* https://psee.io/742h7z

Auyeung, M. S. (2014, November 15). Fo daai suk se ji jau daai maa jin mei [Smell of marijuana suspected in HKUST dorms]. *Wenweipo.* http://paper.wenweipo.com/2014/11/15/HK1411150037.htm

Auyeung, T. S. (2018, September 11). "Cing seoi beng", daai hok cing seoi fu dou zing caak bei dung, "Ceot dou fu dou sat jaa mut jan bong dou ngo" ["Emotional Disorders". University emotional counseling policy is passive, "No one can help me even when I go out to the counseling room"]. *HK01.* https://www.hk01.com/article/233558?utm_source=01articlecopy&utm_medium=referral

Braaten, A., Huta, V., Tyrany, L., & Thompson, A. (2019). Hedonic and eudaimonic motives toward university studies: How they relate to each other and to well-being derived from school. *Journal of Positive Psychology and Wellbeing, 3*(2), 179–196.

Chau, T. Y. (2015, April 20). Leng daai jam ngok wui ging coeng juk ging cou hau go [LU concert sings foul-mouthed song insulting police officers]. *Wenweipo.* http://paper.wenweipo.com/2015/04/20/YO1504200007.htm

Deci, E. L., & Ryan, R. M. (2008). Hedonia, eudaimonia, and well-being: An introduction. *Journal of Happiness Studies, 9*, 1–11. https://doi.org/10.1007/s10902-006-9018-1

Fawcett, E. (2022, November 1). The pandemic generation goes to college. It has not been easy. *The New York Times.* https://www.nytimes.com/2022/11/01/us/covid-college-students.html

Felce, D., & Perry, J. (1995). Quality of life: Its definition and measurement. *Research in Developmental Disabilities, 16*(1), 51–74. https://doi.org/10.1016/0891-4222(94)00028-8

Foxe, K. (2022, September 27). At least 1,500 students at Irish universities reported for cheating, plagiarism, or use of 'essay mills'. *Irish Examiner.* https://www.irishexaminer.com/news/arid-40970204.html

Gou, G. (2022, September 13). Biu cim tung hok daai sau han, lau man sau saang je gung fan [Labeling classmates with hatred, "rogue hostel student" causes public outcry]. *Wenweipo.* https://www.wenweipo.com/a/202209/13/AP631f9aa9e4b033218a624850.html

Hall, R. (2022a, November 14). Pandemic still affecting UK students' mental health, says helpline. *The Guardian.* https://www.theguardian.com/education/2022/nov/14/pandemic-still-affecting-uk-students-mental-health-says-helpline-covid

Hall, R. (2022b, June 28). Warnings of mental health crisis among 'Covid generation' of students. *The Guardian.* https://www.theguardian.com/society/2022/jun/28/warnings-of-mental-health-crisis-among-covid-generation-of-students

HKET. (2016, March 07). Daai hok saang wut naan sik jing, 15% hok saang sau aat [University life is difficult to adapt, 15% of students are under pressure]. *HKET.* https://topick.hket.com/article/1384087

HKET. (2023a, October 06). "O camp fung bo" gong daai: mei faat jin jau hok saang kap duk, coi joek lin jiu kau daai hok zik si aat waai fung ["O camp storm" in HKU: No students found to

have taken drugs, Caroline Choi asked the university to curb the trend immediately]. *HKET*. https://dynamic.hket.com/article/xFV3LK9a62ECb4rd9?r=cpsdlc
HKET. (2023b, May 02). "Gung uk gaa ting" gong neoi wat geoi gung uk jyu dai tung fong taan mou si jan hung gaan, mong man kung jan sang zai m zi nam mat ["Public Housing Family". A Hong Kong woman living in public housing with her younger brother sighed that she had no private space. Netizens: poor people living in public housing do not know how to take care of their children]. *HKET*. https://topick.hket.com/article/3517212?r=cpsdlc
Joseph, S. (2019, August 30). Depression, anxiety rising among U.S. college students. *Reuters*. https://www.reuters.com/article/us-health-mental-undergrads-idUSKCN1VJ25Z
Kawakami, A. (2023, August 08). 'I just can't stop': Online porn addiction becoming serious issue in Japan. *The Mainichi*. https://mainichi.jp/english/articles/20230808/p2a/00m/0na/025000c
Kwok Lai, Y. C. S. (2019, May 24). Enhancing University students' well-being and positive learning experiences—Application of positive education [Paper presentation]. Learning and Teaching@ EdUHK Festival 2019: "Excellence in Learning and Teaching in the Digital Era", Hong Kong, China. https://scholars.cityu.edu.hk/en/publications/publication(203275d9-49e1-49f3-ad20-34f1dfe5b531).html
Kwok, C., Leung, P. Y., Poon, K. Y., & Fung, X. C. (2021). The effects of internet gaming and social media use on physical activity, sleep, quality of life, and academic performance among university students in Hong Kong: A preliminary study. *Asian Journal of Social Health and Behavior, 4*(1), 36. https://doi.org/10.4103/shb.shb_81_20
Lam, C. W. (2019, September 23). Hoeng gong kong ji zung dik gaa ting si lit: ceot zau dik ji zi wo soeng si sau fuk gwaan hai dik mou can [Families torn apart in Hong Kong protests: runaway sons and mothers trying to repair relationships]. *BBC News Chinese*. https://www.bbc.com/zhongwen/simp/chinese-news-49792207
Lau, T. W. (2016, March 18). Fan sik: hoeng gong wai ho hok saang zi saat si gin bat dyun [Analysis: Why do student suicides continue in Hong Kong?]. *BBC News Chinese*. https://www.bbc.com/zhongwen/trad/china/2016/03/160318_ana_hong_kong_youth_suicide
Lee, H. Z. (2007, December 21). Zam daai neoi sang zeoi sei, daai hok se kwai sau gwaan zyu [Drunken death of Baptist University girl, university dormitory rules under scrutiny]. *Wenweipo*. http://paper.wenweipo.com/2007/12/21/HK0712210080.htm
Limaye, Y. (2023, June 5). Afghan women in mental health crisis over bleak future. *BBC News*. https://www.bbc.com/news/world-asia-65765399
Lun, K. W., Chan, C. K., Ip, P. K., Ma, S. Y., Tsai, W. W., Wong, C. S., Wong, C. H., Wong, T. W., & Yan, D. (2018). Depression and anxiety among university students in Hong Kong. *Hong Kong Medical Journal, 24*(5), 466–472. https://doi.org/10.12809/hkmj176915
Mafolo, K. (2019, October 16). SRC elections: Students see little value in campus politics. *Daily Maverick*. https://www.dailymaverick.co.za/article/2019-10-16-src-elections-students-see-little-value-in-campus-politics/
McShane, J., Burke, M., & Helsel, P. (2023, May 05). Ex-UC Davis student arrested in fatal stabbings near campus, police say. *NBC News*. https://pse.is/745lra
Mingpao-Health. (2018, January 08). Din wun sat tiu, jing hoeng gan tung kap duk? Zi liu daa gei jan, sin gaai sam git [Is a video game disorder like drug addiction? The first step in treating video game addiction is to untie the knot in your heart]. *Mingpao-Health*. https://rb.gy/62wkd1
Morris, A., Hastings, C., Mitchell, E., Ramia, G., & Wilson, S. (2020, August 12). 'No one would even know if I had died in my room': Coronavirus leaves international students in dire straits. *The Conversation*. https://theconversation.com/no-one-would-even-know-if-i-had-died-in-my-room-coronavirus-leaves-international-students-in-dire-straits-144128
Oriental D. (2013, September 04). Gan jat sing gong daai saang, suk se dong paau fong [Nearly 10% of HKU students use the dormitory as a "booty call room"]. *Oriental Daily*. https://orientaldaily.on.cc/cnt/news/20130904/00176_054.html

On.cc. (2017, May 20). Taam se dang: daai hok suk se leon mou jim gai lung je je sang go [Searchlights: University dormitories degenerate into "uncovered chicken cages" for nightly entertainment]. *On.cc.* https://hk.on.cc/hk/bkn/cnt/news/20170520/bkn-20170520045941305-0520_00822_001.html

Paúl, M. L. (2021, September 13). College students reported record-high marijuana use and record-low binge drinking in 2020, study says. *The Washington Post.* https://www.washingtonpost.com/health/2021/09/13/college-students-use-more-marijuana-and-less-alcohol/

Prince, M., Patel, V., Saxena, S., Maj, M., Maselko, J., Phillips, M. R., & Rahman, A. (2007). No health without mental health. *The Lancet, 370*(9590), 859–877. https://doi.org/10.1016/S0140-6736(07)61238-0

Shek, D. T. L. (2010). Nurturing holistic development of university students in Hong Kong: Where are we and where should we go? *The Scientific World Journal, 10*, 563–575. https://doi.org/10.1100/tsw.2010.62

Shek, D. T. L. (2020). Protests in Hong Kong (2019–2020): A perspective based on quality of life and well-being. *Applied Research in Quality of Life, 15*(3), 619–635. https://doi.org/10.1007/s11482-020-09825-2

Shek, D. T. L. (2021). COVID-19 and quality of life: Twelve reflections. *Applied Research in Quality of Life, 16*(1), 1–11. https://doi.org/10.1007/s11482-020-09898-z

Shek, D. T. L., Chai, W. Y., & Zhou, K. (2023a). Risk factors and protective factors of internet addiction in university students during the pandemic: Implications for prevention and treatment. *International Journal of Environmental Research and Public Health, 20*(11), Article 5952. https://doi.org/10.3390/ijerph20115952

Shek, D. T. L., Chai, W. Y., Wong, T., & Zhou, K. (2023b). Stress and depressive symptoms in university students in Hong Kong under the pandemic: Moderating effect of positive psychological attributes. *Frontiers in Psychology, 14*, Article 1071938. https://doi.org/10.3389/fpsyg.2023.1071938

Shek, D. T. L., Chai, W. Y., Li, X., & Dou, D. Y. (2023c). Profiles and predictors of mental health of university students in Hong Kong under the COVID-19 pandemic. *Frontiers in Psychology, 14*, Article 1211229. https://doi.org/10.3389/fpsyg.2023.1211229

Shek, D. T. L., & Cheung, B. P. M. (2013). Developmental issues of university students in Hong Kong. *International Journal of Adolescent Medicine and Health, 25*(4), 345–351. https://doi.org/10.1515/ijamh-2013-0032

Shek, D. T. L., Dou, D. Y., Zhu, X. Q., & Chai, W. Y. (2019). Positive youth development: Current perspectives. *Adolescent Health, Medicine and Therapeutics, 10*, 131–141. https://doi.org/10.2147/AHMT.S179946

Shek, D. T. L., & Sun, R. C. F. (2013). The Project PATHS in Hong Kong: Development, training, implementation, and evaluation. *Journal of Pediatric and Adolescent Gynecology, 26*(3), S2–S9. https://doi.org/10.1016/j.jpag.2013.03.009

Shek, D. T. L., & Wong, K. K. (2011). Do adolescent developmental issues disappear overnight? Reflections about holistic development in university students. *The Scientific World Journal, 11*, 353–361. https://doi.org/10.1100/tsw.2011.5

Singtao. (2020, April 26). Maa si hang pai jau daai hok saang bat dung zyun si zung dou, coeng zung si ban gaak [Frederick Ma criticized some university students for not knowing how to respect teachers and advocated emphasizing character]. *Singtao.* https://std.stheadline.com/realtime/article/1255900/%E5%8D%B3%E6%99%82-%E6%B8%AF%E8%81%9E-%E9%A6%AC%E6%99%82%E4%BA%A8%E6%89%B9%E6%9C%89%E5%A4%A7%E5%AD%B8%E7%94%9F%E4%B8%8D%E6%87%82%E5%B0%8A%E5%B8%AB%E9%87%8D%E9%81%93-%E5%80%A1%E9%87%8D%E8%A6%96%E5%93%81%E6%A0%BC

Sun, D. (2020, March 19). Coronavirus: NUS students allegedly abuse Covid-19 measures to cheat on exam. *The Straits Times.* https://www.straitstimes.com/singapore/education/coronavirus-nus-students-allegedly-abuse-covid-19-measures-to-cheat-on-exam

Syal, A. (2022, September 09). COVID-19 at college: Shaming and blaming students can make it worse, experts say. *NBC News*. https://www.nbcnews.com/health/health-news/covid-19-college-shaming-blaming-students-can-make-it-worse-n1239582

Tatarkiewicz, W. (1976). Analysis of happiness. Martinus Nijhoff.

Teotonio, I., & Yousif, N. (2021, September 13). Arrests made as Western University tightens campus security after reports of sexual violence, student death. *The Toronto Star*. https://www.thestar.com/news/gta/arrests-made-as-western-university-tightens-campus-security-after-reports-of-sexual-violence-student-death/article_ea22b1ed-5439-5f09-a95c-306b9e71d7d6.html

Tielemans, J. (2021, June 22). Three out of four KU Leuven students lonely as result of coronavirus, survey finds. *The Brussels Times*. https://www.brusselstimes.com/174768/three-out-of-four-ku-leuven-students-lonely-as-result-of-coronavirus-survey-finds

Wenweipo. (2017, May 16). "Gaai taam mong ji." Laam king ji zaap gong, jau sai lou hang zyut lou ["Street Talk." "Blue Whale" is suspected of attacking Hong Kong, luring the smallest road to extinction]. *Wenweipo*. http://paper.wenweipo.com/2017/05/16/HK1705160010.htm

Wong, R., Ho, A., Ngai, A., Chan, S.-c., Yuen, A., & Cheung, S. (2017). *How young people cope with stress*. The Hong Kong Federation of Youth Groups. https://yrc.hkfyg.org.hk/wp-content/uploads/sites/56/2017/05/YI022_Report.pdf

Wu, K. Y. (2020, August 25). Se wui si gin jyu jik cing ling daai zyun sang sau aat, zam daai teoi mong soeng fu dou gai waak goi sin sam lei gin hong [Social events and epidemics stress tertiary students, HKBU launches online counseling program to improve mental health]. *HK01*. https://www.hk01.com/article/515100?utm_source=01articlecopy&utm_medium=referral

Yeung, K. L., & Chiu, P. L. (2021, August 19). Ging dou gam nin zeoi daai duk cong, gung haa gim 1. 95 jik jyun bing duk hoi lok jing, 22 seoi naam daai hok saang lok mong [The police cracked down on the largest drug warehouse this year, a 22-year-old male university student was caught in the industrial building. The police seized 195 million yuan of methamphetamine heroin]. *HK01*. https://www.hk01.com/article/665701?utm_source=01articlecopy&utm_medium=referral

Chapter 2
Institutional Learning Outcomes and Desired Graduate Attributes in Higher Education

Daniel T. L. Shek and Lindan Tan

Abstract As employers commonly perceive skills gaps in university graduates and there are studies highlighting well-being issues in university students, it is essential to ask whether universities nurture holistic development in university students. However, there is a lack of comprehensive analysis of institutional learning outcomes (ILOs) and/or desired graduate attributes (DGAs) in universities. In this chapter, we analyzed publicly available information from the top 100 universities in the Times Higher Education (THE) rankings 2023. We used a framework consisting of 29 indicators across 12 domains to assess the ILOs and/or DGAs, particularly in terms of non-cognitive skills and psychosocial competencies in these areas. Results revealed that 47% of the surveyed universities explicitly stated ILOs and/or DGAs at the university (39%) or faculty (8%) level, while 31% expressed similar expectations without providing specific ILOs and/or DGAs. Besides, most universities prioritize the development of discipline-specific "hard" employability skills, such as professionalism or discipline knowledge, scientific literacy, applied skills, and global awareness. In contrast, there is a notable neglect of the development of "soft" personal competencies, such as resilience, reflection, empathy, and respect. In view of the developmental issues faced by university students, we argue that there is a need to reflect on how to nurture holistic development in university students with particular reference to the inclusion of non-cognitive personal competencies and interpersonal skills into university education, particularly via credit-bearing subjects.

Keywords Graduate attributes · Institutional learning outcomes (ILOs) · Desired graduate attributes (DGAs) · Intrapersonal competence · Interpersonal skill · Employability · Times Higher Education (THE) · Holistic development

2.1 Introduction

Higher education has been valued through the lens of human capital theory (Gillies, 2015), which recognizes it as primarily an economic device and its indispensable role in global economic development (Bridgstock, 2009). Knapper and Cropley (1985) argued that higher education institutions are obliged to equip students with the

D. T. L. Shek, *Promoting Holistic Development in University Students*, Quality of Life in Asia 17, https://doi.org/10.1007/978-981-96-0251-3_2

essential skills to bolster their employability, aligning with the traditional perception of universities as institutions that foster vocational and professional competencies. However, with the increasing global trend toward "vocationalism, mass education, marketisation" (Green et al., 2009, p. 18), universities are now expected to assume broader responsibilities (Kalfa & Taksa, 2015; Shek & Yu, 2017; Shek et al., 2017c). These responsibilities extend beyond simply imparting discipline-specific knowledge and fostering students' professional skills (Green et al., 2009; Kember et al., 2020) but also nurture a comprehensive set of attributes that align with the demands of a knowledge-based economy in an age of "supercomplexity" (Barnett, 2000, p. 1), encompassing interpersonal skills, adaptability, problem-solving abilities to tackle global challenges, and the capacity to navigate uncertainties, among others. In short, university graduates are expected to acquire 21st-century skills in their undergraduate study.

Unfortunately, employers and academics are raising concerns about whether universities are effectively equipping graduates with the qualities they deem essential for making meaningful contributions to their own lives and society (Kember et al., 2017; Shek et al., 2017d). Critics have raised two primary concerns. Firstly, they argue that there exists a significant mismatch between the skill sets possessed by college graduates and the skills demanded by employers (Osmani et al., 2015). Secondly, there is an overemphasis on the development of cognitive skills and academic achievement, neglecting the promotion of mental health competencies as well as quality of life (Shek et al., 2017d).

2.1.1 Employers' Dissatisfaction with Higher Education Graduates

Obtaining a degree is merely the initial step, as contemporary employers now place value on a diverse set of qualities and accomplishments (Yorke & Harvey, 2005). Finch et al. (2013) identified 17 factors that influence the employability of college graduates by employing interview data from 30 employers and quantitative data from 115 employers. Their findings showed that employers placed the lowest value on academic reputation, including academic performance and institutional reputation, while soft skills, including interpersonal skills, verbal communication skills, and listening skills, were given the highest significance. Unfortunately, numerous studies have consistently highlighted a discrepancy between the expectations of employers and the knowledge taught in undergraduate programs. In the United States, Dewey et al. (2008) examined the convergence and divergence between the competencies developed by job seekers during school and the competencies sought and valued by employers by surveying 53 job seekers and 47 employers. Results indicated a consensus between employers and job seekers regarding the significance of certain competencies, such as quantitative analysis and data management. However, there were notable discrepancies between the skills valued by employers, including interpersonal abilities, presentation skills, project management competencies, and the skills typically acquired by job seekers during their school experience. In addition, over 36,000 graduates from 11 European countries perceived that their competences when they graduated were lower than those required in their jobs. Specifically, the Mediterranean countries exhibited deficiencies in competencies related to working under pressure and computer skills. In contrast, the United Kingdom faced challenges primarily in assertiveness, persistence, teamwork, and adaptability, while the Czech Republic exhibited significant deficits in competencies related to coordination, organization, problem-solving abilities, and broad general knowledge (García-Aracil & Van der Velden, 2008).

In fact, the significant disparity between the competencies of graduates and skills imparted through university education has generated substantial discontent among employers. In Portugal, Suleman and Laranjeiro (2018) revealed that nearly all of the employers under study expressed dissatisfaction with the graduates' inadequacy in terms of soft skills and other personal traits. Similarly, Hong Kong's education system has faced criticism for its heavy reliance on examination-driven competition, resulting in graduates lacking a comprehensive and diverse learning experience and a sense of lifelong learning (Shek et al., 2017a). Besides, the business sector has expressed dissatisfaction with local university graduates, citing their proficiency in examination techniques but a notable deficiency in creativity, innovation, and the ability to make well-informed decisions in professional settings (Hanstedt, 2010).

2.1.2 Student Mental Health Crisis in Higher Education

Besides the deficit mentioned above in non-cognitive skills, concerns have been raised about the potential harm to students' well-being that may arise from the neglect of social, emotional, and interpersonal skills by educators. Shek (2012) argued that the instrumental approach prevalent in higher education places excessive emphasis on academic achievement and the development of professional competence solely for employment purposes, which is accompanied by considerable neglect of the importance of fostering a sense of purpose and self-actualization among students. This neglect has contributed to mental health issues among university students. According to the American College Health Association (2023), a considerable proportion of university students in the United States faced significant mental health challenges, with nearly nine out of ten students (87.9%) who faced academic challenges experiencing moderate to high distress, 36.1% of college students experienced feelings of anxiety that overwhelmed them while approximately 28.4% of students reported depression experience that hindered their daily functioning. Additionally, 2.7% of college students disclosed having attempted suicide within the last 12 months. The World Health Organization's (WHO) "World Mental Health International College Student Initiative" (WMH-ICS) surveyed first-year university students at 24 universities across nine countries. It revealed that 93.7% of students reported varying degrees of stress, with financial burdens, health-related issues, and managing interpersonal relationships being important sources of stress during college (Karyotaki et al., 2020).

Psychological well-being issue is particularly pronounced in East Asia, which has been criticized for overvaluing academic achievement at the cost of neglecting holistic development. Drawing upon an extensive analysis of quantitative and qualitative data gathered from over 100 universities across 11 East Asian countries and territories, Yee (1989) demonstrated that students in Hong Kong, Japan, and Taiwan experienced chronic stress and were prone to severe socio-emotional issues. Furthermore, their cognitive abilities and academic values were significantly impaired primarily because of the immense pressure imposed on them from an early age to excel academically and gain admission to prestigious universities.

In Hong Kong, there is a significant lack of youth prevention and positive youth development programs specifically tailored to university students. Hence, although university graduates in Hong Kong may excel in intellectual growth, their emotional, interpersonal, and social skills are frequently overlooked by both educators and students themselves (Shek et al., 2017d). A study ($N = 978$) revealed that a significant proportion of Hong Kong university students experienced mental health challenges, with 61.3% classified as having mild to severe anxiety and 41.2% exhibiting clinically significant symptoms of depression. Additionally, a substantial majority of participants (78.4%) reported problems related to Internet addiction, while 12.2% disclosed having thoughts of suicide (Shek et al., 2023a). In mainland China, Liu et al. (2021) conducted a survey involving 1,266 medical students to examine the prevalence and impact of test anxiety. They revealed that medical students experienced varying degrees of test anxiety, with 28.6% reporting mild test anxiety, 37.7% experiencing moderate test anxiety, and 33.7% dealing with severe test anxiety.

Furthermore, the lack of holistic university education creates struggles for graduates to adapt to the transition between college and the professional world when they enter the workforce. Research has shown that many graduates struggle with managing their emotions in a professional setting (Delaney, 2003), building professional relationships (Love et al., 2001), and effectively navigating workplace dynamics (Duchscher, 2009). Therefore, citing a misalignment between their acquired knowledge and skills and the level of competence demanded by their jobs, some senior university students and graduates have voiced their discontent with the education offered by the university (García-Aracil, 2009; Milton-Wildey et al., 2014).

2.1.3 Institutional Learning Outcome and Desired Graduate Attributes as a Response

Acknowledging the increased demand from different stakeholders for desired graduates and in response to the evolving role of universities in equipping students for success in the knowledge economy, several countries, such as Australia, the United States, and the United Kingdom, have made public funding for universities partly contingent on the demonstrable learning outcomes of their graduates (Bridgstock, 2009; Su, 2014). Faced with pressure, a majority of universities across the globe, since the 1990s (Bitzer & Withering, 2020), have developed lists of graduate attributes focusing on the expected qualities of graduates and outlining the specific competencies, skills, and qualities that universities strive for their students to acquire by the time they complete their university education.

The notion of "Graduate Attributes" refers to "the qualities, skills, and understandings a university community agrees its students would desirably develop during their time at the institution and, consequently, shape the contribution they are able to make to their profession and as a citizen" (Bowden et al., 2000, p. 1), has gained widespread acceptance globally. In parallel, "Institutional Learning Outcomes (ILOs)" further "provides a guide to gauge an institution's achievement of the mission and delivery of instruction" (Judd & Keith, 2017, p. 69).

However, insufficient attention has been directed toward the identification of common elements intrinsic to ILOs and/or DGAs, as well as the identification of the potential gaps within these inventories (Bridgstock, 2009). An initial exploratory review conducted by Osmani et al. (2015) identified 53 widely used graduate traits by analyzing 39 studies. Interestingly, they found a significant disparity between the content of academic programs that are supposed to match the graduate attribute list and the skills required for success in the professional realm.

To address the gaps mentioned above, we examined the ILOs and/or DGAs of the top 100 universities as ranked by THE 2023 with reference to the following three key questions:

- Research Question 1: What are the institutional ILOs and/or DGAs in the 100 universities under study?
- Research Question 2: What is the relative emphasis of the ILOs and/or DGAs with reference to cognitive (intellectual) skills and non-cognitive skills?
- Research Question 3: Do the ILOs and/or DGAs cover the holistic development of university students, particularly in terms of fostering interpersonal skills and intrapersonal competence?

2.2 Review of Institutional Learning Outcomes and/or Desired Graduate Attributes

The research sample comprised the top 100 universities in the THE 2023 rankings. The THE World University Rankings is widely regarded as a widely cited, comprehensive, and authoritative source of information on higher education institutions throughout the world (Hazelkorn, 2016; Pavel, 2015), giving it an appropriate basis upon which to select a sample of universities that demonstrate high performance in preparing graduates with the desired attributes.

Primarily, we assessed the ILOs and/or DGAs in terms of discipline-based employment capabilities, including generic skills, discipline knowledge, specialist skills, research literacy, application skills, literacy in different domains, and global awareness, among others, which are intellectual skills commonly expected. We also assessed intrapersonal and interpersonal competencies in the strategic plans, curricula, and programs of these universities, which is an essential area of research because these skills and competencies are increasingly recognized as critical not only for success in academics (Liu et al., 2023; Smithers et al., 2018) and professional settings (de Boer & Van Rijnsoever, 2022). They are also commonly regarded as protective factors for mental health as well as well-being (Lamboy et al., 2022; Morales-Rodríguez et al., 2020; Shek & Liang, 2018; Smithers et al., 2018) of college students.

Existing research has provided valuable insights into the framework and categorization of graduate attributes or learning outcomes. Wagner (2010) identified seven essential survival skills that students should possess: "critical thinking and problem-solving," "collaboration across networks and leading by influence," "agility and adaptability," "initiative and entrepreneurialism," "effective oral and written communication," "accessing and analyzing information," and "curiosity and imagination" (p. 90). Expanding on this notion, O'Donnell (2014) presented a bundle of desirable attributes from the perspectives of students, employers, and society, encompassing two domains: "discipline-specific knowledge" and "transferable skills," covering 14 attributes such as "critical thinking," "public speaking," "ethical awareness," "leadership," among others (p. 61). Similarly, Kember et al. (2017) proposed an assessment framework consisting of 13 graduate attributes categorized into three types: "cognitive attributes," which pertain to higher-order intellectual abilities; "social attributes," involving the capability to interact with others effectively; and "affective attributes" related to an individual's values or beliefs (p. 810). Building upon these existing frameworks and through a comprehensive review of the literature (e.g., Bochner & Kelly, 1974; Bridgstock, 2009; Shek & Lin, 2015; Star & Hammer, 2008; Yorke & Harvey, 2005), we established an assessment system containing 29 indicators in 12 domains, including:

(1) Generic Skills/Competence/Broad-based independence
(2) Professionalism/Discipline knowledge
(3) Specialism/Specialist skills
(4) Research/Scientific literacy
(5) Application
(6) Intrapersonal attributes (Cognitive)
(7) Intrapersonal attributes (Non-cognitive)
(8) Intrapersonal attributes (Character and citizenship)
(9) Interpersonal competence
(10) Environmental/global awareness
(11) Entrepreneurship
(12) Literacy in different domains.

Among these 12 domains, Domain 6 (Intrapersonal attributes—Cognitive) covers three indicators, including "Creativity/Innovation (6a)," "Problem-solving

(6b)," and "Critical thinking (6c)." Domain 7 (Intrapersonal attributes—Non-cognitive) covers five indicators, including "Resilience (7a)," "Self-awareness/Self-regulated/Self-direct/Self-management/Sense of self /Self-confidence (7b)," "Well-being (7c)," "Leadership (7d)," and "Reflection (7e)." Domain 8 (Intrapersonal attributes—Character and citizenship) covers four indicators, including "Accountability/Responsibility (8a)," "Morality and ethics (8b)," "Character and integrity (8c)," and "Citizenship/Civic and community (8d)." For Domain 9 (Interpersonal competence), it covers four indicators, including "Communication (9a)," "Cultivate connections to others (9b)," "Empathy (9c)," and "Respect (9d)." Lastly, "Literacy in different domains" (Domain 12) covers "Lifelong learning (12a)."

A qualitative approach was employed in the present study. We used documentary analysis (Bowen, 2009) to review publicly accessible data from all 100 universities. In our analysis, we focused on examining the outward-facing web pages of institutions, along with the accessible policies, curriculum documents, and strategic plans that are readily available on the Internet. The scope of Internet search related to both ILOs and/or DGAs. We collected and analyzed data between November 2022 and January 2023. Five research staff gathered data on university policies, curricula, and other available documents via the Internet. To uphold the accuracy and reliability of the collected data, the researchers implemented a rigorous protocol of repeated visits to the websites to cross-check and verify the information. This approach aimed to minimize any potential errors and inconsistencies that may have arisen during the data collection process.

By adopting this method, the researchers generated a comprehensive and reliable dataset that could be used for further analysis and interpretation. In instances where the information available was not sufficient to directly identify the ILOs and/or DGAs, the researchers in this study classified such situations as "special cases." These special cases are defined as follows:

- *Special Case 1a*: no particular ILOs/DGAs were provided, but related information was provided, such as "mission and culture," "education commitment," "competence framework," "strategic priorities," etc.;
- *Special Case 1b*: no particular ILOs/DGAs were provided, and only scattered and slightly relevant information was obtainable from the university's publicly available policy documents, such as "core value," "motto," "about the university," etc.;
- *Special Case 2*: it pertained to situations where no university-level ILOs/DGAs were provided, but ILOs/DGAs from the department/college/faculty were provided.

Based on the measurement index system with 12 domains covering 29 indicators, we analyzed the collected documentary text and coded the data. When coding the text, we searched for direct references to particular concepts (e.g., global awareness, interpersonal attributes, resilience, etc.) but also indirect references to the related concepts (e.g., international insights, good social relationships, flexibility, etc.). Subsequently, the number of ILOs and/or DGAs that matched the indicator system for the attributes constructed in the present study was calculated for each university. In case there were different views, discussion among the research staff was conducted to reach a consensus.

2.3 Observations

2.3.1 Composition of the Universities Under Study

Among the 100 universities analyzed, 23 were private universities, while the remaining 77 were public universities (Table 2.1). In addition, the sample was geographically diverse, with 38 from North America, 36 from Europe, 19 from Asia, and 7 from Australasia (Table 2.2). Furthermore, an exploration of the national origins of the universities revealed a variety of countries or economies represented (see Table 2.3). The United States had the highest number of institutions in the sample, with 34 universities, followed by the United Kingdom (10), Germany (9), the Netherlands (7), Australia (7), Mainland China (7), Hong Kong (5), Canada (4), France (4), Switzerland (4), South Korea (3), Japan (2), Singapore (2), Belgium (1), and Sweden (1).

2.3.2 Institutional Learning Outcomes and/or Desired Graduate Attributes in 100 Universities

Regarding Research Question 1 on the ILOs and/or DGAs, out of the 100 universities analyzed, only 39 institutions explicitly outlined ILOs and/or DGAs at the university level (Table 2.3). Among the surveyed universities in Hong Kong, all five institutions (100%) developed ILOs and/or DGAs. Similarly, both universities in Singapore (100%) also constructed ILOs and/or DGAs. In Australia, six out of the seven universities examined (85.71%) implemented ILOs and/or DGAs. In the United Kingdom, six out of the ten universities surveyed (60.00%) constructed ILOs and/or DGAs. Among the thirty-four universities in the United States, sixteen institutions (47.06%) developed ILOs and/or DGAs. In Canada, two out of the four universities assessed (50.00%) constructed ILOs and/or DGAs. In mainland China, only one out of the seven universities under study (14.29%) implemented ILOs and/or DGAs. Similarly, one out of the seven universities in the Netherlands (14.29%) constructed ILOs and/or DGAs.

Additionally, we identified three distinct special cases among the universities. The first special case, labeled as "Special Case 1a," comprises 31 universities that did not provide specific ILOs/DGAs, but related information was provided, such as "mission and culture," "education commitment," "competence framework," "strategic priorities," etc. The second special case, denoted as "Special Case 1b," includes 22 universities where no explicit ILOs/DGAs were provided and with only limited and fragmented information in different university policy documents, some of which are only marginally relevant to the DGAs. Finally, the third special case, known as "Special Case 2," consists of 8 universities that lacked university-level ILOs/DGAs but provided ILOs and/or DGAs at the department, college, or faculty level (Table 2.3). These observations revealed differences in the construction and articulation of graduate attribute inventories at the surveyed universities, and there were still many higher education institutions that did not develop specific ILOs/DGAs to guide pedagogical practices.

2.3.3 Format of Institutional Learning Outcomes and/or Desired Graduate Attributes Statement in 100 Universities

Our review showed that there were three predominant formats in the articulation of the ILOs and/or DGAs in the top 100 universities. These included integrated statements, cluster statements, and a mixed approach.

- *Integrated Statements*: The term "integration" was first defined from the confluence of Political science and Economics (Cohen Orantes, 1981), representing "a systemic process of the combination of different individual elements is what makes up a coherent whole when they are brought together" (Tonon, 2019, p. 682). Building upon this notion, the "integrated statement" refers to a statement that combines, incorporates, and synthesizes multiple and diverse components, perspectives, or elements into a unified, coherent expression. It is characterized by presenting a holistic view by incorporating various elements into a single cohesive statement.
- *Cluster Statements*: Originally emerged within the discipline of economic geography (Vorley, 2008), the term "cluster" refers to "a geographically proximate group of interconnected institutions in a particular field, linked by commonalities and complementarities" (Porter, 2000, p. 17). As a corollary, a "cluster statement" is defined as a cohesive grouping of related ideas, concepts, or elements that are organized based on shared characteristics, themes, or relationships, involving identifying commonalities and connections among the elements within the cluster.
- *Mixed Approach*: While the "cluster statement" organizes related elements at each point, and the "integrated statement" synthesizes and unifies multiple components in a cohesive expression, the "mixed statement" combines elements from both the cluster and integrated forms. It blends and interweaves diverse components to create a comprehensive statement, acknowledging relationships and commonalities while synthesizing and unifying multiple components. This approach enables a nuanced and integrated presentation.

Of the surveyed universities, 45 institutions (45%) adopted an integrated statement format, where each attribute is presented as a comprehensive statement. In contrast,

22 universities (22%) employed a cluster format, grouping related outcomes together. The remaining 33 universities (33%) utilized a mixed method, combining elements of both integrated and cluster statements (Table 2.3). Some excerpted examples are as follows:

- *Integrated Statement*: [Chinese University of Hong Kong] "Expected Graduate Attributes: Our graduates will have a growth mindset, adaptive, creative, and strong ethical character with a deep concern for human welfare, contributing to the betterment of humanity. Graduates should have a broad range of intellectual disciplines and general knowledge; a depth of knowledge within a specialty; bilingual proficiency in Chinese and English, and a basket of skills including numeracy, analytic skills, and IT capability; the ability of life-long learning and professional development; be critical and independent; be effective in communication and working in a team; understand Chinese culture and with it a sense of national identity and pride; appreciation of other cultures with inter-cultural sensitivity, tolerance, and a global perspective; an attitude of compassion, honesty, and integrity in relation to self, family, and society, and the ability to contribute as citizens and leaders; a sense of purpose, responsibility and commitment in life, a desire to serve and taste in their pursuits."
- *Cluster Statement*: [University of Cambridge] "Cambridge learner attributes: (1) Confident, secure in their knowledge; ready to take intellectual risks; structured, critical and analytical; communicate and defend views as well as respect those of others; (2) Responsible for themselves, responsive to others, set targets and insist on intellectual integrity; collaborative and supportive; understand their actions' impacts on others/environment; appreciate culture and community; (3) Reflective as learners and become lifelong learners; (4) Innovative, curious, welcoming, and equipped for future challenges, and capable of applying knowledge to solve unfamiliar problems. They can adapt flexibly to new situations; (5) Engaged intellectually and socially, work well independently but also with others, and participate constructively in society locally, nationally, and globally."
- *Mixed Statement*: [University of British Columbia]: "Academic Learning Outcomes (UBC Learner)

  - Identity as a UBC Learner: Curiosity and a sense of belonging to UBC and the wider community.
  - Membership in the Academy: Identify their strengths for contribution to the academy and/or within a particular discipline.
  - Networks and Relationships: Connect to members of the community and build friendship networks.
  - Academic Culture: Cultivate practices that encourage self-directed learning and develop skills for academic success and well-being; Develop academic and personal integrity, rights, and responsibilities; Peer collaborations and team learning; Interact respectfully with peers and faculty; Professional Communication; Learning Management (or Academic Strategies)."

2.3.4 Clustering and Variations of Institutional Learning Outcomes and/or Desired Graduate Attributes

The range of ILOs and/or DGAs presented by the universities in our study varied from 6 to 29, with the median number of attributes across the sample being 21 (Tables 2.3 and 2.4). Among the 100 universities surveyed, four universities demonstrated a relatively low number of ILOs and/or DGAs or related statements that aligned with the 29 indicators proposed in this study, including the University of Bonn (6) in Germany, Sorbonne University (6) and Université Paris-Saclay (7) in France, and the Korea Advanced Institute of Science and Technology (7) in South Korea.

Among the sub-indicators analyzed in this study, the 100 universities' ILOs and/or DGAs and related statements varied. The most emphasized attribute was "generic skills," with a substantial 98% of institutions placing a particular focus on fostering these skills among their graduates. In addition, "citizenship" was highlighted in 85% of the ILOs/DGAs and related statements, while "professionalism/discipline knowledge" was emphasized by 84% of the universities. The attributes of "creativity/innovation" (80%) and "environmental/global awareness" (79%) also received notable attention. Furthermore, institutions highlighted the importance of fostering attributes such as "cultivating connections to others" (78%), "critical thinking" (77%), "research/scientific literacy" (72%), "communication" (72%), and "morality and ethics" (68%), which mainly were falling under the category of discipline-based attributes (Table 2.1).

Conversely, several attributes received relatively less attention. Notably, "empathy" registered a mere 32% emphasis. Similarly, "entrepreneurship" followed with an endorsement of 37%. "Resilience" (41%) and "lifelong learning" (42%) were also among the least emphasized attributes. In addition, "reflection" (45%), "respect" (46%), "specialism/specialist skills" (57%), and "literacy in different domains" (60%) constituted the bottom least emphasized attributes, mostly falling under the category of "non-cognitive intrapersonal competence" and "interpersonal competence" (Table 2.1).

2.3.5 Strong Emphasis on Cognitive (Intellectual) and Disciplinary Skills

To address Research Question 2 concerning the relative emphasis of ILOs and/or DGAs on cognitive (intellectual) skills and non-cognitive skills, our analysis began by examining the indicators categorized as discipline-based attributes and cognitive intrapersonal attributes.

Within the indicators categorized as discipline-based attributes, the analysis revealed the extent to which universities' ILOs and/or DGAs and related statements emphasize certain skills. For example, 98% of universities' ILOs and/or DGAs and related statements prioritized the development of "generic skills," emphasizing their importance in preparing graduates for a wide range of professional contexts. Besides, 84% of universities highlighted the significance of fostering "professionalism/discipline knowledge," recognizing the need for graduates to possess expertise in their respective fields. Additionally, four of the indicators addressed new skills demanded in the 21st-century knowledge economy; 79% of universities' ILOs and/or DGAs and related statements placed emphasis on fostering "environmental/global awareness," and 37% of universities focused on fostering "entrepreneurship." Finally, 60% of universities highlighted the importance of fostering "literacy in different domains," emphasizing the ability to comprehend effectively across different disciplines; 42% of universities emphasized the value of fostering a commitment to lifelong learning, recognizing the necessity for graduates to continually update their knowledge and skills throughout their careers (Table 2.1).

Besides disciplinary skills, the focus on "cognitive intrapersonal attributes" (intellectual skills) was high (96%). Specifically, 80% of universities prioritized fostering "creativity/innovation," recognizing the importance of nurturing students' ability to think outside the box and generate novel ideas. Besides, 64% of universities' ILOs and/or DGAs and related statements emphasized fostering "problem-solving skills," highlighting the significance of equipping graduates with the ability to analyze challenges and develop effective solutions. Finally, 77% of universities emphasized fostering "critical thinking," acknowledging the value of developing graduates' ability to evaluate information, make reasoned judgments, and engage in analytical reasoning (Table 2.1).

2.3.6 *Relatively Weaker Emphasis on Non-cognitive Intrapersonal Attributes*

Moving forward, we explored the domain of "non-cognitive intrapersonal attributes" to provide an answer to Research Question 2. Among the various indicators analyzed in this study, relatively fewer universities focused on non-cognitive intrapersonal attributes. Specifically, just 41% of the institutions surveyed demonstrated a focus on fostering "resilience" in their ILOs and/or DGAs and related statements, which suggested that the development of the ability to bounce back from setbacks and adapt to challenges (Shek & Leung, 2016) was not adequately addressed in the majority of universities' educational frameworks. Furthermore, the attribute of "reflection" was only emphasized by 45% of the universities (Table 2.1), signifying that a considerable number of institutions may not spend much emphasis on the ability to learn from past experiences.

In addition, 66% of the universities emphasized "self-management/self-confidence," while 65% emphasized "well-being," and 64% prioritized "leadership" (Table 2.1). While they represented relatively higher percentages, it still indicated that roughly one-third of universities might not prioritize the cultivation of these attributes, which are crucial for holistic personal growth and, thus, are vital for success in various professional contexts. As an illustration, Table 2.5 shows the ILOs and/or DGAs for the top 11 universities and the bottom 9 universities in the sample that placed the highest and lowest value on "intrapersonal attributes—non-cognitive" (Domain 7), "intrapersonal attributes—character and citizenship" (Domain 8), and "interpersonal competence" (Domain 9).

2.3.7 Relatively Weaker Emphasis on Intrapersonal Attributes (Character and Citizenship) and Interpersonal Competence

In response to Research Question 3, which investigates the coverage of holistic development in university students' ILOs and/or DGAs, particularly in terms of fostering interpersonal skills and intrapersonal competence, our analysis uncovered several noteworthy observations. When examining the sub-indicators of intrapersonal attributes (character and citizenship), it was observed that universities surveyed were not sufficiently aware of the importance of fostering these attributes compared to that paid to discipline-based attributes and cognitive intrapersonal attributes. Only around two-thirds (66%) of the universities' ILOs and/or DGAs and related statements placed emphasis on fostering "accountability/responsibility." Similarly, 68% of universities prioritized fostering "morality and ethics," and 67% of universities' ILOs and/or DGAs and related statements reflected a focus on fostering "character and integrity." On the other hand, the majority of universities, standing at 85%, emphasized developing "citizenship/civic and community" (Table 2.1), which indicated a widespread understanding among education institutes of the significance of actively participating in and contributing to the betterment of the community.

Finally, universities' attention to developing specific interpersonal competence was still limited. Among the sub-indicators, 72% of universities' ILOs and/or DGAs and related statements placed importance on fostering "communication." Similarly, 78% of universities' ILOs and/or DGAs highlighted the cultivation of "connections to others," which indicated a stronger recognition of the value of effective communication and building meaningful relationships and networks. However, again, there was still a portion that may not sufficiently emphasize this aspect. In contrast, a mere 32% of universities' ILOs and/or DGAs emphasized fostering "empathy," and only 46% focused on fostering "respect" (Table 2.1), which suggests a significant gap in recognizing and prioritizing the importance of understanding others and relating to diverse perspectives and experiences. To facilitate the readers to understand the landscape in this area, the desired graduate attributes in the different universities are presented in Table 2.4. In short, these observations suggested that while a majority of the surveyed universities had a focus on interpersonal competence, there was room for improvement in terms of emphasizing specific aspects, particularly empathy and respect.

2.4 Discussion

Our findings revealed that 47% of the surveyed universities explicitly outlined ILOs and/or DGAs at either the university or department level. Additionally, 31% of the universities did not provide specific ILOs/DGAs but presented similar statements such as "Mission and Culture," "Educational Commitment," "Competency Framework," and "Strategic Priorities," among others, through which we can extract the desired attributes of graduates. However, for the remaining 22% of universities, the information provided was limited, fragmented, and only marginally relevant to the desired attributes of graduates. In general, the increasing recognition of graduate attributes as crucial assets in an era characterized by rapid technological and social changes led to more universities focusing on developing graduate attributes not only competent in their academics but also prepared for the evolving workforce (Barrie, 2006; Bowden et al., 2000). This trend aligns with Hammer et al.'s (2021) findings that "There is increasing use of graduate attributes statements to 'brand' or differentiate universities from competitors" (p. 518).

This shift is partly driven by governments, particularly in Australia, the United Kingdom, Hong Kong, and Singapore, which prioritize the development of high-quality graduates as a crucial task in higher education (Green et al., 2009) and linking graduate outcomes with public funding for education (Barrie, 2005). In Australia, the concept of graduate attributes is widely accepted and implemented in higher education curricula, responding to the demands of employers and government initiatives since the 1990s (Bitzer & Withering, 2020; Hill et al., 2016). In Europe, the "Bologna Process," prompted by industry demands and technological advancements, urged universities to cultivate specific competencies and skills crucial to employment (Leoni, 2014). Similarly, universities in Hong Kong, such as The Hong Kong Polytechnic University (PolyU), have introduced the "General University Requirements" (GUR) program to foster the growth of essential attributes in their undergraduates, encompassing critical thinking, creative problem-solving, ethical leadership, and a commitment to lifelong learning (Shek et al., 2017b). Furthermore, to reinforce the implementation of "Outcome-Based Learning" (OBE), PolyU has, since 2008, identified a set of desirable graduate attributes that correspond to undergraduate degree programs and further articulated as ILOs, which are included in the strategic plan. Other Hong Kong universities have also expressed their commitment to cultivating desirable attributes in their graduates. However, our study highlights that a notable proportion of the institutions surveyed do not explicitly establish graduate attribute statements. As advocated by Bowden et al. (2000) and Star and Hammer (2008), the agenda of graduate attributes presents an opportunity for universities to focus on developing qualities that are not only pertinent to employment but also represent higher education's civic mission. Moving forward, establishing a broader agenda for graduate attributes is an intriguing topic.

The present study highlighted the strong emphasis placed by universities on developing discipline-based employability skills and work readiness, which is uncontroversial and widely acknowledged. This focus has long been instrumental in shaping and driving the development of graduate attributes in higher education. It aligns with the historically acknowledged and well-documented shift toward "vocationalism" (García, 2016), with the well-developed generic skills that have been widely demonstrated to enhance graduate employability (Garcia-Aracil et al., 2004). Additionally, the emphasis on 21st-century skills, such as global awareness and diverse literacy, is reflected in some institutional statements. In particular, information and communication technology skills are regarded as a crucial aspect of diverse literacy. The ability to adapt to technology is perceived to be a way for graduates to advance their employability and makes them more competitive in the workplace by continually developing their skills, which employers value (Finch et al., 2013; Garcia-Aracil et al., 2004).

However, our research uncovered a tendency where universities may prioritize the development of discipline-related "hard" employability skills, such as professionalism, scientific literacy, application, and global awareness, while neglecting the cultivation of "soft" personal competencies, in particular resilience and reflection classified as non-cognitive intrapersonal competence, as well as empathy and respect among interpersonal competence, which are vital for students to thrive in not only the workplace but also their life. In parallel, a growing body of scholarly work underscores the importance of promoting the holistic development of university students, with a specific focus on nurturing their character (Brooks et al., 2019), non-cognitive skills (García, 2016), and psychosocial competence (Shek, 2012) integrated into the curriculum. In fact, there is growing evidence showing the importance of nurturing the psychosocial competencies of university students, which can help them better cope with stressful social events and the COVID-19 pandemic (Shek, 2020, 2021; Shek et al., 2022; Shek et al., 2023a, 2023b, 2023c).

On the one hand, intrapersonal competencies refer to "process information about the self, involving a wide range of abilities related to self-understanding and self-management" (Shek & Lin, 2015, p. 255). According to Cox et al. (2013), self-management is reflected in graduates' willingness to take responsibility, resilience, adaptability, time management abilities, and self-confidence, as well as their willingness to improve their performance by actively engaging in feedback and reflective learning practices. Self-management is closely linked to self-efficacy, which signifies the graduates' belief in their ability to navigate personal and professional challenges effectively (Jackson, 2014). Higher self-esteem has been linked to improved job performance, as individuals with elevated levels of self-esteem exhibit a greater propensity for resilience and persistence in the face of failure (Baumeister et al., 2003). Moreover, individuals who have a strong sense of self-esteem tend to have better social relationships, be more popular among peers (Battistich et al., 1993), and establish better rapport with coworkers in the workplace (Frone, 2000). Importantly, self-esteem is closely tied to well-being, with high self-esteem serving as a protective buffer to mitigate the adverse impacts of stress (Baumeister et al., 2003). The capacity to perform effectively under stress and pressure is a crucial prerequisite for the majority of employers, with employees with resilience to stress demonstrating greater adaptability to new work environments, effective management of challenging tasks, and increased well-being (Kuntz et al., 2017). Additionally, leadership (Hosain et al., 2021; Shek et al., 2019) and reflection (Pool, 2017) are highly valued qualities in job candidates. Employers expect graduates with these attributes to demonstrate organizational skills and efficiency when taking on responsibilities or performing assigned tasks, as well as transform experiences into learning through reflection.

On the other hand, interpersonal skills encompass an individual's capacity to communicate, collaborate, and interact effectively with others while contributing value to the organization. These skills are associated with various factors, such as relationship building, teamwork, and active listening (Finch et al., 2013). Bochner and Kelly (1974) emphasized the importance of respect and empathy within the framework of interpersonal competencies. Research conducted by Dewey et al. (2008) highlighted that graduates with insufficient interpersonal ability leave a detrimental impression on employers during job searches, as employers prioritize these skills over other competencies. Furthermore, interpersonal skills serve as a strong predictor of graduates' future career success and overall life satisfaction. Firstly, interpersonal skills are recognized as fundamental strategies for career advancement, playing a crucial role not only in upward mobility but also in the long-term career success of those who are already in leadership positions (Laud & Johnson, 2012). Secondly, interpersonal skills, including emotional intelligence and political acumen, not only enhance job performance but also positively impact leaders' well-being (Mencl et al., 2016). Therefore, aligning with the recommendations of employers and scholars, incorporating interpersonal skills development into college programs will enable graduates to cultivate the ability to inspire and motivate both themselves and others (Mihail & Kloutsiniotis, 2014; Shek et al., 2015).

In the present analysis, we used document analysis, which offers significant advantages in terms of "availability," "stability," and "coverage." In other words, the documents are accessible from the public domain, the content is stable and allows for repeated review (Merriam, 1988), and the documents cover a wide range of periods, events, and contexts, providing a comprehensive scope for the study (Yin, 1994). These qualities have established document analysis as a widely recognized and useful qualitative research method (Bowen, 2009). However, it is important to acknowledge the limitation of "low retrievability" associated with document analysis, as some documents may be difficult to retrieve or intentionally blocked (Yin, 1994). In the present study, the placement of many university documents within institutional firewalls may result in incomplete information regarding the attributes of desirable graduates for certain institutions. Besides, as ILOs/DGAs in universities have changed over time, a snapshot may not be able to assess the dynamic picture in this area. Despite these limitations, "Given its efficiency and cost-effectiveness in particular, document analysis offers advantages that clearly outweigh the limitations" (Bowen, 2009, p. 32). Additionally, we recognize that the findings of this qualitative study represent an initial exploration of desirable graduate qualities in academia, which enables us to explore the question of what universities should do to nurture their students. Moving forward, the next phase of research could involve investigating these attributes across a broader spectrum of disciplines and campus cultures, accompanied by utilizing quantitative survey instruments that build upon the categories identified in this study.

Finally, the findings of this study are based on documentary analysis of web documents, which serve as literal statements of institutional goals but may not fully reflect and guarantee their actual implementation in real-world scenarios (Hammer et al., 2021). Oliver and Jorre de St Jorre (2018) also remarked that "these claims about attributes sometimes bleed into the marketing of courses" (p. 823), but most may not, which is the particular aspect that was not explored in this study. Future research can explore how the development of graduate attributes becomes integrated into the curriculum. Moreover, while existing research has predominantly focused on objectively examining institutional understanding and formulation of graduate attributes, it would be intriguing to investigate the subjective perspectives of teachers and students regarding the actual implementation of the process to attain desirable graduate attributes and the effectiveness of the associated learning processes.

Acknowledgements The preparation of this chapter is financially supported by The Hong Kong Polytechnic University (ZZ4U and ZZUE), Li and Fung Endowed Professorship in Service Leadership Education, Wofoo Foundation, and the Matching Fund of Research Grants Council (ZECL and ZH4Q).

Appendix

Table 2.1 Number and percentage of top 100 universities in THE 2023 with the attributes by funding ($N = 100$)

Attributes	Private universities ($N = 23$)		Public universities ($N = 77$)		Total ($N = 100$)	
	n	%	*n*	%	*n*	%
1. Generic skills/Competence/Broad-based independence	23	100.00	75	97.40	98	98.00
2. Professionalism/Discipline knowledge	19	82.61	65	84.42	84	84.00
3. Specialism/Specialist skills	15	65.22	42	54.55	57	57.00
4. Research/Scientific literacy	17	73.91	55	71.43	72	72.00
5. Application	15	65.22	51	66.23	66	66.00
6. Intrapersonal attributes (Cognitive)	21	91.30	75	97.40	96	96.00
6a. Creativity/Innovation	19	82.61	61	79.22	80	80.00
6b. Problem-solving	17	73.91	47	61.04	64	64.00
6c. Critical thinking	16	69.57	61	79.22	77	77.00
7. Intrapersonal attributes (Non-cognitive)	22	95.65	68	88.31	90	90.00
7a. Resilience	10	43.48	31	40.26	41	41.00
7b. Self-awareness/Self-regulated/Self-direct/Self-management/Sense of self/Self-confidence	19	82.61	47	61.04	66	66.00
7c. Well-being	20	86.96	45	58.44	65	65.00
7d. Leadership	15	65.22	49	63.64	64	64.00
7e. Reflection	12	52.17	33	42.86	45	45.00
8. Intrapersonal attributes (Character and citizenship)	22	95.65	73	94.81	95	95.00
8a. Accountability/Responsibility	13	56.52	53	68.83	66	66.00
8b. Morality and ethics	18	78.26	50	64.94	68	68.00
8c. Character and integrity	18	78.26	49	63.64	67	67.00
8d. Citizenship/Civic and community	21	91.30	64	83.12	85	85.00
9. Interpersonal competence	21	91.30	63	81.82	84	84.00
9a. Communication	18	78.26	54	70.13	72	72.00
9b. Cultivate connections to others	19	82.61	59	76.62	78	78.00
9c. Empathy	11	47.83	21	27.27	32	32.00
9d. Respect	14	60.87	32	41.56	46	46.00
10. Environmental/global awareness	22	95.65	57	74.03	79	79.00
11. Entrepreneurship	8	34.78	29	37.66	37	37.00
12. Literacy in different domains	16	69.57	44	57.14	60	60.00
12a. Lifelong learning	8	34.78	34	44.16	42	42.00

Table 2.2 Number and percentage of top 100 universities in THE 2023 with the attributes by region ($N = 100$)

Attributes	Asia ($N = 19$)		Australasia ($N = 7$)		Europe ($N = 36$)		North America ($N = 38$)	
	n	%	*n*	%	*n*	%	*n*	%
1. Generic Skills/Competence/ Broad-based independence	18	94.74	7	100.00	35	97.22	38	100.00
2. Professionalism/Discipline knowledge	17	89.47	7	100.00	30	83.33	30	78.95
3. Specialism/Specialist skills	14	73.68	4	57.14	19	52.78	20	52.63
4. Research/Scientific literacy	11	57.89	5	71.43	28	77.78	28	73.68
5. Application	11	57.89	7	100.00	23	63.89	25	65.79
6. Intrapersonal attributes (Cognitive)	19	100.00	7	100.00	34	94.44	36	94.74
6a. Creativity/Innovation	17	89.47	7	100.00	26	72.22	30	78.95
6b. Problem-solving	7	36.84	7	100.00	23	63.89	27	71.05
6c. Critical thinking	12	63.16	7	100.00	29	80.56	29	76.32
7. Intrapersonal attributes (Non-cognitive)	17	89.47	6	85.71	31	86.11	36	94.74
7a. Resilience	8	42.11	4	57.14	14	38.89	15	39.47
7b. Self-awareness/Self-regulated/ Self-direct/Self-management/Sense of self /Self-confidence	13	68.42	6	85.71	22	61.11	25	65.79
7c. Well-being	11	57.89	3	42.86	21	58.33	30	78.95
7d. Leadership	14	73.68	4	57.14	18	50.00	28	73.68
7e. Reflection	5	26.32	5	71.43	15	41.67	20	52.63
8. Intrapersonal attributes (Character and citizenship)	18	94.74	7	100.00	33	91.67	37	97.37
8a. Accountability/Responsibility	14	73.68	6	85.71	23	63.89	23	60.53
8b. Morality and ethics	14	73.68	6	85.71	20	55.56	28	73.68
8c. Character and integrity	15	78.95	4	57.14	20	55.56	28	73.68
8d. Citizenship/Civic and community	17	89.47	7	100.00	25	69.44	36	94.74
9. Interpersonal competence	13	68.42	7	100.00	27	75.00	37	97.37
9a. Communication	12	63.16	6	85.71	23	63.89	31	81.58
9b. Cultivate connections to others	12	63.16	6	85.71	25	69.44	35	92.11
9c. Empathy	6	31.58	3	42.86	4	11.11	19	50.00
9d. Respect	6	31.58	6	85.71	14	38.89	20	52.63
10. Environmental/global awareness	17	89.47	7	100.00	22	61.11	33	86.84
11. Entrepreneurship	5	26.32	4	57.14	15	41.67	13	34.21
12. Literacy in different domains	9	47.37	6	85.71	21	58.33	24	63.16
12a. Lifelong learning	7	36.84	3	42.86	16	44.44	16	42.11

Table 2.3 Number of attributes of top 100 universities in THE 2023 ($N = 100$)

THE 2023 rank	University	Country/ Economy	No. of attributes ($N = 29$)	No. of attributes in domains 7, 8, 9 ($N = 16$)	Format	Special case report
1	University of Oxford (Oxon.)	United Kingdom	20	9	Integrated	Special case 1a
2	Harvard University	United States	17	10	Integrated	Special case 1a
3	University of Cambridge (Cambridge)	United Kingdom	23	12	Cluster	Normal
3	Stanford University (Stanford)	United States	26	14	Mixed	Special case 1a
5	Massachusetts Institute of Technology (MIT)	United States	18	11	Integrated	Special case 1b
6	California Institute of Technology (Caltech)	United States	24	14	Mixed	Normal
7	Princeton University (Princeton)	United States	19	10	Mixed	Special case 1a
8	University of California, Berkeley (UC Berkeley)	United States	16	11	Integrated	Special case 1a
9	Yale University (Yale)	United States	21	10	Integrated	Normal
10	Imperial College London (Imperial)	United Kingdom	18	8	Mixed	Normal
11	Columbia University (Columbia)	United States	24	13	Cluster	Special case 1a
11	ETH Zurich (ETHZ)	Switzerland	24	14	Cluster	Special case 1a
13	The University of Chicago (UChicago)	United States	20	12	Integrated	Special case 1a
14	University of Pennsylvania (UPenn)	United States	12	3	Integrated	Special case 1b
15	Johns Hopkins University (JHU)	United States	24	16	Mixed	Normal
16	Tsinghua University (THU)	Mainland China	12	5	Integrated	Special case 1b
17	Peking University (PKU)	Mainland China	20	12	Integrated	Special case 1a
18	University of Toronto (U of T)	Canada	19	12	Cluster	Normal
19	National University of Singapore (NUS)	Singapore	22	9	Integrated	Normal
20	Cornell University (Cornell)	United States	25	14	Mixed	Normal
21	University of California, Los Angeles (UCLA)	United States	19	9	Integrated	Special case 1a

(continued)

Table 2.3 (continued)

THE 2023 rank	University	Country/ Economy	No. of attributes ($N = 29$)	No. of attributes in domains 7, 8, 9 ($N = 16$)	Format	Special case report
22	University College London (UCL)	United Kingdom	17	9	Cluster	Special case 1b
23	University of Michigan-Ann Arbor (UMich)	United States	23	14	Mixed	Normal
24	New York University (NYU)	United States	20	13	Mixed	Normal
25	Duke University (Duke)	United States	19	9	Cluster	Special case 2
26	Northwestern University (NorthwesternU)	United States	27	16	Cluster	Normal
26	University of Washington (UW)	United States	22	15	Mixed	Special case 1a
28	Carnegie Mellon University (CMU)	United States	22	12	Mixed	Special case 1a
29	University of Edinburgh (UoE)	United Kingdom	23	14	Cluster	Normal
30	Technical University of Munich (TUM)	Germany	21	12	Integrated	Special case 1b
31	University of Hong Kong (HKU)	Hong Kong	26	14	Cluster	Normal
32	University of California, San Diego (UCSD)	United States	22	12	Mixed	Normal
33	LMU Munich (LMU)	Germany	11	3	Integrated	Special case 1b
34	University of Melbourne (UniMelb)	Australia	29	16	Integrated	Normal
35	King's College London (KCL)	United Kingdom	21	10	Integrated	Normal
36	Nanyang Technological University (NTU)	Singapore	23	13	Mixed	Normal
37	London School of Economics and Political Science (LSE)	United Kingdom	8	4	Integrated	Special case 1b
38	Georgia Institute of Technology (Georgia Tech)	United States	21	10	Mixed	Normal
39	The University of Tokyo (UTokyo)	Japan	21	13	Integrated	Special case 1a
40	University of British Columbia (UBC)	Canada	16	11	Mixed	Normal
41	École Polytechnique Fédérale de Lausanne (EPFL)	Switzerland	13	7	Integrated	Special case 1b
42	KU Leuven	Belgium	22	12	Integrated	Special case 1a

(continued)

Table 2.3 (continued)

THE 2023 rank	University	Country/ Economy	No. of attributes ($N = 29$)	No. of attributes in domains 7, 8, 9 ($N = 16$)	Format	Special case report
43	Universität Heidelberg (Uni-Heidelberg)	Germany	23	12	Integrated	Special case 1a
44	Monash University (Monash)	Australia	18	6	Mixed	Normal
45	Chinese University of Hong Kong (CUHK)	Hong Kong	22	14	Integrated	Normal
46	McGill University (McGill)	Canada	24	11	Cluster	Special case 2
47	Paris Sciences et Lettres—PSL Research University Paris (PSL)	France	11	4	Integrated	Special case 1b
48	University of Illinois at Urbana-Champaign (U of I)	United States	21	12	Mixed	Normal
49	Karolinska Institute (KI)	Sweden	18	8	Mixed	Special case 2
50	University of Texas at Austin (UT-Austin)	United States	22	12	Integrated	Special case 1a
51	Fudan University (FDU)	Mainland China	11	7	Integrated	Special case 1b
52	Shanghai Jiao Tong University (SJTU)	Mainland China	25	14	Mixed	Normal
53	The University of Queensland (UQ)	Australia	22	11	Cluster	Normal
54	University of Manchester (Manchester)	United Kingdom	25	13	Mixed	Normal
54	University of Sydney (USYD)	Australia	25	14	Cluster	Normal
56	Seoul National University (SNU)	South Korea	22	12	Integrated	Special case 1a
57	Washington University in St Louis (WUSTL)	United States	25	15	Mixed	Special case 1a
58	The Hong Kong University of Science and Technology (HKUST)	Hong Kong	22	14	Cluster	Normal
59	Wageningen University & Research (WUR)	Netherlands	27	14	Integrated	Special case 1a
60	University of Amsterdam (UvA)	Netherlands	21	11	Integrated	Special case 1a
61	Brown University (Brown)	United States	21	13	Integrated	Special case 1a
62	Australian National University (ANU)	Australia	23	13	Mixed	Special case 1a
63	University of California, Davis (UC Davis)	United States	21	13	Cluster	Normal

(continued)

Table 2.3 (continued)

THE 2023 rank	University	Country/ Economy	No. of attributes ($N = 29$)	No. of attributes in domains 7, 8, 9 ($N = 16$)	Format	Special case report
64	University of California, Santa Barbara (UCSB)	United States	17	8	Mixed	Normal
65	University of Southern California (USC)	United States	20	12	Integrated	Special case 1b
66	Utrecht University (UU)	Netherlands	24	13	Mixed	Special case 2
67	Zhejiang University (ZJU)	Mainland China	13	8	Integrated	Special case 1b
68	Kyoto University (KyotoU)	Japan	23	14	Mixed	Special case 1a
69	University of North Carolina at Chapel Hill (UNC)	United States	22	15	Integrated	Special case 1a
70	Delft University of Technology (TU Delft)	Netherlands	25	14	Cluster	Normal
71	Boston University (BU)	United States	27	15	Mixed	Normal
71	UNSW Sydney (UNSW)	Australia	22	11	Mixed	Normal
73	Charité—Universitätsmedizin Berlin (Charité)	Germany	20	10	Integrated	Special case 1a
74	University of Science and Technology of Mainland China (USTC)	Mainland China	17	8	Integrated	Special case 1a
75	University of Groningen (UG)	Netherlands	18	11	Mixed	Special case 2
76	University of Bristol (Bristol)	United Kingdom	25	15	Cluster	Special case 1a
77	Leiden University (LEI)	Netherlands	16	9	Cluster	Special case 1a
78	Yonsei University (Seoul campus) (Yonsei)	South Korea	15	8	Integrated	Special case 1a
79	The Hong Kong Polytechnic University (PolyU)	Hong Kong	24	12	Cluster	Normal
80	Erasmus University Rotterdam (EUR)	Netherlands	21	10	Integrated	Special case 1b
81	University of Wisconsin-Madison (UW)	United States	19	7	Cluster	Normal
82	Emory University (Emory)	United States	13	5	Mixed	Special case 2
82	University of Glasgow (UofGlasgow)	United Kingdom	27	15	Mixed	Normal

(continued)

Table 2.3 (continued)

THE 2023 rank	University	Country/ Economy	No. of attributes ($N = 29$)	No. of attributes in domains 7, 8, 9 ($N = 16$)	Format	Special case report
82	University of Zurich (UZH)	Switzerland	12	5	Mixed	Special case 1b
85	McMaster University (McMaster)	Canada	20	10	Mixed	Special case 2
86	Humboldt University of Berlin (HU Berlin)	Germany	18	10	Integrated	Special case 1b
86	University of Tübingen (Uni Tuebingen)	Germany	25	14	Integrated	Special case 1a
88	University of Adelaide (UniofAdelaide)	Australia	25	15	Cluster	Normal
89	University of Bonn (Uni Bonn)	Germany	6	2	Mixed	Special case 1b
90	Sorbonne University (Sorbonne)	France	6	0	Integrated	Special case 1b
91	Free University of Berlin (FU Berlin)	Germany	23	11	Integrated	Special case 1a
91	Korea Advanced Institute of Science and Technology (KAIST)	South Korea	7	3	Integrated	Special case 1b
93	Université Paris-Saclay (UPSaclay)	France	7	2	Integrated	Special case 1b
94	University of Bern (Unibe)	Switzerland	10	5	Integrated	Special case 1b
95	University of California, Irvine (UCI)	United States	24	14	Mixed	Normal
95	Institut Polytechnique de Paris (IP Paris)	France	10	5	Integrated	Special case 1b
95	Nanjing University (NJU)	Mainland China	22	11	Integrated	Special case 2
98	Vanderbilt University (Vandy)	United States	25	15	Cluster	Normal
99	City University of Hong Kong (CityU)	Hong Kong	12	4	Cluster	Normal
99	RWTH Aachen University (RWTH Aachen)	Germany	17	8	Integrated	Special case 1b

Note Normal = There were particular ILOs/DGAs provided
Special case 1a = No particular ILOs/DGAs were provided, but related information was provided, such as "mission and culture," "education commitment," "competence framework," "strategic priorities," etc.;
Special case 1b = No particular ILOs/DGAs were provided, and only less scattered and slightly relevant information was obtained;
Special case 2 = No university-level ILOs/DGAs were provided, but ILOs/DGAs from the department/college/faculty were provided.

Table 2.4 ILOs and/or DGAs of top 100 universities in THE 2023 ($N = 100$)

Attributes	1	2	3	4	5	6	7	8	9	10	11	12	13	14	15	16	17	18	19	20	21	22	23	24	25	26
1. Generic skills/Competence/Broad-based independence	√	√	√	√	√	√	√	√	√	√	√	√	√	√	√	√	√	√	√	√	√	√	√	√	√	√
2. Professionalism/Discipline knowledge	√	√	√	√	√	√	√		√	√	√	√		√		√	√		√	√	√		√	√	√	√
3. Specialism/Specialist skills	√			√	√	√		√	√		√	√		√		√	√		√	√			√	√	√	√
4. Research/Scientific literacy	√		√	√		√	√		√		√	√		√	√	√	√	√	√	√	√		√		√	√
5. Application	√	√	√	√		√			√	√		√	√	√				√	√	√	√	√		√	√	√
6. Intrapersonal attributes (Cognitive)	√	√	√	√	√	√	√	√	√	√	√	√	√	√	√	√	√	√	√	√	√	√	√		√	√
6a. Creativity/Innovation		√	√	√	√	√	√	√	√	√	√	√	√	√	√	√	√	√	√	√	√	√	√			√
6b. Problem-solving	√	√	√		√	√	√			√		√	√		√			√	√	√	√	√			√	√
6c. Critical thinking	√		√	√			√		√	√	√	√	√	√			√	√	√	√	√	√	√		√	√
7. Intrapersonal attributes (Non-cognitive)	√	√	√	√	√	√	√	√	√	√	√	√	√		√		√	√	√	√	√	√	√	√	√	√
7a. Resilience	√		√	√		√		√			√	√	√		√			√		√		√				√
7b. Self-awareness/Self-regulated/ Self-direct/Self-management/Sense of self / Self-confidence	√	√	√	√	√	√				√	√	√	√		√		√	√		√		√	√	√	√	√
7c. Well-being	√	√		√	√	√	√	√	√	√	√	√	√		√	√	√		√	√	√	√	√	√		√
7d. Leadership		√			√	√		√	√			√			√		√	√	√		√	√	√	√		√
7e. Reflection			√	√			√	√				√	√		√		√			√			√	√		√
8. Intrapersonal attributes (Character and citizenship)	√	√	√	√	√	√	√	√	√	√	√	√	√	√	√	√	√	√	√	√	√		√	√	√	√
8a. Accountability/Responsibility			√	√		√			√		√	√			√	√	√			√			√		√	√
8b. Morality and ethics		√		√	√	√	√		√			√	√		√		√	√		√			√	√	√	√
8c. Character and integrity		√	√	√	√	√	√	√	√	√	√	√	√		√	√		√	√	√	√			√		√

(continued)

Table 2.4 (continued)

Attributes	1	2	3	4	5	6	7	8	9	10	11	12	13	14	15	16	17	18	19	20	21	22	23	24	25	26
8d. Citizenship/Civic and community	√	√	√	√	√	√	√	√	√		√	√	√	√	√	√	√	√	√	√	√		√		√	√
9. Interpersonal competence	√	√	√	√	√	√	√	√	√	√	√	√	√		√		√	√	√	√	√	√	√	√	√	√
9a. Communication	√	√	√	√	√	√		√			√	√			√		√	√		√		√	√	√	√	√
9b. Cultivate connections to others	√		√	√		√	√	√	√	√	√	√	√		√		√	√	√	√	√	√	√	√	√	√
9c. Empathy				√							√		√	√	√			√	√		√	√	√	√		√
9d. Respect			√		√	√	√			√	√				√					√			√	√		√
10. Environmental/global awareness	√	√	√	√	√	√	√	√	√	√	√		√	√	√	√	√		√	√	√		√	√	√	√
11. Entrepreneurship	√		√	√						√	√		√						√			√	√	√		
12. Literacy in different domains	√			√		√	√		√	√	√	√			√				√	√		√		√	√	√
12a. Lifelong learning			√	√					√		√				√				√		√					
Total attributes per university	20	17	23	26	18	24	19	16	21	18	24	24	20	12	24	12	20	19	22	25	19	17	23	20	19	27
Percentage of attributes per university (%)	69	59	79	90	62	83	66	55	72	62	83	83	69	41	83	41	69	66	76	86	66	59	79	69	66	93
Attributes	27	28	29	30	31	32	33	34	35	36	37	38	39	40	41	42	43	44	45	46	47	48	49	50	51	52
1. Generic skills/Competence/ Broad-based independence	√	√	√	√	√	√	√	√	√	√	√	√	√	√	√	√	√	√	√	√	√	√	√	√	√	√
2. Professionalism/Discipline knowledge		√		√	√	√	√	√	√	√		√	√	√	√	√	√	√	√	√	√	√	√	√	√	√
3. Specialism/Specialist skills		√		√	√		√	√	√	√		√	√			√	√	√		√		√	√		√	√
4. Research/Scientific literacy			√		√	√	√	√	√	√		√		√		√	√	√		√	√		√	√		√
5. Application		√	√	√	√			√				√	√	√	√		√	√		√		√	√			√
6. Intrapersonal attributes (Cognitive)	√	√	√	√	√	√	√	√	√	√	√	√	√	√	√	√	√	√	√	√	√	√	√	√	√	√
6a. Creativity/Innovation	√		√	√	√	√	√	√	√	√	√		√					√	√	√	√	√		√		√
6b. Problem-solving	√	√	√		√	√		√	√	√		√			√	√	√	√		√		√	√	√		

(continued)

Table 2.4 (continued)

Attributes	27	28	29	30	31	32	33	34	35	36	37	38	39	40	41	42	43	44	45	46	47	48	49	50	51	52
6c. Critical thinking	√	√	√		√	√		√	√		√	√				√	√	√	√	√	√	√	√	√		√
7. Intrapersonal attributes (Non-cognitive)	√	√	√	√	√	√		√	√	√	√	√	√	√	√	√	√		√	√	√	√		√	√	√
7a. Resilience	√		√	√	√			√	√				√						√						√	√
7b. Self-awareness/Self-regulated/ Self-direct/Self-management/Sense of self/ Self-confidence	√		√		√			√	√	√			√	√		√	√			√					√	√
7c. Well-being	√	√		√			√	√	√	√		√		√			√		√	√		√		√		√
7d. Leadership	√	√	√		√	√		√		√	√	√	√		√	√			√	√	√	√		√		√
7e. Reflection	√	√	√		√	√		√				√				√	√					√			√	
8. Intrapersonal attributes (Character and citizenship)	√	√	√	√	√	√	√	√	√	√	√	√	√	√	√	√	√	√	√	√	√	√	√	√	√	√
8a. Accountability/Responsibility	√		√	√	√	√		√		√			√	√	√	√	√	√	√	√		√	√	√		√
8b. Morality and ethics		√	√	√	√	√		√	√	√		√			√	√		√	√	√		√	√	√	√	√
8c. Character and integrity	√		√	√	√	√	√	√	√	√			√	√			√		√		√	√	√	√	√	√
8d. Citizenship/Civic and community	√	√	√	√	√	√		√	√	√	√	√	√	√	√	√	√	√	√	√		√		√		√
9. Interpersonal competence	√	√	√	√	√	√		√	√	√		√	√	√	√	√	√	√	√	√		√	√	√		√
9a. Communication	√	√	√	√	√	√		√		√		√	√	√		√	√	√	√	√			√	√		√
9b. Cultivate connections to others	√	√	√	√	√	√		√	√	√		√	√	√		√	√		√	√		√	√	√		√
9c. Empathy	√	√						√					√			√			√			√				√
9d. Respect	√	√	√	√	√	√		√		√			√	√			√		√				√	√		
10. Environmental/global awareness		√	√	√	√	√	√	√	√	√		√	√				√	√	√	√		√		√		√
11. Entrepreneurship				√		√		√	√	√						√		√		√	√					

(continued)

Table 2.4 (continued)

Attributes	27	28	29	30	31	32	33	34	35	36	37	38	39	40	41	42	43	44	45	46	47	48	49	50	51	52
12. Literacy in different domains	√	√			√	√	√	√				√	√			√	√	√	√	√			√	√		√
12a. Lifelong learning	√	√	√	√	√			√	√	√		√			√	√	√		√	√			√	√		√
Total attributes per university	22	22	23	21	26	22	11	29	21	23	8	21	21	16	13	22	23	18	22	24	11	21	18	22	11	25
Percentage of attributes per university (%)	76	76	79	72	90	76	38	100	72	79	28	72	72	55	45	76	79	62	76	83	38	72	62	76	38	86
Attributes	53	54	55	56	57	58	59	60	61	62	63	64	65	66	67	68	69	70	71	72	73	74	75	76	77	78
1. Generic skills/Competence/ Broad-based independence	√	√	√	√	√	√	√	√	√	√	√	√	√	√	√	√	√	√	√	√	√	√	√	√	√	√
2. Professionalism/Discipline knowledge	√	√	√	√		√	√	√		√	√	√	√	√		√		√	√	√	√	√	√	√		√
3. Specialism/Specialist skills	√	√	√	√		√	√						√	√		√		√	√		√	√				
4. Research/Scientific literacy	√	√		√	√	√	√	√	√	√	√	√	√	√		√		√	√	√	√	√	√	√	√	
5. Application	√	√	√	√	√		√	√	√	√		√		√		√	√	√	√	√	√	√	√			
6. Intrapersonal attributes (Cognitive)	√	√	√	√	√	√	√	√	√	√	√	√		√	√	√	√	√	√	√	√	√	√	√	√	√
6a. Creativity/Innovation	√	√	√	√	√		√	√	√	√	√	√	√	√	√	√		√	√	√		√	√	√		√
6b. Problem-solving	√	√	√		√		√		√	√					√		√	√	√	√	√	√		√	√	√
6c. Critical thinking	√	√	√	√	√	√	√	√		√	√	√		√		√	√	√	√	√	√		√	√	√	√
7. Intrapersonal attributes (Non-cognitive)	√	√	√	√	√	√	√	√	√	√	√	√	√	√	√	√	√	√	√	√	√	√	√	√	√	√
7a. Resilience			√		√	√	√			√	√					√	√	√	√			√		√	√	
7b. Self-awareness/Self-regulated/ Self-direct/Self-management/Sense of self/ Self-confidence	√	√	√	√	√	√	√	√	√	√			√	√		√	√	√	√	√		√	√	√	√	√
7c. Well-being		√	√	√	√		√	√	√	√			√	√	√	√	√		√		√		√	√		√
7d. Leadership		√	√		√	√	√		√		√	√	√		√	√	√	√	√	√	√		√	√		√
7e. Reflection	√			√	√		√	√	√	√				√			√	√	√	√			√	√	√	

(continued)

Table 2.4 (continued)

Attributes	53	54	55	56	57	58	59	60	61	62	63	64	65	66	67	68	69	70	71	72	73	74	75	76	77	78
8. Intrapersonal attributes (Character and citizenship)	√	√	√	√	√	√	√	√	√	√	√	√	√	√	√	√	√	√	√	√	√	√	√	√	√	√
8a. Accountability/Responsibility	√	√	√	√	√	√	√		√		√			√	√	√	√	√	√	√	√	√	√	√		
8b. Morality and ethics	√	√	√	√	√	√	√	√			√		√	√	√	√	√	√	√	√		√	√	√		√
8c. Character and integrity		√	√	√	√	√		√	√	√	√	√		√	√	√	√	√	√		√	√		√		√
8d. Citizenship/Civic and community	√	√	√	√	√	√	√		√	√	√	√	√	√	√	√	√	√	√	√	√	√		√	√	√
9. Interpersonal competence	√	√	√	√	√	√	√	√	√	√	√	√	√	√		√	√	√	√	√	√		√	√	√	
9a. Communication	√	√	√	√	√	√	√	√	√	√	√	√	√	√		√		√	√		√		√	√	√	
9b. Cultivate connections to others	√	√	√	√	√	√	√	√	√	√	√	√	√	√		√	√	√	√	√	√		√	√	√	
9c. Empathy					√	√		√		√	√		√				√									
9d. Respect	√	√	√			√	√		√	√	√		√	√		√	√	√	√	√				√		
10. Environmental/global awareness	√	√	√	√	√	√	√	√	√	√	√	√	√	√	√	√		√	√	√		√		√	√	√
11. Entrepreneurship		√					√		√				√	√			√			√				√		
12. Literacy in different domains	√	√	√	√	√	√	√	√		√		√	√				√	√	√		√			√	√	
12a. Lifelong learning			√		√		√	√			√			√					√	√	√					
Total attributes per university	22	25	25	22	25	22	27	21	21	23	21	17	20	24	13	23	22	25	27	22	20	17	18	25	16	15
Percentage of attributes per university (%)	76	86	86	76	86	76	93	72	72	79	72	59	69	83	45	79	76	86	93	76	69	59	62	86	55	52

Attributes	79	80	81	82	83	84	85	86	87	88	89	90	91	92	93	94	95	96	97	98	99	100	Total (*N* = 100)	
																							n	%
1. Generic skills/ Competence/ Broad-based independence	√	√	√	√	√	√	√	√	√	√	√		√		√	√	√	√	√	√	√	√	98	98

(continued)

Table 2.4 (continued)

Attributes	79	80	81	82	83	84	85	86	87	88	89	90	91	92	93	94	95	96	97	98	99	100	Total (N = 100)	
																							n	%
2. Professionalism/ Discipline knowledge	√	√	√	√	√		√	√	√	√	√	√	√		√		√	√	√	√	√	√	84	84
3. Specialism/ Specialist skills	√		√		√							√	√		√			√	√	√		√	57	57
4. Research/ Scientific literacy		√	√	√	√	√		√	√		√		√		√		√		√	√		√	72	72
5. Application	√	√	√		√		√	√	√	√			√	√			√		√		√	√	66	66
6. Intrapersonal attributes (Cognitive)	√	√	√	√	√	√	√	√	√	√		√	√	√		√	√	√	√	√	√	√	96	96
6a. Creativity/ Innovation	√	√	√	√	√		√	√	√	√		√	√	√		√		√	√		√	√	80	80
6b. Problem-solving	√	√	√	√	√	√	√		√	√			√				√			√		√	64	64
6c. Critical thinking	√	√	√	√	√	√	√	√	√	√			√			√	√		√	√	√	√	77	77
7. Intrapersonal attributes (Non-cognitive)	√	√		√	√	√	√	√	√	√			√	√		√	√	√	√	√		√	90	90
7a. Resilience					√				√	√			√							√			41	41
7b. Self-awareness/ Self-regulated/ Self-direct/ Self-management/ Sense of self / Self-confidence	√	√		√	√	√	√		√	√			√				√		√	√			66	66

(continued)

Table 2.4 (continued)

Attributes	79	80	81	82	83	84	85	86	87	88	89	90	91	92	93	94	95	96	97	98	99	100	Total (N = 100)	
																							n	%
7c. Well-being	√	√			√		√	√	√							√	√			√		√	65	65
7d. Leadership	√	√			√		√		√	√				√			√	√	√	√		√	64	64
7e. Reflection	√	√			√				√	√							√			√			45	45
8. Intrapersonal attributes (Character and citizenship)	√	√	√		√	√	√	√	√	√			√		√	√	√	√	√	√	√	√	95	95
8a. Accountability/ Responsibility	√		√		√	√		√	√	√			√			√	√	√	√	√		√	66	66
8b. Morality and ethics	√	√	√		√		√	√	√	√			√				√		√			√	68	68
8c. Character and integrity					√			√		√			√				√		√	√		√	67	67
8d. Citizenship/Civic and community	√	√	√		√		√	√		√			√		√	√	√	√	√	√	√	√	85	85
9. Interpersonal competence	√	√	√	√	√		√	√	√	√	√		√				√		√	√	√		84	84
9a. Communication	√		√	√	√		√	√	√	√	√		√				√		√	√	√		72	72
9b. Cultivate connections to others	√	√	√	√	√	√	√	√	√	√							√		√	√			78	78

(continued)

Table 2.4 (continued)

Attributes	79	80	81	82	83	84	85	86	87	88	89	90	91	92	93	94	95	96	97	98	99	100	Total (*N* = 100)	
																							n	%
9c. Empathy									√	√				√			√			√			32	32
9d. Respect					√				√	√			√							√			46	46
10. Environmental/ global awareness	√	√	√		√		√	√		√		√	√		√	√	√		√	√	√		79	79
11. Entrepreneurship	√	√		√			√		√	√		√		√			√		√				37	37
12. Literacy in different domains	√	√	√		√	√			√	√	√		√				√		√	√			60	60
12a. Lifelong learning	√		√		√	√	√		√				√							√	√		42	42
Total attributes per university	24	21	19	13	27	12	20	18	25	25	6	6	23	7	7	10	24	10	22	25	12	17		
Percentage of attributes per university (%)	83	72	66	45	93	41	69	62	86	86	21	21	79	24	24	34	83	34	76	86	41	59		

Note 1 = Oxon.; 2 = Harvard; 3 = Cambridge; 4 = Stanford; 5 = MIT; 6 = Caltech; 7 = Princeton; 8 = UC Berkeley; 9 = Yale; 10 = Imperial; 11 = Columbia; 12 = ETHZ; 13 = UChicago; 14 = UPenn; 15 = JHU; 16 = THU; 17 = PKU; 18 = U of T; 19 = NUS; 20 = Cornell; 21 = UCLA; 22 = UCL; 23 = UMich; 24 = NYU; 25 = Duke; 26 = NorthwesternU; 27 = UW; 28 = CMU; 29 = UoE; 30 = TUM; 31 = HKU; 32 = UCSD; 33 = LMU; 34 = UniMelb; 35 = KCL; 36 = NTU; 37 = LSE; 38 = Georgia Tech; 39 = UTokyo; 40 = UBC; 41 = EPFL; 42 = KU Leuven; 43 = Uni-Heidelberg; 44 = Monash; 45 = CUHK; 46 = McGill; 47 PSL; 48 = U of I; 49 = KI; 50 = UT-Austin; 51 = FDU; 52 = SJTU; 53 = UQ; 54 = Manchester; 55 = USYD; 56 = SNU; 57 = WUSTL; 58 = HKUST; 59 = WUR; 60 = UvA; 61 = Brown; 62 = ANU; 63 = UC Davis; 64 = UCSB; 65 = USC; 66 = UU; 67 = ZJU; 68 = KyotoU; 69 = UNC; 70 = TU Delft; 71 = BU; 72 = UNSW; 73 = Charité; 74 = USTC; 75 = UG; 76 = Bristol; 77 = LEI; 78 = Yonsei; 79 = PolyU; 80 = EUR; 81 = UW; 82 = Emory; 83 = UofGlasgow; 84 = UZH; 85 = McMaster; 86 = HU Berlin; 87 = Uni Tuebingen; 88 = UniofAdelaide; 89 = Uni Bonn; 90 = Sorbonne; 91 = FU Berlin; 92 = KAIST; 93 = UPSaclay; 94 = Unibe; 95 = UCI; 96 = IP Paris; 97 = NJU; 98 = Vandy; 99 = CityU; 100 = RWTH Aachen

Table 2.5 Selected excerpted ILOs and/or DGAs of the top 100 universities in THE 2023 based on their emphasis on Domains 7, 8, and 9*

THE 2023 rank	15	26	34	26	57
University	Johns Hopkins University (JHU)	Northwestern University (NorthwesternU)	University of Melbourne (UniMelb)	University of Washington (UW)	Washington University in St Louis (WUSTL)
Funding	Private	Private	Public	Public	Private
Format	Mixed	Cluster	Integrated	Mixed	Mixed
Special case#	Normal	Normal	Normal	Special case 1a	Special case 1a
No. of Attributes in Domains 7, 8, 9 ($N = 16$)	16	16	16	15	15
ILOs and/or DGAs	"**Aspirations for Student Learning** 1. Curiosity: Explore new ideas; Dream big and develop talents to support healthy communities where everyone thrives; Integrative thinkers and lifelong learners	"**Division Student Learning Outcomes** *1. Personal Development* • Ethics, integrity, accountability • Personal identity; Positive sense of self (Adaptability, persistence, dependability, resilience; Self-reflection; Act independently; Emotional intelligence)	"***Graduate Attributes & Educational Objectives*** - Academic Distinction: Well-rounded; Specialist disciplines and skills, multiple disciplinary perspectives; Research and reasoning skills; Critically apply knowledge to solve practical problems; Effective oral and written Communicators; Entrepreneurial and innovative thought-leaders; Lifelong learners	"**Values of Undergraduate Academic Affairs** • Make humane and informed decisions • Independent judgment • Critical thinking and effective articulation of thinking • Collaboration • Compassion, care for self and others • Curiosity and engage humbly and creatively	"**Goals** - Cultivate students' habits of lifelong learning and ethical thinking as productive members and leaders of a global society - Equip them with life skills, academic skills/academic experiences, self-reflection/values exploration/self-awareness - Adopt qualities of curious, creative, concern for others, and support one another

(continued)

Table 2.5 (continued)

THE 2023 rank	15	26	34	26	57
	2. Self-awareness 3. Collaboration: Expand local and global consciousness; Embrace diverse perspectives and foster compassion 4. Confidence: Promote emotional strength and healthy self-esteem; Grow academically and emotionally; Build tenacity, determination, and resilience 5. Responsible Leadership: Ethical decision-making; Address complex issues	*2. Interpersonal Competence* • Leadership (Respect others' perspectives; Maintain healthy relationships with others) • Civic Engagement (Care for others' welfare) • Interdependence (Works collaboratively; Resolve interpersonal conflicts) *3. Social Responsibility* • Social Justice (Foster inclusive communities) • Civic Engagement (global awareness)	- Active Citizenship: Ethics deep respect; Socially responsible; Collaboration (work cooperatively with others from diverse linguistic backgrounds), working effectively across disciplines and cultures; Influential citizens with high leadership potential; Engaging with national and global issues Integrity, Self-awareness, Self-direction: Reflective; Personal and professional integrity; Confident; Flexible and adaptable; Empathy; Value their well-being."	• Equity, integrity, and reflecting on their values • Transformative learning (push students beyond the familiar to shape their sense of self and develop attitudes and skills to uniquely contribute to society)	

(continued)

Table 2.5 (continued)

THE 2023 rank	15	26	34	26	57
	Ensure Instruction in Foundational Abilities • Value language and complex creative expressions • Scientific, numerical, and algorithmic reasoning; Use computational and analytical methods • Cultivate intellectual and emotional responses to aesthetic and cultural experiences • Engage effectively as citizens • Reflective, effective, ethical agents • Independently conceptualize and complete large-scale projects."	*4. Cognitive and Practical Skills* • Critical thinking, applying theories to creatively solve practical problems) • Life Skills • Career development (Apply professional strengths, skills/competencies; Utilize career management tools/skills; Apply academic experiences) • Promote health and wellness • Communication skills and technological literacy."	Link(s): 1. https://melbourne-cshe.unimelb.edu.au/resources/categories/teaching-and-learning/teaching-in-practice/the-melbourne-way 2.https://handbook.unimelb.edu.au/2023/courses/b-arts/attributes-outcomes-skills	**Build Core Employ Skills** • Manage Self (Accountability; Adaptability—Learn emerging tools and methodologies, and view setbacks as opportunities) • Engage Others (Communication; Collaboration with empathy and curiosity; Respectfully negotiate differences; Confidently lead) • Produce Results (Critical Thinking; Creative Problem-Solving; Continuous Improvement; Reflect and self-evaluate)."	**Leadership Initiative Competencies and Learning Outcomes** – Apply innovative solutions for positive change – Utilize technology to communicate and engage in meaningful interactions with others – Develop critical thinking skills for decision-making, solve problems, develop confidence and resilience – Ethics and integrity – Connection and collaboration – Socially responsible."

(continued)

Table 2.5 (continued)

THE 2023 rank	15	26	34	26	57
	Link(s): 1.https://studentaffairs.jhu.edu/viceprovost/aspirations-for-student-learning/ 2. https://provost.jhu.edu/education/second-commission-on-undergraduate-education/	Link(s): https://www.northwestern.edu/studentaffairs/assessment/learning-outcomes/division-student-learning-outcomes/		Link(s): 1.https://www.washington.edu/admin/rules/policies/BRG/RP1.html 2. https://www.washington.edu/uaa/about/vision-mission-and-values/ 3. https://careers.uw.edu/channels/build-skills/	Link(s): 1. https://wustl.edu/about/mission-statement/ 2. https://admissions.wustl.edu/building-our-community/ 3. https://cpb-us-w2.wpmucdn.com/sites.wustl.edu/dist/d/3840/files/2016/01/CE-2014-Full-rszp7t.pdf (pp. 20–21)
THE 2023 rank	69	71	76	82	88
University	University of North Carolina at Chapel Hill (UNC)	Boston University (BU)	University of Bristol (Bristol)	University of Glasgow (UofGlasgow)	University of Adelaide (UniofAdelaide)
Funding	Public	Private	Public	Public	Public
Format	Integrated	Mixed	Cluster	Mixed	Cluster
Special case[#]	Special case 1a	Normal	Special case 1a	Normal	Normal
No. of Attributes in Domains 7, 8, 9 ($N = 16$)	15	15	15	15	15

(continued)

Table 2.5 (continued)

THE 2023 rank	69	71	76	82	88
ILOs and/or DGAs	"**Educational Priority** 1. Students will be engaged community members 2. Resilience—students can employ positive adaptive skillset to address challenges and build and maintain positive relationships 3. Diversity and inclusion—students will apply a personal framework, that will drive how they engage globally and inform individual self-reflection, which helps with their development in critical consciousness and inclusive leadership practices 4. Develop a sense of belonging and empower students to design a fulfilling life that enables them to apply strategies for decision-making	"**Learning Outcomes and Essential capacities** Lifelong learning, professional training, and leading for students to become leaders who are reflective and adaptive 1. Philosophical inquiry (life's meaning) 2. Curiosity, identify and apply 3. Quantitative reasoning: personal self-sufficiency, responsible citizenship, solve complex problems 4. Global citizenship: participate respectfully, ethical reasoning, social responsibility, engaged citizenship, and intercultural literacy 5. Communication: digital/ multimedia expression as effective writers	"**Skills Framework** 1. Focus on the academic skills, personal effectiveness, and well-being 2. Self-management, e.g., work-life balance, Time management 3. Personal well-being, self-reflection, self-awareness, self-confidence, resilience 4. Personal effectiveness, e.g., responsibility, integrity & ethical awareness, enthusiasm 5. Engagement, e.g., collaboration, community engagement, enterprise 6. Teamwork, e.g., respect for diversity, collaboration, leadership 7. Communication	"**Graduate attributes** 1. Subject specialists: Possess discipline-relevant professional skills, knowledge and competencies 2. Independent and critical thinkers: Constructing meaning, apply creative, and innovative ideas to problem-solving 3. Resourceful and responsible: Self-directed learning, authentic research-led enquiry, and accountability 4. Effective communicators: Communicate in written and spoken English confidently 5. Confident: Excellent interpersonal and social skills, leadership and positively influence on others	"**Graduate Attributes** 1. Deep discipline knowledge and intellectual breadth; Ability to apply their knowledge and multidisciplinary 2. Creative and critical thinking, and problem-solving 3. Collaborative teamwork and communication skills 4. Professionalism and leadership readiness 5. Potential to be entrepreneurial role and recognize personal values

(continued)

Table 2.5 (continued)

THE 2023 rank	69	71	76	82	88
	Committed to Personal and Collective Ethics – Integrity – Accountability—e.g., Justice – Community—e.g., Mutual respect – Empathy." Link(s) 1. https://studentaffairs.unc.edu/about-us/curricular-approach/ 2. https://www.unc.edu/about/mission/ 3. https://ethicspolicy.unc.edu/about/statement-of-ethics/	6. Intellectual toolkit: critical thinking; self-discipline; research literacy: use discipline-specific information sources to communicate findings; Creative/innovation; life skills regarding their physical and mental well-being 7. A broad range of knowledge and disciplines 8. Stronger personal connections with others and thrive in their civic lives." Link(s): 1. https://www.bu.edu/hub/about-the-hub/why-the-bu-hub/ 2. https://www.bu.edu/hub/about-the-hub/what-is-the-hub/ 3. https://www.bu.edu/academics/hub/learning-outcomes/	8. Knowledge, e.g., academic subject knowledge, academic integrity, quantitative skills 9. Intellectual attitudes, e.g., analysis, synthesis & evaluation, Problem-solving 10. Creativity and innovation 11. Future thinking 12. Global citizenship." Link(s): 1. https://issuu.com/bristolsu/docs/pdp_guide 2. https://www.bristol.ac.uk/media-library/sites/university/documents/governance/university-strategy.pdf (pp. 5–6)	6. Adaptable: Multidisciplinary learning, adapt skills and knowledge, resilience, and positivity 7. Experienced collaborators: Respect others when working in a team 8. Ethically and Socially Aware: Social and global responsibilities 9. Reflective learners: Continuing development." Link(s): https://www.gla.ac.uk/myglasgow/students/attributes/yourattributes/	6.Intercultural and ethical competency 7. Global citizens, responsible members of society 8. Cultural competency 9. Digital capabilities 10. Self-awareness and emotional intelligence Reflective, resilient, accept and give constructive feedback, integrity and responsibility." Link(s): https://www.adelaide.edu.au/learning/resources-for-educators/graduate-attributes-attribute-1-deep-discipline-knowledge-and-intellectual-breadth

(continued)

Table 2.5 (continued)

THE 2023 rank	98	37	47	99	14
University	Vanderbilt University (Vandy)	London School of Economics and Political Science (LSE)	Paris Sciences et Lettres—PSL Research University Paris (PSL)	City University of Hong Kong (CityU)	University of Pennsylvania (UPenn)
Funding	Private	Public	Public	Public	Private
Format	Cluster	Integrated	Integrated	Cluster	Integrated
Special case[#]	Normal	Special case 1b	Special case 1b	Normal	Special case 1b
No. of Attributes in Domains 7, 8, 9 ($N = 16$)	15	4	4	4	3
ILOs and/or DGAs	"**Associate Learning Outcomes** Technical operations, sense of self, and sharpen interpersonal skills 1. Problem-Solving; Adaptability; Critical Thinking 2. **Technical Operations; Audio/visual equipment; Digital Technology** 3. **Personal Development; Promote well-being; Self-awareness—reflection**	"**LSE 2030 Strategy—Educate for impact** Fostering fearless intellects: We will equip students with the insights and skills to become independent thinkers, critical investigators, and the thought-leaders of tomorrow Think, learn, lead: innovate and create real change within LSE and beyond."	"**Education Features and CPES Degree Learning Outcomes** 1. Cross-disciplinarity to stimulate curiosity, an open mind, and innovation at the crossroads of culture, knowledge, and methodology 2. Learning through research, creation, and entrepreneurship to develop critical thinking, creativity, and daring 3. Foster decision-makers, academic researchers, and entrepreneurs for the economic, academic, and cultural spheres."	"**CityU graduate outcomes** for **Undergraduate Students** 1. Globally minded professional 2. Innovative and critical thinker 3. Effective communicator 4. Lifelong learner 5. Civically-oriented individual (e.g., create applicable knowledge for social and economic advancement)."	"**Undergraduate Education** 1. Penn education informed by inclusivity, intellectual rigor, research, and the impetus to create new knowledge to the benefit of individuals and communities around the world 2. Penn integrates a liberal arts education with professional training and encourages undergraduates to apply knowledge in ways that benefit the public good

(continued)

Table 2.5 (continued)

THE 2023 rank	98	37	47	99	14
	4. **Interpersonal Skills; Professionalism, Collaboration—build relationships; Communication; Hospitality; Inclusion** 5. **Leadership Skills. e.g., Expertise and address society's challenges** 6. Lifelong journey, intellectual knowledge, curiosity and humility 7. Scholarly exploration, empower global neighborhood 8. Persevering in adversity 9. Honesty, accountability, and respectful." Link(s): 1. https://www.vanderbilt.edu/studentcenters/wp-content/uploads/sites/151/Learning-Outcomes.pdf (pp. 1–2) 2. https://www.vanderbilt.edu/this-is-vanderbilt/ 3. https://www.vanderbilt.edu/student_handbook/print-handbook/	Link(s): https://www.lse.ac.uk/2030/assets/pdf/LSE-2030-booklet.pdf (p. 3) (Source: https://www.lse.ac.uk/2030)	Link(s): 1. https://psl.eu/en/education 2. https://psl.eu/en/education/multidisciplinary-undergraduate-degree-cpes	Link(s): 1. https://www.cityu.edu.hk/qac/city_university_graduate_outcomes.htm 2. https://libguides.library.cityu.edu.hk/il/goal	3. Students experience critical learning experiences, pursue original research, and apply their learning to environments beyond the campus." Link(s): 1. https://provost.upenn.edu/education/undergraduate 2. https://www.upenn.edu/about

(continued)

Table 2.5 (continued)

THE 2023 rank	33	91	89	93	90
University	LMU Munich (LMU)	Korea Advanced Institute of Science and Technology (KAIST)	University of Bonn (Uni Bonn)	Université Paris-Saclay (UPSaclay)	Sorbonne University (Sorbonne)
Funding	Public	Public	Public	Public	Public
Format	Integrated	Integrated	Integrated	Integrated	Integrated
Special case#	Special case 1b	Special case 1b	Special case 1b	Special case 1b	Special case 1b
No. of Attributes in Domains 7, 8, 9 ($N = 16$)	3	3	2	2	0
ILOs and/or DGAs	“**About LMU and Research-oriented teaching** At LMU, we thrive on the specialist knowledge, the diverse perspectives, and the curiosity of our students LMU offers Scientific training, Interdisciplinary Program, Internationalization and Digitalization learning, helping develop students’ talents (including skills in data science methods) to achieve successful personal and professional development.”	“**Mission and Vision 2023: Global Value-Creative Leading University** KAIST will provide education to foster creative leaders who are creativity, embrace challenges, and possess caring minds in creating knowledge and translating knowledge into transformative innovation.”	“**Additional Qualifications** Key competences, academic training, specialist knowledge, presentation, language skills.”	“**Training and An Undergraduate Programme with Strong Student Support** Develop their knowledge in various scientific and economic sectors, academic laboratories and in the socio-economic world or specific professional sectors Acquiring skills and knowledge in their discipline Responsible citizens, open to the world.”	“**The Strategic Plan (2019–2023)** Fostering more students’ mobility in a global world Entrepreneurship Knowledge, expertise and flexible; innovation.”

(continued)

Table 2.5 (continued)

THE 2023 rank	33	91	89	93	90
	Link(s): 1. https://www.lmu.de/en/about-lmu/index.html 2. https://www.lmu.de/en/about-lmu/lmu-at-a-glance/awards/excellence-strategy/university-of-excellence/research-oriented-teaching/index.html	Link(s): 1. https://www.kaist.ac.kr/en/html/kaist/01.html 2. https://www.kaist.ac.kr/en/html/kaist/011301.html	Link(s): https://www.uni-bonn.de/en/studying/organizing-your-studies/during-your-studies/additional-qualifications	Link(s): 1. https://www.universite-paris-saclay.fr/en/education 2. https://www.universite-paris-saclay.fr/en/news/undergraduate-studies-universite-paris-saclay-engaging-stimulating-and-innovative-training-courses-ledition-13-june-2020	Link(s): https://www.sorbonne-universite.fr/en/university/about-us/strategic-plan

Note *Domain 7 = Intrapersonal attributes—Non-cognitive; Domain 8 = Intrapersonal attributes—Character and citizenship; Domain 9 = Interpersonal competence;
#Normal = The particular ILOs/DGAs were provided. Special case 1a = No particular ILOs/DGAs were provided, but related information was provided, such as "mission and culture," "education commitment," "competence framework," "strategic priorities," etc.; Special case 1b = No particular ILOs/DGAs were provided, and only less scattered and slightly relevant information was obtained; Special case 2 = No university-level ILOs/DGAs were provided, but ILOs/DGAs from the department/college/faculty were provided

References

American College Health Association. (2023). *American college health association-national college health assessment III: Undergraduate student reference group executive summary spring 2023*. American College Health Association. https://sairo.ucla.edu/file/1c288221-aa6a-426c-9a59-c24a3f25f936

Barnett, R. (2000). University knowledge in an age of supercomplexity. *Higher Education, 40*, 409–422. https://doi.org/10.1023/A:1004159513741

Barrie, S. C. (2005). Rethinking generic graduate attribute. *HERDSA News, 27*(1), 1–6.

Barrie, S. C. (2006). Understanding what we mean by the generic attributes of graduates. *Higher Education, 51*(2), 215–241. https://doi.org/10.1007/s10734-004-6384-7

Battistich, V., Solomon, D., & Delucchi, K. (1993). Interaction processes and student outcomes in cooperative learning groups. *The Elementary School Journal, 94*(1), 19–32. https://doi.org/10.1086/461748

Baumeister, R. F., Campbell, J. D., Krueger, J. I., & Vohs, K. D. (2003). Does high self-esteem cause better performance, interpersonal success, happiness, or healthier lifestyles? *Psychological Science in the Public Interest, 4*(1), 1–44. https://doi.org/10.1111/1529-1006.01431

Bitzer, E., & Withering, M. (2020). Graduate attributes: How some university students experience and learn them. *South African Journal of Higher Education, 34*(3), 13–31. https://doi.org/10.20853/34-3-3504

Bochner, A. P., & Kelly, C. W. (1974). Interpersonal competence: Rationale, philosophy, and implementation of a conceptual framework. *The Speech Teacher, 23*(4), 279–301. https://doi.org/10.1080/03634527409378103

Bowden, J., Hart, G., King, B., Trigwell, K., & Watts, O. (2000). *Generic capabilities of ATN university graduates*. https://webarchive.nla.gov.au/awa/20030402040510/http://www.clt.uts.edu.au/ATN.grad.cap.project.index.html

Bowen, G. A. (2009). Document analysis as a qualitative research method. *Qualitative Research Journal, 9*(2), 27–40. https://doi.org/10.3316/QRJ0902027

Bridgstock, R. (2009). The graduate attributes we've overlooked: Enhancing graduate employability through career management skills. *Higher Education Research & Development, 28*(1), 31–44. https://doi.org/10.1080/07294360802444347

Brooks, E., Brant, J., & Lamb, M. (2019). How can universities cultivate leaders of character? Insights from a leadership and character development program at the University of Oxford. *International Journal of Ethics Education, 4*(2), 167–182. https://doi.org/10.1007/s40889-019-00075-x

Cohen Orantes, I. (1981). El concepto de integración. *Revista de la CEPAL*, 149–159. https://hdl.handle.net/11362/10232

Cox, A. M., Al Daoud, M., & Rudd, S. (2013). Information management graduates' accounts of their employability: A case study from the University of Sheffield. *Education for Information, 30*(1–2), 41–61. https://doi.org/10.3233/efi-130929

de Boer, T., & Van Rijnsoever, F. (2022). In search of valid non-cognitive student selection criteria. *Assessment & Evaluation in Higher Education, 47*(5), 783–800. https://doi.org/10.1080/02602938.2021.1958142

Delaney, C. (2003). Walking a fine line: Graduate nurses' transition experiences during orientation. *Journal of Nursing Education, 42*(10), 437–443. https://doi.org/10.3928/0148-4834-20031001-05

Dewey, J. D., Montrosse, B. E., Schröter, D. C., Sullins, C. D., & Mattox, J. R., II. (2008). Evaluator competencies: What's taught versus what's sought. *American Journal of Evaluation, 29*(3), 268–287. https://doi.org/10.1177/1098214008321152

Duchscher, J. E. B. (2009). Transition shock: The initial stage of role adaptation for newly graduated registered nurses. *Journal of Advanced Nursing, 65*(5), 1103–1113. https://doi.org/10.1111/j.1365-2648.2008.04898.x

Finch, D. J., Hamilton, L. K., Baldwin, R., & Zehner, M. (2013). An exploratory study of factors affecting undergraduate employability. *Education + Training, 55*(7), 681–704. https://doi.org/10.1108/ET-07-2012-0077

Frone, M. R. (2000). Interpersonal conflict at work and psychological outcomes: Testing a model among young workers. *Journal of Occupational Health Psychology, 5*(2), 246–255. https://doi.org/10.1037/1076-8998.5.2.246

García, E. (2016). The need to address non-cognitive skills in the education policy agenda. In M. S. Khine & S. Areepattamannil (Eds.), *Non-cognitive skills and factors in educational attainment* (pp. 31–64). Brill.

García-Aracil, A. (2009). European graduates' level of satisfaction with higher education. *Higher Education, 57*(1), 1–21. https://doi.org/10.1007/s10734-008-9121-9

Garcia-Aracil, A., Mora, J. G., & Vila, L. E. (2004). The rewards of human capital competences for young European higher education graduates. *Tertiary Education and Management, 10*(4), 287–305. https://doi.org/10.1080/13583883.2004.9967133

García-Aracil, A., & Van der Velden, R. (2008). Competencies for young European higher education graduates: Labor market mismatches and their payoffs. *Higher Education, 55*(2), 219–239. https://doi.org/10.1007/s10734-006-9050-4

Gillies, D. (2015). Human capital theory in education. In M. Peters (Ed.), *Encyclopedia of educational philosophy and theory* (pp. 1–5). Springer. https://doi.org/10.1007/978-981-287-532-7_254-1

Green, W., Hammer, S., & Star, C. (2009). Facing up to the challenge: Why is it so hard to develop graduate attributes? *Higher Education Research & Development, 28*(1), 17–29. https://doi.org/10.1080/07294360802444339

Hammer, S., Ayriss, P., & McCubbin, A. (2021). Style or substance: How Australian universities contextualise their graduate attributes for the curriculum quality space. *Higher Education Research & Development, 40*(3), 508–523. https://doi.org/10.1080/07294360.2020.1761304

Hanstedt, P. (2010). Hong Kong's experiment in integrative teaching and learning. *Liberal Education, 96*(4), 18–23.

Hazelkorn, E. (2016). *Global rankings and the geopolitics of higher education: Understanding the influence and impact of rankings on higher education, policy and society*. Routledge.

Hill, J., Walkington, H., & France, D. (2016). Graduate attributes: Implications for higher education practice and policy. *Journal of Geography in Higher Education, 40*(2), 155–163. https://doi.org/10.1080/03098265.2016.1154932

Hosain, M. S., Mustafi, M. A. A., & Parvin, T. (2021). Factors affecting the employability of private university graduates: An exploratory study on Bangladeshi employers. *PSU Research Review, 7*(3), 163–183. https://doi.org/10.1108/PRR-01-2021-0005

Jackson, D. (2014). Testing a model of undergraduate competence in employability skills and its implications for stakeholders. *Journal of Education and Work, 27*(2), 220–242. https://doi.org/10.1080/13639080.2012.718750

Judd, T., & Keith, B. (2017). Implementing undergraduate student learning outcomes assessment at the program and institutional levels. In C. Secolsky & D. B. Denison (Eds.), *Handbook on measurement, assessment, and evaluation in higher education* (pp. 69–86). Routledge.

Kalfa, S., & Taksa, L. (2015). Cultural capital in business higher education: Reconsidering the graduate attributes movement and the focus on employability. *Studies in Higher Education, 40*(4), 580–595. https://doi.org/10.1080/03075079.2013.842210

Karyotaki, E., Cuijpers, P., Albor, Y., Alonso, J., Auerbach, R. P., Bantjes, J., Bruffaerts, R., Ebert, D. D., Hasking, P., Kiekens, G., Lee, S., McLafferty, M., Mak, A., Mortier, P., Sampson, N. A., Stein, D. J., Vilagut, G., & Kessler, R. C. (2020). Sources of stress and their associations with mental disorders among college students: Results of the World Health Organization world mental health surveys international college student initiative. *Frontiers in Psychology, 11*, Article 1759. https://doi.org/10.3389/fpsyg.2020.01759

Kember, D., Hong, C., Yau, V. W. K., & Ho, S. A. (2017). Mechanisms for promoting the development of cognitive, social and affective graduate attributes. *Higher Education, 74*(5), 799–814. https://doi.org/10.1007/s10734-016-0077-x

Kember, D., Webster, B. J., & Chan, W. S. C. (2020). Refocusing the 3P model to incorporate a learning and teaching environment and graduate attributes. *Educational Psychology, 40*(5), 592–607. https://doi.org/10.1080/01443410.2020.1732304

Knapper, C., & Cropley, A. J. (1985). *Lifelong learning in higher education.* Croom Helm.

Kuntz, J. R. C., Malinen, S., & Näswall, K. (2017). Employee resilience: Directions for resilience development. *Consulting Psychology Journal: Practice and Research, 69*(3), 223–242. https://doi.org/10.1037/cpb0000097

Lamboy, B., Beck, F., Tessier, D., Williamson, M.-O., Fréry, N., Turgon, R., Tassie, J.-M., Barrois, J., Bessa, Z., & Shankland, R. (2022). The key role of psychosocial competencies in evidence-based youth mental health promotion: Academic support in consolidating a national strategy in France. *International Journal of Environmental Research and Public Health, 19*(24), Article 16641. https://doi.org/10.3390/ijerph192416641

Laud, R. L., & Johnson, M. (2012). Upward mobility: A typology of tactics and strategies for career advancement. *Career Development International, 17*(3), 231–254. https://doi.org/10.1108/13620431211241072

Leoni, R. (2014). Graduate employability and the development of competencies. The incomplete reform of the "Bologna Process." *International Journal of Manpower, 35*(4), 448–469. https://doi.org/10.1108/ijm-05-2013-0097

Liu, Y., Afari, E., & Khine, M. S. (2023). Effect of non-cognitive factors on academic achievement among students in Suzhou: Evidence from OECD SSES data. *European Journal of Psychology of Education. 38*(4), 1643–1657. https://doi.org/10.1007/s10212-022-00660-7

Liu, Y., Pan, H., Yang, R., Wang, X., Rao, J., Zhang, X., & Pan, C. (2021). The relationship between test anxiety and emotion regulation: The mediating effect of psychological resilience. *Annals of General Psychiatry, 20*, Article 40. https://doi.org/10.1186/s12991-021-00360-4

Love, P. E. D., Haynes, N. S., & Irani, Z. (2001). Construction managers' expectations and observations of graduates. *Journal of Managerial Psychology, 16*(8), 579–593. https://doi.org/10.1108/EUM0000000006301

Mencl, J., Wefald, A. J., & Van Ittersum, K. W. (2016). Transformational leader attributes: Interpersonal skills, engagement, and well-being. *Leadership & Organization Development Journal, 37*(5), 635–657. https://doi.org/10.1108/lodj-09-2014-0178

Merriam, S. B. (1988). *Case study research in education: A qualitative approach.* Jossey-Bass.

Mihail, D. M., & Kloutsiniotis, P. V. (2014). The impact of an MBA on managerial skills and career advancement: The Greek case. *The International Journal of Management Education, 12*(3), 212–222. https://doi.org/10.1016/j.ijme.2014.04.002

Milton-Wildey, K., Kenny, P., Parmenter, G., & Hall, J. (2014). Educational preparation for clinical nursing: The satisfaction of students and new graduates from two Australian universities. *Nurse Education Today, 34*(4), 648–654. https://doi.org/10.1016/j.nedt.2013.07.004

Morales-Rodríguez, F. M., Espigares-López, I., Brown, T., & Pérez-Mármol, J. M. (2020). The relationship between psychological well-being and psychosocial factors in university students. *International Journal of Environmental Research and Public Health, 17*(13), Article 4778. https://doi.org/10.3390/ijerph17134778

O'Donnell, R. (2014). What do graduate attributes have to do with political economy? In S. K. Schroeder, & L. Chester (Eds.), *Challenging the orthodoxy: Reflections on Frank Stilwell's contribution to political economy* (pp. 57–76). Springer. https://doi.org/10.1007/978-3-642-36121-0_5

Oliver, B., & de St Jorre, T. J. (2018). Graduate attributes for 2020 and beyond: Recommendations for Australian higher education providers. *Higher Education Research & Development*, *37*(4), 821–836. https://doi.org/10.1080/07294360.2018.1446415

Osmani, M., Weerakkody, V., Hindi, N. M., Al-Esmail, R., Eldabi, T., Kapoor, K., & Irani, Z. (2015). Identifying the trends and impact of graduate attributes on employability: A literature review.

Tertiary Education and Management, 21(4), 367–379. https://doi.org/10.1080/13583883.2015.1114139
Pavel, A.-P. (2015). Global university rankings: A comparative analysis. *Procedia Economics and Finance, 26*, 54–63. https://doi.org/10.1016/S2212-5671(15)00838-2
Pool, L. D. (2017). Developing graduate employability: The career EDGE model and the importance of emotional intelligence. In M. Tomlinson & L. Holmes (Eds.), *Graduate employability in context: theory, research and debate* (pp. 317–338). Palgrave Macmillan. https://doi.org/10.1057/978-1-137-57168-7_15
Porter, M. E. (2000). Location, competition, and economic development: Local clusters in a global economy. *Economic Development Quarterly, 14*(1), 15–34. https://doi.org/10.1177/089124240001400105
Shek, D. T. L. (2012). Development of a positive youth development subject in a university context in Hong Kong. *International Journal on Disability and Human Development, 11*(3), 173–179. https://doi.org/10.1515/ijdhd-2012-0036
Shek, D. T. L. (2020). Protests in Hong Kong (2019–2020): A perspective based on quality of life and well-being. *Applied Research in Quality of Life, 15*(3), 619–635. https://doi.org/10.1007/s11482-020-09825-2
Shek, D. T. L. (2021). COVID-19 and quality of life: Twelve reflections. *Applied Research in Quality of Life, 16*(1), 1–11. https://doi.org/10.1007/s11482-020-09898-z
Shek, D. T. L., Chai, W., Li, X., & Dou, D. (2023a). Profiles and predictors of mental health of university students in Hong Kong under the COVID-19 pandemic. *Frontiers in Psychology, 14*, Article 1211229. https://doi.org/10.3389/fpsyg.2023.1211229
Shek, D. T. L., Chai, W., Wong, T., & Zhou, K. (2023b). Stress and depressive symptoms in university students in Hong Kong under the pandemic: Moderating effect of positive psychological attributes. *Frontiers in Psychology, 14*, Article 1071938. https://doi.org/10.3389/fpsyg.2023.1071938
Shek, D. T. L., Chai, W., & Zhou, K. (2023c). Risk factors and protective factors of internet addiction in university students during the pandemic: Implications for prevention and treatment. *International Journal of Environmental Research and Public Health, 20*(11), Article 5952. https://doi.org/10.3390/ijerph20115952
Shek, D. T. L., Ngai, G., & Chan, S. C. F. (2019). *Service-learning for youth leadership: The case of Hong Kong*. Springer.
Shek, D. T. L., Dou, D., Zhu, X., Wong, T., & Tan, L. (2022). Need satisfaction and depressive symptoms among university students in Hong Kong during the COVID-19 pandemic: Moderating effects of positive youth development attributes. *Frontiers in Psychiatry, 13*, Article 931404. https://doi.org/10.3389/fpsyt.2022.931404
Shek, D. T. L., & Leung, H. (2016). Resilience as a focus of a subject on leadership and intrapersonal development. *International Journal on Disability and Human Development, 15*(2), 149–155. https://doi.org/10.1515/ijdhd-2016-0704
Shek, D. T. L., & Liang, L. Y. (2018). Psychosocial factors influencing individual well-being in Chinese adolescents in Hong Kong: A six-year longitudinal study. *Applied Research in Quality of Life, 13*(3), 561–584. https://doi.org/10.1007/s11482-017-9545-4
Shek, D. T. L., & Lin, L. (2015). Intrapersonal competencies and service leadership. *International Journal on Disability and Human Development, 14*(3), 255–263. https://doi.org/10.1515/ijdhd-2015-0406
Shek, D. T. L., & Yu, L. (2017). General university requirements and holistic development in university students in Hong Kong. *International Journal of Adolescent Medicine and Health, 29*(1), 41–48. https://doi.org/10.1515/ijamh-2017-3006
Shek, D. T. L., Yu, L., & Chai, W. (2017a). Evaluation of the general university requirements: What did students say? *International Journal of Adolescent Medicine and Health, 29*(1), 75–82. https://doi.org/10.1515/ijamh-2017-3010

Shek, D. T. L., Yu, L., & Chi, X. (2017b). Focus group evaluation of teachers' views on a new general education program in Hong Kong. *International Journal of Adolescent Medicine and Health, 29*(1), 67–74. https://doi.org/10.1515/ijamh-2017-3009

Shek, D. T. L., Yu, L., & Siu, A. M. H. (2015). Interpersonal competence and service leadership. *International Journal on Disability and Human Development, 14*(3), 265–274. https://doi.org/10.1515/ijdhd-2015-0407

Shek, D. T. L., Yu, L., Wu, F. K. Y., Ng, C. S. M., & Chai, W. (2017c). Qualitative evaluation of general university requirements in a new 4-year university curriculum: Findings based on experiences of students. *International Journal of Adolescent Medicine and Health, 29*(1), 91–102. https://doi.org/10.1515/ijamh-2017-3012

Shek, D. T. L., Yu, L., & Xie, Q. (2017d). Student feedback on a pioneer subject on leadership and intrapersonal development in Hong Kong. *International Journal of Adolescent Medicine and Health, 29*(1), 83–89. https://doi.org/10.1515/ijamh-2017-3011

Smithers, L. G., Sawyer, A. C. P., Chittleborough, C. R., Davies, N. M., Davey Smith, G., & Lynch, J. W. (2018). A systematic review and meta-analysis of effects of early life non-cognitive skills on academic, psychosocial, cognitive and health outcomes. *Nature Human Behaviour, 2*(11), 867–880. https://doi.org/10.1038/s41562-018-0461-x

Star, C., & Hammer, S. (2008). Teaching generic skills: Eroding the higher purpose of universities, or an opportunity for renewal? *Oxford Review of Education, 34*(2), 237–251. https://doi.org/10.1080/03054980701672232

Su, Y. (2014). Self-directed, genuine graduate attributes: The person-based approach. *Higher Education Research & Development, 33*(6), 1208–1220. https://doi.org/10.1080/07294360.2014.911255

Suleman, F., & Laranjeiro, A. M. C. (2018). The employability skills of graduates and employers' options in Portugal. *Education + Training, 60*(9), 1097–1111. https://doi.org/10.1108/ET-10-2017-0158

Tonon, G. (2019). Integrated methods in research. In P. Liamputtong (Ed.), *Handbook of research methods in health social sciences* (pp. 681–694). Springer. https://doi.org/10.1007/978-981-10-5251-4_96

Vorley, T. (2008). The geographic cluster: A historical review. *Geography Compass, 2*(3), 790–813. https://doi.org/10.1111/j.1749-8198.2008.00108.x

Wagner, T. (2010). *The global achievement gap: Why even our best schools don't teach the new survival skills our children need and what we can do about it*. Basic Books.

Yee, A. H. (1989). Cross-cultural perspectives on higher education in East Asia: Psychological effects upon Asian students. *Journal of Multilingual and Multicultural Development, 10*(3), 213–232. https://doi.org/10.1080/01434632.1989.9994375

Yin, R. K. (1994). *Case study research: Design and methods* (2nd ed.). SAGE.

Yorke, M., & Harvey, L. (2005). Graduate attributes and their development. *New Directions for Institutional Research, 2005*(128), 41–58. https://doi.org/10.1002/ir.162

Chapter 3
Developmental Issues of University Students in Hong Kong

Daniel T. L. Shek and Tiffany T. Y. Wong

Abstract The current scoping review covers 29 articles in five categories of Hong Kong university students' developmental issues. These include 17 articles on depression, anxiety, and stress, 3 articles on non-suicidal self-injury, suicidal ideation, and suicidal behavior, 6 articles on addictive behavior, 7 articles on sleep problems and eating disorders, and 2 articles on physical assault and interpersonal violence, with some articles covering multiple issues. This chapter first analyzed the prevalence rates of Hong Kong university students' developmental issues and compared them with studies based on other populations. Then, this chapter examined whether students' holistic development, well-being, and quality of life were emphasized in the Institutional Learning Outcomes (ILOs) of 11 public and private institutions in Hong Kong. The results showed that Hong Kong university students had higher prevalence rates of non-suicidal self-injury, suicidal ideation and behavior, and physical assault perpetration against dating partners when compared to the international samples of college students. For ILOs, Hong Kong higher education institutions had a stronger emphasis on employment capability and cognitive skills, moderate emphasis on character and citizenship, and a minor emphasis on non-cognitive skills and interpersonal competence. These findings suggest that local higher education institutions may not adequately address students' holistic development.

Keywords University students · Developmental issues · Hong Kong · Institutional learning outcomes (ILOs) · Desired graduate attributes (DGAs)

3.1 Introduction

In Chap. 1, we present news on university students' developmental issues globally and locally. In Chap. 2, we briefly highlight university students' developmental issues in the global context. We also present materials on whether strengthening student holistic development (such as promotion of well-being) is embedded in the institutional learning outcomes (ILOs) and desired graduate attributes (DGAs) of the universities ranked in the first 100 places in THE ranking system. Our impression is that the promotion of holistic development (particularly psychosocial competence,

D. T. L. Shek, *Promoting Holistic Development in University Students*, Quality of Life in Asia 17, https://doi.org/10.1007/978-981-96-0251-3_3

mental well-being, and quality of life) is not a top priority in many globally renowned universities.

In this chapter, we focus on university students' developmental issues in Hong Kong. Shek (2010) and Shek and Wong (2011) pointed out that Hong Kong university students face many alarming developmental issues. To deepen our understanding, we conducted a scoping review of Hong Kong university students' developmental problems. Scoping review is a strategy to synthesize knowledge in an existing body of knowledge with several steps: asking research questions, finding relevant studies, selecting studies for the review, charting and synthesizing the data, and lastly, reporting the findings (Mak & Thomas, 2022).

To conduct the scoping review, we searched two databases in June 2023, including the Web of Science and Scopus. The keywords for this scoping review were chosen based on a preliminary review of literature on adolescents' developmental issues, which showed that mental distress, suicidal behavior, and addiction problems were the main developmental challenges of Hong Kong adolescents (Shek & Wong, 2011). On the Web of Science database, we searched within the topic (title, abstract, author keywords, and Keywords Plus) with the keywords: "prevalence" and ("mental illness" or "mental disorders" or "anxiety" or "depression or suicide" or "self-harm" or "addiction") and "Hong Kong" and (postsecondary OR college OR university* or undergraduate) and "student"*, which resulted in 78 citations. In the second database (i.e., Scopus), we searched within the "article title, abstract, and keywords" fields with the keywords: "prevalence" and ("mental illness" or "mental disorders" or "anxiety" or "depression" or "suicide" or "self-harm" or "addiction") and "Hong Kong" and (postsecondary OR college OR university* or undergraduate) and "student"*, which resulted in 27 citations. The total number of citations from the two databases was 105.

Subsequently, four criteria were set in the selection of these articles: (1) the study's sampled population was Hong Kong university students, (2) the study was an empirical study, (3) the study analyzed the prevalence of university students' developmental issues, and (4) full-text of the study was available. First of all, 19 duplicated articles were removed. Second, after reviewing the titles and abstracts, 46 articles were excluded, resulting in 40 potential articles to be considered. Lastly, after reading the full-text documents, the 40 citations were further reduced to 29 articles, including 4 articles selected from reviewing reference list of the articles. Please see Fig. 3.1 in the Appendix for the PRISMA flow diagram for the selection of these articles (Page et al., 2021).

3.2 Developmental Issues of University Students in Hong Kong: A Scoping Review

This scoping review revealed five categories of developmental issues in Hong Kong university students, including (1) depression, anxiety, and stress; (2) non-suicidal self-injury, suicidal ideation, and suicidal behavior; (3) addictive behavior; (4) sleep and eating problems; (5) interpersonal problems. This section reviews the articles identified from this scoping review, summarizes the prevalence rate of Hong Kong university students' development issues, and compares the prevalence rates with studies based on other populations.

3.2.1 Prevalence of Depression, Anxiety, and Stress

Researchers have applied various scales to measure the severity of depression, anxiety, and stress among Hong Kong college students. The scales used included the DASS-21 (short form), DASS-42 (full form), CES-D, CESD-R, Patient Health Questionnaire, Generalized Anxiety Disorder Scale, and the Beck Depression Inventory-II. This scoping review showed that different scales yielded different prevalence rates of depression, anxiety, and stress.

First, the majority of the articles (10 out of 17) used the DASS-21 or DASS-42 scale to measure Hong Kong college students' depression, anxiety, and stress (Chan & Cheung, 2022; Cheung et al., 2016, 2020; Hung et al., 2022; Leung & Pong, 2021; Li et al., 2021; Shek et al., 2022b; Sze et al., 2021; Wong et al., 2006, 2021). Using the DASS-21 and DASS-42 scales, a wide range of prevalence rates of depression, anxiety, and stress were found. For moderate or above levels of depression, anxiety, and stress, this scoping review showed that the prevalence rates ranged from 2% to 60% for depression, 3% to 73.3% for anxiety, and 1.2% to 60% for stress. Additionally, using the DASS-21 scale, the mean scores for depression and anxiety were in the mild to moderate range (depression mean score: 5.16 to 8.9; anxiety mean score: 4.18 to 6.53), and the mean score for stress was in the normal to moderate range (stress mean score: 6.72 to 12.94).

Second, two studies used the CES-D or CESD-R scale to measure the prevalence of depression in Hong Kong college students (Shek et al., 2022a; Song et al., 2008), and one study utilized the Beck Depression Inventory-II (Li et al., 2020). The prevalence of depression found by CES-D, CESD-R, and Beck Depression Inventory-II resulted in relatively high prevalence rates. Shek et al. (2022a) and Song et al. (2008) found that 43.9% to 48.4% of university students were clinically depressed, and 17.6% were severely depressed. Li et al. (2020) used the Beck Depression Inventory-II and found a high depression prevalence rate of 41%.

Third, two studies utilized the 9-item Patient Health Questionnaire (PHQ-9) and the 7-item Generalized Anxiety Disorder Scale (GAD-7) to measure Hong Kong college students' severity of depression and anxiety. Lun et al. (2018) revealed that 27% and 20% of students had moderate or above levels of depression and anxiety, respectively. Additionally, Yu and Luo (2021) found that the mean depression score was within the minimal depression range (mean depression score = 1.95). These figures showed that studies using the PHQ-9 and the GAD-7 scales to assess depression and anxiety yielded lower prevalence rates.

Fourth, under the social unrest and the COVID-19 pandemic in Hong Kong, researchers have utilized self-constructed scales to measure college students' level of worry about social events and the pandemic. Guo et al. (2022) found that 60.5% of the students were worried about social unrest in 2019, and 55.3% of the students were worried about being infected by the virus. Besides, Park et al. (2022) reported that 13.7% of Hong Kong college students had a high level of stress because of various social issues or life events.

Fifth, researchers investigated the severity of depression, anxiety, and stress of first-year Hong Kong university students with different student statuses. Cheung et al. (2020) revealed that, for moderate or above levels of depression, the overall prevalence rate was 11.9%, with student-athletes having the highest (21.1%) and international students having the lowest prevalence rate (2.7%). For moderate or above levels of anxiety, the overall prevalence rate was 29.1%, with community college transfer students having the highest (30.9%) and student-athletes having the lowest prevalence rate (16.7%). Also, for moderate or above levels of stress, the overall prevalence rate was 8.8%, with community college transfer students having the highest (13.6%) and international students having the lowest prevalence rate (2.8%). This study demonstrated that prevalence rates of depression, anxiety, and stress in Hong Kong university students vary in students with different student statuses.

Recent studies also found that Hong Kong university students' mental health has deteriorated over the years. When compared with the DASS scores of Hong Kong college students revealed by Wong et al. (2006), Li et al. (2021) observed that the mean scores had moved from "normal" to "mild" for depression, from "mild" to "moderate" for anxiety, and stayed at the "normal" level for stress. Besides, the prevalence rate for moderate or above levels of depression increased from 21% in Wong et al. (2006) to 32.7% in Li et al. (2021), and the same applied to anxiety (increased from 41% in Wong et al., 2006 to 44.7% in Li et al., 2021). Li et al. (2021) argued that Hong Kong university students' level of psychological morbidity had worsened after 2014, which was a time when the civil disobedience campaign "Umbrella Movement" happened in Hong Kong. Lun et al. (2018) also found that Hong Kong university students' levels of depression and anxiety had deteriorated significantly when compared to the findings by Wong et al. (2006). They argued that socio-political factors had an important influence on college students' mental health. Moreover, during the pandemic, the prevalence rates for Hong Kong university students' mental distress (depression: 40.0%, anxiety: 50.7%, stress: 22.2%; Shek et al., 2022b) were much higher than the rates before the pandemic, revealing the significant influence of the pandemic on university students' mental health.

Compared to the Hong Kong general population, research findings showed that Hong Kong college students had more severe mental problems. A large-scale mental morbidity survey on the Hong Kong general population found that the one-week prevalence of Common Mixed Mental Disorders (CMD) was 13.3%, with the mixed anxiety and depressive disorder (MADD) being the most common condition (Lam et al., 2015). Studying depression and anxiety levels of the Hong Kong general public in 2020, Choi et al. (2020) also found that only 14.0% and 19.8% of the respondents had depression and anxiety, respectively. These figures showed that mental distress prevalence rates for Hong Kong general population were much lower than the prevalence rates for Hong Kong university students.

Compared with university students in the international context, Hong Kong college students had a comparable prevalence of mental distress. For example, examining Latina or Latino university students residing near the US-Mexico border, Camacho et al. (2016) revealed that the prevalence rates for at least moderate level of depression, anxiety, and stress (female: 18% depression; 33.1% anxiety; 16.4% stress; male: 15.9% depression; 34.1% anxiety; 12.9% stress). Also, Asif et al. (2020) showed that college students in Pakistan had a relatively higher prevalence of mental problems (59% depression; 84% anxiety; 51.4% stress), while Ramón-Arbués et al. (2020) illustrated that Spanish college students' prevalence rates of mental distress (18.4% depression; 23.6% anxiety; 34.5% stress). These figures show that the prevalence rates of mental distress in Hong Kong university students were comparable to university students in the international context.

When compared with Macau and Mainland China university students, Hong Kong college students showed higher prevalence rates of depression. Li et al. (2020) showed that the overall prevalence rate for depression was 28.9% in Hong Kong, Macau, and Mainland China university students, with Hong Kong students (41.0%) having more severe depression problems than students in Macau (35.2%) and Mainland China (16.8%). Previous studies also investigated the difference in depression prevalence rates among Hong Kong and Mainland China university students and found similar results (Hong Kong: 43.9%; Mainland China: 24.8%; Song et al., 2008).

3.2.2 Prevalence of Suicidal Behavior and Non-suicidal Self-injury

This scoping review found two articles that investigated Hong Kong college students' prevalence of suicidal ideation and behavior (Chan et al., 2007; Ong & Thompson, 2019). These studies used the Personal and Relationship Profile or the Suicidal Behaviors Questionnaire-Revised to estimate the prevalence rates for suicidal ideation, suicide risk, and suicide attempt. These studies found that 41.2% of students experienced lifetime suicidal ideation, 40.17% had a high risk of suicide, and 4.24% had at least one suicide attempt.

Compared to international samples of university students, Hong Kong college students had a higher prevalence of suicidal ideation and behavior. The meta-analysis conducted by Mortier et al. (2018) showed that the pooled estimates of the lifetime prevalence of college students' suicidal ideation, suicidal plans, and suicidal attempts were 22.3%, 6.1%, and 3.2%, respectively. A more recent meta-analysis conducted by Crispim et al. (2021) found that the pooled prevalence estimates of college students' lifetime suicidal ideation, past-year suicidal ideation, and lifetime attempted suicide were 27.1%, 14.1%, and 3.1%, respectively. In Norway, Sivertsen et al. (2019) revealed that the prevalence rates of lifetime suicidal thoughts in college students were 21.0% and past-year suicidal thoughts were 7.2%; while lifetime suicide attempt was 4.2% and past-year suicide attempt was 0.4%. In Uganda,

Kaggwa et al. (2022) showed that the past-year suicidal ideation prevalence rate was 31.85%, suicide plans were 8.15%, and suicide attempts were 6.11% among undergraduate students. In Bangladesh, Rasheduzzaman et al. (2022) reported that the prevalence rates for university students' past-year suicidal ideation, lifetime suicide plans, and suicide attempts were 13.4%, 6.0%, and 4.4%, respectively. In Mainland China, a meta-analysis of university students' suicidal ideation showed that the prevalence rate of past-year suicidal ideation was 10.72% (Li et al., 2014). An empirical study on university students in Mainland China also found that the suicide ideation prevalence rate for the previous months and years was 13.03% (Huang et al., 2019). These figures showed that Hong Kong college students had a relatively high risk of suicide when compared to international samples of college students.

Furthermore, this scoping review found one article that studied Hong Kong college students' risk of non-suicidal self-injury (NSSI). Wong and Chung (2023) applied the Functional Assessment of Self-Mutilation (FASM) and found that 22% of students in two Hong Kong universities were identified as non-suicidal self-injurers. Compared to international samples of university students, Hong Kong college students' NSSI prevalence was relatively high. The prevalence rate found by Wong and Chung (2023) was slightly higher than the global estimates of NSSI (18.0%) and deliberate self-harm (DSH) (16.1%) among adolescents (Muehlenkamp et al., 2012). Besides, Paul et al. (2015) used a self-developed scale and found that the NSSI prevalence rate of US college students was 14%. Using the Deliberate Self-harm Inventory (DSHI), Tresno et al. (2012) revealed that the prevalence rate of self-injurious behavior was 38% among Indonesian college students, but the rate was lower among Japanese college students (10%) (Tresno et al., 2013). A high rate of self-injurious behavior was also observed among Indian college students (31.2%) by Kharsati and Bhola (2016) using the FASM as the instrument. These figures showed that the prevalence rate of self-injurious behavior differed significantly by country or region, but the rate for Hong Kong university students was relatively high.

3.2.3 Prevalence of Addictive Behavior

This scoping review found six articles on the addictive behavior of Hong Kong college students. Out of the six articles, four of them examined students' addiction to the Internet, gaming, and online social networking (Poon, 2018; Tang et al., 2018; Wong et al., 2020; Yu & Luo, 2021). To assess college students' Internet addiction, Young's Internet Addiction Test was applied in these studies. However, various scales were used to measure problematic gaming (e.g., Internet Gaming Disorder Scales-Short Form (IGDS-SF9), 12-item Problematic Online Gaming Questionnaire Short-Form), and online social networking addiction (e.g., Bergen Social Media Addiction Scale (BSMAS), Bergen Facebook Addiction Scale, Social Media Disorder Scale (SMD)). In terms of prevalence rates, these studies found that the prevalence rates ranged from 5.7% to 18.3% for Internet addiction, from 23.3% to 25.7% for online gaming addiction or Internet gaming disorder, and from 21.5% to 42.2% for online social networking addiction or social media addiction.

Compared to international samples of students, Hong Kong university students had comparable prevalence rates of addiction to the Internet, gaming, and online social networking. Studying college students in the US and six Asian countries/regions, Tang et al. (2018) revealed that the overall prevalence rate of Internet use addiction was 8.9%, online gaming addiction was 19.0%, and online social networking addiction was 33.1%. Other empirical studies examined college students' addiction to the Internet, gaming, or online social networking, respectively. For Internet addiction, Young's Internet Addiction Test was commonly used. Chi et al. (2016) showed that the prevalence rate for Mainland Chinese university students' Internet addiction was 15.2%; Babakr et al. (2019) found that the rate was 36.5% among Kurdistan university students; while Bisen and Deshpande (2020) revealed that the rate was 12.52% among Indian college students. For social media addiction, Kircaburun and Griffiths (2018) used the Instagram Addiction Scale and found that 33.5% of Turkish university students were risky Instagram users; Jaradat and Atyeh (2017) used the social media addiction scale by Hong et al. (2014) and the Obsessive Compulsive Foundation (OCF)'s diagnosis criteria and revealed that 7.9% college students in Jordan were addicted to social media and 62.1% were classified as belonging to the alert group; while Tang et al. (2017) used the Bergen Facebook Addiction Scale and found that 44.5% Mainland Chinese college students were addicted to online social networking. For gaming disorder, Borges et al. (2019) used the Diagnostic and Statistical Manual of Mental Disorders (DSM-5) criteria. They showed that 5.2% of Mexican university students had Internet gaming disorder in the past year, while Li et al. (2016) applied the Online Game Cognition Addiction Scale (OGCAS) and revealed that 4.7% of Mainland Chinese college students had online gaming addiction. The considerable variation in the prevalence rates might be caused by the use of different addiction scales. In general, Hong Kong college students' prevalence of addiction to the Internet, gaming, and online social networking was comparable to university students in the international context.

Additionally, this scoping review found two studies that examined Hong Kong college students' alcohol, tobacco, or substance abuse. Griffiths et al. (2006) revealed that 62% of college students drank alcohol before, 7% experienced binge-drinking, and 0.8% had alcohol-related problems, while Abdullah et al. (2002) revealed that 61% and 13% had current and past use of alcohol and tobacco, respectively. Only a small percentage of students used marijuana (2%) or other illicit drugs (0.4%) currently or in the past.

Compared to general Hong Kong adults and international samples of college students, Hong Kong college students showed less severe alcohol and substance addiction problems. Hong Kong university students' rates of problematic alcohol consumption were lower than Hong Kong adults aged 18 to 20 (59.0% ever drinking; 12.33% past-month binge-drinking; 2.1% past-year alcohol abuse; 1.4% alcohol dependence) and Hong Kong adults aged 21 to 30 (78.5% ever drinking; 23.3% past-month binge-drinking; 7.2% past-year alcohol abuse; 3.1% alcohol dependence; Kim et al., 2008). Besides, international samples of college students suffered from more severe problematic alcohol consumption than Hong Kong college students. For example, Tavolacci et al. (2016) found that 51.3% and 13.8% French college students were occasional and frequent binge-drinkers, respectively; Wilczyński et al. (2013) revealed that, in Poland, 95.5% of university students tended to overuse alcohol, 28.86% had more than three times excessive drinking in the past month, and 46% experienced alcoholic palimpsest more than once; while Mekonen et al. (2017) found that 11.4% Ethiopia university students were problematic alcohol users. For illicit drug use, the prevalence rate for Hong Kong college students was also lower than the rate for college students in the international context. For example, a report from the US Department of Health and Human Services (2014) stated that 22.3% of full-time college students were illicit drug users in 2013. In the UK, Bennett and Holloway (2015) showed that 20.7% of college students used illicit drugs in the past year, while El Ansari et al. (2015) revealed that 25% of students used illicit drugs occasionally, and 5% were regular illicit drug users. In Turkey, Bakar et al. (2013) reported that 6.3% of college students had at least one illicit drug use in their lifetime.

3.2.4 Prevalence of Sleep and Eating Problems

There were seven articles that analyzed Hong Kong college students' sleep and eating problems, six articles of which examined their sleep problems (Guo et al., 2022; Huen et al., 2007; Sing & Wong, 2010; Suen et al., 2008; Wong et al., 2020; Yeung et al., 2008). Three out of these six studies utilized the Pittsburgh Sleep Quality Index (PSQI), one article applied Wing et al.'s (2002) Sleep Questionnaire, and two articles used a self-designed scale to measure participants' sleep quality. Using the PSQI scale, the three articles showed that the prevalence of sleep problems ranged from 57.5% to 68.6% (Sing & Wong, 2010; Suen et al., 2008), and the mean PSQI scores ranged from 5.20 to 6.63 (Suen et al., 2008; Wong et al., 2020), which were above the cutoff score of 5. Guo et al. (2022) used self-constructed measures and reported that 38.6% of students slept fewer than 7 hours per day, and 25.6% had insomnia symptoms. Among medical students, Yeung et al. (2008) used a self-constructed scale and found that 21.2% of the students had "very bad" or "fairly bad" sleep quality, while Huen et al. (2007) used Wing et al.'s (2002) Sleep Questionnaire and reported that 70% had sleep deprivation, with no significant gender and age differences.

The sleep problem of Hong Kong university students was comparable to international samples of college students. A number of studies used the PSQI scale to measure college students' sleep problems. For example, two studies on US college students showed that 62% to 65.9% had poor sleep quality (Becker et al., 2018; Lund et al., 2010); a study on Turkish university students found that 52.4% of college students had poor sleep quality (Ozcan & Acimis, 2021); while a study on college students in Taiwan revealed that 33.8% had poor sleep quality (Kang & Chen, 2009). Moreover, Naito et al. (2021) measured the percentage of students having less than 7 hours of sleep per day and found that 58.1% of Malaysian undergraduate students had sleep deprivation. Using a self-developed measure, Peltzer and Pengpid (2015) investigated the sleep problem of university students in 26 countries. The study revealed that the severity of sleep problems differed by country or region, and the prevalence rates ranged from 32.9% in Indonesia, 7.5% in South Africa, to 3.0% in Thailand. Within China, the study found that 4.6% of the students in Chengdu had sleep problems, while 8.1% of students in Hong Kong had sleep problems.

A large variation in prevalence rates of sleep problems between studies was found, which could be caused by the use of different measurement scales. For example, a study on German university students used the International Classification of Sleep Disorders-Second Edition (ICSD-2) and found that 7.7% suffered from insomnia (Schlarb et al., 2012). However, another study on German college students using the PSQI scale found that 42.9% had impaired sleep, and 17.7% suffered from severe sleep problems (Schlarb et al., 2017). The use of different scales to measure sleep problems may be the reason for the large variation in the prevalence rates.

This scoping review found one article that examined Hong Kong college students' eating disorders (Sze et al., 2021). Sze et al. (2021) utilized the 13-item Emotional Eating Subscale of the Dutch Eating Behavior Questionnaire (DEBQ) and found that the prevalence of emotional eating was 9.9%. Compared to college students in the international context, the prevalence rate for Hong Kong university students was lower. For example, a latent class analysis of US undergraduate students showed that the prevalence rates of having both emotional over- and under-eating was 18.3%, emotional over-eating was 18.2%, and emotional under-eating was 27.8% (Dixit et al., 2023). Similarly, a latent class analysis of Mainland Chinese undergraduate students revealed that the prevalence rates of emotional over- and under-eating was 15.4%, emotional over-eating was 14.7%, and emotional under-eating was 31.0% (He et al., 2020). In Spain, Carlos et al. (2020) showed that 29% of university students suffered from emotional eating. Examining university students in Bahrain, Alalwan et al. (2019) revealed that a considerable percentage of students increased their food intake because of loneliness (32.0%), happiness (39.6%), and boredom (71.6%). These figures showed that the prevalence of emotional eating among Hong Kong university students was less severe than among college students in the international context.

3.2.5 *Prevalence of Interpersonal Problems*

This scoping review found two articles that examined the severity of interpersonal violence perpetration and victimization of Hong Kong college students. First, using the Revised Conflict Tactics Scales (CTS2), Chan et al. (2007) found that the lifetime and preceding-year prevalence rates of physical assault perpetration against dating partners among students in three Hong Kong universities were 56.7% and 46.1%, respectively.

Compared to university students in the international context, Hong Kong university students had higher prevalence rates of violence perpetration in romantic relationships. Chan et al. (2008) examined violence against dating partners among university students in 21 countries or regions. The rates ranged from 17% to 44%, with Hong Kong students having a perpetration rate of 36.9%, showing that the severity of Hong

Kong students' dating violence was relatively high. Chan and Strauss (2008) also compared Hong Kong and US college students' prevalence rates of physical assault perpetration in romantic relationships and revealed that the preceding year's prevalence rate for Hong Kong students was higher than for US students (46.08% vs. 29.50%). Moreover, for Spanish university students, physical aggression in dating relationships prevalence rates were 30.4% in female and 32.2% in male students (Muñoz-Rivas et al., 2007). Besides, in a US university, Baker and Stith (2008) reported that 31.8% of male and 41.4% of female students were physically violent toward their dating partner at least once in the past year. These studies showed that compared with international figures, Hong Kong college students had more severe violence perpetration in dating relationships.

Second, this scoping review found one article that examined intimate partner sexual violence (IPSV) victimization of Hong Kong college students. Using the Chinese Revised Conflict Tactics Scale (CTS2), Wong et al. (2021) showed that 12.1% of college students from four Hong Kong universities suffered from IPSV victimization. Compared to international studies, the prevalence rate for Hong Kong college students was much lower. For example, 33.1% of Canadian university students suffered from at least one IPSV victimization in the past year (Jeffrey & Barata, 2021), and 22% of US female college students reported being victims of physical violence threats, physical abuse, or sexual abuse in romantic relationships (Grimmett et al., 2015; Knowledge Networks, 2011). For Iranian college students, the lifetime prevalence of IPSV victimization was 43.5% for men and 49.3% for women (Kamimura et al., 2016). These figures showed that Hong Kong college students had less severe problems in IPSV when compared to international samples of students.

3.2.6 Summary

First, in terms of Hong Kong university students' depression, anxiety, and stress, this scoping review found a large variation in prevalence rates, which could be attributed to the use of different assessment scales employed in different studies. Researchers also used self-constructed scales to measure Hong Kong college students' level of worry about the social unrest in 2019 and the COVID-19 pandemic. Besides, studies have analyzed Hong Kong college students' mental health status over the years and found that the situation worsened in recent years, especially during the pandemic. Moreover, compared to the Hong Kong general population and university students in Macau and Mainland China, Hong Kong university students had more serious mental problems. However, Hong Kong university students had a comparable prevalence of mental distress when compared to college students in the international context.

Second, for non-suicidal self-injury, suicidal ideation, and suicidal behavior, Hong Kong college students had relatively higher prevalence rates than university students in other places. Moreover, figures from the literature show that the prevalence rates of self-injurious behavior and suicidal ideation and behavior differed significantly by country or region.

Third, for addiction problems, this study found that Hong Kong university students had comparable prevalence rates of addiction to the Internet, gaming, and online social networking with reference to college students in the international context. A considerable variation in the prevalence rates was also observed in the literature, which could be caused by the use of different addiction scales in the studies. In terms of alcohol and substance addiction, Hong Kong college students showed less severe problems than Hong Kong adults of similar age or college students internationally.

Fourth, this scoping review analyzed Hong Kong college students' sleep and eating problems. It was found that the prevalence rates of Hong Kong university students' sleep problems were comparable to the rates for international samples of college students. The literature also showed a significant variation in sleep problem prevalence rates, which could be caused by the use of different scales to measure sleep quality or insomnia symptoms. For emotional eating, compared to university students in the international context, Hong Kong college students had a lower prevalence rate.

Lastly, in terms of interpersonal violence, compared to university students in the international context, Hong Kong university students had higher prevalence rates of physical assault perpetration against dating partners. However, in terms of intimate partner sexual violence victimization, the prevalence rate for Hong Kong college students was much lower than the prevalence rates for university students in the international context.

3.3 Institutional Learning Outcomes Related to Hong Kong University Students' Mental Health and Well-Being

In view of the severity of Hong Kong university students' developmental issues, as described above, it is vital to understand whether Hong Kong higher education institutions have initiatives to improve the mental health and well-being of their students. One strategy is to understand local universities' ILOs and/or DGAs related to their students' and graduates' holistic development. ILOs are important for higher education institutions because they represent institutional values and goals, which could turn into various long- or short-term plans and operate through the application of specific objectives, goals, or programs. Organizational effectiveness could also be measured by examining whether the institutions meet their ILOs (Serban, 2004).

In this study, the ILOs of 11 public and private universities in Hong Kong were examined using the framework we adopted in Chap. 2. Again, we examined whether employment capability, cognitive skills, non-cognitive skills, and psychosocial competencies were emphasized in the ILOs of these 11 Hong Kong higher education institutions. These attributes are essential to adolescents' quality of life. Studies argued that attributes related to psychosocial competencies, stress management, interpersonal relationships, conflict resolution, self-leadership, and problem-solving are critical to enhancing children's and adolescents' holistic development (Ando, 2011; Lamboy et al., 2022; Philips et al., 2022). Besides, some attributes, such as resilience and psychosocial competence, are fundamental to individuals' mental health. Analyzing whether local universities emphasize these attributes in their ILOs enables us to understand further the degree to which student mental well-being is being prioritized at the institutional level.

Specifically, 29 indicators were used to measure 12 domains of DGAs in the learning outcomes of these 11 universities at the institutional level. We visited the websites of the 11 universities to search for information related to these DGAs in the ILOs. Tables 3.1 and 3.2 summarize the findings from this analysis. For employment capability, 8 domains of DGAs were identified, including generic skills, professionalism, specialism, scientific literacy, application, global awareness, entrepreneurship, and literacy in different domains. Furthermore, cognitive skills refer to intrapersonal attributes, including creativity, problem-solving, and critical thinking, while non-cognitive skills refer to other intrapersonal attributes, including resilience, self-awareness, well-being, leadership, and reflection. Other psychosocial competencies were also measured, including interpersonal competence and intrapersonal competence on character and citizenship.

Table 3.1 shows the results of each institution's emphases in terms of the 12 domains of DGAs. In Table 3.2, we divided the 11 institutions into public or private universities and showed the number and percentage of each DGA in each of the category. Table 3.2 shows no significant difference between public and private universities in terms of institutional emphases. For Table 3.1, the discussion on the percentage of institutions emphasizing each attribute is as follows.

For employment capability, all 11 institutions emphasized generic skills and professionalism in their ILOs. The majority of the institutions emphasized global awareness (90.91%), while fewer institutions focused on literacy in different domains (72.73%), specialism (63.64%), application (63.64%), and scientific literacy (54.55%). Only three institutions highlighted entrepreneurship (27.27%). This shows that Hong Kong higher education institutions placed a relatively high emphasis on their graduates' employment capacity.

For cognitive skills, this study found that local institutions also placed heavy emphasis on these attributes. It was found that all institutions emphasized critical thinking in their ILOs, while the majority of them highlighted creativity/innovation (81.82%), and roughly half of the universities emphasized problem-solving (54.55%).

In terms of non-cognitive skills, not all institutions highlighted these attributes in their ILOs: 63.64% of the institutions stressed leadership, 54.55% emphasized self-awareness, 45.45% focused on resilience and well-being, and only 36.36% highlighted reflection. Results show that relatively fewer institutions emphasized the importance of non-cognitive skills in their graduates.

For intrapersonal attributes in terms of character and citizenship, this study found that a relatively large proportion of institutions highlighted these attributes in their ILOs. First, all institutions stressed citizenship, and the majority of them highlighted accountability (90.91%). Comparatively speaking, fewer institutions focused on morality (72.73%) and character (63.64%). These results show that character and citizenship were still regarded as important graduate attributes by the majority of higher education institutions in Hong Kong. However, the question of whether there is a conscious effort to nurture such attributes still needs to be answered.

Regarding interpersonal competence, relatively few institutions emphasized it in their ILOs. All institutions emphasized communication in their ILOs, and the majority highlighted connecting with others (72.73%). However, very few institutions focused on respect (36.36%) and empathy (27.27%). These results show that Hong Kong higher education institutions placed less emphasis on their graduates' interpersonal competence.

There are several observations when we compare the findings in Hong Kong with those reported in Chap. 2. First, there is wide variation in the ILOs/DGAs across universities in Hong Kong. Second, the current analysis show that Hong Kong higher education institutions strongly emphasized employment capability and cognitive skills in their ILOs. A moderate level of emphasis was placed on intrapersonal attributes in terms of character and citizenship. Third, non-cognitive skills and interpersonal competence received the least attention from the local institutions. Although employment capability and cognitive skills are essential to adolescents' well-being, a lower emphasis on their non-cognitive skills and interpersonal competence may put university students and graduates at greater risk of having deteriorated mental health and developmental problems. This deficiency also means that the graduates may not function well in the service economy, where all of these attributes are needed in the workplace (Kennedy & Sundberg, 2020). Finally, it should be realized that enhancement of psychosocial competence of students is very important to help them cope with the stress arising from social change (Shek, 2020) as well as the COVID-19 pandemic (Shek, 2021; Shek et al., 2022a, 2022b, 2023a, 2023b, 2023c).

3.4 Conclusion

Similar to Chap. 2, the scoping review conducted in this chapter suggests that Hong Kong university students have several developmental problems deserving our concern. These include mental health morbidity, addiction problems, lifestyle issues, and interpersonal problems. In view of these concerns, we ask whether the promotion of holistic development (such as psychosocial competence) is intrinsic to the ILOs of 11 Hong Kong higher education institutions. In line with our observation in Chap. 2, we found that despite Hong Kong university students having various developmental issues, the promotion of well-being and psychosocial competence does not occupy an important role in higher education policies in Hong Kong. As such, we have to ask two questions. First, what holistic development attributes should be nurtured in university students? Second, what strategies should be designed to promote Hong Kong university students' holistic well-being? To answer the first question, we highlight the importance of the development of 21st-century skills and make a comprehensive analysis based on the OECD Learning Compass 2030 in Chap. 4. Moreover, we discuss the concept of developmental assets and positive youth development in Chap. 5 and the role of leadership and Service-Learning in nurturing university students' well-being in Chap. 6. To answer the second question, we highlight the importance of having leadership and Service-Learning subjects in the formal curriculum to strengthen university students' holistic development in Chap. 7.

Acknowledgements The preparation of this chapter is financially supported by The Hong Kong Polytechnic University (ZZ4U and ZZUE), Li and Fung Endowed Professorship in Service Leadership Education, Wofoo Foundation, and the Matching Fund of Research Grants Council (ZECL and ZH4Q).

Appendix

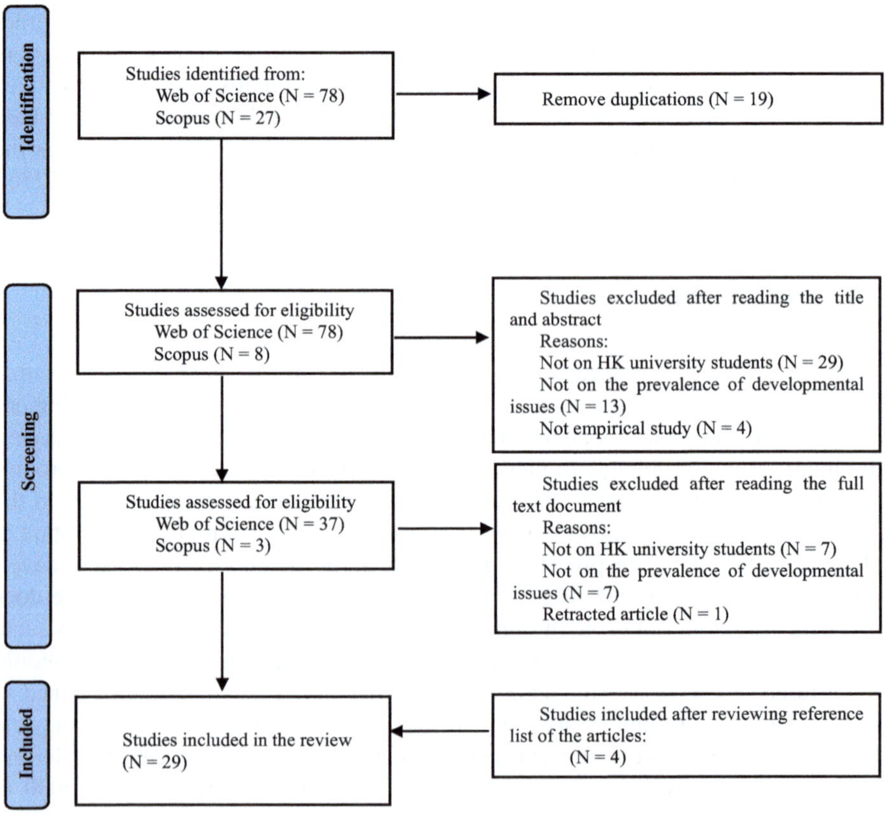

Fig. 3.1 PRISMA flow diagram for article selection

Table 3.1 Desired graduate attributes (DGAs) of Hong Kong universities ($N = 11$)

Attributes	HKU	CUHK	HKUST	PolyU	CityU	HKBU	LU	EdUHK	HSUHK	HKSYU	HKMU	Total	Percentage (%)
1. Generic skills/Competence/ Broad-based independence	√	√	√	√	√	√	√	√	√	√	√	11	100.00
2. Professionalism/Discipline knowledge	√	√	√	√	√	√	√	√	√	√	√	11	100.00
3. Specialism/Specialist skills	√		√	√		√		√	√	√		7	63.64
4. Research/Scientific literacy	√		√			√	√	√			√	6	54.55
5. Application	√			√	√	√	√	√		√		7	63.64
6. Intrapersonal attributes (Cognitive)	√	√	√	√	√	√	√	√	√	√	√	11	100.00
6a. Creativity/Innovation	√	√		√	√	√	√	√		√	√	9	81.82
6b. Problem-solving	√			√		√	√	√	√			6	54.55
6c. Critical thinking	√	√	√	√	√	√	√	√	√	√	√	11	100.00
7. Intrapersonal attributes (Non-cognitive)	√	√	√	√		√	√	√	√	√	√	10	90.91
7a. Resilience	√	√	√				√	√				5	45.45
7b. Self-awareness/ Self-regulated/Self-direct/ Self-management/Sense of self / Self-confidence	√		√	√		√			√	√		6	54.55
7c. Well-being		√		√		√		√	√			5	45.45

(continued)

Table 3.1 (continued)

Attributes	HKU	CUHK	HKUST	PolyU	CityU	HKBU	LU	EdUHK	HSUHK	HKSYU	HKMU	Total	Percentage (%)
7d. Leadership	√	√	√	√		√			√		√	7	63.64
7e. Reflection	√			√		√		√				4	36.36
8. Intrapersonal attributes (Character and citizenship)	√	√	√	√	√	√	√	√	√	√	√	11	100.00
8a. Accountability/Responsibility	√	√	√	√		√	√	√	√	√	√	10	90.91
8b. Morality and ethics	√	√	√	√		√		√	√	√		8	72.73
8c. Character and integrity	√	√	√			√	√	√	√			7	63.64
8d. Citizenship/Civic and community	√	√	√	√	√	√	√	√	√	√	√	11	100.00
9. Interpersonal competence	√	√	√	√	√	√	√	√	√	√	√	11	100.00
9a. Communication	√	√	√	√	√	√	√	√	√	√	√	11	100.00
9b. Cultivate their connections to others	√	√	√	√		√		√	√		√	8	72.73
9c. Empathy		√	√					√				3	27.27
9d. Respect	√	√	√			√						4	36.36
10. Environmental/Global awareness	√	√	√	√	√	√	√	√		√	√	10	90.91
11. Entrepreneurship				√			√	√				3	27.27
12. Literacy in different domains	√	√	√	√		√	√	√	√			8	72.73
12a. Lifelong learning	√	√		√	√	√	√	√	√	√	√	10	90.91
Total attributes per university	26	22	22	24	12	26	20	26	20	17	16		
Percentage of attributes per university (%)	89.66	75.86	75.86	82.76	41.38	89.66	68.97	89.66	68.97	58.62	55.17		

Note HKU = University of Hong Kong; CUHK = Chinese University of Hong Kong; HKUST = The Hong Kong University of Science and Technology; PolyU = The Hong Kong Polytechnic University; CityU = City University of Hong Kong; HKBU = Hong Kong Baptist University; LU = Lingnan University; EdUHK = The Education University of Hong Kong; HSUHK = Hang Seng University of Hong Kong; HKSYU = Hong Kong Shue Yan University; HKMU = Hong Kong Metropolitan University

Table 3.2 Number and percentage of Hong Kong public and private universities with the desired graduate attributes (DGAs)

Attributes	Public universities ($N = 8$)		Private universities ($N = 3$)		Total ($N = 11$)	
	n	%	*n*	%	*n*	%
1. Generic skills/Competence/Broad-based independence	8	100.00	3	100.00	11	100.00
2. Professionalism/Discipline knowledge	8	100.00	3	100.00	11	100.00
3. Specialism/Specialist skills	5	62.50	2	66.67	7	63.64
4. Research/Scientific literacy	5	62.50	1	33.33	6	54.55
5. Application	6	75.00	1	33.33	7	63.64
6. Intrapersonal attributes (Cognitive)	8	100.00	3	100.00	11	100.00
6a. Creativity/Innovation	7	87.50	2	66.67	9	81.82
6b. Problem-solving	5	62.50	1	33.33	6	54.55
6c. Critical thinking	8	100.00	3	100.00	11	100.00
7. Intrapersonal attributes (Non-cognitive)	7	87.50	3	100.00	10	90.91
7a. Resilience	5	62.50	0	0.00	5	45.45
7b. Self-awareness/Self-regulated/Self-direct/ Self-management/Sense of self /Self-confidence	4	50.00	2	66.67	6	54.55
7c. Well-being	4	50.00	1	33.33	5	45.45
7d. Leadership	5	62.50	2	66.67	7	63.64
7e. Reflection	4	50.00	0	0.00	4	36.36
8. Intrapersonal attributes (Character and citizenship)	8	100.00	3	100.00	11	100.00
8a. Accountability/Responsibility	7	87.50	3	100.00	10	90.91
8b. Morality and ethics	6	75.00	2	66.67	8	72.73
8c. Character and integrity	6	75.00	1	33.33	7	63.64
8d. Citizenship/Civic and community	8	100.00	3	100.00	11	100.00
9. Interpersonal competence	8	100.00	3	100.00	11	100.00
9a. Communication	8	100.00	3	100.00	11	100.00
9b. Cultivate their connections to others	6	75.00	2	66.67	8	72.73
9c. Empathy	3	37.50	0	0.00	3	27.27
9d. Respect	4	50.00	0	0.00	4	36.36
10. Environmental/Global awareness	8	100.00	2	66.67	10	90.91
11. Entrepreneurship	3	37.50	0	0.00	3	27.27

(continued)

Table 3.2 (continued)

Attributes	Public universities (*N* = 8)		Private universities (*N* = 3)		Total (*N* = 11)	
	n	%	*n*	%	*n*	%
12. Literacy in different domains	7	87.50	1	33.33	8	72.73
12a. Lifelong learning	7	87.50	3	100.00	10	90.91

Note Public universities include University of Hong Kong (HKU), Chinese University of Hong Kong (CUHK), The Hong Kong University of Science and Technology (HKUST), The Hong Kong Polytechnic University (PolyU), City University of Hong Kong (CityU), Hong Kong Baptist University (HKBU), Lingnan University (LU), and The Education University of Hong Kong (EdUHK); Private universities include Hang Seng University of Hong Kong (HSUHK), Hong Kong Shue Yan University (HKSYU), and Hong Kong Metropolitan University (HKMU)

References[1]

*Abdullah, A. S. M., Fielding, R., & Hedley, A. J. (2002). Patterns of cigarette smoking, alcohol use and other substance use among Chinese university students in Hong Kong. *The American Journal on Addictions, 11*(3), 235–246. https://doi.org/10.1080/10550490290088018

*Chan, C. Y., & Cheung, K. L. (2022). Exploring the gender difference in relationships between narcissism, competitiveness, and mental health problems among college students. *Journal of American College Health, 70*(4), 1169–1178. https://doi.org/10.1080/07448481.2020.1788565

*Chan, K. L., Tiwari, A., Leung, W. C., Ho, H. W., & Cerulli, C. (2007). Common correlates of suicidal ideation and physical assault among male and female university students in Hong Kong. *Violence and Victims, 22*(3), 290–303. https://doi.org/10.1891/088667007780842766

*Cheung, K., Tam, K. Y., Tsang, M. H., Zhang, L. W., & Lit, S. W. (2020). Depression, anxiety and stress in different subgroups of first-year university students from 4-year cohort data. *Journal of Affective Disorders, 274*, 305–314. https://doi.org/10.1016/j.jad.2020.05.041

*Cheung, T., Wong, S. Y., Law, L. Y., Ng, K., Tong, M. T., Wong, K. Y., Ng, M. Y., & Yip, P. S. F. (2016). Depression, anxiety and symptoms of stress among baccalaureate nursing students in Hong Kong: A cross-sectional study. *International Journal of Environmental Research and Public Health, 13*(8), 779. https://doi.org/10.3390/ijerph13080779

*Griffiths, S., Lau, J. T., Chow, J. K., Lee, S. S., Kan, P. Y., & Lee, S. (2006). Alcohol use among entrants to a Hong Kong University. *Alcohol and Alcoholism, 41*(5), 560–565. https://doi.org/10.1093/alcalc/agl047

*Guo, N., Luk, T. T., Wu, Y., Lai, A. Y. K., Li, Y., Cheung, D. Y. T., et al. (2022). Between-and within-person associations of mobile gaming time and total screen time with sleep problems in young adults: Daily assessment study. *Addictive Behaviors, 134*, 107408. https://doi.org/10.1016/j.addbeh.2022.107408

*Huen, L. L. E., Chan, T. W. G., Yu, W. M. M., & Wing, Y. K. (2007). Do medical students in Hong Kong have enough sleep? *Sleep and Biological Rhythms, 5*, 226–230. https://doi.org/10.1111/j.1479-8425.2007.00278.x

*Hung, M. S. Y., Ng, W. W. M., & Choi, E. K. Y. (2022). The impacts of the COVID-19 pandemic on Hong Kong nursing students' mental health and quality of life. *International Journal of Environmental Research and Public Health, 19*(22), 15117. https://doi.org/10.3390/ijerph192215117

[1] References marked with an asterisk indicate studies included in the scoping review.

*Leung, C. H., & Pong, H. K. (2021). Cross-sectional study of the relationship between the spiritual wellbeing and psychological health among university students. *PLoS One, 16*(4), Article e0249702. https://doi.org/10.1371/journal.pone.0249702

*Li, L., Lok, G. K., Mei, S. L., Cui, X. L., An, F. R., Li, L., Cheung, T., Ungvari, G. S., & Xiang, Y. T. (2020). Prevalence of depression and its relationship with quality of life among university students in Macau, Hong Kong and mainland China. *Scientific Reports, 10*(1), 15798. https://doi.org/10.1038/s41598-020-72458-w

*Li, X., Shek, D. T. L., & Shek, E. Y. (2021). Psychological morbidity among university students in Hong Kong (2014–2018): Psychometric properties of the Depression Anxiety Stress Scales (DASS) and related correlates. *International Journal of Environmental Research and Public Health, 18*(16), 8305. https://doi.org/10.3390/ijerph18168305

*Lun, K. W., Chan, C. K., Ip, P. K., Ma, S. Y., Tsai, W. W., Wong, C. S., Wong, C. H., Wong, T. W., & Yan, D. (2018). Depression and anxiety among university students in Hong Kong. *Hong Kong Medical Journal, 24*(5), 466–472. https://doi.org/10.12809/hkmj176915

*Ong, E., & Thompson, C. (2019). The importance of coping and emotion regulation in the occurrence of suicidal behavior. *Psychological Reports, 122*(4), 1192–1210. https://doi.org/10.1177/0033294118781855

*Park, J., Choi, S., Hong, H. C., Lee, H., & Cho, A. (2022). A latent class analysis of life stress among female East Asian college students: A multi-country study. *Journal of Affective Disorders, 310*, 310–317. https://doi.org/10.1016/j.jad.2022.05.053

*Poon, K. T. (2018). Unpacking the mechanisms underlying the relation between ostracism and internet addiction. *Psychiatry Research, 270*, 724–730. https://doi.org/10.1016/j.psychres.2018.10.056

*Shek, D. T. L., Dou, D. Y., Zhu, X. Q., Wong, T., & Tan, L. (2022a). Need satisfaction and depressive symptoms among university students in Hong Kong during the COVID-19 pandemic: Moderating effects of positive youth development attributes. *Frontiers in Psychiatry, 13*, 931404. https://doi.org/10.3389/fpsyt.2022.931404

*Shek, D. T. L., Dou, D. Y., & Zhu, X. Q. (2022b). Prevalence and correlates of mental health of university students in Hong Kong: What happened one year after the occurrence of COVID-19? *Frontiers in Public Health, 10*, 857147. https://doi.org/10.3389/fpubh.2022.857147

*Sing, C. Y., & Wong, W. S. (2010). Prevalence of insomnia and its psychosocial correlates among college students in Hong Kong. *Journal of American College Health, 59*(3), 174–182. https://doi.org/10.1080/07448481.2010.497829

*Song, Y., Huang, Y., Liu, D., Kwan, J. S., Zhang, F., Sham, P. C., & Tang, S. W. (2008). Depression in college: Depressive symptoms and personality factors in Beijing and Hong Kong college freshmen. *Comprehensive Psychiatry, 49*(5), 496–502. https://doi.org/10.1016/j.comppsych.2008.02.005

*Suen, L. K. P., Ellis Hon, K. L., & Tam, W. W. S. (2008). Association between sleep behavior and sleep-related factors among university students in Hong Kong. *Chronobiology International, 25*(5), 760–775. https://doi.org/10.1080/07420520802397186

*Sze, K. Y., Lee, E. K., Chan, R. H., & Kim, J. H. (2021). Prevalence of negative emotional eating and its associated psychosocial factors among urban Chinese undergraduates in Hong Kong: A cross-sectional study. *BMC Public Health, 21*, 583. https://doi.org/10.1186/s12889-021-10531-3

*Tang, C. S. K., Wu, A. M. S., Yan, E. C. W., Ko, J. H. C., Kwon, J. H., Yogo, M., Gan, Y. Q., & Koh, Y. Y. W. (2018). Relative risks of Internet-related addictions and mood disturbances among college students: A 7-country/region comparison. *Public Health, 165*, 16–25. https://doi.org/10.1016/j.puhe.2018.09.010

*Wong, H. Y., Mo, H. Y., Potenza, M. N., Chan, M. N. M., Lau, W. M., Chui, T. K., Pakpour, A. H., & Lin, C.-Y. (2020). Relationships between severity of internet gaming disorder, severity of problematic social media use, sleep quality and psychological distress. *International Journal of Environmental Research and Public Health, 17*(6), 1879. https://doi.org/10.3390/ijerph17061879

*Wong, J. G., Cheung, E. P., Chan, K. K., Ma, K. K., & Tang, S. W. (2006). Web-based survey of depression, anxiety and stress in first-year tertiary education students in Hong Kong. *Australian & New Zealand Journal of Psychiatry, 40*(9), 777–782. https://doi.org/10.1080/j.1440-1614.2006.01883.x

*Wong, J. Y., Choi, E. P., Lo, H. H., Wong, W., Chio, J. H., Choi, A. W., & Fong, D. Y. (2021). Intimate partner sexual violence and mental health indicators among Chinese emerging adults. *Journal of Interpersonal Violence, 36*(19–20), NP10229-NP10254. https://doi.org/10.1177/0886260519872985

*Wong, S. L., & Chung, M. C. (2023). Child abuse and non-suicidal self-injury among Chinese university students: The role of emotion dysregulation and attachment style. *Current Psychology, 42*, 4862–4872. https://doi.org/10.1007/s12144-021-01832-2

*Yeung, W. F., Chung, K.-F., & Cy Chan, T. (2008). Sleep-wake habits, excessive daytime sleepiness and academic performance among medical students in Hong Kong. *Biological Rhythm Research, 39*(4), 369–377. https://doi.org/10.1080/09291010701425124

*Yu, L., & Luo, T. (2021). Social networking addiction among Hong Kong university students: Its health consequences and relationships with parenting behaviors. *Frontiers in Public Health, 8*, 555990. https://doi.org/10.3389/fpubh.2020.555990

Alalwan, T. A., Hilal, S. J., Mahdi, A. M., Ahmed, M. A., & Mandeel, Q. A. (2019). Emotional eating behavior among University of Bahrain students: A cross-sectional study. *Arab Journal of Basic and Applied Sciences, 26*(1), 424–432. https://doi.org/10.1080/25765299.2019.1655836

Ando, M. (2011). An intervention program focused on self-understanding and interpersonal interactions to prevent psychosocial distress among Japanese university students. *Journal of Adolescence, 34*(5), 929–940. https://doi.org/10.1016/j.adolescence.2010.12.003

Asif, S., Mudassar, A., Shahzad, T. Z., Raouf, M., & Pervaiz, T. (2020). Frequency of depression, anxiety and stress among university students. *Pakistan Journal of Medical Sciences, 36*(5), 971–976. https://doi.org/10.12669/pjms.36.5.1873

Babakr, Z. H., Majeed, K., Mohamedamin, P., & Kakamad, K. (2019). Internet addiction in Kurdistan university students: prevalence and association with self-control. *European Journal of Educational Research, 8*(3), 867–873. https://doi.org/10.12973/eu-jer.8.3.867

Bakar, C., Gündogar, D., Ozisik Karaman, H. I., & Maral, I. (2013). Prevalence and related risk factors of tobacco, alcohol and illicit substance use among university students. *The European Journal of Psychiatry, 27*(2), 97–110. https://doi.org/10.4321/S0213-61632013000200003

Baker, C. R., & Stith, S. M. (2008). Factors predicting dating violence perpetration among male and female college students. *Journal of Aggression, Maltreatment & Trauma, 17*(2), 227–244. https://doi.org/10.1080/10926770802344836

Becker, S. P., Jarrett, M. A., Luebbe, A. M., Garner, A. A., Burns, G. L., & Kofler, M. J. (2018). Sleep in a large, multi-university sample of college students: Sleep problem prevalence, sex differences, and mental health correlates. *Sleep Health, 4*(2), 174–181. https://doi.org/10.1016/j.sleh.2018.01.001

Bennett, T. H., & Holloway, K. R. (2015). Drug use among college and university students: Findings from a national survey. *Journal of Substance Use, 20*(1), 50–55. https://doi.org/10.3109/14659891.2013.878762

Bisen, S. S., & Deshpande, Y. (2020). Prevalence, predictors, psychological correlates of internet addiction among college students in India: A comprehensive study. *Anatolian Journal of Psychiatry/Anadolu Psikiyatri Dergisi, 21*(2). https://doi.org/10.5455/apd.47328

Borges, G., Orozco, R., Benjet, C., Martínez Martínez, K. I., Contreras, E. V., Jiménez Pérez, A. L., Peláez Cedrés, A. J., Hernández Uribe, P. C., Díaz Couder, M. A. C., Gutierrez-Garcia, R. A., Quevedo Chavez, G. E., Albor, Y., Mendez, E., Medina-Mora, M. E., Mortier, P., & Rumpf, H. J. (2019). DSM-5 Internet gaming disorder among a sample of Mexican first-year college students. *Journal of Behavioral Addictions, 8*(4), 714–724. https://doi.org/10.1556/2006.8.2019.62

Camacho, Á., Cordero, E. D., & Perkins, T. (2016). Psychometric properties of the DASS-21 among Latina/o college students by the US-Mexico border. *Journal of Immigrant and Minority Health, 18*, 1017–1023. https://doi.org/10.1007/s10903-016-0415-1

Carlos, M., Elena, B., & Teresa, I. M. (2020). Are adherence to the Mediterranean diet, emotional eating, alcohol intake, and anxiety related in university students in Spain? *Nutrients, 12*(8), 2224. https://doi.org/10.3390/nu12082224

Chan, K. L., & Straus, M. A. (2008). Prevalence and correlates of physical assault on dating partners. *The Open Social Science Journal, 2008*(1), 5–14. https://doi.org/10.2174/1874945300801010005

Chan, K. L., Straus, M. A., Brownridge, D. A., Tiwari, A., & Leung, W. C. (2008). Prevalence of dating partner violence and suicidal ideation among male and female university students worldwide. *Journal of Midwifery and Women's Health, 53*(6), 529–537. https://doi.org/10.1016/j.jmwh.2008.04.016

Chi, X., Lin, L., & Zhang, P. (2016). Internet addiction among college students in China: Prevalence and psychosocial correlates. *Cyberpsychology, Behavior, and Social Networking, 19*(9), 567–573. https://doi.org/10.1089/cyber.2016.0234

Choi, E. P. H., Hui, B. P. H., & Wan, E. Y. F. (2020). Depression and anxiety in Hong Kong during COVID-19. *International Journal of Environmental Research and Public Health, 17*, 3740. https://doi.org/10.3390/ijerph17103740

Crispim, M. D. O., Santos, C. M. R. D., Frazão, I. D. S., Frazão, C. M. F. D. Q., Albuquerque, R. C. R. D., & Perrelli, J. G. A. (2021). Prevalence of suicidal behavior in young university students: A systematic review with meta-analysis. *Revista Latino-Americana de Enfermagem, 29*, e3495. https://doi.org/10.1590/1518-8345.5320.3495

Dixit, U., He, J., Whited, M., Ellis, J. M., & Zickgraf, H. F. (2023). Negative emotional eating patterns among American university students: A replication study. *Appetite, 186*, 106554. https://doi.org/10.1016/j.appet.2023.106554

El Ansari, W., Vallentin-Holbech, L., & Stock, C. (2015). Predictors of illicit drug/s use among university students in Northern Ireland, Wales and England. *Global Journal of Health Science, 7*(4), 18–29. https://doi.org/10.5539/gjhs.v7n4p18

Grimmett, J., Lewis, W. S., Schuster, S. K., Sokolow, B. A., Swinton, D. C., & Van Brunt, B. (2015). *The challenge of title ix responses to campus relationship & intimate partner violence*. Association of Title IX Administrators. https://cdn1.sportngin.com/attachments/document/0128/6286/Challenge-of-TIX-with-Author-Photos.pdf

He, J., Chen, G., Wu, S., Niu, R., & Fan, X. (2020). Patterns of negative emotional eating among Chinese young adults: A latent class analysis. *Appetite, 155*, 104808. https://doi.org/10.1016/j.appet.2020.104808

Hong, F. Y., Huang, D. H., Lin, H. Y., & Chiu, S. L. (2014). Analysis of the psychological traits, Facebook usage, and Facebook addiction model of Taiwanese university students. *Telematics and Informatics, 31*(4), 597–606.

Huang, Y., Kuang, L., Wang, W., Cao, J., & Xu, L. (2019). Association between personality traits and risk of suicidal ideation in Chinese university students: Analysis of the correlation among five personalities. *Psychiatry Research, 272*, 93–99. https://doi.org/10.1016/j.psychres.2018.12.076

Jaradat, M. I. R. M., & Atyeh, A. J. (2017). Do personality traits play a role in social media addiction? Key considerations for successful optimized model to avoid social networking sites addiction: A developing country perspective. *International Journal of Computer Science and Network Security, 17*(8), 120–131.

Jeffrey, N. K., & Barata, P. C. (2021). Intimate partner sexual violence among Canadian university students: Incidence, context, and perpetrators' perceptions. *Archives of Sexual Behavior, 50*(5), 2123–2138. https://doi.org/10.1007/s10508-021-02006-8

Kaggwa, M. M., Arinaitwe, I., Muwanguzi, M., Nduhuura, E., Kajjimu, J., Kule, M., Najjuka, S. M., Nkola, R., Ajuna, N., Wamala, N. K., Machacha, I., Mamun, M. A., Ho, C. S., Griffiths, M. D., & Rukundo, G. Z. (2022). Suicidal behaviours among Ugandan university students: A cross-sectional study. *BMC Psychiatry, 22*, 234. https://doi.org/10.1186/s12888-022-03858-7

Kamimura, A., Nourian, M. M., Assasnik, N., & Franchek-Roa, K. (2016). Depression and intimate partner violence among college students in Iran. *Asian Journal of Psychiatry, 23*, 51–55. https://doi.org/10.1016/j.ajp.2016.07.014

Kang, J. H., & Chen, S. C. (2009). Effects of an irregular bedtime schedule on sleep quality, daytime sleepiness, and fatigue among university students in Taiwan. *BMC Public Health, 9*(1), 1–6. https://doi.org/10.1186/1471-2458-9-248

Kennedy, T. J., & Sundberg, C. W. (2020). 21st century skills. In B. Akpan & T. J. Kennedy (Eds.), *Science education in theory and practice* (pp. 479–496). Springer.

Kharsati, N., & Bhola, P. (2016). Self-injurious behavior, emotion regulation, and attachment styles among college students in India. *Industrial Psychiatry Journal, 25*(1), 23–28. https://doi.org/10.4103/0972-6748.196049

Kim, J. H., Lee, S., Chow, J., Lau, J., Tsang, A., Choi, J., & Griffiths, S. M. (2008). Prevalence and the factors associated with binge drinking, alcohol abuse, and alcohol dependence: A population-based study of Chinese adults in Hong Kong. *Alcohol and Alcoholism, 43*(3), 360–370. https://doi.org/10.1093/alcalc/agm181

Kircaburun, K., & Griffiths, M. D. (2018). Instagram addiction and the Big Five of personality: The mediating role of self-liking. *Journal of Behavioral Addictions, 7*(1), 158–170. https://doi.org/10.1556/2006.7.2018.15

Knowledge Networks for Liz Claiborne Inc. (2011). *College dating violence and abuse poll.* Break the Cycle. https://www.breakthecycle.org/dating-violence-research/college-dating-violence-and-abuse-poll/

Lam, L. C. W., Wong, C. S. M., Wang, M. J., Chan, W. C., Chen, E. Y. H., Ng, R. M. K., Hung, S. F., Cheung, E. F. C., Sham, P. C., Chiu, H. F. K., Lam, M., Chang, W. C., Lee, E. H. M., Chiang, T. P., Lau, J. T. F., van Os, J., Lewis, G., & Bebbington, P. (2015). Prevalence, psychosocial correlates and service utilization of depressive and anxiety disorders in Hong Kong: The Hong Kong Mental Morbidity Survey (HKMMS). *Social Psychiatry and Psychiatric Epidemiology, 50*, 1379–1388. https://doi.org/10.1007/s00127-015-1014-5

Lamboy, B., Beck, F., Tessier, D., Williamson, M. O., Fréry, N., Turgon, R., Tassie, J. M., Barrois, J., Bessa, Z., & Shankland, R. (2022). The key role of psychosocial competencies in evidence-based youth mental health promotion: Academic support in consolidating a national strategy in France. *International Journal of Environmental Research and Public Health, 19*(24), 16641. https://doi.org/10.3390/ijerph192416641

Li, H., Zou, Y., Wang, J., & Yang, X. (2016). Role of stressful life events, avoidant coping styles, and neuroticism in online game addiction among college students: A moderated mediation model. *Frontiers in Psychology, 7*, 1794. https://doi.org/10.3389/fpsyg.2016.01794

Li, Z.-Z., Li, Y.-M., Lei, X.-Y., Zhang, D., Liu, L., Tang, S.-Y., & Chen, L. (2014). Prevalence of suicidal ideation in Chinese college students: A meta-analysis. *PLoS ONE, 9*(10), Article e104368. https://doi.org/10.1371/journal.pone.0104368

Lund, H. G., Reider, B. D., Whiting, A. B., & Prichard, J. R. (2010). Sleep patterns and predictors of disturbed sleep in a large population of college students. *Journal of Adolescent Health, 46*(2), 124–132. https://doi.org/10.1016/j.jadohealth.2009.06.016

Mak, S., & Thomas, A. (2022). Steps for conducting a scoping review. *Journal of Graduate Medical Education, 14*(5), 565–567. https://doi.org/10.4300/JGME-D-22-00621.1

Mekonen, T., Fekadu, W., Chane, T., & Bitew, S. (2017). Problematic alcohol use among university students. *Frontiers in Psychiatry, 8*, 86. https://doi.org/10.3389/fpsyt.2017.00086

Mortier, P., Cuijpers, P., Kiekens, G., Auerbach, R. P., Demyttenaere, K., Green, J. G., Kessler, R. C., Nock, M. K., & Bruffaerts, R. (2018). The prevalence of suicidal thoughts and behaviours among college students: A meta-analysis. *Psychological Medicine, 48*(4), 554–565. https://doi.org/10.1017/S00.29717002215

Muehlenkamp, J. J., Claes, L., Havertape, L., & Plener, P. L. (2012). International prevalence of adolescent non-suicidal self-injury and deliberate self-harm. *Child and Adolescent Psychiatry and Mental Health, 6*, 10. https://doi.org/10.1186/1753-2000-6-10

Muñoz-Rivas, M. J., Graña Gómez, J. L., O'Leary, D. K., & González Lozano, P. (2007). Physical and psychological aggression in dating relationships in Spanish university students. *Psicothema, 19*(1), 102–107.

Naito, R., Yun Low, W., & Wan Yuen, C. (2021). Sleep deprivation and its associated factors among undergraduate students in Malaysia. *Asia Pacific Journal of Public Health, 33*(5), 530–538. https://doi.org/10.1177/1010539521101993

Ozcan, B., & Acimis, N. M. (2021). Sleep Quality in Pamukkale University Students and its relationship with smartphone addiction. *Pakistan Journal of Medical Sciences, 37*(1), 206–211. https://doi.org/10.12669/pjms.37.1.3130

Page, M. J., McKenzie, J. E., Bossuyt, P. M., Boutron, I., Hoffmann, T. C., Mulrow, C. D., Shamseer, L., Tetzlaff, J. M., Akl, E. A., Brennan, S. E., Chou, R., Glanville, J., Grimshaw, J. M., Hróbjartsson, A., Lalu, M. M., Li, T., Loder, E. W., Mayo-Wilson, E., McDonald, S., ... Moher, D. (2021). The PRISMA 2020 statement: An updated guideline for reporting systematic reviews. *BMJ, 372*, n71. https://doi.org/10.1136/bmj.n71

Paul, E., Tsypes, A., Eidlitz, L., Ernhout, C., & Whitlock, J. (2015). Frequency and functions of non-suicidal self-injury: Associations with suicidal thoughts and behaviors. *Psychiatry Research, 225*(3), 276–282. https://doi.org/10.1016/j.psychres.2014.12.026

Peltzer, K., & Pengpid, S. (2015). Nocturnal sleep problems among university students from 26 countries. *Sleep and Breathing, 19*, 499–508. https://doi.org/10.1007/s11325-014-1036-3

Phillips, T. K., Rose, A. L., & Strickland, M. L. (2022). The mediating role of self-leadership in the link between racial identity attitudes, mental health outcomes, and race related stress. *International Journal of Systemic Therapy, 33*(3), 175–195. https://doi.org/10.1080/2692398X.2022.2084316

Ramón-Arbués, E., Gea-Caballero, V., Granada-López, J. M., Juárez-Vela, R., Pellicer-García, B., & Antón-Solanas, I. (2020). The prevalence of depression, anxiety and stress and their associated factors in college students. *International Journal of Environmental Research and Public Health, 17*(19), 7001. https://doi.org/10.3390/ijerph17197001

Rasheduzzaman, M., Al-Mamun, F., Hosen, I., Akter, T., Hossain, M., Griffiths, M. D., & Mamun, M. A. (2022). Suicidal behaviors among Bangladeshi university students: Prevalence and risk factors. *PLoS ONE, 17*(1), Article e0262006. https://doi.org/10.1371/journal.pone.0262006

Schlarb, A. A., Claßen, M., Grünwald, J., & Vögele, C. (2017). Sleep disturbances and mental strain in university students: Results from an online survey in Luxembourg and Germany. *International Journal of Mental Health Systems, 11*, 24. https://doi.org/10.1186/s13033-017-0131-9

Schlarb, A. A., Kulessa, D., & Gulewitsch, M. D. (2012). Sleep characteristics, sleep problems, and associations of self-efficacy among German university students. *Nature and Science of Sleep, 4*, 1–7. https://doi.org/10.2147/NSS.S27971

Serban, A. M. (2004). Assessment of student learning outcomes at the institutional level. *New Directions for Community Colleges, 2004*(126), 17–27. https://doi.org/10.1002/cc.151

Shek, D. T. L. (2010). Nurturing holistic development of university students in Hong Kong: Where are we and where should we go? *The Scientific World Journal, 10*, 563–575. https://doi.org/10.1100/tsw.2010.62

Shek, D. T. L. (2020). Protests in Hong Kong (2019–2020): A perspective based on quality of life and well-being. *Applied Research in Quality of Life, 15*(3), 619–635. https://doi.org/10.1007/s11482-020-09825-2

Shek, D. T. L. (2021). COVID-19 and quality of life: Twelve reflections. *Applied Research in Quality of Life, 16*(1), 1–11. https://doi.org/10.1007/s11482-020-09898-z

Shek, D. T. L., Chai, W. Y., Wong, T., & Zhou, K. (2023a). Stress and depressive symptoms in university students in Hong Kong under the pandemic: Moderating effect of positive psychological attributes. *Frontiers in Psychology, 14*, 1071938. https://doi.org/10.3389/fpsyg.2023.1071938

Shek, D. T. L., Chai, W., Li, X., & Dou, D. (2023b). Profiles and predictors of mental health of university students in Hong Kong under the COVID-19 pandemic. *Frontiers in Psychology, 14*, 1211229. https://doi.org/10.3389/fpsyg.2023.1211229

Shek, D. T. L., Chai, W., & Zhou, K. (2023c). Risk factors and protective factors of internet addiction in university students during the pandemic: Implications for prevention and treatment. *International Journal of Environmental Research and Public Health, 20*(11), 5952. https://doi.org/10.3390/ijerph20115952

Shek, D. T. L., & Wong, K. K. (2011). Do adolescent developmental issues disappear overnight? Reflections about holistic development in university students. *The Scientific World Journal, 11*, 353–361. https://doi.org/10.1100/tsw.2011.5

Sivertsen, B., Hysing, M., Knapstad, M., Harvey, A. G., Reneflot, A., Lønning, K. J., & O'Connor, R. C. (2019). Suicide attempts and non-suicidal self-harm among university students: Prevalence study. *Bjpsych Open, 5*(2), e26. https://doi.org/10.1192/bjo.2019.4

Tang, C. S. K., Koh, Y. W., & Gan, Y. (2017). Addiction to Internet use, online gaming, and online social networking among young adults in China, Singapore, and the United States. *Asia Pacific Journal of Public Health, 29*(8), 673–682. https://doi.org/10.1177/1010539517739558

Tavolacci, M. P., Boerg, E., Richard, L., Meyrignac, G., Dechelotte, P., & Ladner, J. (2016). Prevalence of binge drinking and associated behaviours among 3286 college students in France. *BMC Public Health, 16*, 178. https://doi.org/10.1186/s12889-016-2863-x

Tresno, F., Ito, Y., & Mearns, J. (2012). Self-injurious behavior and suicide attempts among Indonesian college students. *Death Studies, 36*(7), 627–639. https://doi.org/10.1080/07481187.2011.604464

Tresno, F., Ito, Y., & Mearns, J. (2013). Risk factors for non-suicidal self-injury in Japanese college students: The moderating role of mood regulation expectancies. *International Journal of Psychology, 48*(6), 1009–1017. https://doi.org/10.1080/00207594.2012.733399

U.S. Department of Health and Human Services. (2014). *Results from the 2013 national survey on drug use and health: Summary of national findings*. https://www.samhsa.gov/data/sites/default/files/NSDUHresultsPDFWHTML2013/Web/NSDUHresults2013.pdf

Wilczyński, K., Witowski, L., Pawlik, A., Krysta, K., & Krupka-Matuszczyk, I. (2013). Consumption of alcohol and risk of alcohol addiction among students in Poland. *Psychiatria Danubina, 25*(2), 78–82.

Wing, Y. K., Li, R. H. Y., Lam, C. W., Ho, C. K. W., Fong, S. Y. Y., & Leung, T. (2002). The prevalence of narcolepsy among Chinese in Hong Kong. *Annals of Neurology, 51*(5), 578–584. https://doi.org/10.1002/ana.10162

Chapter 4
Development of 21st-Century Skills: A Comprehensive Analysis Based on the OECD Learning Compass 2030

Daniel T. L. Shek, Ginger C. C. Chau, and Britta M. Lee

Abstract The landscape of education and skills is undergoing significant transitions in the new era of globalization and technological advances. As such, future-ready young people need to equip themselves with interdisciplinary competencies, creativity, innovation, and other skills in their daily lives and respond to challenges and opportunities in this changeable world. In particular, education should be personalized and adaptable to address the diverse profiles and personal goals of students. This chapter delves into the Organization for Economic Co-operation and Development (OECD)'s view on 21st-century skills, particularly in the context of the OECD Learning Compass 2030. The framework acts as a roadmap for educators and practitioners to cultivate students' holistic development, help adolescents thrive and flourish in future world, and influence the well-being of the world. This chapter first gives the background of the OECD's Future of Education and Skills 2030 project, including the challenges and opportunities in the new era of the digital world and the call for an educational revolution. Then, this chapter explores the essential concepts in the Learning Compass 2030 and investigates why they are needed for students to navigate the future world. In the final part, the challenges and difficulties in teaching 21st-century skills will be discussed, and some thriving examples in the universities will be presented as well.

Keywords 21st-century skills · Organization for Economic Co-operation and Development (OECD) · Learning compass 2030 · Personalized education · Challenges and opportunities · Educational revolution · Holistic development

4.1 Introduction and Background

The Organization for Economic Co-operation and Development (OECD) is an international body that aims to improve the economic and social well-being of people worldwide. Established in 1961, the OECD encourages governments to cooperate, share experiences, and tackle common problems, from economic and environmental issues to education and skills development. Today, 38 member countries have joined the OECD, and it has formed collaborative partnerships with other non-member

D. T. L. Shek, *Promoting Holistic Development in University Students*, Quality of Life in Asia 17, https://doi.org/10.1007/978-981-96-0251-3_4

countries globally. For example, when the Program for International Student Assessment (PISA) was launched in 2018, 80 countries and economies joined. China has cooperated as a non-member state since 1995 (OECD, n.d.).

The OECD has been recognized as a "global education policy shaper" (Ydesen, 2019, p. 2) and is collaborating with the United Nations in developing global indicators to monitor the process of achieving Goal 4 of the Sustainable Development Goals (OECD, 2016). Specifically, Goal 4 emphasizes "inclusive and equitable quality education and promotes lifelong learning opportunities for all" (United Nations, 2015). Now, the OECD also compares the design of educational systems and paradigms and implements indicators for educational measurement (Martens & Jakobi, 2010; Schmelzer, 2016). Its most central goal is not education itself but enabling learners to acquire skills, competence, and character qualities through education that make them thrive and develop (OECD, 2016). When the Future of Education and Skills 2030 project was initiated in 2015, the OECD aimed to build a knowledge base to guide curricula redesign and educational development worldwide (Marope et al., 2017). With this guidance, education can prepare students to be ready for future jobs, technologies, opportunities, and challenges in the 2030 world.

4.2 The Need for an Education Revolution

As the world is changing dramatically in every aspect, young people need to be prepared to embrace a broader goal of becoming active and responsible citizens with essential skills, especially non-cognitive skills (OECD, 2018a). Some people criticize the educational systems nowadays for not responding well to the digital revolution, saying that "today's students are living in a digital world while studying in the nineteenth century" (OECD, 2019k, p. 23). Crucially, a profound education revolution is not about the replication of past practices and models but about an orientation to the future (Dobryakova et al., 2023). Education needs to fulfill two purposes: learn from the past and be ready for future challenges, which inspire students to cultivate their agency, develop a sense of purpose and responsibility, build competencies, and influence the people around them and the world they live in (OECD, 2018a).

Nowadays, the terms "competencies," "competences," "21st-century skills," "soft skills," "transversal skills," "non-cognitive skills," "transferrable skills," and "new literacy" are always used interchangeably by many people or institutions (Care, 2017). Technical skills will no longer be sufficient, and the demand for soft skills is increasing. Thomas Friedman, an MIT columnist, mentioned that "It is the Age of Global Accelerations, where technology is powerfully reshaping social and economic life, and humans are experiencing disruptive forces from all aspects." Although the challenges are enormous, he stressed that the opportunities are open to all human beings, as anyone can be a stakeholder in the global conversation (Dizikes, 2018). Artificial intelligence (AI) performs better than human beings when doing routine manual work and routine cognitive tasks. However, human beings can outperform AI in abstract tasks, interpersonal communication, complex contextual tasks, and ethical judgments. Moreover, human beings can set goals, embrace a sense of responsibility, and initiate changes to influence the world, namely "agency" (Luckin & Issroff, 2018). These challenges and opportunities suggest a revolution in education.

4.3 The Future of Education and Skills 2030 Project

The Future of Education and Skills 2030 is based on the OECD's Definition and Selection of Competencies Project (DeSeCo). DeSeCo operated from 1996 to 2003 to initiate curricula and educational reform in many countries. In the first stage, DeSeCo explored competencies that could "contribute to valued outcomes for societies and individuals; help individuals meet important demands in a wide variety of contexts; and be important not just for specialists but for all individuals" (OECD, 2005, p. 4). Nevertheless, this initiative did not generate satisfactory results as many member countries were changing their curricula quickly and did not spend enough time doing research and reflecting on the effectiveness of their curricula (Dobryakova et al., 2023). In 2017, The OECD revised DeSeCo and proposed the "Future of Education and Skills 2030" project, emphasizing an evidence-based and systematic curriculum redesign and regarding the needs of students as the priority (OECD, 2019k).

There are two phases in the project. In Phase One (2015–2019), the main focus was on "what" questions, namely "What kinds of competencies (knowledge, skills, attitudes, and values) do students need to propel humankind to a prosperous future?" These attributes also provide a knowledge base for different stakeholders to do effective communication and foster an innovative learning future. Additionally, Phase One initiates an International Curriculum Analysis to provide guidelines for countries to design their curriculum more systematically. When it comes to Phase Two (2019 and beyond), the OECD's Learning Compass 2030 was proposed to initiate principles and instructional curriculum designs. Instead of merely knowing what attributes are needed, Phase Two extends its mission to explore "How do we make changes in the learning environments and curriculum to nurture the competencies of students?" (OECD, 2018a, p. 2). Teachers are encouraged to take up the role of coaches, mentors, and facilitators to help learners achieve their goals. Furthermore, strategies will be developed to improve teacher competencies, such as teacher training programs (Schleicher, 2018). Notably, the framework is about the orientation of best practices during which experts, educators, and practitioners are able to exchange their knowledge and learn from each other. It acts as a learning compass to guide individuals' goals and aspirations, enables the development of competence in the learning cycle, and promotes lifelong learning for all groups of people (OECD, 2018a).

4.4 Basic Concepts in the Learning Compass 2030

Learning does not necessarily happen in school because it can take place in a variety of contexts. The Compass provides guidance for learners to go through challenging and unfamiliar circumstances and achieve positive development through meaningful, purposeful, and responsible actions. Equally importantly, it empowers students to develop "student agency" to make their own choices directly instead of receiving instructions from others (OECD, 2019g). In this sense, the Compass values the intrinsic motivation of learning. Moreover, different stakeholders take part in students' learning as "co-agency." The components in the Compass include "core foundations," "knowledge, skills, attitudes, and values," "transformative competencies," and the "Anticipation-Action-Reflection cycle (AAR cycle)." Individual well-being contributes to societal well-being as a whole, which also enriches individual well-being.

The Compass values that each individual has a unique learning compass as it is created by one's competencies, knowledge, experiences, family background, and culture. Therefore, each student will follow their own way of learning and be directed to paths that are different from others. Nevertheless, they share a common goal to enhance societal well-being (OECD, 2019g). More importantly, the Compass proposes that students take up an active role in the education system, where they can propel changes in society. Therefore, only a dynamic and flexible education system can address students' needs and maximize their strengths and well-being (OECD, 2019b).

4.4.1 Core Foundations

With information technology, routine skills are no longer as essential as they were, and people who can exhibit complex, creative, strategic, analytical skills and high-level competencies are valued (Burbules et al., 2020). The world has shifted emphasis from the 3Rs (Reading, Writing, and Arithmetic) to the 4Cs (Critical thinking, Creativity, Communication, and Collaboration) (National Education Association, 2012). Core foundations are defined as the "core skills, knowledge, and attitudes and values that can prepare individuals for future learning in their lifespan" (p. 4). It builds the basis for developing student agency and transformative competencies that individuals need. There are three essential foundations in the framework: cognitive foundations, health foundations, and social and emotional foundations. More importantly, the core foundations propose more competencies for the 2030 world, such as financial literacy, global competence, and media literacy (OECD, 2019e).

4.4.1.1 Cognitive Foundations

Cognitive foundations include literacy and numeracy. Literacy can be understood as people's relationship with various information under different contexts (OECD, 2019e). For instance, people can understand verbal or non-verbal clues from others and make effective and meaningful conversations for diverse purposes. Numeracy is defined as "the ability to access, use, interpret, and communicate mathematical information and ideas to engage in and manage mathematical demands of a range of situations" (PIAAC Numeracy Expert Group, 2009, p. 6). With numeracy, people can apply mathematical tools for diverse objectives. Being able to read and write is far from enough to function effectively nowadays. Numeracy is quite essential in the era of digitalization when all sorts of data and digital clues are being bombarded (OECD, 2019e). Literacy and numeracy require individuals to utilize different types of information through all sorts of channels. Basic understandings of AI concepts, data and digital literacy, media literacy, financial literacy, cyber safety, and the ethics of utilization of AI are essential (Luckin & Issroff, 2018).

Data and Digital Literacy

Human interactions and communications have been transformed by digitalization. The labor market is reacting quickly to this new trend; more and more jobs are hiring employees who are competent in digital marketing and AI programming. Some traditional jobs are at stake (L. Yu et al., 2019, S. Yu et al., 2019). To fulfill one's full potential, one needs to develop data and digital literacy. Data and digital literacy refer to the ability to know "What data mean, including how to read charts appropriately, draw correct conclusions from data, and recognize when data are being used in misleading or inappropriate ways" (Carlson et al., 2011, p. 5). Data can be managed to be meaningful and beneficial for human beings. An increasing number of companies are applying digital technology to manage marketing, human resources, financing, and budgeting. Data and digital literacy have become one of the basic requirements of the labor market.

The digital products are transforming our daily lives enormously. For example, thousands of different types of apps on our mobile phones receive and analyze personal data. People utilize apps to get news and information all around the world. There is no need to read the newspaper the next day; breaking news pops up immediately on cell phones. Smart home products free people from tedious housework. Digital technology is making life more convenient and creating a new way of interpersonal communication. Nonetheless, the conveniences may show disadvantages in terms of privacy, safety, and poor mental and physical health (Malik et al., 2021). For example, online gaming and social media can affect adolescents' creativity and logical thinking. Moreover, big data comes from various platforms, such as searching history on web pages, chat history, or purchasing of products, which will increase concerns about personal privacy.

The population of digital users is increasing at an unprecedented pace. It is reported that 4.95 billion people (61.4% of the world population) are using social media in 2023, and there were only 2.07 billion users in 2015. Over 80.8% of users are aged over 18 years old (Dean, 2023). Moreover, every user may use an average of 6.7 social media platforms. Twitter has 353 million followers worldwide in 2023; 42% of Americans aged 12–34 are using Twitter; and 48% of Twitter users rely on Twitter to get the latest news. Users send out more than 500 million Tweets on a daily basis (Martin, 2023). Many people regard young people as "digital natives" (Prensky, 2001). Although young people nowadays have easy access to the Internet and smartphones, which are often known as conventional technologies, a deeper level of skills to adopt and apply technology should be cultivated among youngsters (Lee & Hidayat, 2019). With the advancement of digital technology, the digital divide has become more evident among different countries and regions, and it has become one of the most concerning social inequality issues nowadays (Hoffman et al., 2001). The digital divide cannot be diminished by merely acquiring access to technology (Bonfadelli, 2002).

As Jones and Flannigan (2006) stated, "Being void of digital or visual literacy is akin to being handicapped. And the problem is accelerated further in the field of education" (p. 4). A more extensive and more profound perspective on applying technology effectively and efficiently is needed (Hargittai, 2001). True digital literacy involves the use of technology effectively and efficiently to facilitate students to live with technology in their daily lives and apply technology to create new technologies (Huedo-Martínez et al., 2018). It is necessary to think about how to implement technology into education. For instance, technology can be meaningful when it is utilized to facilitate online learning, share information, and create an interactive learning environment. Concerning the above issues, adolescents need to develop data and digital literacy to know how to apply and implement technology to improve their well-being. They should be learners, providers, and sharers of resources in digital learning (Lee & Hidayat, 2019). Crucially, education curricula and teachers should prepare students to embrace a positive attitude toward technology and the challenges brought about by technological evolution. Equally important, the government should not only enhance the digital infrastructures but also offer appropriate education for people to develop their data and digital literacy.

Digital Financial Competence

Digital financial literacy is a critical competence in the era of digitalization. Cryptocurrency, for example, has become a hot investment among adolescents and young investors (Ryan, 2023). Cryptocurrency is an encrypted digital or virtual currency created by algorithms and monitored and organized by a blockchain (Micro, n.d.). There are over 20,000 types of cryptocurrencies in the market as of 2023, while over 9,000 types are active. Adolescents regard cryptocurrency as a payment tool, a value of freedom (Gagarina et al., 2019), a desire for financial autonomy, a criterion for their economic socialization, or merely choosing cryptocurrency for "competition" or "novelty" (Ramesh, 2012).

Nevertheless, adolescents are not fully aware of its risks and are vulnerable to cryptocurrency scams and a devastating loss due to cryptocurrency investment. It is reported that nearly 8% of teenagers aged 13–16 in the U.K. have invested in cryptocurrency, and 15% of them are planning to. Influencers and celebrities are promoting cryptocurrencies through all sorts of social media platforms (Matters, 2023). In 2021, members of the popular esports organization FaZe Clan promoted a new cryptocurrency named "Save the Kids" with the idea of building a bright future for kids. Millions of their fans, most of them young, were not knowledgeable about cryptocurrency and its risks in investing their money. The value of this cryptocurrency dropped 60% a few months later, resulting in a massive loss of money for the investors (Ramesh, 2012). Young people need to develop digital financial literacy, which enables them to evaluate the information available and conduct comprehensive analysis regarding the risks and returns of cyber currencies and their transactions.

Cyber Security Competence

Another crucial competence in the age of digitalization is cyber security competence. Global cyber connects the world in a new manner and brings about conveniences as well as risks of various cyber threats. Cyber security threats, like cyber addiction, online fraud, racial abuse, gaming, online gambling, cybersex, and personal information exposure, are alerting (Rahman et al., 2020). Developing cyber security competence not only applies to professionals but should also be regarded as a civic skill for youngsters (Lehto, 2015).

As such, cyber security education should be embedded in education curricula to equip adolescents with the competence to assess the threats of the cyber world. The government should also provide relevant resources to train young people in cyber security competence. In Germany, research in cybersecurity, as well as research centers in universities, is supported by the government. In Korea, the government and universities are cooperating in carrying out curricula that cover different technical aspects, including networks, new technologies, and cyber law. Moreover, new majors such as privacy, financial security, cybersecurity, and public security policy are implemented to facilitate competence-building and decision-making level training through professional training (Radunović & Rüfenacht, 2016). Aalto University in Finland provides a wide range of cyber security education and research, including risk analysis, modeling, and any related topics of cyber security in public administration and legislation. The Digital Agenda for Finlan 2011–2020 emphasized that IT skills, communication skills, media literacy, and social media application are fundamental skills in the era of digital services. ICT education has been included as an integral part of school education and in primary and supplementary training for teaching staff (Lehto, 2015).

Digital Media Literacy

The OECD highlights that digital media literacy is also essential, which is defined as "the ability to get, comprehend, evaluate, and generate content through digital media" (Penman & Turnbull, 2007, p. 1). Compared with traditional media, which is mainly used to receive information, digital media requires people to generate ideas and evaluate content. Therefore, creativity and critical thinking skills are involved in forming digital media literacy. Park (2012) emphasized that in the era of digitalization, information poverty is a crucial indicator of social exclusion.

It is worrying that AI technology can produce misinformation and disinformation quickly nowadays, such as realistic-looking images and videos, which increases the risks and challenges of sorting information (Metz, 2022). Moreover, hurtful biases and stereotypes can be strengthened by the open-ended nature of the AI system. All kinds of information are being spread all over the world at an unparalleled speed. Influencers and users are producing fake news to catch the attention of others (Britt & Rouet, 2020; Riesmeyer et al., 2019). Personal bloggers or Internet celebrities are selling or promoting products for their benefit.

The revolution of Information technology, AI, algorithms, and big data are transforming all walks of life nowadays. The unprecedented rate of data and information in the age of mass media is bringing about a big pool of opportunities but also creates challenges, ethical dilemmas, and risks for people. People need to learn how to evaluate the source of information and its reliability. Education in this technologically revolutionary world is not just about sitting in front of computers in the classroom or studying digital textbooks or devices. The OECD (2019l) highlighted that the complexity and speed of change call for schools, teachers, students, and society to equip themselves with competencies and connect education to react efficiently to the changes (Burbules et al., 2020). More importantly, combining knowledge creatively and efficiently and forming interdisciplinary thinking styles become as important as receiving proper education (Borgonovi & Pál, 2016).

4.4.1.2 Health Foundations

Good physical and mental health is another core foundation that students need, which is highly related to people's quality of life and the well-being of society (World Health Organization [WHO], 2018). Health literacy refers to individuals' knowledge and competence to understand factors that influence their health and know effective ways to address them. Healthy literate individuals will take active responsibility for their health and that of others (Sørensen et al., 2012). Health foundations are closely interlinked with cognitive, social, and emotional foundations. Individuals need cognitive foundations to learn, understand, and explore health-related information and knowledge to stay healthy. In order to improve physical and mental well-being, individuals need to apply their knowledge to make valid judgments in their daily lives, which, in return, strengthen their cognitive foundations. On the other hand, health also influences people's social and emotional foundations, which further affects students' willingness and opportunities to achieve academic development at school and their participation in the workplace and society (OECD, 2018d).

Apart from physical health, good mental health is one of the determining factors for adolescents to live productive and fulfilling lives (OECD, 2018b). Poor mental well-being of adolescents impairs physical and mental health. Shek and Leung (2013) identified several developmental issues of adolescents, such as substance abuse, addiction to the Internet, problematic sexual attitudes and behaviors, and school bullying and cyberbullying. WHO (2021) revealed that around 13% of young people are suffering from mental disorders and that suicide has become the fourth highest cause of death among adolescents. Moreover, depression, anxiety, and behavioral disorders are the most prevalent factors that affect the mental health of adolescents.

Effective school education has been widely identified as one of the most crucial factors in improving the well-being of students (McGill, 2016). Sun and Shek (2010) argued that students' well-being is related to their mental and physical health status and their experience in school. They urged schools to consider non-academic achievement, such as the level of students' well-being, as educational objectives. To improve the psychological well-being of adolescents, WHO (2021) proposed that schools and society promote Social-Emotional Learning (SEL) programs and provide adequate resources and support for adolescents to get mental health care. OECD (2018b) adopted the Mental Health Performance Framework to address mental illness and promote the psychological well-being of adolescents.

One topic concerning the physical and mental health of adolescents is sex education. WHO (2010) emphasized that informal and formal sexual education should be provided to young people in schools. It is reported that some adolescents get "sex education" from pornography. Rothman et al. (2021) surveyed U.S. teenagers aged 14–24 and found that around 25% of them regarded pornography as the most helpful source to get information regarding sex, other than from parents, schools, partners, or friends. Teenagers' early and unregulated exposure to pornography has deleterious effects on their sexual maturation, sexual behavior, and addiction to the Internet (Jones, 2018). They are more likely to engage in unhealthy, illegal, or extreme sexual activities, which are harmful to their mental and physical health. Moreover, there are legal consequences for sharing or downloading those materials, which could potentially be a criminal act (Martellozzo et al., 2016). In Japan, an average of 6000 girls are choosing to be actresses in the sex film industry annually, and most of them are young girls from ordinary families (Simonitch, 2012). It is worrying that most pornography does not convey healthy sex information to young adults.

Promoting multifaceted and healthy sex education in schools and colleges can prevent young people from developing the wrong concepts of sexuality (Adarsh & Sahoo, 2023). Rothman et al. (2018) suggested that implementing a pornography literacy curriculum in a non-school setting might have a positive impact on adolescents. Some European countries, such as the Netherlands and Sweden, require schools to provide school-based sex education to help students understand different aspects of sex. Around 76–93% of teenagers regard school as their primary source of information regarding sexuality, and only 0.2–3.4% of them regard pornography as their information guide (Ketting et al., 2018). In U.S. schools, sex education requirements in different states are different. Not all states require sex education in school. As a result, a more significant percentage of youth in the U.S. turn to seek information from other channels, such as pornography (Rothman et al., 2021). Therefore, formal sex education should be provided for students to help them get helpful information regarding sex or their perceptions of sex, which enhances their physical and mental well-being.

4.4.1.3 Social and Emotional Foundations

Social and emotional foundations, including emotional management, interpersonal communication, and relationship building with others, have a significant impact on adolescents' engagement with others and the environment (OECD, 2019e). Social and emotional skills may affect academic achievement at schools, future careers, performance in the workforce, and interpersonal and intrapersonal relationships (Kankaraš, 2017; Schoon et al., 2015). The definition of social-emotional skills is diversified, and some terms are used interchangeably, such as "21st-century competencies," "employability skills," "character strengths," "non-cognitive skills," "soft skills," "transformative skills," and "lifelong learning skills" (Jones & Doolittle, 2017).

In the recent survey of the National Association of Colleges and Employers (2023), the importance of communication (95.6%), critical thinking (94.4%), and teamwork (92.3%) are rated as the three leading career readiness competencies rated by the employers, which are more important than the quality of hard skills, technology (74%). The survey indicated that these soft skills are fundamental for graduates to enter the workforce. Nevertheless, employers responded that recent graduates lack proficiency in these competencies that only 46.9% of them possess communication skills, 55.9% show critical thinking competence, and 73.3% display proficiency in teamwork attributes. Another report conducted by the American Association of Colleges and Universities showed that the skills of liberal education are viewed as very important by employers, teamwork (93%), ethical judgment and reasoning (91%), interpersonal communication with people from diverse backgrounds (89%), communication skills (93%), and civic engagement (83%) (Finley, 2021). Shah et al. (2015) revealed that communication, teamwork, integrity, intellectual ability, and confidence are the most desired attributes of graduates from the perspective of employers. Apart from intellectual ability, the other four qualities belong to the dimension of social-emotional skills. Steponavičius et al. (2023) concluded that emotional intelligence and empathy are positively related to academic achievement, job performance, and quality of life. Moreover, social problem-solving skills are fundamental to health and prosocial behavior.

Malleability and plasticity of social-emotional traits are identified during adolescence, and youth are capable of learning and developing complex social-emotional skills (Kankaraš, 2017). There are many social-emotional competency frameworks for adolescents to learn social-emotional skills. Berg et al. (2017) identified 136 frameworks in their research. They found that one of the most popular frameworks is

Positive Youth Development, which includes the "Five Cs model: competence, confidence, connection, character, and caring," "Social-Emotional Learning (SEL): self-awareness, social awareness, self-management, relationship skills, and responsible decision-making," and "Developmental Assets model: internal assets and external assets." OECD (2018c) emphasized the "Big Five model: openness to experience, conscientiousness, emotional stability, extraversion, and agreeableness" to show how social and emotional skills should be organized. When analyzing transversal skills, Shek et al. (2023a, 2023b, 2023c, 2023d) made a comparison among six famous frameworks of transversal skills and concluded that social-emotional related skills are emphasized in many frameworks. For instance, collaboration and teamwork skills are mentioned by all six frameworks, communication is mentioned by five of them, empathy and sympathy are highlighted by five frameworks, and three frameworks emphasize the quality of self-awareness and self-control.

Nevertheless, the education of soft skills in a formal curriculum is far from enough for students' holistic development and future careers (Shek et al., 2021). Shek et al. (2023a, 2023b, 2023c, 2023d) proposed that an evolution of university education that integrates non-cognitive skills into formal university curricula is needed. For instance, universities should adopt student-centered approaches, such as implementing experiential learning pedagogies to develop soft skills. Moreover, Service-Learning (SL) courses enable students to learn and practice non-cognitive skills through providing services and reflecting on their experiences. Crosbie (2005) suggested that people can acquire soft skills by getting strategic and meaningful skill-building training programs that require active involvement and incorporate kinesthetic learning elements. Watson and Burr (2018) identified several transversal skills that are needed for medical training programs and initiated the redesign of curricula. Rosa et al. (2022) encouraged universities to integrate the elements of interpersonal skills, socioemotional competence, and citizen-oriented skills into their health and social care disciplines.

Specifically, universities in Hong Kong have made significant attempts to integrate the element of soft skills into their formal curriculum. For example, at The Hong Kong Polytechnic University (PolyU), experiential learning elements are embedded into their major courses. Students can learn knowledge in the classroom by participating in various forms of lectures, group projects, seminars, and workshops to practice their skills and consolidate their learning. Moreover, SL courses provided by different disciplines facilitate students' development of soft skills by providing multifaceted forms of services to needy communities. Additionally, elements of innovation, communication skills, and teamwork are increasingly emphasized in general education programs (e.g., Shek & Yu, 2016; Shek et al., 2015b; Shek et al., 2017a; Shek et al., 2017b).

In conclusion, integrating non-cognitive skills into formal university curricula can empower young people to explore their potential and thrive in future. Instead of focusing on "doing things right," education should focus on "doing the right things" and "everyone can be a leader" (Shek et al., 2023a, 2023b, 2023c, 2023d). More importantly, when biases, risks, and limitations take place, soft skills enable individuals to resolve conflict and tension, which also highlights the attributes of transferrable competencies (OECD, 2018a).

4.4.2 *Transformative Competencies*

The Learning Compass 2030 identifies three transformative competencies, including "creating new value," "reconciling tensions and dilemmas," and "taking responsibility" (OECD, 2019j). Transformative competencies inspire people to take adventures and try out new possibilities without hesitation (Grayling, 2017). Firstly, "creating new value" signifies the processes of making, formulating, innovating, and bringing about fresh and original ways of thinking, initiating positive worth, and shaping the future. This competence will be the milestone in bringing about changes in social, political, and cultural models (Dizikes, 2018), which is essential in the age of drastic changes and innovation. Specifically, the subdomains in this competency are "adaptability," "creativity," "curiosity," and "open-mindedness." To be ready for the challenges in the 2030 world, learners need to think creatively with a set of new products, ideas, services, jobs, methods, ways of thinking and living, business models, and social models. In education, creativity and novelty enable learners to pave the way to learning skills, understanding new concepts, trying different methods, experimenting with right and wrong, and solving problems. Therefore, grading and assessment may not be the only indicators of a good learner, and individuals need to take responsibility for their learning and be evaluators of themselves. Additionally, creating value also entails resilience, as people need to develop adaptability when trying different means to complete a task (Grayling, 2017).

The competence of "reconciling conflicts and dilemmas" is needed as young people are living in a world of growing complexity, interdependency, transition, and conflict. Mobility, connection, and communication take place at an unprecedented pace. People, ideas, services, and information are moving abound, and the complexity of information and networks brings about conflicts and dilemmas (Grayling, 2017). For instance, students may meet classmates from different cultural backgrounds, and they need to acquire information to solve cultural conflicts effectively. Additionally, people need to adhere to their moral standards in the face of complex and uncertain ethical dilemmas where opportunities and temptations conflict. Young people who value "reconciling conflicts and dilemmas" can develop an integrated way of thinking that leads to mature and concrete conclusions and value interconnections (OECD, 2018a). Specifically, the subdomains under this competence include "empathy," "communication and collaboration skills," "perspective-taking," "resilience," and "trust" (Bentley, 2017). The ability to navigate and solve conflicts effectively can determine an individual's well-being and success to a large extent. Thus, cognitive, pre-cognitive, meta-cognitive, and psychosocial skills are involved in developing this competence (Grayling, 2017).

Steinberg (2014) stressed that developing the quality of taking responsibility can be a critical factor in determining whether one is successful or not in future. The subdomains of "taking responsibility" include "critical thinking," "meta-learning," "mindfulness," "problem-solving," "risk management," and "self-regulation" (Grayling, 2017). "Taking responsibility" acts as a prerequisite of the above two transformative competencies. Creativity and novelty suggest that people can "think for themselves," and problem-solving ability also requires individuals to consider future consequences of their behaviors, assess uncertainties and benefits, and take personal responsibility for their actions and work. With this competency, people can reflect on their personal experiences and evaluate the values and moral and ethical standards in society. The crux of this competency is being able to regulate and take responsibility at personal, interpersonal, and societal levels (OECD, 2019j).

4.4.3 Knowledge, Skills, and Attitudes and Values

Students who want to create value and thrive in the 2030 world need to integrate knowledge, skills, attitudes, and values, which have evolved interdependently (OECD, 2019f).

4.4.3.1 Knowledge

Firstly, knowledge is a significant factor in the learning framework. In the theory of Powerful Knowledge, Young and Muller (2016) specified that the best knowledge human beings have is fallible and open to challenge. In the Compass, there are four categories of knowledge, namely, "disciplinary knowledge," "interdisciplinary knowledge," "epistemic knowledge," and "procedural knowledge" (OECD, 2019f).

Disciplinary knowledge, which is also referred to as subject-specific knowledge and contents with details, lays the foundation for understanding and developing other forms of intelligence (Gardner, 2011). A basic level of disciplinary knowledge enables students to specialize their knowledge further or create new areas of knowledge. Subject-specific concepts are changing with time as well. For example, AI is changing disciplinary knowledge; students need to learn different forms of knowledge and concepts related to AI, such as data literacy, online safety, and basic AI programming.

By acquiring interdisciplinary knowledge, people can identify similarities and differences between different concepts and knowledge, and integrate and create new understanding. In return, it integrates interdisciplinary knowledge into curricula and supports project-based learning. Transferring key concepts deepens learning and enables an effective transfer of knowledge and skills. The framework presents five ways in curricula design to enable students to receive interdisciplinary knowledge, including "transferring key concepts," "identifying interconnectedness," "thematic learning," "combining related subjects or creating new subjects," and "project-based learning" (OECD, 2019f).

Epistemic knowledge requires students to explore the process of thinking and take action attentively, which enhances people's experience as learners and active thinkers. Students explore the interest and purpose of learning and know how to apply knowledge to go beyond and deepen their understanding. Epistemic knowledge enables students to apply their disciplinary knowledge effectively and achieve future outcomes, which ultimately enhances their well-being. Young and Muller (2016) suggested that faculties integrate various domains of knowledge and pedagogies in their curriculum to develop students' critical thinking, problem-solving, and learning-to-learn competence. For example, apart from merely teaching engineering students to solve technical problems, schools also need to inspire students to reflect on what kind of challenges they are facing.

Lastly, procedural knowledge enables students to figure out the procedure of a task and reflect on the processes, which is beneficial for students to tackle problems and issues effectively (OECD, 2019f). Benander (2018) emphasized that transferring disciplinary knowledge and procedural knowledge helps students explore ill-defined systems in their daily lives. Procedural knowledge can be related to a specific domain or interrelated to different disciplines. Systematic thinking and design thinking are always involved in procedural knowledge, which can enable students to form thought patterns and structured processes to solve problems and investigate whether it is socially or culturally appropriate to have this solution (Pourdehnad et al., 2011). Students with system thinking could explore how the system is organized (Mobus, 2018). In another sense, design thinking involves tackling comprehensive problems. Kelley et al. (2015) revealed that systems thinking and design thinking programs enable students to explore various ways to solve unfamiliar and tricky problems. Benander (2018) stated that students with design thinking have a holistic understanding of the problem, but they also focus on some specific areas.

Notably, the four categories of knowledge intertwine with each other and enable students to enhance their learning and make changes in their daily lives. Suitable training and resources are helpful for students to form a more profound understanding by connecting both disciplinary and procedural knowledge. Moreover, they should be connected to skills, attitudes, and the ability to facilitate the process of knowledge transfer.

4.4.3.2 Skills

It is unrealistic to talk about knowledge and skills separately as they are connected and grow together (OECD, 2019h). Klieme (2004) noted that "the increasing proceduralization of knowledge characterizes higher competency levels, so, at higher levels, knowledge is converted to skills" (p. 70). Scott (2015) emphasized that learning to know is an essential requirement as a learner, while learning to do (problem-solving, critical thinking, and collaboration), learning to be (psychosocial skills, taking personal responsibility, and self-management), and learning to live together (teamwork, citizenship, and global and cultural competence) are equally important.

Although the demand for routine work has declined drastically due to technological advancement, there are more job opportunities for people with interpersonal skills, creativity, and cognitive skills (Bialik & Fadel, 2018). Being able to "come up with new ideas and plans" and have the "willingness to challenge different views" distinguish people from others (OECD, 2019h). Berger and Frey (2016) pointed out that new jobs, such as robotics engineers, statisticians, and video game designers, are emerging. They emphasized that "fusion skills" such as creativity, entrepreneurship, and technical skills are needed for individuals to be competent in the job market. Students need to develop new skills to increase their competitiveness in the labor market and adopt positive attitudes and a strong commitment to lifelong learning.

Three types of skills are stressed in the framework (OECD, 2019h). Firstly, cognitive skills and meta-cognitive skills are the thinking strategies that one can apply, such as verbal, non-verbal, higher-order thinking, executive functioning, problem-solving, learning to learn, and self-management. Meta-cognitive skills denote the capacity to identify one's knowledge, skills, attitudes, and values. Second, social and emotional skills show one's ability to display thoughts, feelings, and behaviors consistently. For instance, students with empathy, self-awareness, and effective communication can respond to problems effectively, ethnically, and culturally. Individuals with self-efficacy, a sense of responsibility, curiosity, and emotional stability may have a higher chance of achieving better performance both at school and at work. Berger and Frey (2016) stated that AI cannot take up jobs that need complex interpersonal communications. For example, people who work as helping professionals should do complex assessments and provide tangible and emotional support to the clients and their family members. Empathy and empowerment are needed, while AI is not good at empowering clients through verbal and non-verbal communication.

Finally, physical and practical skills include manual skills, life skills, professional skills, and mobilization skills. The skills needed to thrive in this digital world have been changed drastically, and the ability to utilize information and AI tools is also included. Besides, art skills are also emphasized, which enhances students' empathy, emotional engagement, commitment, and persistence (OECD, 2019h). Foundational skills are the skills to know "how," including reading and writing, numbering, translating, and exchanging information and data. The ability to be creative, take responsibility, and learn to learn are emphasized. To remain competitive, individuals need to learn new skills, be flexible, and develop lifelong learning commitments.

There are several prerequisites for individuals to transfer knowledge and skills from one context to another successfully. Abuzour et al. (2018) found that students should possess appropriate basic knowledge and get guidelines from others. Moreover, reinforcement can motivate students to apply their skills to new environments. Playing or project-based learning is identified as effective in facilitating the transferability of knowledge and skills (Lee & Tsai, 2004).

4.4.3.3 Attitudes and Values

Attitudes and values will act as mediators in the usage of knowledge and skills (OECD, 2018a). Eagly and Chaiken (1993) defined attitudes as "a psychological tendency that is expressed by evaluating a particular entity with some degree of favor or disfavor" (p. 1). Attitudes can change according to specific circumstances, which are more flexible and moldable than individual values, traits, or characteristics (Haste, 2018). Halstead and Taylor (2000) defined values as "guiding principles by which particular beliefs, behaviors, and actions are judged to be suitable or desirable" (p. 1). Young people are guided by their values to take action, make judgments, evaluate their experiences, and define their belief systems. Both attitudes and values are influenced by personal, local, community, societal, and global domains. Young people need to strike a balance between tensions and conflicts, recognize universal values and norms, and acknowledge personal diversity (OECD, 2019d).

There are four types of values in the framework: personal, social, societal, and human values. Firstly, personal values show how a person defines life and how to achieve one's aspirations. Social values are the principles and rules that are closely related to interpersonal relationships. Societal values are principles or beliefs that are shared by societies or cultures. Sometimes, social structures, policies, and democratic practices are influenced by societal values. Human values share some commonality with societal values, but they are not constrained to specific cultures or communities, which defines the well-being of humankind.

Many countries have incorporated the elements of values into their curriculum. For example, in Singapore, a subject titled "Character and Citizenship Education" is included in its twenty-first century competencies framework to nurture students' qualities of social responsibility, civic engagement, resilience, moral competence, and empathy. In the age of globalization and technological advances, students can be more self-directed learners and responsible citizens in future. In China, a holistic approach, the "trinity" model, is adopted in the curriculum. It emphasizes "Five Ways of Life (DE—'Moral,' Zhi—'Wisdom,' Ti—'Body,' Qun—'Collectivity,' and Mei—'Aesthetics')" (OECD, 2019a, p. 111). Moreover, Chinese cultures also emphasize collective values as individuals live in society and interact with the collective group. Additionally, the understanding of aesthetics is also beneficial for the heritage of human cultures. Therefore, cultivating positive attitudes and values can be achieved by education (OECD, 2018a).

4.4.4 Student Agency

Young people who are ready to react to challenges and opportunities in future world can be effective change agents. Student agency refers to the ability to establish a goal, reflect actively on one's actions, and take responsible actions to bring about changes. It is developed on the belief that students will actively shape the world instead of being shaped (OECD, 2019i). In this sense, developing student agency is a learning goal. Equally important, student agency can be a learning process (Schoon, 2018). In the decision-making process, the students will develop a higher level of determination and willingness to learn and explore the meaning of their learning. The agency enables students to tackle challenges and obstacles effectively. Students' affective, cognitive, and behavioral development are crucial and meaningful. The development of agency is a continuous process, and it evolves over students' life span, which highlights the value of lifelong learning in developing agency (OECD, 2019i).

Graduating from university does not mean the end of the learning journey. Instead, learning comes from all types of interactions and experiences outside school, anytime and anywhere. Traditional education is mainly institution-driven. However, lifelong learning represents individualized learning where personal needs, interests, and aspirations are taken into account (Dabbagh & Castaneda, 2020). In this regard, the commitment to lifelong learning enables learners to follow their learning path by taking a more open and flexible learning approach. Developing agency is one of the objectives of education and a critical element in the learning process. Su (2011) argued that with a higher sense of autonomy and responsibility, the agency acts as an internal drive for the achievement of lifelong learning throughout one's life span. Students should be recognized as lifelong learners and treated as human beings instead of "knowing beings" (Barnett, 2005). Learners are capable of creating their own learning experiences and searching for meaning in life.

Agency does not mean a personality trait; it can be learned, acquired, and shaped. The development of agency is influenced by many factors, such as the family background, the education level of the parents, and whether the family is financially well off (Brooks-Gunn & Duncan, 1997). Davis-Kean (2005) revealed that when the family plays a responsible and positive role in engaging with school, the student will display a positive development in terms of academic performance. Students from disadvantaged families or communities will encounter more difficulty in achieving their agency, and parents will be less likely to provide an effective learning environment for their children. Children from well-off households have more resources to get quality education and access to achieve their goals (Schoon, 2018). Nevertheless, children from disadvantaged families or backgrounds need additional assistance in building foundation skills, psychosocial skills, writing, reading, or speaking skills to develop agency and realize their potential (Talreja, 2017).

Another critical element is the community. When a community is actively involved in sharing the responsibility of children's education, the children have more opportunities to realize their potential, be responsible citizens, and contribute to shaping the future. In return, the community may develop a concrete view of the needs and concerns of the young people (OECD, 2019i). Young people should practice agency in school, communities, or society. They should be involved in society actively and exert positive influence on others, the community, and society to achieve their personal goals (OECD, 2018a). In this way, they could not only acquire the knowledge and skills needed, but they could utilize internal resources to meet complex social needs.

The above discussion denotes the concept of co-agency, which emphasizes the collaborative, interactive, mutually beneficial, and supportive relationships between students, teachers, parents, and communities (OECD, 2019i). The process of interaction with peers, teachers, and families continues and develops throughout one's life (Schoon, 2018). To enable co-agency for young people, an individualized learning environment is needed to support their learning, nurture their passions, motivate them to learn from different practices, and inspire them to develop their aspirations (OECD, 2018a). Equally important, not only are the students the stakeholders of education goals, but teachers, parents, and the community also share the education goals (Salmela-Aro, 2009). For instance, to be effective co-agents, teachers need to make efforts to develop their professional growth, students' growth, and colleagues' growth (Calvert, 2016). Moreover, additional support and resources, such as professional training and education, are needed to create an effective learning environment for students to realize their potential. Therefore, every individual is a learner and stakeholder in the learning compass.

Notably, the agency is essential in all aspects of life: moral, social, economic, and creativity. For instance, moral agency helps students distinguish right from wrong, make ethical decisions, and consider the rights of others. Social agency enables students to interact with others with social competence. Students can achieve long-term goals (Leadbeater, 2017). Nevertheless, it does not mean that there are no limits or boundaries for students to practice their agency; students need to respect social norms instead of merely doing things along with their self-interest and wishes (OECD, 2019i). A well-developed sense of agency is related to the identity and sense of belonging of students. To develop a sense of citizenship, young people should pursue social justice, shoulder social responsibility, and make active contributions to society and the community. Motivation, aspiration, self-assurance, and the desire and belief that abilities can be developed motivate adolescents to pursue the fullness of life (Leadbeater, 2017). Notably, learning to be capable learners with agency and developing learning-to-learn skills have lifelong benefits for students and society (OECD, 2019i).

4.4.5 Anticipation-Action-Reflection (AAR) Cycle

The Anticipation-Action-Reflection (AAR) cycle refers to an interactive learning process in which learners continuously plan, experience, and reflect on their thoughts and behaviors and make continuous efforts to improve their thinking and actions (OECD, 2019c). The AAR cycle usually takes place when the individual interacts with others or the community (Vygotsky & Cole, 1978). Through this cycle, learners could explore a deeper level of understanding and thinking and broaden their worldview, which benefits the well-being of individuals and society. There are three phases: anticipation, action, and reflection, which inform, complement, and enhance each other. It can build the future of learners and contribute to the well-being of society.

Individuals can carry out the AAR process in their daily lives as part of their daily and social routines, which can enhance their lifelong learning process (OECD, 2019c).

In the anticipation phase, learners can forecast the results of behaviors in the short and long run. They can have a clear understanding of their motives and those of others. Instead of simply asking questions, individuals should foresee the results and impact of one specific action (OECD, 2019c). Anticipation means that an individual can pre-experience the future through the process of prospection, which can connect themselves firmly to their future selves (Gilbert & Wilson, 2007). In this way, individuals can be motivated to carry out actions that will contribute to their well-being in future (Prabhakar et al., 2016). Students can apply the ability of anticipation to recognize problems, consider a variety of outcomes, resolve conflicts and dilemmas, and perceive the direct and durable consequences of one's actions. More importantly, individuals can determine a goal and recognize what kind of actions should be carried out (OECD, 2019c).

In the action phase, learners take responsible actions to achieve specific objectives and enhance their well-being. Actions can lead to positive or negative outcomes for individuals, the community, and the whole world; it is necessary to take intentional and responsible actions. Therefore, anticipation should be placed before action takes place, and reflection should be followed after action (OECD, 2019c). Learners set goals and objectives for specific actions. Action links the knowledge of one individual to what they want to achieve (Leadbeater, 2017). Jensen and Schnack (1997) emphasized that actions can be goal-oriented, responsibility-oriented, or change-initiated. In this regard, individuals should take responsible actions to create new perspectives, solve conflicts, and improve the well-being of individuals and society.

Reflection is a systematic, structured, and disciplined way of thinking. Dewey (1994) defined reflection as "the meaning-making process that moves a learner from one experience into the next with a deeper understanding of its relationships with and connections to other experiences and ideas" (p. 21). Learners should recognize the perspectives of individuals and others, therefore combining comprehensive thinking into their actions. In this way, they can develop their understanding to a deeper level and improve their competence to carry out behaviors that are consistent with mutual values and intentions. Additionally, individuals can adapt to changing environments and take action effectively in future, which may bring about the positive development of the individual agency. Canto-Sperber and Dupuy (2001) proposed that self-oriented skills and creative thinking should be utilized in the reflection process, and transformative competencies can be cultivated and strengthened through reflection.

Crucially, different competencies are required in the AAR cycle: proactive, perspective-taking, critical thinking, and reflective thinking (Rolheiser et al., 2000). Anticipation, action, and reflection are intertwined with each other, and they reinforce each other. Firstly, anticipation leads the learner to take informed actions, and taking actions without anticipation results in unclear consequences. Equally important, anticipation without action increases uncertainties about the future. Therefore, goal setting and prospection can actively link these two phases. Moreover, reflection-on-action shows that individuals actively reflect while carrying out some behaviors (Schön, 2017).

In the learning compass, the AAR cycle is interdependent on other concepts, and they develop together (OECD, 2019c). Firstly, learners can develop a sense of responsibility as they feel empowered to recognize the challenges and solve them, which strengthens the belief that they can bring about positive changes in society. In this way, learners can express and develop their agency in diverse situations and even gain lifelong benefits (OECD, 2019c). Besides, transformative competencies require individuals to be adaptive and reflective and take effective actions. Additionally, taking responsibility requires individuals to foresee the impact of their actions and take different perspectives from stakeholders and others, which is related to anticipation and reflection in the AAR cycle. Moreover, reconciling conflicts means individuals are able to explore appropriate solutions to make changes. Lastly, creating new values facilitates learners' carrying out actions that are beneficial to the well-being of others and society, which also requires individuals to take different perspectives and carry out innovative actions. Therefore, the AAR cycle enables the development of both transformative competencies and individual agency.

4.5 Cultivation of Soft Skills in Higher Education

In Chaps. 2 and 3, we reviewed the institutional learning outcomes and desired graduate attributes in universities in different parts of the world, including Hong Kong. Our observation is that the coverage of soft skills or psychosocial competencies in the formal curriculum varies among universities. Besides, some essential skills such as resilience, empathy, and purpose highlighted in the OECD framework are not strongly emphasized in many universities.

Besides, although it is universally recognized that soft skills are essential for enriching personal development, employability, and social engagement, it is hard to utilize the single best approach to teach soft skills in the classroom. Teachers in universities feel that it is challenging to teach soft skills in formal classrooms (Adams, 2014). Kechagias (2011) analyzed and presented several issues in teaching and developing soft skills that contribute to the difficulty. One issue is that soft skills are not universally defined and implemented. For instance, the skill of critical thinking is always regarded as a desired attribute of students. However, different disciplines have their own focus on teaching and implementing the skills. Humanities students are trained to evaluate the problem instead of solving it, while management students are trained with case studies to solve the problem with critical thinking in practice. Therefore, there is confusion about the undefined skills and approaches among the disciplines. Additionally, there is discussion regarding the generalists and specificists of teaching and development of soft skills. The generalist approach suggested that soft skills are generic, which can be taught independently and can be applied universally. In contrast, specificists proposed that soft skills cannot be taught independently from their professional knowledge and thus should be learned contextually (Moore, 2004).

Kechagias (2011) noted that teaching and assessing soft skills is more challenging than hard skills. He also highlighted that social-emotional learning programs are effective. Vogler et al. (2018) proposed that case studies or project-based learning are involved in the teaching of soft skills. Other studies also showed that project-based learning experiences have a positive impact on the development of soft skills and employability after graduation (e.g., Jollands et al., 2012; Lima et al., 2007). Eyler et al. (2001) viewed SL as an effective tool in cultivating the soft skills of students. Shek et al. (2023a, 2023b, 2023c, 2023d) proposed that curricula reform, teacher training, and policy changes are needed. Ngai and Shek (2022) proposed that "teamwork and effective communication belong to the social and emotional domain of soft skills" and "applying knowledge to deal with real-life complex issues and problem-solving skills are cognitive and meta-cognitive skills" (p. 83), which is in line with the soft skills recommended by OECD (2019a). Besides, studies have shown that soft skills and non-cognitive skills are important resources for young people to cope with changing social circumstances such as political turbulences and pandemic (Shek, 2020, 2021; Shek et al., 2022, 2023a, 2023b, 2023c).

Specifically, in Hong Kong, reform in higher education has brought about more changes in the curricula. Universities are putting more resources and focus on general education, and there is an increase in the subjects aiming at training leadership qualities and enhancing students' mental health. Additionally, SL subjects are gaining more popularity. Hong Kong Education Commission (2000) initiated educational reform to promote lifelong learning and the holistic development of university students. Apart from equipping students with professional knowledge and skills, university education should provide more resources and platforms for students to gain knowledge beyond their professions. Equally important, university students should develop a sense of "integrity, positive attitude, a broad vision, and important generic skill" (p. 9). To enrich students' learning experiences and holistic development, PolyU proposes six major desired attributes for graduates, including "professional competence, critical thinking, effective communication, problem-solving, lifelong learning, and ethical leadership" (Shek et al., 2015a, 2015b), which are in line with the agenda of the Learning Compass 2030. For instance, general education courses, especially the SL subjects, are implemented in the undergraduate curriculum as compulsory courses to promote intrapersonal and interpersonal competencies, ethical leadership, and lifelong learning commitment of university students (Shek & Chak, 2019). In the following few chapters, we will present four credit-bearing subjects responding to the emphases highlighted in the OECD 2030 model.

4.6 Conclusion

The OECD Learning Compass 2030 framework exhibits a comprehensive and systematic approach to education and curriculum redesign, which facilitates learners to respond to challenges and opportunities in the new era. This chapter first introduces the background of the OECD and the need for an education revolution. Then, this chapter delves into the Future of Education and Skills 2030 project and the Learning Compass 2030 framework. There are essential concepts in the learning compass. Not only cognitive development but also twenty-first century skills can prepare individuals to thrive and contribute to the well-being of society. The rapid advancement of information technology requires an education revolution, and the way students learn has been significantly reshaped. Hence, this chapter explores the changes and their implications for future education. Students in the twenty-first century are expected to develop both technical and soft skills. The OECD Learning Compass 2030 emphasizes the ability of lifelong learning and student agency, which help students achieve holistic development and thrive in future. With the guidance of the Learning Compass and the framework, educators can integrate this framework into their curriculum to cultivate students' knowledge, competence, skills, and values that are needed to navigate the complexities in future world effectively and successfully. In the following few chapters, we will present four credit-bearing subjects responding to the emphases of the OECD Learning Compass 2030.

Acknowledgements The preparation of this chapter is financially supported by The Hong Kong Polytechnic University (ZZ4U and ZZUE), Li and Fung Endowed Professorship in Service Leadership Education, Wofoo Foundation, and the Matching Fund of Research Grants Council (ZECL and ZH4Q).

References

Abuzour, A. S., Lewis, P. J., & Tully, M. P. (2018). Practice makes perfect: A systematic review of the expertise development of pharmacist and nurse independent prescribers in the United Kingdom. *Research in Social and Administrative Pharmacy, 14*(1), 6–17. https://doi.org/10.1016/j.sapharm.2017.02.002

Adams, S. (2014, November 12). The 10 skills employers most want in 2015 graduates. *Forbes.* https://www.forbes.com/sites/susanadams/2014/11/12/the-10-skills-employers-most-want-in-2015-graduates/?sh=351e885c2511

Adarsh, H., & Sahoo, S. (2023). Pornography and its impact on adolescent/teenage sexuality. *Journal of Psychosexual Health, 5*(1), 35–39. https://doi.org/10.1177/26318318231153984

Barnett, R. (2005). Recapturing the universal in the university. *Educational Philosophy and Theory, 37*(6), 785–797. https://doi.org/10.1111/j.1469-5812.2005.00158.x

Benander, R. (2018). *A literature summary for research on the transfer of learning.* OECD Publishing. https://www.oecd.org/education/2030-project/about/documents/A-Literature-Summary-for-Research-on-the-Transfer-of-Learning.pdf

Bentley, T. (2017). *Brief comments on "creating new value" and "taking responsibility" section of education 2030-Conceptual learning framework: Background papers.* https://www.oecd.org/education/2030-project/contact/Conceptual_learning_framework_Conceptual_papers.pdf

Berg, J., Osher, D., Same, M. R., Nolan, E., Benson, D., & Jacobs, N. (2017). Identifying, defining, and measuring social and emotional competencies. *American Institutes for Research.* https://www.air.org/sites/default/files/downloads/report/Identifying-Defining-and-Measuring-Social-and-Emotional-Competencies-December-2017-rev.pdf

Berger, T., & Frey, C. B. (2016). *Structural transformation in the OECD: Digitalisation, deindustrialisation and the future of work.* OECD Publishing. https://doi.org/10.1787/5jlr068802f7-en

Bialik, M., & Fadel, C. (2018). Knowledge for the age of artificial intelligence: What should students learn? *Center for Curriculum Redesign*. https://curriculumredesign.org/wp-content/uploads/CCR_Knowledge_FINAL_January_2018.pdf

Bonfadelli, H. (2002). The Internet and knowledge gaps: A theoretical and empirical investigation. *European Journal of Communication, 17*(1), 65–84. https://doi.org/10.1177/026732310201700 1607

Borgonovi, F., & Pál, J. (2016). A framework for the analysis of student well-being in the PISA 2015 study: Being 15 in 2015. *OECD Education Working Papers*. https://doi.org/10.1787/199 39019

Britt, M. A., & Rouet, J. (2020). Multiple document comprehension. *Oxford Research Encyclopedia of Education*. https://doi.org/10.1093/acrefore/9780190264093.013.867

Brooks-Gunn, J., & Duncan, G. J. (1997). The effects of poverty on children. *The Future of Children, 7*(2), 55–71. https://doi.org/10.2307/1602387

Burbules, N. C., Fan, G., & Repp, P. (2020). Five trends of education and technology in a sustainable future. *Geography and Sustainability, 1*(2), 93–97. https://doi.org/10.1016/j.geosus.2020.05.001

Calvert, L. (2016). Moving from compliance to agency: What teachers need to make professional learning work. *Learning Forward and NCTAF*. https://learningforward.org/wp-content/uploads/2017/08/moving-from-compliance-to-agency.pdf

Canto-Sperber, M., & Dupuy, J.-P. (2001). Competencies for the good life and the good society. In D. S. Rychen, & L. H. Salganik (Eds.), *Defining and selecting key competencies* (pp. 67–92). Hogrefe & Huber. https://www.deseco.ch/bfs/deseco/en/index/02.parsys.69356.downloadList.26477.DownloadFile.tmp/2000.desecocontrib.inesg.a.pdf

Care, E. (2017). Global initiative around assessment of 21st century skills. *UNESCO*. Retrieved February 24, 2024, from https://www.unesco.org/en/articles/global-initiative-around-assess ment-21st-century-skills

Carlson, J., Fosmire, M., Miller, C., & Nelson, M. S. (2011). Determining data information literacy needs: A study of students and research faculty. *Johns Hopkins University Press, 11*(2), 629–657. https://doi.org/10.1353/pla.2011.0022

Crosbie, R. (2005). Learning the soft skills of leadership. *Industrial and Commercial Training, 37*(1), 45–51. https://doi.org/10.1108/00197850510576484

Dabbagh, N., & Castaneda, L. (2020). The PLE as a framework for developing agency in lifelong learning. *Educational Technology Research and Development, 68*, 3041–3055. https://doi.org/10.1007/s11423-020-09831-z

Davis-Kean, P. E. (2005). The influence of parent education and family income on child achievement: The indirect role of parental expectations and the home environment. *Journal of Family Psychology, 19*(2), 294–304. https://doi.org/10.1037/0893-3200.19.2.294

Dean, B. (2023, December 19). Social network usage & growth statistics: How many people use social media in 2024? *Back Linko*. https://backlinko.com/social-media-users

Dewey, J. (1994). How we think: A restatement of the relation of reflective thinking to the educative process. A seminar on critical thinking, Petaling Jaya.

Dizikes, P. (2018, October 2). Thomas Friedman examines impact of global "accelerations". *MIT News*. https://news.mit.edu/2018/thomas-friedman-impact-global-accelerations-1003

Dobryakova, M., Froumin, I., Barannikov, K., Moss, G., Remorenko, I., & Hautamäki, J. (2023). *Key competences and new literacies: From slogans to school reality*. Springer Cham. https://doi.org/10.1007/978-3-031-23281-7

Eagly, A. H., & Chaiken, S. (1993). *The psychology of attitudes*. Harcourt Brace Jovanovich College Publishers.

Eyler, J., Giles Jr, D. E., Stenson, C. M., & Gray, C. J. (2001). At a glance: What we know about the effects of service-learning on college students, faculty, institutions and communities, 1993–2000. *Higher Education*. https://digitalcommons.unomaha.edu/slcehighered/139

Finley, A. (2021). How college contributes to workforce success. Employer views on what matters most. *American Association of Colleges and Universities*. https://dgmg81phhvh63.cloudfront.net/content/user-photos/Research/PDFs/AACUEmployerReport2021.pdf

Gagarina, M., Nestik, T., & Drobysheva, T. (2019). Social and psychological predictors of youths' attitudes to cryptocurrency. *Behavioral Sciences, 9*(12), 118. https://doi.org/10.3390/bs9120118

Gardner, H. (2011). Five minds for the future: An overview. *Journal of Educational Sciences and Psychology, 1*(2), 1–11. https://proquest.com/openview/008e2e384bfcba98ae9bccc4910d205c/1?pq-origsite=gscholar&cbl=786381

Gilbert, D. T., & Wilson, T. D. (2007). Prospection: Experiencing the future. *Science, 317*(5843), 1351–1354. https://doi.org/10.1126/science.1144161

Grayling, A. (2017). *"Creating New Value" section of Future and Education and Skills 2030: Reflections on transformative competencies 2030*. OECD Publishing. https://www.oecd.org/education/2030-project/contact/EDU-EDPC(2017)16-ANN5.pdf

Halstead, J. M., & Taylor, M. J. (2000). Learning and teaching about values: A review of recent research. *Cambridge Journal of Education, 30*(2), 169–202. https://doi.org/10.1080/713657146

Hargittai, E. (2001). Second-level digital divide: Mapping differences in people's online skills. *First Monday*. https://doi.org/10.48550/arXiv.cs/0109068

Haste, H. (2018). Attitudes and values and the OECD learning framework 2030: A critical review of definitions, concepts and data. *OECD Publishing, 20*, 30. https://www.oecd.org/education/2030-project/contact/Draft_Papers_supporting_the_OECD_Learning_Framework_2030.pdf

Hoffman, D. L., Novak, T. P., & Schlosser, A. E. (2001). The evolution of the digital divide: Examining the relationship of race to Internet access and usage over time. In B. M. Compaine (Ed.), *The digital divide: Facing a crisis or creating a myth* (pp. 47–98). The MIT Press.

Hong Kong Education Commission. (2000). *Learning for life, learning through life: Reform proposals for the education system in Hong Kong. Education blueprint for the 21st century*. Hong Kong. https://www.e-c.edu.hk/doc/en/publications_and_related_documents/education_reform/Edu-reform-eng.pdf

Huedo-Martínez, S., Molina-Carmona, R., & Llorens-Largo, F. (2018). Study on the attitude of young people towards technology. In P. Zaphiris, & A. Ioannou (Eds.), *Learning and collaboration technologies. Learning and teaching. LCT 2018. Lecture notes in computer science* (Vol. 10925, pp. 26–43). Springer. https://doi.org/10.1007/978-3-319-91152-6_3

Jensen, B. B., & Schnack, K. (1997). The action competence approach in environmental education. *Environmental Education Research, 3*(2), 163–178. https://doi.org/10.1080/1350462970030205

Jollands, M., Jolly, L., & Molyneaux, T. (2012). Project-based learning as a contributing factor to graduates' work readiness. *European Journal of Engineering Education, 37*(2), 143–154. https://doi.org/10.1080/03043797.2012.665848

Jones, B., & Flannigan, S. L. (2006). Connecting the digital dots: Literacy of the 21st century. *Educause Quarterly, 29*(2), 8–10. https://citeseerx.ist.psu.edu/document?repid=rep1&type=pdf&doi=c2fbd52466a35cd62d1476a9840e5064e88118c4

Jones, M. (2018, February 7). What teenagers are learning from online porn. *The New York Times*. https://www.nytimes.com/2018/02/07/magazine/teenagers-learning-online-porn-literacy-sex-education.html

Jones, S. M., & Doolittle, E. J. (2017). Social and emotional learning: Introducing the issue. *The Future of Children, 27*(1), 3–11. https://www.jstor.org/stable/44219018

Kankaraš, M. (2017). Personality matters: Relevance and assessment of personality characteristics. *OECD Publishing*. https://doi.org/10.1787/8a294376-en

Kechagias, K. (2011). *Teaching and assessing soft skills*. Second Chance School of Thessaloniki. https://web.archive.org/web/20150807162639/http://mass.educational-innovation.org/attachments/396_MASS%20wp4%20final%20report%20part-1.pdf

Kelley, T. R., Capobianco, B. M., & Kaluf, K. J. (2015). Concurrent think-aloud protocols to assess elementary design students. *International Journal of Technology and Design Education, 25*, 521–540. https://doi.org/10.1007/s10798-014-9291-y

Ketting, E., Brockschmidt, L., Renner, I., Luyckfasseel, L., & Ivanova, O. (2018). Sexuality education in Europe and Central Asia: Recent developments and current status. In R. A. Benavides-Torres, D. J. Onofre-Rodriguez, M. A. Marquez-Vega, & R. d. C. Barbosa-Martinez (Eds.), *Sex*

education. Global perspectives, effective programs and socio-cultural challenges (pp. 75–120). Nova Science Publishers.
Klieme, E. (2004). Assessment of cross-curricular problem-solving competencies. In J. Moskowitz, & M. Stephens (Eds.), *Comparing learning outcomes. International assessments and education policy* (pp. 81–107). Routledge.
Leadbeater, C. (2017). *"Student Agency" section of Education 2030—Conceptual learning framework: Background papers.* OECD Publishing. http://www.oecd.org/education/2030-project/contact/Conceptual_learning_framework_Conceptual_papers.pdf
Lee, C. I., & Tsai, F. Y. (2004). Internet project-based learning environment: The effects of thinking styles on learning transfer. *Journal of Computer Assisted Learning, 20*(1), 31–39. https://doi.org/10.1111/j.1365-2729.2004.00063.x
Lee, J. Y., & Hidayat, D. N. (2019). Digital technology for Indonesia's young people: The significance of SNS use and digital literacy for learning. *MedienPädagogik: Zeitschrift für Theorie und Praxis der Medienbildung, 35*, 20–35. https://doi.org/10.21240/mpaed/35/2019.10.17.X
Lehto, M. (2015). Cyber security competencies: Cyber security education and research in Finnish universities. In N. Abouzakhar (Ed.), *ECCWS2015-Proceedings of the 14th European conference on cyber warfare & security: ECCWS* (Vol. 2015, pp. 179–188). Academic Conferences and Publishing International Limited. https://jyx.jyu.fi/bitstream/handle/123456789/46540/lehtoeccws2015.pdf?sequence=1
Lima, R. M., Carvalho, D., Assunção Flores, M., & Van Hattum-Janssen, N. (2007). A case study on project led education in engineering: Students' and teachers' perceptions. *European Journal of Engineering Education, 32*(3), 337–347. https://doi.org/10.1080/03043790701278599
Luckin, R., & Issroff, K. (2018). Education and AI: Preparing for the future & AI, attitudes and values. In *8th Informal Working Group (IWG) Meeting.* https://www.oecd.org/education/2030/Education-and-AI-preparing-for-the-future-AI-Attitudes-and-Values.pdf
Malik, S., Bansal, R., & Tyagi, A. K. (2021). *Impact and role of digital technologies in adolescent lives.* IGI Global.
Marope, M., Griffin, P., & Gallagher, C. (2017). Future competences and the future of curriculum: A global reference for curricula transformation. *International Bureau of Education.* https://fundaciobofill.cat/uploads/docs/9/s/a/p/n/m/m/c/0/book_complete_future_competences_and_the_future_of_curriculum.pdf
Martellozzo, E., Monaghan, A., Adler, J. R., Davidson, J., Leyva, R., & Horvath, M. A. (2016). *"I wasn't sure it was normal to watch it…" A quantitative and qualitative examination of the impact of online pornography on the values, attitudes, beliefs and behaviours of children and young people.* O. Middlesex University: NSPCC. https://learning.nspcc.org.uk/media/1187/mdx-nspcc-occ-pornography-report.pdf
Martens, K., & Jakobi, A. P. (2010). *Mechanisms of OECD governance: International incentives for national policy-making?* Oxford University Press.
Martin, M. (2023, March 13). Twitter stats that matter to marketers in 2024. *Hootsuite.* https://blog.hootsuite.com/twitter-statistics/
Matters, I. (2023, July 5). Report reveals concerns over children being targeted by online cryptocurrency scams. *Internet Matters.* https://www.internetmatters.org/hub/press-release/report-children-targeted-by-online-cryptocurrency-scams/
McGill, N. (2016). Education attainment linked to health throughout lifespan: Exploring social determinants of health. *The Nation's Health, 46*(6), 1–19. https://www.thenationshealth.org/content/46/6/1.3
Metz, R. (2022, August 2). AI made these stunning images. Here's why experts are worried. *CNN Business.* https://edition.cnn.com/2022/06/30/tech/openai-google-realistic-images-bias/index.html
Micro, T. (n.d.). *Cryptocurrency.* Retrieved February 19, 2024, from https://www.trendmicro.com/vinfo/us/security/definition/cryptocurrency
Mobus, G. E. (2018). Teaching systems thinking to general education students. *Ecological Modelling, 373*, 13–21. https://doi.org/10.1016/j.ecolmodel.2018.01.013

Moore, T. (2004). The critical thinking debate: How general are general thinking skills? *Higher Education Research and Development, 23*(1), 3–18. https://doi.org/10.1080/0729436032000168469

National Association of Colleges and Employers. (2023). Job outlook 2023. https://wwwcdn.ithaca.edu/file-download/download/public/63317

National Education Association. (2012). Preparing 21st century students for a global society: An educator's guide to "the four Cs". https://dl.icdst.org/pdfs/files3/0d3e72e9b873e0ef2ed780bf53a347b4.pdf

Ngai, G., & Shek, D. T. L. (2022). How Hong Kong university teachers assess students in service-learning: An exploratory study. In G. Ngai, & D. T. L. Shek (Eds.), *Service-learning capacity enhancement in Hong Kong higher education* (pp. 71–97). Springer. https://doi.org/10.1007/978-981-19-2437-8_5

OECD. (2005). *The definition and selection of key competencies*. OECD Publishing. https://www.oecd.org/pisa/definition-selection-key-competencies-summary.pdf

OECD. (2016). *Education at a glance 2016: OECD indicators* (Vol. 90). OECD Publishing. http://edukacjaidialog.pl/_upload/file/2016_10/education_at_a_glance_2016.pdf

OECD. (2018a). *The future of education and skills: Education 2030*. OECD Publishing. https://www.oecd.org/content/dam/oecd/en/publications/reports/2018/06/the-future-of-education-and-skills_5424dd26/54ac7020-en.pdf

OECD. (2018b). *OECD mental health performance framework*. OECD Publishing. https://www.oecd.org/health/OECD-Mental-Health-Performance-Framework-2019.pdf

OECD. (2018c). *OECD study on social and emotional skills*. OECD Publishing.

OECD. (2018d). *Physical health and well-being in children and youth: Review of the literature* . OECD Publishing. https://www.oecd-ilibrary.org/docserver/102456c7-en.pdf?expires=1709339968&id=id&accname=guest&checksum=3356B4D4B00819100D67515FA5C131DE

OECD. (2019a). *OECD future of education and skills 2030. OECD Learning Compass 2030. A series of concept notes*. OECD Publishing. https://issuu.com/oecd.publishing/docs/e2030-learning_compass_2030-concept_notes

OECD. (2019b). *OECD future of education and skills 2030: Project background*. OECD Publishing. https://www.oecd.org/content/dam/oecd/en/about/projects/edu/education-2040/publications/Project%20background%20E2030%20Introduction_FINAL_rev.pdf

OECD. (2019c). *OECD learning compass 2030 concept notes: Anticipation-action-reflection cycle for 2030*. OECD Publishing. https://www.oecd-ilibrary.org/content/dam/oecd/en/about/projects/edu/education-2040/concept-notes/AAR_Cycle_concept_note.pdf

OECD. (2019d). *OECD learning compass 2030 concept notes: Attitudes and values for 2030*. OECD Publishing. https://www.oecd.org/content/dam/oecd/en/about/projects/edu/education-2040/concept-notes/Attitudes_and_Values_for_2030_concept_note.pdf

OECD. (2019e). *OECD learning compass 2030 concept notes: Core foundations for 2030*. OECD Publishing. https://www.oecd.org/content/dam/oecd/en/about/projects/edu/education-2040/concept-notes/Core_Foundations_for_2030_concept_note.pdf

OECD. (2019f). *OECD learning compass 2030 concept notes: Knowledge for 2030*. OECD Publishing. https://www.oecd.org/content/dam/oecd/en/about/projects/edu/education-2040/concept-notes/Knowledge_for_2030_concept_note.pdf

OECD. (2019g). *OECD learning compass 2030 concept notes: Learning compass 2030*. OECD Publishing. https://www.oecd.org/content/dam/oecd/en/about/projects/edu/education-2040/concept-notes/OECD_Learning_Compass_2030_concept_note.pdf

OECD. (2019h). *OECD learning compass 2030 concept notes: Skills for 2030*. OECD Publishing. https://www.oecd.org/content/dam/oecd/en/about/projects/edu/education-2040/concept-notes/Skills_for_2030_concept_note.pdf

OECD. (2019i). *OECD learning compass 2030 concept notes: Student agency for 2030*. OECD Publishing. https://www.oecd.org/education/2030-project/teaching-and-learning/learning/student-agency/Student_Agency_for_2030_concept_note.pdf

OECD. (2019j). *OECD learning compass 2030 concept notes: Transformative competencies for 2030*. OECD Publishing. https://www.oecd.org/content/dam/oecd/en/about/projects/edu/education-2040/concept-notes/Transformative_Competencies_for_2030_concept_note.pdf

OECD. (2019k). An OECD learning framework 2030. In G. Bast, E. G. Carayannis, & D. F. J. Campbell (Eds.), *The future of education and labor* (pp. 23–35). Springer. https://doi.org/10.1007/978-3-030-26068-2_3

OECD. (2019l). *Trends shaping education 2019*. OECD Publishing. https://doi.org/10.1787/trends_edu-2019-en

OECD. (n.d.). *About OECD*. Organisation for Economic Co-operation and Development. https://www.oecd.org/about/

Park, S. (2012). Dimensions of digital media literacy and the relationship with social exclusion. *Media International Australia, 142*(1), 87–100. https://doi.org/10.1177/1329878X1214200111

Penman, R., & Turnbull, S. (2007). *Media literacy: Concepts, research and regulatory issues*. https://apo.org.au/sites/default/files/resource-files/2007-07/apo-nid2871.pdf

PIAAC Numeracy Expert Group (2009). *PIAAC numeracy: A conceptual framework*. OECD Publishing. https://doi.org/10.1787/220337421165

Pourdehnad, J., Wexler, E. R., & Wilson, D. V. (2011). Integrating systems thinking and design thinking. *The Systems Thinker*, *22*(9), 2–6. https://thesystemsthinker.com/wp-content/uploads/pdfs/220901pk.pdf

Prabhakar, J., Coughlin, C., & Ghetti, S. (2016). The neurocognitive development of episodic prospection and its implications for academic achievement. *Mind, Brain, and Education, 10*(3), 196–206. https://doi.org/10.1111/mbe.12124

Prensky, M. (2001). Digital natives, digital immigrants part 2: Do they really think differently? *On the Horizon, 9*(6), 1–6. https://doi.org/10.1108/10748120110424843

Radunović, V., & Rüfenacht, D. (2016). *Cybersecurity competence building trends*. DiPLO. https://www.diplomacy.edu/wp-content/uploads/2019/02/Cybersecurity20Full20Report.pdf

Rahman, N. A. A., Sairi, I. H., Zizi, N. A. M., & Khalid, F. (2020). The importance of cybersecurity education in school. *International Journal of Information and Education Technology, 10*(5), 378–382. https://www.ijiet.org/vol10/1393-JR419.pdf

Ramesh, A. (2012, August 13). How 'The youths' are being scammed by influencers into investing in cryptocurrency. *Biometrica*. https://www.biometrica.com/how-the-youths-are-being-scammed-by-influencers-into-investing-in-cryptocurrency/

Riesmeyer, C., Naab, T., Camerini, A.-L., Festl, R., & Dallmann, C. (2019). Media literacy as intergenerational project: Skills, norms, and mediation. *MedienPädagogik: Zeitschrift für Theorie und Praxis der Medienbildung, 35*, i–v. https://doi.org/10.21240/mpaed/35/2019.10.15.X

Rolheiser, C., Bower, B., & Stevahn, L. (2000). *The portfolio organizer: Succeeding with portfolios in your classroom*. ASCD.

Rosa, N., Benet, M., & Carrió, M. (2022). Integrating transversal skills into higher education in health and social care. In *8th International Conference on Higher Education Advances (HEAd'22)*. Editorial Universitat Politècnica de València. https://doi.org/10.4995/HEAd22.2022.14570

Rothman, E. F., Adhia, A., Christensen, T. T., Paruk, J., Alder, J., & Daley, N. (2018). A pornography literacy class for youth: Results of a feasibility and efficacy pilot study. *American Journal of Sexuality Education, 13*(1), 1–17. https://doi.org/10.1080/15546128.2018.1437100

Rothman, E. F., Beckmeyer, J. J., Herbenick, D., Fu, T.-C., Dodge, B., & Fortenberry, J. D. (2021). The prevalence of using pornography for information about how to have sex: Findings from a nationally representative survey of US adolescents and young adults. *Archives of Sexual Behavior, 50*, 629–646. https://doi.org/10.1007/s10508-020-01877-7

Ryan, E. (2023). Save the kids: The need for regulation of cryptocurrency to protect adolescents from fraud. *Family Court Review, 61*(3), 650–664. https://doi.org/10.1111/fcre.12729

Salmela-Aro, K. (2009). Personal goals and well-being during critical life transitions: The four C's—Channelling, choice, co-agency and compensation. *Advances in Life Course Research, 14*(1–2), 63–73. https://doi.org/10.1016/j.alcr.2009.03.003

Schleicher, A. (2018). *World class: How to build a 21st-century school system.* OECD Publishing. https://doi.org/10.1787/9789264300002-en

Schmelzer, M. (2016). *The crisis before the crisis: The 'problems of modern society' and the OECD. 1968–74.* Routledge.

Schön, D. A. (2017). *The reflective practitioner: How professionals think in action.* Routledge. https://doi.org/10.4324/9781315237473

Schoon, I. (2018). Conceptualising learner agency: A socio-ecological developmental approach. *LLAKES Research Paper, 64.* https://discovery.ucl.ac.uk/id/eprint/10048718/1/LLAKES%20Research%20Paper%2064%20-%20Schoon%2C%20Learner%20Agency.pdf

Schoon, I., Nasim, B., Sehmi, R., & Cook, R. (2015). The impact of early life skills on later outcomes: Report for the OECD (Early childhood education and care). *University College London.* https://discovery.ucl.ac.uk/id/eprint/10051902

Scott, C. L. (2015). The futures of learning 2: What kind of learning for the 21st century? *UNESCO.* https://unesdoc.unesco.org/ark:/48223/pf0000242996

Shah, M., Grebennikov, L., & Nair, C. S. (2015). A decade of study on employer feedback on the quality of university graduates. *Quality Assurance in Education, 23*(3), 262–278. https://doi.org/10.1108/QAE-04-2014-0018

Shek, D. T. L. (2020). Protests in Hong Kong (2019–2020): A perspective based on quality of life and well-being. *Applied Research in Quality of Life, 15*(3), 619–635. https://doi.org/10.1007/s11482-020-09825-2

Shek, D. T. L. (2021). COVID-19 and quality of life: Twelve reflections. *Applied Research in Quality of Life, 16*(1), 1–11. https://doi.org/10.1007/s11482-020-09898-z

Shek, D. T. L., Chai, W., Li, X., & Dou, D. (2023a). Profiles and predictors of mental health of university students in Hong Kong under the COVID-19 pandemic. *Frontiers in Psychology, 14,* 1211229. https://doi.org/10.3389/fpsyg.2023.1211229

Shek, D. T. L., Chai, W. Y., Wong, T., & Zhou, K. (2023b). Stress and depressive symptoms in university students in Hong Kong under the pandemic: Moderating effect of positive psychological attributes. *Frontiers in Psychology, 14,* 1071938. https://doi.org/10.3389/fpsyg.2023.1071938

Shek, D. T. L., Chai, W., & Zhou, K. (2023c). Risk factors and protective factors of internet addiction in university students during the pandemic: Implications for prevention and treatment. *International Journal of Environmental Research and Public Health, 20*(11), 5952. https://doi.org/10.3390/ijerph20115952

Shek, D. T. L., & Chak, Y. L. Y. (2019). Perceived changes and benefits of a service-learning subject for underprivileged children in Shanghai: Views of university students. In D. T. L. Shek, G. Ngai, & S. C. F. Chan (Eds.), *Service-learning for youth leadership: The case of Hong Kong* (pp. 33–47). Springer. https://doi.org/10.1007/978-981-13-0448-4_3

Shek, D. T. L., Chau, C. C., Zhou, K., Chu, C. K. M., Chu, K., & Li, A. (2023d). Nurturing holistic development of university students: The role of non-cognitive skills. *International Journal of Child and Adolescent Health, 16*(2), 111–122. https://web-p-ebscohost-com.ezproxy.lb.polyu.edu.hk/ehost/pdfviewer/pdfviewer?vid=0&sid=7315a185-0b0e-4e1d-bb39-1932cf1b0477%40redis

Shek, D. T. L., Dou, D., Zhu, X., Wong, T., & Tan, L. (2022). Need satisfaction and depressive symptoms among university students in Hong Kong during the COVID-19 pandemic: Moderating effects of positive youth development attributes. *Frontiers in Psychiatry, 13,* 931404. https://doi.org/10.3389/fpsyt.2022.931404

Shek, D. T. L., & Leung, J. T. Y. (2013). Adolescent developmental issues in Hong Kong: Phenomena and implications for youth service. In D. T. L. Shek, & R. Sun (Eds.), *Development and evaluation of positive adolescent training through holistic social programs (P.A.T.H.S.).* (pp. 1–13). Springer. https://doi.org/10.1007/978-981-4451-54-3_1

Shek, D. T. L., Lin, L., Ma, C. M. S., Yu, L., Leung, J. T. Y., Wu, F. K. Y., Leung, H., & Dou, D. (2021). Perceptions of adolescents, teachers and parents of life skills education and life skills in

high school students in Hong Kong. *Applied Research in Quality of Life, 16*, 1847–1860. https://doi.org/10.1007/s11482-020-09848-9
Shek, D. T. L., & Yu, L. (2016). Student feedback on a subject on leadership and intrapersonal development for university students in Hong Kong. *International Journal on Disability and Human Development, 15*(3), 339–346. https://doi.org/10.1515/ijdhd-2015-6002
Shek, D. T. L., Yu, L., & Chai, W. Y. (2017a). Evaluation of the general university requirements: What did students say? *International Journal of Adolescent Medicine and Health, 29*(1), 75–82. https://doi.org/10.1515/ijamh-2017-3010
Shek, D. T. L., Yu, L., Wu, F. K. Y., & Chai, W. Y. (2015a). General university requirements at Hong Kong Polytechnic University: Evaluation findings based on student focus groups. *Assessment and Evaluation in Higher Education, 40*(8), 1017–1031. https://doi.org/10.1080/02602938.2014.960362
Shek, D. T. L., Yu, L., Wu, F. K. Y., & Ng, C. S. M. (2015b). General education program in a new 4-year university curriculum in Hong Kong: Findings based on multiple evaluation strategies. *International Journal on Disability and Human Development, 14*(4), 377–384. https://doi.org/10.1515/ijdhd-2015-0459
Shek, D. T. L., Yu, L., & Xie, Q. Z. (2017b). Student feedback on a pioneer subject on leadership and intrapersonal development in Hong Kong. *International Journal of Adolescent Medicine and Health, 29*(1), 83–89. https://doi.org/10.1515/ijamh-2017-3011
Simonitch, S. (2012, September 13). Japan sees surge in aspiring adult film actresses; 6000 said to debut each year. *Japan Today*. https://japantoday.com/category/features/japan-sees-surge-in-aspiring-adult-film-actresses-6000-said-to-debut-each-year
Sørensen, K., Van den Broucke, S., Fullam, J., Doyle, G., Pelikan, J., Slonska, Z., Brand, H., & European, C. H. L. P. (2012). Health literacy and public health: A systematic review and integration of definitions and models. *BMC Public Health, 12*, Article 80. https://doi.org/10.1186/1471-2458-12-80
Steinberg, L. D. (2014). *Age of opportunity: Lessons from the new science of adolescence*. Houghton Mifflin Harcourt.
Steponavičius, M., Gress-Wright, C., & Linzarini, A. (2023). Social and emotional skills: Latest evidence on teachability and impact on life outcomes. *OECD Education Working Papers, 304*. https://one.oecd.org/document/EDU/WKP(2023)19/en/pdf
Su, Y.-H. (2011). The constitution of agency in developing lifelong learning ability: The 'being' mode. *Higher Education, 62*(4), 399–412. https://doi.org/10.1007/s10734-010-9395-6
Sun, R. C. F., & Shek, D. T. L. (2010). Life satisfaction, positive youth development, and problem behaviour among Chinese adolescents in Hong Kong. *Social Indicators Research, 95*, 455–474. https://doi.org/10.1007/s11205-009-9531-9
Talreja, V. (2017). *"Learner agency: The impact of adversity" section of Education 2030—Conceptual learning framework: Background papers*. OECD Publishing. https://www.oecd.org/education/2030-project/contact/Conceptual_learning_framework_Conceptual_papers.pdf
United Nations. (2015). *Sustainable development goals-Goal 4*. Department of Economic and Social Affairs. Retrieved February 26, 2024, from https://sdgs.un.org/goals/goal4
Vogler, J. S., Thompson, P., Davis, D. W., Mayfield, B. E., Finley, P. M., & Yasseri, D. (2018). The hard work of soft skills: Augmenting the project-based learning experience with interdisciplinary teamwork. *Instructional Science, 46*, 457–488. https://doi.org/10.1007/s11251-017-9438-9
Vygotsky, L. S., & Cole, M. (1978). *Mind in society: Development of higher psychological processes*. Harvard University Press.
Watson, H. R., & Burr, S. (2018). Twelve tips for teaching twelve transferable skills. *MedEdPublish, 7*, 177. https://doi.org/10.15694/mep.2018.0000177.1
World Health Organization. (2010). *Who regional office for Europe and BZgA-standards for sexuality education in Europe: A framework for policy makers, educational and health authorities and specialists*. Federal Centre for Health Education.
World Health Organization. (2018). *The Global burden of disease: 2004 update*. http://www.who.int/healthinfo/global_burden_disease/2004_report_update/en/

World Health Organization. (2021). *Mental health of adolescents*. Retrieved from January 5. https://www.who.int/news-room/fact-sheets/detail/adolescent-mental-health

Ydesen, C. (2019). Introduction: What can we learn about global education from historical and global policy studies of the OECD? In C. Ydesen (Ed.), *The OECD's historical rise in Education: The formation of a global governing complex* (pp. 1–14). Global Histories of Education. https://doi.org/10.1007/978-3-030-33799-5_1

Young, M., & Muller, J. (2016). *Curriculum and the specialization of knowledge: Studies in the sociology of education*. Routledge.

Yu, L., Shek, D. T. L., & Xing, K. Y. (2019). Impact of a service-learning programme in Mainland China: Views of different stakeholders. In D. T. L. Shek, G. Ngai, & S. C. F. Chan (Eds.), *Service-learning for youth leadership: The case of Hong Kong* (pp. 49–63). Springer. https://doi.org/10.1007/978-981-13-0448-4_4

Yu, S., Niemi, H., & Mason, J. (2019). *Shaping future schools with digital technology. An international handbook*. Springer. https://doi.org/10.1007/978-981-13-9439-3.pdf

Chapter 5
Positive Youth Development Approach

Daniel T. L. Shek, Diya Dou, and Ginger C. C. Chau

Abstract This chapter provides an overview of the positive youth development (PYD) approach, its impact on youth development, and its implementation in studies and programs across China. Manifesting through various models, such as the "40 Developmental Assets," "5Cs and 6Cs Models," "15 PYD Constructs," "Social-Emotional Learning (SEL) Model," and "the 'Being' perspective," the PYD approach views adolescents as productive individuals and valuable societal assets, emphasizing their potential and strengths rather than merely focusing on their problems. Research indicates that PYD programs enhance developmental assets, foster positive outcomes, reduce problematic behaviors, and improve adolescent well-being, supported by empirical evidence from studies throughout China. The chapter also discusses future research directions, including the application of meta-analytic designs for evaluation studies. Additionally, it highlights Project P.A.T.H.S., a notable PYD program for secondary school students, detailing its success in promoting PYD attributes and reducing negative developmental outcomes through curriculum development, training for teachers and youth practitioners, and comprehensive program implementation and evaluation. Further research is necessary to explore the impact of PYD programs under different cultural contexts and their long-term effectiveness. Collaborative efforts among researchers, practitioners, educators, organizations, communities, youth workers, parents, and youths are recommended to enhance PYD intervention programs, policies, and practices.

Keywords Positive youth development (PYD) approach · PYD studies and programs · Impact and evaluation · China · Project P.A.T.H.S.

5.1 Overview of Positive Youth Development Approach

Since early times, adolescent psychology has been dominated by the "deficit" views on adolescence, focusing on the problematic sides of adolescence. In particular, Hall (1904) regarded adolescence as a period of "storm and stress," highlighting the inevitability of disturbances and problems during this period. Hall's framework significantly shaped the landscape of adolescent psychology in the past century (Damon, 2004). Furthermore, Steinberg and Lerner (2004) commented that the initial

D. T. L. Shek, *Promoting Holistic Development in University Students*, Quality of Life in Asia 17, https://doi.org/10.1007/978-981-96-0251-3_5

phase of research on adolescence was mainly theoretical and descriptive (Erikson, 1968; Freud, 1958; Hall, 1904), and there was a huge gap between theory and empirical research.

In contrast, the PYD approach focuses on developmental plasticity and diversity in adolescents. Proposed by Hamilton (1999), PYD is a novel, healthy, positive, and strength-based approach for understanding adolescents and adopting a more affirmative and positive perspective on youth (Damon, 2004). According to this approach, young people are "not problems to be fixed" (Roth et al., 1998), and adolescent problems are viewed through an ecological and positive lens (Lerner et al., 2005a). Additionally, young people are regarded as resources in society that can be developed, nurtured, and cultivated, and they have potential and capacities (Lerner & Benson, 2003). To help young people thrive in their environments, PYD focuses more on fostering youth's health, developmental potential, and developmental plasticity through more developmental opportunities (Damon, 2004).

According to Benson (2006), the PYD perspective has many roots, including the emergence of PYD research, the call of youth workers, the enactment of policy initiatives, the support of community-based organizations, and the promotion of social welfare programs that protect and facilitate the healthy development of youth and their families. There are also many versions of the PYD approach. However, although PYD frameworks have been used in different contexts, some similarities were identified among them. Tolan et al. (2016) concluded that most models had similar emphases, such as "(a) the potentials and abilities of adolescents, (b) developmental plasticity, (c) internal developmental assets (e.g., social-emotional competence), and (d) external developmental assets, such as the support of family and peers." In the following section, we outline some of the prominent PYD models, including Benson's "40 Developmental Assets," Lerner's "5Cs and 6Cs Models," Catalano's "15 PYD constructs," "Social-Emotional Learning (SEL)," and "the 'being' perspective" (Shek et al., 2019), with a view to providing insights into future research directions of PYD programs.

5.1.1 Benson's 40 Developmental Assets

In the late 1980s, the relationship between individual needs, external environments, and other determinants for young people to achieve effective functioning was highlighted (Steinberg & Lerner, 2004). Researchers recognized that adolescent problems are interrelated, and it is crucial to train adolescents with consciousness and the necessary skills to help them achieve healthy and whole-person development. The Search Institute proposed a range of valuable qualities and competencies of children and youth. As one of the models, first initiated in 1990 and then revised in 1995, the Developmental Assets Framework was presumed to show the qualities young people need to achieve effective functioning and thriving (Benson et al., 2011; O'Connor et al., 2014).

Benson (1992) defined individual strengths and environmental resources as "developmental assets." The Search Institute further identified 40 crucial factors for the development of adolescents and the skills, energies, strengths, and constructive interests that adolescents have (Damon, 2004). The 40 assets, including internal and external assets, show the contributing roles that adolescents themselves, families, schools, neighbors, organizations, and agencies in the communities play in young people's positive development (O'Connor et al., 2014).

The 20 external assets focus on "the positive experiences that adolescents gain from the outside world," which can be categorized into four dimensions (Benson, 2006). Students "feel cared for and cared about" when they recognize that they possess these assets (Rose, 2006).

(1) "*Support.*" The experience of all sorts of support, care, acceptance, and love from other people, communities, organizations, and institutions surrounding young people is needed, which includes "family support," "positive family communication," "other adult relationships," "caring neighborhood," "caring school climate," and "parents' involvement in schooling."
(2) "*Empowerment.*" Adolescents seek the chance to develop their capacities, help others, and make contributions to the community. They must feel safe and secure before they can be empowered. In this way, their identity can be recognized, and their value can be fulfilled. Empowerment includes "community values youth," "youth as resources," "service to others," and "safety."
(3) "*Boundaries and expectations.*" Knowing the expectations of others, the boundaries, and the consequences of engaging in activities and behaviors that are out of bounds is essential for young people. These assets involve "family boundaries," "school boundaries," "neighborhood boundaries," "adult role models," "positive peer influence," and "high expectations."
(4) "*Constructive use of time.*" Adolescents can develop their skills through constructive and enriching activities, youth programs, and quality time with others. These assets include "creative activities," "youth programs," "religious community," and "time at home."

Equally important, promoting internal qualities helps adolescents make healthy decisions and establish a strong sense of commitment and values (O'Connor et al., 2014). The 20 internal assets represent positive personal characteristics of young people, which include the following four categories:

(1) "*Commitment to learning.*" Young people need to value the significance of lifelong education and learning, igniting their potential and abilities to achieve their goals. Instead of merely achieving success in school, commitments and beliefs, including "achievement," "motivation," "school engagement," "homework," "bonding to school," and "reading for pleasure," are vital for youth development.
(2) "*Positive values.*" Guiding principles are also essential for adolescents to make healthy decisions. These principles include "caring," "equality and social justice," "integrity," "honesty," "responsibility," and "self-control."

(3) "*Social competencies.*" Practical interpersonal competencies are helpful for youth to make positive decisions, establish interpersonal relationships, and adapt to the changing environment (Scales & Leffert, 1999). The competencies include "planning and decision-making," "interpersonal competence," "cultural competence," "resistance skills," and "peaceful conflict resolution."
(4) "*Positive identity.*" Developing a solid feeling of power, purpose, worth, strengths, and capacities is essential. The identities include "personal power," "self-esteem," "sense of purpose," and "positive view of personal future." Adolescents feel a sense of purpose and robust control and are optimistic when they possess these assets (Rose, 2006).

Researchers widely regarded these assets as tools to support the needs of adolescents and facilitate the constructive use of these assets (Scales, 1999). Specifically, the Search Institute developed instruments for individual assets, evaluated studies and publications related to each asset, and conducted surveys in more than 2000 communities. The findings have revealed positive relationships between assets and developmental outcomes (Scales, 1999). Specifically, research showed that when young people possess more assets, they will be less involved in risky behaviors and will experience more positive outcomes. Moreover, the results are consistent across different genders, ethnicities, and socioeconomic statuses of the participants under different reviews (Benson et al., 2011; Soares et al., 2019). Additionally, child development literature has also shown that the assets are also relevant to children (Scales, 1999). According to Rose (2006), more youth intervention programs are applying this approach to target different developmental assets.

Under the above circumstances, there is a need to conduct more empirical studies and implement scientific measurement tools for evaluating each asset and its effectiveness in preventing and decreasing behavioral problems, particularly in a cross-cultural context. Additionally, more studies are needed to demonstrate the strategies to improve individual assets (Rose, 2006) and to prove which dimension of individual developmental assets is more important in generating positive and specific outcomes for young people (Scales et al., 2000). Despite these limitations, the Developmental Assets Framework is suggested by many scholars as a group of protective factors that can benefit youth outcomes. This framework also forms a holistic approach to promote the successful development of psychological, physical, and socio-emotional developmental domains (Soares et al., 2019).

5.1.2 Lerner's 5Cs and 6Cs Models

The PYD approach suggests that resources can be developed, nurtured, and cultivated (Lerner et al., 2005a). Social context, which refers to the family, school, and community organizations where young people live, is an essential PYD resource for youth (Abdul Kadir & Mohd, 2021). Based on the Relational-Developmental-Systems approach, PYD emphasizes that individuals and their social context exert mutual influence on each other (Bowers et al., 2015). Moreover, researchers emphasized the positive influence of community interventions on the development of adolescents (National Research Council & Institute of Medicine, 2002). Specifically, researchers reported that PYD programs emphasizing youth's strengths could be enhanced and practiced by promoting five qualities: "competence, confidence, connection, character, and caring" (Roth & Brooks-Gunn, 2003). Lerner et al. (2005a) asserted that programs involving healthy interpersonal relationships, skill-training sessions, and chances for leadership training activities could result in the development of these 5Cs, and the achievement of 5Cs may lead to the attainment of the sixth C, "Contribution."

As one of the key PYD conceptual frameworks, the 5Cs Model mainly emphasizes the positive elements that facilitate youth in enjoying healthy lives and contributing to society, which, in turn, benefits themselves, their families, their communities, and society (Bowers et al., 2015). Specifically, the 5Cs include:

(1) "*Competence*" is the abilities and skills to confront challenges and stressors in life, which include "cognitive, social, academic, health, and vocational competencies" (Lerner et al., 2005b). Specifically, abilities like problem-solving, logical thinking, and decision-making are denoted as cognitive competence. Social competence represents interpersonal abilities, such as dealing with conflicts. Developing working habits and exploring career choices can be regarded as vocational competence, such as practical entrepreneurial skills (Shek et al., 2019).
(2) "*Confidence*" refers to an internal sense of firm belief in one's value and abilities. Confident youth strongly believe that they can utilize their own abilities to overcome challenges and further influence society.
(3) "*Connection*" denotes the positive bonds between individuals and others, such as their family members, peers, and communities. Youth can experience positive development when they feel valued and further develop a strong sense of belongingness in their communities. The positive connections facilitate youth in improving their own lives and the lives of those around them.
(4) "*Character*" shows the societal and cultural norms and standards of positive behaviors that promote social functioning in societies, which include a well-formed sense of morality, integrity, and internal value standards. Youth can adhere to internal values and moral standards regardless of whether others are around.
(5) "*Caring*" means that youth will not only care about their interests but also show sympathy and empathy for the feelings and experiences of others (Lerner et al., 2005b). More importantly, thriving youth strongly believe that caring for others can influence other people's lives.

Although promoting PYD does not mean eliminating risky behaviors in young people, researchers found that thriving youth with the 5Cs have a lower chance of engaging in risky and problematic behaviors (Lerner et al., 2005a). Remarkably, the 5Cs are essential for the successful development of young people if they want to succeed in their lives and contribute to society. To address this, Lerner et al. (2005a) suggested that "Contribution" (the sixth C) would emerge when the 5Cs are achieved. Specifically, "Contribution" refers to "positively contributing to oneself, family, community, and society." The "Contribution" domain shows a relationship between adolescents and their environment. That is, the supportive environment facilitates the cultivation of PYD among youth. In return, thriving youth would be motivated to engage in and contribute to society.

Many researchers, youth workers, practitioners, and parents use the 5Cs to depict the qualities of adolescents who are full of vigor and vitality (King et al., 2005). Researchers have conducted a wide range of qualitative and quantitative evaluations to measure the effectiveness of the 5Cs model. In terms of assessment, some measurement tools have been designed, such as "the 5Cs Questionnaire" (Lerner et al., 2005b), the "PYD 34-item short form" (PYD-SF), and a "17-item very short form" (PYD-VSF) (Geldhof et al., 2015). Nevertheless, it was argued that the lack of diversity and contextual specificity may limit the applicability of these measurements because the individual C may vary in different contexts (Bowers et al., 2015). Moreover, these tools were primarily used for research and evaluation purposes rather than to facilitate the development of mentor-oriented programs, and some programs may inappropriately apply the tools (Bowers et al., 2014). To fill the gaps, the Thrive Foundation for Youth further developed the "Growth Grids Rubrics" with a unique feature of flexibility and can link the activities in the program to foster the 6Cs qualities. Nonetheless, to ensure accuracy and reliability, applying the Growth Grids effectively also requires consistent training and scoring (Napolitano et al., 2014).

Some studies have examined how individual C influence problem/risk behaviors (Bowers et al., 2015). Heck and Subramaniam (2009) compared a variety of PYD models in terms of validity, utility, and universality in their review. Five models were examined, including "Targeting Life Skills" (Hendricks, 1996), "Developmental Assets" (Benson, 2006), "The Four Essential Elements" (Brendtro et al., 2009), "The 5Cs Model" (Lerner et al., 2005b), and "The Community Action Framework for Youth Development" (Gambone et al., 2003). It was argued that, although the 5Cs model is effective in examining the PYD process, the ways to convert the vital elements into specific programs need further demonstration (Heck & Subramaniam, 2009). Notwithstanding the arguments, they suggested that the 5Cs and 6Cs Models are supported by considerable empirical evidence nowadays, and this model has good psychometric properties. Apart from this review, other research has also shown that the 5Cs and 6Cs Models can indicate youth development, and follow-up studies showed that the scores of the youth on each dimension remain consistent across the adolescent period (Geldhof et al., 2014). More importantly, Bowers et al. (2015) also cautioned that each youth's pathway may not be generalized as the influence of others and the environment can shape it.

In conclusion, findings demonstrated that the 5Cs and 6Cs Models are functional and practical for practitioners to measure and evaluate PYD. Bowers et al. (2015) made several suggestions to practitioners. Firstly, as a multi-faceted and comprehensive measurement of youth development, the 5Cs and 6Cs Models should be promoted. Moreover, the programs should consider youth-adult partnerships to ensure that each of the 5Cs and Contribution is achieved. Additionally, PYD programs should consider both positive and negative outcomes for adolescents, and researchers should examine how individual and contextual factors influence youth development. As every youth has unique strengths and abilities, researchers should address the influence of each level of the "5Cs and Contribution" on adolescents (Lerner et al., 2005b). To fully enhance adolescents' strengths and facilitate PYD among youth, more comprehensive models that consider the ecological, individual, and demographic characteristics of youth should be implemented (Bowers et al., 2014).

5.1.3 15 Positive Youth Development Constructs

Although many PYD programs have emerged in the past decades, the definition of PYD still needs to be well specified. As discussed before, the PYD programs showed that different factors usually promote positive outcomes (e.g., creating a thriving pathway) and mitigate negative ones (e.g., prevention of the occurrence of risk behaviors and problems) for youth. To analyze PYD programs and their effectiveness, Catalano et al. (2004) conducted a comprehensive review based on both published and unpublished PYD programs in the United States. They summarized the outcomes of their evaluations and identified 77 programs that met the criteria. As a result, 25 programs were recognized as effective in terms of good evaluation designs, acceptable standards, adequate methodological details, and significant effects on promoting PYD. More importantly, researchers proposed 15 developmental constructs underlying effective PYD programs (Shek et al., 2019). The review demonstrated that the PYD programs that address PYD constructs are effective in enhancing children's positive behaviors or reducing problematic activities. The promotion of the 15 positive development constructs is outlined below:

(1) "*Promotion of bonding.*" A child's emotional connection and commitment to maintaining interpersonal relationships with families, peers, schools, communities, and culture are crucial. Studies have shown that the bonding between the child and their caregivers influences the child's relationship with other people (Bowlby, 1979). Positive bonding helps the child build trust, adapt to changes effectively, and develop healthy and functional habits and behaviors. In contrast, inadequate and poor bonding results in insecurity, self-doubt, mistrust in self and others, and finally, behavioral problems (Braucht et al., 1978). More importantly, Caplan et al. (1992) demonstrated that programs promoting positive bonding and developmental skills reduce antisocial behaviors in adolescents.

(2) "*Fostering of resilience.*" Resilience denotes one's capacity to react to sudden transitions and transformations, risk factors, and stressors in a healthy way (Catalano et al., 2004). Chalk and Phillips (1996) noted that resilience can prevent adolescents from engaging in risky activities under unexpected circumstances.

(3) "*Promotion of social competence.*" The skills the youth can utilize to achieve social and interpersonal goals are denoted as social competence (Caplan et al., 1992). It includes receiving and understanding social cues, developing strategies to solve interpersonal problems, foreseeing the consequences of interpersonal challenges, and putting decisions into practical actions (The Consortium on the School-Based Promotion of Social Competence, 1996).
(4) "*Promotion of emotional competence.*" Although researchers have proposed different definitions of emotional competence, it commonly refers to "the ability to recognize the feelings and emotions of oneself and others and generate suitable responses to the emotions" (Catalano et al., 2004). According to Salovey and Mayer (1990), emotional competence includes understanding and managing emotions, motivating oneself, identifying others' emotions, and dealing with interpersonal relationships.
(5) "*Promotion of cognitive competence.*" Cognitive competence refers to "the ability to engage in self-talk, problem-solving, decision-making, logical and analytical thinking, and abstract reasoning" (Grant, 1992).
(6) "*Promotion of behavioral competence.*" Behavioral competence represents the practical actions to make nonverbal and verbal communication and take effective actions (Grant, 1992), such as saying "no" to smoking and engaging in antisocial behaviors.
(7) "*Promotion of moral competence.*" It shows one's skills to evaluate and react to a situation ethically. Moral development consists of several stages during which children understand standards of right and wrong in society and react to moral dilemmas (Kohlberg, 1969). Moreover, Hoffman (1981) emphasized that empathetic arousal is the foundation of morality and helps build the quality of altruism.
(8) "*Nurturance of self-determination.*" It denotes the skills to consider oneself and consistently respond to that thought, such as making independent decisions. Ewalt and Mokuau (1995) argued that individual development may be overemphasized, which may de-emphasize group-oriented values. At the same time, Deci and Ryan (1994) asserted that self-determination is related to one's need for competence, autonomy, and relatedness.
(9) "*Promotion of spirituality.*" Researchers propose different definitions of spirituality (Shek, 2012). Houghton Mifflin (1999) defined spiritual as "relating to, consisting of, or having the nature of spirit, soul, or God." Stark and Bainbridge (2012) associated spirituality with "youth's moral reasoning and commitment or belief in the social order." Benson (1992) demonstrated that religiosity promoted prosocial values and activities and prevented risk and problematic behaviors.
(10) "*Fostering of self-efficacy.*" It represents one's capacity to achieve desired goals through actions. Bandura (1986) stated that self-efficacy strategies such as personal goal setting are affected by one's evaluation of one's own abilities. Locke et al. (1984) demonstrated that stronger perceived self-efficacy was related to higher goal-setting and firmer commitment to goals.

(11) "*Fostering a clear and positive identity.*" It shows a coherent sense of self, and it helps explain how children build their identities in various cultural and social contexts (Catalano et al., 2004). Erikson (1968) defined identity as "a self-structure constructed by one's understanding of the usual crises and challenges at different developmental stages." He further stated that an unhealthy identity might result in role confusion and that successful resolution of an earlier stage of the child generates successful identity achievement.

(12) "*Fostering belief in future.*" Belief in future shows hope and optimism toward possible future outcomes. Holding this belief enables the youth to try their best and value their lives. Wyman et al. (1993) also showed that having confidence in future facilitates the youth to adjust to social and emotional changes better in school and protects the child from a negative evaluation of one's competence.

(13) "*Providing recognition for positive behavior.*" Positive reactions to desired behaviors can reinforce such positive behaviors. Reward and avoidance of punishment can strengthen behaviors, and aversive stimuli and loss of reward can weaken behaviors. Reinforcement can affect one's desire to be involved in similar future behaviors (Akers et al., 1995).

(14) "*Providing opportunities for prosocial involvement.*" It denotes increasing the chances for youth under different contexts and encouraging them to join in prosocial activities (Catalano et al., 2004). Positive opportunities for interaction enable a child to obtain essential interpersonal skills. In adolescence, having the opportunity to interact with peers, groups, family, school, and community can facilitate youth's development.

(15) "*Fostering prosocial norms.*" It encourages adolescents to develop positive beliefs and standards for behaviors. For instance, Hawkins et al. (1992) suggested that programs involving older youth acting as facilitators could be effective in fostering prosocial norms. In this way, they can convey positive and healthy standards and encourage younger children to build standards for themselves.

Catalano et al. (2004) also provided some suggestions for further studies. Firstly, evaluators should agree on using standardized measurement tools, especially for positive constructs, to ensure the results of PYD programs are applicable. Moreover, the impact of the PYD programs should be evaluated with a comprehensive measurement package. Furthermore, they also suggested that the field could reach a greater consensus in program design, measurement, and information to enrich the database for PYD program evaluations.

5.1.4 Social-Emotional Learning

An increasing number of educators call for enhancing social, emotional, and physical development in youth (Elias et al., 1997). Based on the "social information-processing theory," "social cognitive theory," and "emotional intelligence theories,"

Social-Emotional Learning (SEL) was characterized as one of the PYD frameworks focusing on the importance of psychosocial competence (Tolan et al., 2016). Specifically, SEL was defined as "the process by which one develops the necessary skills, attitudes, and values to gain social-emotional competence" (Elias et al., 1997). Social-emotional competence includes being aware of oneself, controlling one's impulsiveness, cooperating with others efficiently, and caring about oneself and others' feelings and emotions. The competencies develop across youth's lives and enable one to manage life tasks successfully, such as developing interpersonal relationships, confronting challenges, and meeting the demands of healthy development (Collaborative for Academic, Social, and Emotional Learning [CASEL], 2012).

SEL can be applied under different circumstances, such as classrooms, extracurricular activities, and community services (Hawkins et al., 2004), and school-based SEL programs are gaining popularity nowadays (CASEL, 2012). The SEL model is one of the major frameworks nowadays and is regarded as a general PYD model that can be applied to developmental stages (Shek et al., 2019). This model conceptualizes SEL in terms of five essential skills that integrate cognitive, affective, and behavioral competencies, which include "self-awareness, social awareness, responsible decision-making, self-management, and relationship skills" (CASEL, 2012).

(1) "*Self-awareness.*" Identifying one's own emotions, thoughts, values, and their influence on actions, along with accurately recognizing personal strengths and weaknesses, includes "identifying emotions," "accurate self-perception," "recognizing strengths," "self-confidence," and "self-efficacy."
(2) "*Self-management.*" Managing one's emotions, thoughts, and behaviors in various contexts and endeavoring successfully to achieve one's aspirations. The abilities are "impulse control," "stress management," "self-discipline," "self-motivation," "goal setting," and "organizational skills."
(3) "*Social awareness.*" Knowing others' situations, showing empathy toward others from different contexts, and being aware of resources available and supportive networks. The competencies include "perspective-taking," "empathy," "appreciating diversity," and "respect for others."
(4) "*Relationship skills.*" Developing and cultivating healthy and productive relationships with others. This domain can be concluded as "communication," "social engagement," "relationship-building," and "teamwork."
(5) "*Responsible decision-making.*" Making clear and productive decisions about personal activities and interpersonal relationships that are grounded on moral, ethical, and social norms, safety concerns, the evaluation of consequences, and the well-being of self and others. The skills include "identifying problems," "analyzing situations," "solving problems," "evaluating," "reflecting," and "taking ethical responsibility."

SEL primarily emerged as an education-focused initiative that cultivates skills and interventions related to school engagement and academic achievement (Tolan et al., 2016). An increasing number of educators and practitioners are dedicated to evaluating the influence of social-emotional competencies and social support on educational achievements (Elias & Haynes, 2008; Walsh et al., 2022). Various studies have proven the importance of SEL programs for children and youth. For instance, Elias and Haynes (2008) suggested that programs addressing students' social-emotional competencies and enhancing teachers' support could help disadvantaged students improve their achievements in school. Research conducted by Rieber and Carton (1987) demonstrated that social interactions in the early stages laid the foundation for children's future development. Essentially, Saarni (2007) recognized that developing social-emotional skills helps build effective interpersonal relationships. Moreover, Elias and Haynes (2008) further examined that social-emotional competencies enable children who come from minority groups, financially disadvantaged households, and urban schools to achieve better outcomes in school. They have a lower risk of engaging in risky and problematic behaviors and a higher potential to demonstrate positive developmental outcomes.

Apart from merely focusing on academic achievement, more researchers are applying the SEL model more generally as a PYD approach (Durlak et al., 2015). Remarkably, Jagers et al. (2018) demonstrated that SEL is a practical prevention framework for delinquency, drug abuse, and problem behaviors. In their review, Trentacosta and Fine (2010) found that embedding core social-emotional skills in prevention programs can promote social competence or prevent risk and problematic behaviors of youth. Similar results can be found in Izard et al. (2008), which stated that it is beneficial to enhance SEL education for children and youth. Equally important, SEL programs also show beneficial effects on teachers. Collie et al. (2012) exhibited that teachers experienced more teaching efficacy and job satisfaction and much less perceived stress after participation in SEL programs. The positive experiences of teachers benefit the teachers and nourish the teacher-student relationship. More importantly, the teachers can develop more profound efficacy to assist and guide the students in developing their social-emotional competencies (Bridgeland et al., 2013).

In conclusion, the SEL model and related studies strongly suggest that adjustments to school environments and curricula could be achieved by cultivating students' psychosocial competence. For instance, Elias and Haynes (2008) suggested that classroom-based interventions, new curricula, and additional assessments are necessary. Moreover, interactions with peers and support from teachers are also essential to enhance youth's social-emotional competencies. SEL's impact on achieving academic success, promoting equity, addressing poverty, and enhancing other life outcomes is remarkable. More research could be done to examine which aspects of SEL programs could be more beneficial in enhancing PYD for children and youth (Trentacosta & Fine, 2010).

5.1.5 The "Being" Perspective

According to Shek et al. (2019), the PYD approach also has its roots in the "being" perspective based on "humanistic psychology," "existential psychology," and "positive psychology." First, humanistic psychology forms the backdrop for the positive conception of youth development. Maslow (1987) highlighted that "fulfilling social needs, esteem and self-esteem needs, and self-actualization needs is fundamentally important," which resonates with the concepts of developmental assets (e.g., bonding and positive self-identity) and 5Cs. The concepts of "positive regard from others" and "unconditional positive self-regard" are also consistent with the concepts of "positive and healthy identity" and "social competence" in the PYD literature. Frankl's (1985) concept of "will to being" also forms the basis of "spirituality" and "values" in the PYD literature. Finally, the PYD approach also emphasizes many essential concepts in the strengths-based perspective and positive psychology, such as optimism, resilience, forgiveness, and well-being. In particular, this perspective focuses on the importance of "being" over "doing." In other words, inner qualities are more critical than sheer possession of psychosocial competence.

5.2 The Impact of Positive Youth Development on Youth Development

A rising number of studies suggest that PYD programs can strengthen developmental assets, foster positive outcomes, reduce problematic behaviors, and improve the well-being of adolescents (Benson & Saito, 2001). At the beginning of the evaluations in this field, Conrad and Hedin (1981) used a survey involving 4000 participants from 30 PYD programs. Results showed that positive outcomes, such as improvements in intrapersonal and interpersonal development, self-esteem, and moral judgment, existed in students in the treatment group. Similarly, Cognetta and Sprinthall (1978) recognized the improvements in ego and moral development, and Newmann and Rutter (1983) observed the enhancement of social responsibility and social competence in PYD programs in their early studies. After entering the millennium, Lerner et al. (2005b) collected data from around 7000 students from the 5th grade and tracked the participants till they reached the 12th grade. This longitudinal sequential design showed that PYD prevention programs could nurture positive qualities and reduce risk and developmental problems of adolescents, which further helped them adapt to developmental challenges and promote healthy functioning. Similar results are revealed in Catalano et al. (2004), in which 77 PYD programs were evaluated for their effects, and 25 of them were identified as effective.

Apart from the studies examining the effectiveness of a number of PYD approaches, some researchers focused on the effectiveness of one or a few PYD programs utilizing some PYD constructs. Such studies showed that PYD programs could promote Contribution and adolescent sexual health or address bullying (Hilliard et al., 2015). Di Fabio and Palazzeschi (2015) asserted that PYD qualities promoted life satisfaction and reduced depression and adolescent misbehavior. Durlak et al. (2011) revealed that SEL programs were effective in enhancing students' social competence, academic performance, and emotional management and adjustment after reviewing over 200 SEL programs in different schools. In another review,

Tolan et al. (2016) showed that promoting PYD qualities and competencies enhanced holistic youth development and decreased developmental problems. Furthermore, Walsh et al. (2022) suggested that PYD programs that build social-emotional skills and interpersonal relationships encourage students to make healthier decisions and reduce problem behaviors during high school. In another meta-analytic review, Taylor et al. (2017) conducted follow-up assessments for 92 SEL programs in school contexts and found that the impact of promoting social and emotional skills and attitudes could be sustained. Zych et al. (2019) revealed that a series of developmental assets are protective factors to protect youth from bullying and violent actions in school.

Specifically, the limitations of current studies regarding the impact of PYD programs should be highlighted. For example, results indicated that not all PYD outcomes could be sustained over time (Gresham, 1997; Gutman et al., 2003; Viadero, 2003; Wade-Mdivanian et al., 2016). As Wade-Mdivanian et al. (2016) suggested, additional year-round follow-up sessions could be added to enhance the positive influence of PYD programs and reinforce the lessons and skills. Hence, more studies with a longitudinal design are needed to testify to the beneficial effect of PYD programs on youth over time. Furthermore, most of the review studies only evaluated PYD programs that have taken place in America, while the need to conduct more reviews regarding other cultures or contexts is highlighted (Shek & Zhu, 2020). More research is needed to fill these gaps.

There are several possibilities for future research. First, more evaluation studies with meta-analysis designs could help explore the impact of PYD programs. Second, research regarding the effectiveness of PYD programs under different cultural contexts is needed. Third, researchers should pay attention to the long-term effectiveness of the PYD programs. The life-span development analysis approach can evaluate the effectiveness of interventions on adolescents' development and provide evidence for an empirically based unified PYD model (Tolan et al., 2016). Fourth, there are many PYD models available, and in-depth studies to compare their validity are essential. Fifth, since some studies only focused on one or a few of PYD qualities, it would be beneficial to employ studies to measure more PYD constructs and compare the relative advantages of different modes of intervention (Shek et al., 2019). Sixth, research and evaluation can help improve PYD intervention programs, policy, and practice. Equally important, the efforts to employ PYD models and constructs among adolescents also emphasize the development of developmentally appropriate prevention policies and programs (Lerner et al., 2005b). Finally, joint efforts among researchers, practitioners, educators, teachers, organizations, communities, youth workers, parents, and youths are also recommended.

All in all, the evidence from the reviews and evaluations suggests that PYD interventions can be practical tools for boosting youths' potential and reducing problem behavior (DuBois et al., 2011; Tolan et al., 2014). However, while most of the PYD programs are implemented in high schools, one outstanding question remains: whether it is possible to develop the "university versions" of PYD programs beneficial for late adolescents or emerging adults.

5.3 Positive Youth Development Studies and Programs in China

In a scientometric study of PYD studies globally, Qi et al. (2022) showed that Tufts University and The Hong Kong Polytechnic University had conducted many PYD studies, with Daniel Shek publishing the highest number of PYD studies. How PYD attributes influence adolescent development has been reported in different Chinese societies. For example, Shek and Chai (2020) showed that "PYD qualities increase academic satisfaction and reduce academic pressure in the long run." Utilizing two periods of longitudinal data, Zhou et al. (2020a) showed that there were concurrent and longitudinal predictions of PYD qualities on life satisfaction and hopelessness. Similarly, Zhou et al. (2020b) revealed that PYD attributes had negative concurrent and longitudinal relationships with depression. In another study, Shek et al. (2022b) exhibited that "PYD attributes mediated the influence of family functioning on adolescent delinquency." Similarly, Shek et al. (2022b) reported that "Family functioning predicted adolescent materialism and egocentrism, with PYD attributes as a mediating factor." Finally, there are studies showing that PYD attributes were negatively related to posttraumatic stress disorder during the pandemic (Shek et al., 2022a, 2022b, 2022c, 2023a, 2023b, 2023c). In fact, Shek (2020, 2021a, 2021b) argued that PYD attributes can help young people to cope with changing circumstances such as social events and the COVID-19 pandemic.

Regarding PYD programs in China, Shek and Yu (2011) conducted a review of PYD programs in Asia and concluded that validated PYD programs in Asia are scarce. Notably, Project P.A.T.H.S., an influential PYD program for high school students, was developed by a team of colleagues from five universities in Hong Kong (Shek & Sun, 2013; Shek & Wu, 2016). Besides developing the curriculum materials, the researchers also trained teachers and youth practitioners (over 10,000 up to now), supported the program implementation process, and evaluated its effectiveness. Multiple methods of evaluation showed that the program significantly promoted the participants' PYD attributes and reduced their negative development. Moreover, different stakeholders, including students and program implementers, also evaluated the program and its benefits positively (Shek et al., 2021a, 2021b). For example, Shek and Zhu (2020) showed that students' psychosocial competencies were enhanced after the programs. Remarkably, the study showed that PYD qualities, such as "resilience," "emotional competence," and "spirituality," can protect adolescents from burnout under stressors in life. The World Health Organization acknowledged Project P.A.T.H.S. as effective in cultivating psychosocial competencies in young people. In 2020, Project P.A.T.H.S. was recognized by the Hong Kong Research Assessment Exercise as a world-leading (4*) project in terms of the social impact, the research, and the benefits to the program participants.

As Project P.A.T.H.S. has gathered remarkably successful experiences in Hong Kong, the Tin Ka Ping Foundation invited the research team to implement the project in mainland China. In the initial stage, the project was implemented in four cities in East China (Shanghai, Suzhou, Changzhou, and Yangzhou). In order to sustain the long-term impact of programs, we spent one year (2014–15 academic year) training the potential program implementers. When it came to the 2015/16 and 2017/18 academic year, the project was fully implemented. Different evaluation studies consistently showed that students and program implementers viewed the activities, instructors, and benefits of the program positively. In another quasi-experimental study, Zhu and Shek (2021) found that students in the programs exhibited more positive development and showed fewer problematic behaviors compared to the control group. Moreover, Shek et al. (2022c) found that teachers considered the program beneficial for both themselves and their students.

One question we should consider is whether PYD attributes are only relevant to adolescents. Theoretically speaking, we argue that PYD attributes and programs are also relevant to all human beings, including university students. First, PYD attributes such as resilience and emotional competence are relevant to people in different age groups, including late adolescents and emerging adults. Second, evidence showed that PYD attributes promote students' psychological well-being. For example, during the COVID-19 pandemic, some findings showed that "PYD attributes, such as 'resilience,' 'emotional competence,' and 'meaning in life,' can buffer the negative influence of the pandemic on adolescents' mental health" (Shek, 2021a, 2021b; Shek et al., 2021c, 2022a). In view of the developmental issues faced by university students (see Chap. 1) and the neglect of life skills in the institutional learning outcomes (Chaps. 2 and 3), we developed Project P.A.T.H.S. for universities under the new undergraduate program implemented in the 2012/13 academic year. In Chap. 8, we will introduce a credit-bearing subject utilizing PYD principles as a university version of the Project P.A.T.H.S. In addition, with the service sector dominating Hong Kong's economy, we also developed a subject on "Service Leadership" that highlights the importance of 3Cs in leaders, namely "competence," "character," and "care." The 3Cs are closely related to PYD attributes. Finally, to enhance students' learning experience and civic engagement, we have also developed two Service-Learning subjects utilizing PYD constructs, which promote empathy and the understanding of the needs of deprived communities.

5.4 Summary and Conclusion

The PYD has been introduced as a strengths-based approach to replace the deficit view (e.g., problematic, broken, and dangerous) of young people. Instead of focusing on adolescent problems, the PYD framework embraces a positive perspective that regards each adolescent as productive and effective at tasks and as a resource for society. PYD models are not merely examinations of qualities that are beneficial for adolescents but are the exploration of ways to acknowledge youth's full potential, like talents, interests, and strengths. Adolescents can learn and thrive in diverse contexts (Damon, 2004). Various themes and highlights are proposed in different PYD models. Professionals are investigating the PYD qualities and their relationship with youth development outcomes.

In this chapter, we first introduce the orientation and development of PYD. Then, several models of PYD are examined, including the "5Cs and 6Cs Models," "40 Developmental Assets," "15 PYD constructs," "Social-Emotional Learning (SEL)," and "the 'being' perspective." Specifically, the originality, detail, effectiveness, and arguments of these models are discussed in each part. Besides, the impact of the PYD framework on adolescents and its implications are addressed. Programs in Western contexts are also highlighted. The discussion showed that PYD programs are beneficial in enhancing youth's developmental qualities and preventing them from risky and problematic actions (Catalano et al., 2012). With the enhancement of PYD, thriving young people can form reciprocal relationships with the people and communities in which they live. In return, healthy interpersonal relationships can benefit individuals, the people around them, their community, and the society (Lerner et al., 2005b). More importantly, adolescents may thrive and develop to achieve their success, and the whole community may prosper.

With particular attention to university students, a leadership subject entitled "Tomorrow's Leaders" was implemented based on different PYD constructs utilized in Project P.A.T.H.S. in Hong Kong. Chapter 9 will give a thorough introduction to this subject and its impact. Furthermore, with reference to the world economy focusing more on the service sector, we also developed a subject entitled "Service Leadership" utilizing PYD constructs, which will be described in Chap. 10. Finally, utilizing experiential learning and focusing on the active learning characteristics of students, we have developed two Service-Learning subjects that attempt to cultivate the holistic development of university students. We will present these two subjects in Chaps. 11 and 12.

Acknowledgements The preparation of this chapter is financially supported by The Hong Kong Polytechnic University (ZZ4U and ZZUE), Li and Fung Endowed Professorship in Service Leadership Education, Wofoo Foundation, and the Matching Fund of Research Grants Council (ZECL and ZH4Q).

References

Abdul Kadir, N. B., & Mohd, R. H. (2021). The 5Cs of positive youth development, purpose in life, hope, and well-being among emerging adults in Malaysia. *Frontiers in Psychology, 12*. Article 641876. https://doi.org/10.3389/fpsyg.2021.641876

Akers, R. L., Krohn, M. D., Lanza-Kaduce, L., & Radosevich, M. (1995). Social learning and deviant behavior: A specific test of a general theory. In J. McCord, & J. H. Laub (Eds.) *Contemporary Masters in Criminology,* (pp. 187–214). Springer. https://doi.org/10.1007/978-1-4757-9829-6_12

Bandura, A. (1986). *Social foundations of thought and action: A social cognitive theory*. Prentice-Hall.

Benson, P. L. (1992). Religion and substance use. In J. F. Schumaker (Ed.), *Religion and mental health* (pp. 211–220). Oxford University Press.

Benson, P. L. (2006). *All kids are our kids: What communities must do to raise caring and responsible children and adolescents* (2nd ed.) Jossey-Bass.

Benson, P. L., & Saito, R. N. (2001). The scientific foundations of youth development. In P. L. Benson & K. J. Pittman (Eds.), *Trends in youth development: Visions, realities and challenges* (pp. 135–154). Springer. https://doi.org/10.1007/978-1-4615-1459-6_5

Benson, P. L., Scales, P. C., & Syvertsen, A. K. (2011). The contribution of the developmental assets framework to positive youth development theory and practice. *Advances in Child Development and Behavior, 41*, 197–230. https://doi.org/10.1016/B978-0-12-386492-5.00008-7

Bowers, E. P., Geldhof, G. J., Johnson, S. K., Hilliard, L. J., Hershberg, R. M., Lerner, J. V., & Lerner, R. M. (Eds.). (2015). *Promoting positive youth development: Lessons from the 4-H study*. Springer. https://doi.org/10.1007/978-3-319-17166-1

Bowers, E. P., Geldhof, G. J., Johnson, S. K., Lerner, J. V., & Lerner, R. M. (2014). Special issue introduction: Thriving across the adolescent years: A view of the issues. *Journal of Youth and Adolescence, 43*(6), 859–868. https://doi.org/10.1007/s10964-014-0117-8

Bowlby, J. (1979). On knowing what you are not supposed to know and feeling what you are not supposed to feel. *The Canadian Journal of Psychiatry, 24*(5), 403–408. https://doi.org/10.1177/070674377902400506

Braucht, G. N., Kirby, M. W., & Berry, G. J. (1978). Psychosocial correlates of empirical types of multiple drug abusers. *Journal of Consulting and Clinical Psychology, 46*(6), 1463–1475. https://doi.org/10.1037/0022-006X.46.6.1463

Brendtro, L., Brokenleg, M., & Van Bockern S. (2009). *Reclaiming youth at risk: Our hope for the future*. Solution Tree Press.

Bridgeland, J., Bruce, M., & Hariharan, A. (2013). *The missing piece: A national teacher survey on how social and emotional learning can empower children and transform schools*. Civic Enterprises. https://files.eric.ed.gov/fulltext/ED558068.pdf

Caplan, M., Weissberg, R. P., Grober, J. S., Sivo, P. J., Grady, K., & Jacoby, C. (1992). Social competence promotion with inner-city and suburban young adolescents: Effects on social adjustment and alcohol use. *Journal of Consulting and Clinical Psychology, 60*(1), 56–63. https://doi.org/10.1037/0022-006X.60.1.56

Catalano, R. F., Berglund, M. L., Ryan, J. A. M., Lonczak H. S., & Hawkins, J. D. (2004). Positive youth development in the United States: Research findings on evaluations of positive youth development programs. *The ANNALS of the American Academy of Political and Social Science, 591*(1), 98–124. https://doi.org/10.1177/0002716203260102

Catalano, R. F., Fagan, A. A., Gavin, L. E., Greenberg, M. T., Irwin, C. E., Ross, D. A., & Shek, D. T. L. (2012). Worldwide application of prevention science in adolescent health. *The Lancet, 379*(9826), 1653–1664. https://doi.org/10.1016/S0140-6736(12)60238-4

Chalk, R., & Phillips, D. A. (Eds.). (1996). *Youth development and neighborhood influences: Challenges and opportunities*. National Academy Press.

Cognetta, P. V., & Sprinthall, N. A. (1978). Students as teachers: Role taking as a means of promoting psychological and ethical development during adolescence. *Character Potential: A Record of Research, 8*(4), 188–195.

Collaborative for Academic, Social, and Emotional Learning (CASEL). (2012). *Effective social and emotional learning programs: Preschool and elementary school edition*. https://files.eric.ed.gov/fulltext/ED581699.pdf

Collie, R. J., Shapka, J. D., & Perry, N. E. (2012). School climate and social-emotional learning: Predicting teacher stress, job satisfaction, and teaching efficacy. *Journal of Educational Psychology, 104*(4), 1189–1204. https://doi.org/10.1037/a0029356

Conrad, D., & Hedin, D. (1981). National assessment of experiential education: Summary and implications. *Journal of Experiential Education, 4*(2), 6–20. https://doi.org/10.1177/105382598100400202

The Consortium on the School-Based Promotion of Social Competence. (1996). The school-based promotion of social competence: Theory, research, practice, and policy. In R. J. Haggerty, L. R. Sherrod, N. Garmezy, & M. Rutter (Eds.), *Stress, risk, and resilience in children and adolescents: Processes, mechanisms, and interventions* (pp. 268–316). Cambridge University Press.

Damon, W. (2004). What is positive youth development? *The ANNALS of the American Academy of Political and Social Science, 591*(1), 13–24. https://doi.org/10.1177/0002716203260092

Deci, E. L., & Ryan, R. M. (1994). Promoting self-determined education. *Scandinavian Journal of Educational Research, 38*(1), 3–14. https://doi.org/10.1080/0031383940380101

Di Fabio, A., & Palazzeschi, L. (2015). Hedonic and eudaimonic well-being: The role of resilience beyond fluid intelligence and personality traits. *Frontiers in Psychology, 6*, Article 1367. https://doi.org/10.3389/fpsyg.2015.01367

DuBois, D. L., Portillo, N., Rhodes, J. E., Silverthorn, N., & Valentine, J. C. (2011). How effective are mentoring programs for youth? A systematic assessment of the evidence. *Psychological Science in the Public Interest, 12*(2), 57–91. https://doi.org/10.1177/1529100611414806

Durlak, J. A., Domitrovich C. E., Weissberg R. P., & Gullotta T. P. (Eds.). (2015). *Handbook of social and emotional learning: Research and practice.* The Guilford Press.

Durlak, J. A., Weissberg, R. P., Dymnicki, A. B., Taylor, R. D., & Schellinger, K. B. (2011). The impact of enhancing students' social and emotional learning: A meta-analysis of school-based universal interventions. *Child Development, 82*(1), 405–432. https://doi.org/10.1111/j.1467-8624.2010.01564.x

Elias, M., Zins, J. E., Weissberg, R. P., Frey, K., Greenberg, M. T., Haynes, N. M., Kessler, R., Schwab-Stone, M. E., & Shriver, T. P. (1997). *Promoting social and emotional learning guidelines for educators.* Association for Supervision and Curriculum Development.

Elias, M. J., & Haynes, N. M. (2008). Social competence, social support, and academic achievement in minority, low-income, urban elementary school children. *School Psychology Quarterly, 23*(4), 474–495. https://doi.org/10.1037/1045-3830.23.4.474

Erikson, E. H. (1968). *Identity: Youth and crisis* W. W. Norton & Company.

Ewalt, P. L., & Mokuau, N. (1995). Self-determination from a pacific perspective. *Social Work, 40*(2), 168–175. https://doi.org/10.1093/sw/40.2.168

Frankl, V. E. (1985). *Man's search for meaning.* Simon and Schuster.

Freud, A. (1958). Adolescence. *The Psychoanalytic Study of the Child, 13*(1), 255–278. https://doi.org/10.1080/00797308.1958.11823182

Gambone, M., Klem, A., & Connell, J. (2003). *Finding out what matters for youth: Testing key links in a community action framework for youth development.* Youth Development Strategies; Institute for Research and Reform in Education.

Geldhof, G. J., Bowers, E. P., Boyd, M. J., Mueller, M. K., Napolitano, C. M., Schmid, K. L., Lerner, J. V., & Lerner, R. M. (2014). Creation of short and very short measures of the five Cs of positive youth development. *Journal of Research on Adolescence, 24*(1), 163–176. https://doi.org/10.1111/jora.12039

Geldhof, G. J., Bowers, E. P., Mueller, M. K., Napolitano, C. M., Callina, K. S., Walsh, K. J., Lerner, J. V., & Lerner, R. M. (2015). The five Cs model of positive youth development. In E. P. Bowers, G. J. Geldhof, S. K. Johnson, L. J. Hilliard, R. M. Hershberg, J. V. Lerner, & R. M. Lerner (Eds.), *Promoting positive youth development: Lessons from the 4-H study* (pp. 161–186). Springer. https://doi.org/10.1007/978-3-319-17166-1_9

Grant, W. T. (1992). Consortium on the school-based promotion of social competence. Drug and alcohol prevention curricula. In J. D. Hawkins, & R. F. Catalano (Eds.), *Communities that care: Action for drug abuse prevention* (pp. 129–148). Jossey-Bass.

Gresham, F. M. (1997). Social competence and students with behavior disorders: Where we've been, where we are, and where we should go. *Education & Treatment of Children, 20*(3), 233–249. https://www.jstor.org/stable/42900487

Gutman, L. M., Sameroff, A. J., & Cole, R. (2003). Academic growth curve trajectories from 1st grade to 12th grade: Effects of multiple social risk factors and preschool child factors. *Developmental Psychology, 39*(4), 777–790. https://doi.org/10.1037/0012-1649.39.4.777

Hall, G. S. (1904). *Adolescence: Its psychology and its relations to physiology, anthropology, sociology, sex, crime, religion, and education.* Appleton.

Hamilton, S. (1999). *A three-part definition of youth development* [Unpublished manuscript]. Cornell University College of Human Ecology.

Hawkins, J. D., Catalano, R. F., & Miller, J. Y. (1992). Risk and protective factors for alcohol and other drug problems in adolescence and early adulthood: Implications for substance abuse prevention. *Psychological Bulletin, 112*(1), 64–105. https://doi.org/10.1037/0033-2909.112.1.64

Hawkins, J. D., Smith, B. H., & Catalano, R. F. (2004). Social development and social and emotional learning. In J. E. Zins, R. P. Weissberg, M. C. Wang, & H. J. Walberg (Eds.), *Building academic success on social and emotional learning: What does the research say* (pp. 135–150). Teachers College Press.

Heck, K., & Subramaniam, A. (2009). *Youth development frameworks*. 4-H Center for Youth Development.

Hendricks, P. A. (1996). *Developing youth curriculum using the targeting life skills model: Incorporating developmentally appropriate learning opportunities to assess impact of life skill development*. Iowa State University.

Hilliard, L. J., Batanova, M., & Bowers, E. P. (2015). A positive youth development approach to bullying: Promoting thriving and reducing problem behaviors. In E. P. Bowers, G. J. Geldhof, S. K. Johnson, L. J. Hilliard, R. M. Hershberg, J. V. Lerner, & R. M. Lerner (Eds.), *Promoting positive youth development: Lessons from the 4-H study* (pp. 249–272). Springer International Publishing. https://doi.org/10.1007/978-3-319-17166-1_13

Hoffman, M. L. (1981). Is altruism part of human nature? *Journal of Personality and Social Psychology, 40*(1), 121–137. https://doi.org/10.1037/0022-3514.40.1.121

Houghton Mifflin (1999). Spiritual. In Webster's II new college dictionary (3rd ed., p. 1090)

Izard, C. E., King, K. A., Trentacosta, C. J., Morgan, J. K., Laurenceau, J. P., Krauthamer-Ewing, E. S., & Finlon, K. J. (2008). Accelerating the development of emotion competence in Head Start children: Effects on adaptive and maladaptive behavior. *Development and Psychopathology, 20*(1), 369–397. https://doi.org/10.1017/S0954579408000175

Jagers, R. J., Rivas-Drake, D., & Borowski, T. (2018). *Equity & social and emotional learning: A cultural analysis*. Collaborative for Academic, Social, and Emotional Learning (CASEL).

King, P. E., Dowling, E. M., Mueller, R. A., White, K., Schultz, W., Osborn, P., Dickerson, E., Bobek, D. L., Lerner, R. M., Benson, P. L., & Scales, P. C. (2005). Thriving in adolescence: The voices of youth-serving practitioners, parents, and early and late adolescents. *The Journal of Early Adolescence, 25*(1), 94–112. https://doi.org/10.1177/0272431604272459

Kohlberg, L. (1969). Stage and sequence: The cognitive-developmental approach to socialization. In D. A. Goslin (Ed.), *Handbook of socialization theory and research* (pp. 347–480). Rand McNally.

Lerner, R. M., Almerigi, J. B., Theokas, C., & Lerner, J. V. (2005a). Positive youth development: A view of the issues. *The Journal of Early Adolescence, 25*(1), 10–16. https://doi.org/10.1177/0272431604273211

Lerner, R. M., & Benson, P. L. (Eds.). (2003). *Developmental assets and asset-building communities: Implications for research, policy, and practice*. Springer Science & Business Media.

Lerner, R. M., Lerner, J. V., Almerigi, J. B., Theokas, C., Phelps, E., Gestsdottir, S., Naudeau, S., Jelicic, H., Alberts, A., Ma, L., Smith, L. M., Bobek, D. L., Richman-Raphael, D., Simpson, I., Christiansen, E. D., & von Eye, A. (2005b). Positive youth development, participation in community youth development programs, and community contributions of fifth-grade adolescents: Findings from the first wave of the 4-h study of positive youth development. *The Journal of Early Adolescence, 25*(1), 17–71. https://doi.org/10.1177/0272431604272461

Levesque, R. J. (2007). *Advancing responsible adolescent development*. Springer.

Locke, E. A., Frederick, E., Lee, C., & Bobko, P. (1984). Effect of self-efficacy, goals, and task strategies on task performance. *Journal of Applied Psychology, 69*(2), 241–251. https://doi.org/10.1037/0021-9010.69.2.241

Maslow, A. H. (1987). *Motivation and personality* (3rd ed.). Harper & Row Publishers.

Napolitano, C. M., Bowers, E. P., Arbeit, M. R., Chase, P., Geldhof, G. J., Lerner, J. V., & Lerner, R. M. (2014). The GPS to success growth grids: Measurement properties of a tool to promote

intentional self-regulation in mentoring programs. *Applied Developmental Science, 18*(1), 46–58. https://doi.org/10.1080/10888691.2014.866768
National Research Council & Institute of Medicine. (2002). *Community programs to promote youth development*. National Academy Press. https://doi.org/10.17226/10022
Newmann, F. M., & Rutter, R. A. (1983). *The effects of high school community service programs on students' social development*. Wisconsin Center for Educational Research.
O'Connor, A., Hoff, N., & Peterson, R. L. (2014). *Developmental assets. Strategy brief.* Student Engagement Project; University of Nebraska-Lincoln; The Nebraska Department of Education. http://k12engagement.unl.edu/developmental-assets
Qi, S. J., Hua, F. R., Zhou, Z., & Shek, D. T. L. (2022). Trends of positive youth development publications (1995–2020): A scientometric review. *Applied Research in Quality of Life, 17*(1), 421–446. https://doi.org/10.1007/s11482-020-09878-3
Rieber, R. W., & Carton, A. S. (Eds.). (1987). *The collected works of L. S. Vygotsky: Problems of general psychology, including the volume thinking and speech.* Springer. https://doi.org/10.1007/978-1-4613-1655-8
Rose, H. A. (2006). Asset-based development for child and youth care. *Reclaiming Children and Youth, 14*(4), 236–240.
Roth, J. L., & Brooks-Gunn, J. (2003). What exactly is a youth development program? Answers from research and practice. *Applied Developmental Science, 7*(2), 94–111. https://doi.org/10.1207/S1532480XADS0702_6
Roth, J., Brooks-Gunn, J., Murray, L., & Foster, W. (1998). Promoting healthy adolescents: Synthesis of youth development program evaluations. *Journal of Research on Adolescence, 8*(4), 423–459. https://doi.org/10.1207/s15327795jra0804_2
Saarni, C. (2007). The development of emotional competence: Pathways for helping children to become emotionally intelligent. In R. Bar-On, J. G. Maree, & M. J. Elias (Eds.), *Educating people to be emotionally intelligent* (pp. 15–35). Praeger Publishers.
Salovey, P., & Mayer, J. D. (1990). Emotional intelligence. *Imagination, Cognition and Personality, 9*(3), 185–211. https://doi.org/10.2190/DUGG-P24E-52WK-6CDG
Scales, P. C. (1999). Reducing risk and building developmental assets: Essential actions for promoting adolescent health. *The Journal of School Health, 69*(3), 113–119. https://doi.org/10.1111/j.1746-1561.1999.tb07219.x
Scales, P. C., Benson, P. L., Leffert, N., & Blyth, D. A. (2000). Contribution of developmental assets to the prediction of thriving among adolescents. *Applied Developmental Science, 4*(1), 27–46. https://doi.org/10.1207/S1532480XADS0401_3
Scales, P. C., & Leffert, N. (1999). *Developmental assets: A synthesis of the scientific research on adolescent development*. Search Institute
Shek, D. T. L. (2012). Spirituality as a positive youth development construct: A conceptual review. *The Scientific World Journal, 2012*(1), Article 458953. https://doi.org/10.1100/2012/458953
Shek, D. T. L. (2020). Protests in Hong Kong (2019–2020): A perspective based on quality of life and well-being. *Applied Research in Quality of Life, 15*(3), 619–635. https://doi.org/10.1007/s11482-020-09825-2
Shek, D. T. L. (2021a). COVID-19 pandemic and developmental outcomes in adolescents and young adults: In search of the missing links. *Journal of Adolescent Health, 69*(5), 683–684. https://doi.org/10.1016/j.jadohealth.2021.07.035
Shek, D. T. L. (2021b). COVID-19 and quality of life: Twelve reflections. *Applied Research in Quality of Life, 16*(1), 1–11. https://doi.org/10.1007/s11482-020-09898-z
Shek, D. T. L., & Chai, W. Y. (2020). The impact of positive youth development attributes and life satisfaction on academic well-being: A longitudinal mediation study. *Frontiers in Psychology, 11*, Article 2126. https://doi.org/10.3389/fpsyg.2020.02126
Shek, D. T. L., Chai, W., Li, X., & Dou, D. (2023a). Profiles and predictors of mental health of university students in Hong Kong under the COVID-19 pandemic. *Frontiers in Psychology, 14*, Article 1211229. https://doi.org/10.3389/fpsyg.2023.1211229

Shek, D. T. L., Chai, W. Y., Wong, T., & Zhou, K. (2023b). Stress and depressive symptoms in university students in Hong Kong under the pandemic: Moderating effect of positive psychological attributes. *Frontiers in Psychology, 14*, Article 1071938. https://doi.org/10.3389/fpsyg.2023.1071938

Shek, D. T. L., Chai, W., & Zhou, K. (2023c). Risk factors and protective factors of internet addiction in university students during the pandemic: Implications for prevention and treatment. *International Journal of Environmental Research and Public Health, 20*(11), Article 5952. https://doi.org/10.3390/ijerph20115952

Shek, D. T. L., Dou, D. Y., Zhu, X. Q., & Chai, W. Y. (2019). Positive youth development: Current perspectives. *Adolescent Health, Medicine and Therapeutics, 10*, 131–141. https://doi.org/10.2147/AHMT.S179946

Shek, D. T. L., Dou, D. Y., Zhu, X. Q., Wong, T. Q., & Tan, L. D. (2022a). Need satisfaction and depressive symptoms among university students in Hong Kong during the COVID-19 pandemic: Moderating effects of positive youth development attributes. *Frontiers in Psychiatry, 13*, Article 931404. https://doi.org/10.3389/fpsyt.2022.931404

Shek, D. T. L., Leung, K. H., Dou, D. Y., & Zhu, X. Q. (2022b). Family functioning and adolescent delinquency in mainland China: Positive youth development attributes as a mediator. *Frontiers in Psychiatry, 13*, Article 883439. https://doi.org/10.3389/fpsyt.2022.883439

Shek, D. T. L., Li, X., Yu, L., Lin, L., & Chen, Y. K. (2022c). Evaluation of electronic service-learning (e-service-learning) projects in mainland China under COVID-19. *Applied Research in Quality of Life, 17*(5), 3175–3198. https://doi.org/10.1007/s11482-022-10058-8

Shek, D. T. L., Lin, L., Ma, M. S., Yu, L., Leung, T. Y., Wu, K. Y., Leung, H., & Dou, D. Y. (2021a). Perceptions of adolescents, teachers and parents of life skills education and life skills in high school students in Hong Kong. *Applied Research in Quality of Life, 16*(5), 1847–1860. https://doi.org/10.1007/s11482-020-09848-9

Shek, D. T. L., & Sun, R. C. F. (Eds.). (2013). *Development and evaluation of positive adolescent training through holistic social programs (P.A.T.H.S.)* (Vol. 3). Springer.

Shek, D. T. L., & Wu, K. Y. (2016). The Project P.A.T.H.S. in Hong Kong: Work done and lessons learned in a decade. *Journal of Pediatric & Adolescent Gynecology, 29*(1), S3-S11. https://doi.org/10.1016/j.jpag.2015.10.003

Shek, D. T. L., Yang, Z., Ma, C. M. S., & Chai, C. W. Y. (2021b). Subjective outcome evaluation of service-learning by the service recipients: Scale development, normative profiles and predictors. *Child Indicators Research, 14*(1), 411–434. https://doi.org/10.1007/s12187-020-09765-1

Shek, D. T. L., & Yu, L. (2011). A review of validated youth prevention and positive youth development programs in Asia. *International Journal of Adolescent Medicine and Health, 23*(4), 317–324. https://doi.org/10.1515/IJAMH.2011.028

Shek, D. T. L., Zhao, L., Dou, D. Y., Zhu, X. Q., & Xiao, C. (2021c). The impact of positive youth development attributes on posttraumatic stress disorder symptoms among Chinese adolescents under COVID-19. *Journal of Adolescent Health, 68*(4), 676–682. https://doi.org/10.1016/j.jadohealth.2021.01.011

Shek, D. T. L., & Zhu, X. Q. (2020). Promotion of thriving among Hong Kong Chinese adolescents: Evidence from eight-wave data. *Research on Social Work Practice, 30*(8), 870–883. https://doi.org/10.1177/1049731520947156

Soares, A. S., Pais-Ribeiro, J. L., & Silva, I. (2019). Developmental assets predictors of life satisfaction in adolescents. *Frontiers in Psychology, 10*, Article 236. https://doi.org/10.3389/fpsyg.2019.00236

Stark, R., & Bainbridge, W. S. (2012). *Religion, deviance, and social control*. Routledge.

Steinberg, L., & Lerner, R. M. (2004). The scientific study of adolescence: A brief history. *The Journal of Early Adolescence, 24*(1), 45–54. https://doi.org/10.1177/0272431603260879

Taylor, R. D., Oberle, E., Durlak, J. A., & Weissberg, R. P. (2017). Promoting positive youth development through school-based social and emotional learning interventions: A meta-analysis of follow-up effects. *Child Development, 88*(4), 1156–1171. https://doi.org/10.1111/cdev.12864

Tolan, P. H., Henry, D. B., Schoeny, M. S., Lovegrove, P., & Nichols, E. (2014). Mentoring programs to affect delinquency and associated outcomes of youth at risk: A comprehensive meta-analytic review. *Journal of Experimental Criminology, 10*(2), 179–206. https://doi.org/10.1007/s11292-013-9181-4

Tolan, P., Ross, K., Arkin, N., Godine, N., & Clark, E. (2016). Toward an integrated approach to positive development: Implications for intervention. *Applied Developmental Science, 20*(3), 214–236. https://doi.org/10.1080/10888691.2016.1146080

Trentacosta, C. J., & Fine, S. E. (2010). Emotion knowledge, social competence, and behavior problems in childhood and adolescence: A meta-analytic review. *Social Development, 19*(1), 1–29. https://doi.org/10.1111/j.1467-9507.2009.00543.x

Viadero, D. (2003, April 16). *Study finds higher gains in states with high-stakes tests.* Education Week. https://www.edweek.org/leadership/study-finds-higher-gains-in-states-with-high-stakes-tests/2003/04

Wade-Mdivanian, R., Anderson-Butcher, D., Newman, T. J., Ruderman, D. E., Smock, J., & Christie, S. (2016). Exploring the long-term impact of a positive youth development-based alcohol, tobacco and other drug prevention program. *Journal of Alcohol and Drug Education, 60*(3), 67–90. https://www.jstor.org/stable/48511403

Walsh, S., Jenner, E., Qaragholi, N., Henley, C., Demby, H., Leger, R., & Burgess, K. (2022). The impact of a high school-based positive youth development program on sexual health outcomes: Results from a randomized controlled trial. *The Journal of School Health, 92*(12), 1155–1164. https://doi.org/10.1111/josh.13216

Wyman, P. A., Cowen, E. L., Work, W. C., & Kerley, J. H. (1993). The role of children's future expectations in self-system functioning and adjustment to life stress: A prospective study of urban at-risk children. *Development and Psychopathology, 5*(4), 649–661. https://doi.org/10.1017/S0954579400006210

Zhou, Z., Shek, D. T. L., & Zhu, X. Q. (2020a). The importance of positive youth development attributes to life satisfaction and hopelessness in mainland Chinese adolescents. *Frontiers in Psychology, 11*. Article 553313 https://doi.org/10.3389/fpsyg.2020.553313

Zhou, Z., Shek, D. T. L., Zhu, X. Q., & Dou, D. Y. (2020b). Positive youth development and adolescent depression: A longitudinal study based on mainland Chinese high school students. *International Journal of Environmental Research and Public Health, 17*(12), Article 4457. https://doi.org/10.3390/ijerph17124457

Zhu, X. Q., & Shek, D. T. L. (2021). Problem behavior and life satisfaction in early adolescence: Longitudinal findings in a Chinese context. *Journal of Happiness Studies, 22*(7), 2889–2914. https://doi.org/10.1007/s10902-020-00346-1

Zych, I., Farrington, D. P., & Ttofi, M. M. (2019). Protective factors against bullying and cyberbullying: A systematic review of meta-analyses. *Aggression and Violent Behavior, 45*, 4–19. https://doi.org/10.1016/j.avb.2018.06.008

Chapter 6
Leadership Education for University Students

Daniel T. L. Shek, Xiaoqin Zhu, and Ginger C. C. Chau

Abstract Although there are different definitions of leadership, there is a consensus that leadership denotes the ability to lead others as well as oneself to achieve specific goals. Leadership emphasizes multifaceted qualities that can be nurtured and trained by appropriate training and intervention programs (e.g., leadership education). Notably, student leadership programs can enrich students' experiences, empower them to develop a sense of control over their lives and future, and cultivate qualities and competencies for future leadership roles. Generally speaking, effective student leadership programs can be embedded with diversified content and objectives, applying an integrated approach with action, reflection, learning, and practice to cultivate students' inward and outward qualities. Despite diversified leadership theories and models adopted, most effective student leadership programs concentrate on teaching leadership knowledge, building students' various leadership skills (e.g., problem-solving, planning, decision-making, and self-awareness), values, integrity, ethics, and morality, reflecting on one's behaviors, attitudes, beliefs, and values, and providing opportunities for students to perform Service-Learning or community practice under the supervision of mentors.

Keywords Leadership education · University students · Leadership training programs · Empowerment · Essential qualities of leadership · Service-Learning (SL) · Leadership skills

6.1 Introduction

The definition of leadership varies, as the concept has developed rapidly over the past decades, and diverse perspectives on skills, values, and qualities have been addressed (Haber & Komives, 2009). The concept of "leadership" carries different meanings across various professions and among practitioners, as they focus on personal qualities, psychosocial and emotional qualities, dispositions, or group orientations (Karagianni & Montgomery, 2018). Burns (1978) emphasized moral competence and ethical leadership. According to Bennis (1999), leadership is a process of developing self-awareness, learning to communicate effectively, building trustworthy relationships with others, and adopting appropriate behaviors to fulfill leadership capacities.

D. T. L. Shek, *Promoting Holistic Development in University Students*, Quality of Life in Asia 17, https://doi.org/10.1007/978-981-96-0251-3_6

Shankman and Allen (2009) also defined leadership as a process instead of a position, one that works toward or serves a greater good beyond oneself. Moreover, leaders should develop an awareness of themselves and be able to manage both themselves and others (Komives & Wagner, 2016).

To many scholars, leadership is a dynamic process and a comprehensive term emphasizing multifaceted qualities instead of pre-defined personality qualities. Therefore, leadership can be trained by appropriate interventions (Sisk, 2022). Astin and Astin (2000) viewed leaders as catalysts who foster change and help others become responsible citizens. They pointed out that leadership not only refers to the elites, appointed officials, and specific individuals but also includes those engaged in bringing about positive societal changes. Therefore, everyone can be a leader, whether or not they hold a formal title. Moreover, leadership development can enrich students' experiences in school and empower them to develop a sense of control over their lives and future. Although there are different definitions of leadership, it is commonly agreed upon that leadership denotes the ability to lead others to meet certain goals as well as leading oneself (e.g., self-leadership).

Leadership education is gaining popularity worldwide, with an increasing number of institutions and organizations promoting student leadership programs nowadays (Huber, 2002). In particular, higher education institutions are expected to be responsible for training leadership among university students. Cultivating college student leaders has been regarded as one of their primary objectives (Zimmerman-Oster & Burkhardt, 1999). According to Montgomery and Kehoe (2016), school is the first organization where students learn about and experience power, leadership, group dynamics, and self-esteem. Higher education has the power and opportunities to train future leaders through curriculum and co-curricular activities (Astin and Astin, 2000; Roberts, 2007). Nevertheless, Ricketts and Rudd (2002) criticized that university graduates could not be influential leaders and that the university did not provide sufficient and appropriate formal training for the students.

Notably, the skills needed for leaders nowadays have changed dramatically. Employers rated "problem-solving skills," "the ability to work in a team," "strong work ethic," "analytical skills," and "communication skills" as the top five skills, all of which were leadership-related (National Association of Colleges and Employers, 2023). Moreover, this study presented the top ten personal qualities desired by the job market, such as communication, motivation, teamwork, interpersonal skills, adaptability, integrity, ethics, and analytical skills. Besides, students who participated in a formal leadership training curriculum performed better in terms of the top ten personal qualities (Carter & Spotanski, 1989). The studies urged higher education institutions to provide appropriate and effective education and training to students and equip them with personal qualities and practical skills to be influential future leaders.

The early design of leadership programs for students was highly influenced by Chickering (De Larrosa & Butner, 2000). Chickering and Reisser (1993) highlighted the theoretical context for student development and urged higher educational institutions to cultivate human potential. Chickering proposed seven vectors of student development theory to explain how the college environment influences different aspects of students emotionally, interpersonally, physically, cognitively, and in terms of the development of self-identity. The seven vectors include: "developing competence," "managing emotions," "moving through autonomy toward interdependence," "developing mature interpersonal relationships," "establishing identity," "developing purpose," and "developing integrity" (Chickering & Reisser, 1993). Chickering's theory emphasizes that college students develop in a dynamic process, and each student has a unique experience (Zubernis et al., 2011) and characteristics within each vector (De Larrosa & Butner, 2000). This model has been widely recognized as one of the most predominant theories to demonstrate how college students develop and thrive (Zubernis et al., 2011). Chickering applied a comprehensive approach that included individual worldviews and holistic perspectives (Wise, 2017). His theory provided the theoretical foundation of student development in the context and showed how to achieve future success in the long run (Garfield & David, 1986).

For the past few decades, university students' leadership programs have flourished (Karagianni & Montgomery, 2018). Freeman and Goldin (2008) denoted that student leadership development programs have been experiencing a dramatic increase in the past few decades. Most leadership programs highlight two dimensions of student development: psychosocial and cognitive (De Larrosa & Butner, 2000). One aspect emphasizes the importance of acquiring and understanding theory and knowledge in traditional classroom settings. Additionally, competencies such as critical thinking, self-identity, self-efficacy, emotional management, communication skills, empathy, integrity, morality, and team spirit are equally important (Bennis & Nanus, 1985). Most leadership programs aspire to empower students to build self-awareness, explore their potential, form positive attitudes, and motivate them to initiate positive social changes. Komives et al. (2011) asserted that leadership education programs should be constructed to cultivate students' knowledge, attitude, and competence for effective leadership under different contexts. Mukoza and Goodman (2013) also highlighted that leadership programs serve as a supplementary element in many universities to fulfill their goal of training well-rounded students.

Interestingly, the definition of a student leadership program varies as well. Leadership activities can be implemented through formal classroom and extracurricular activities, such as Service-Learning (SL), residential living, community service, and student organizations (Zimmerman-Oster & Burkhardt, 1999), through which students learn how to collaborate to serve the institution or society. Heifetz (1994) advocated a collaborative approach to cultivate effective leadership. Des Marais and Farzanehkia (2000) asserted that several elements should be embedded in student leadership programs, including establishing healthy relationships with others, empowering youth to take responsibility for their actions, providing learning opportunities, and appreciating their experience, knowledge, and competence. Haber (2006) stated that formal leadership programs enrich university students' understanding, competence, and values by providing learning opportunities through different strategies, such as councils, formal courses, retreats, workshops, mentorship, and consulting services. Many models highlight that managing oneself, embracing purpose and commitment, and developing one's value are crucial for university students (Goleman et al., 2001; Haber & Komives, 2009). The programs aim to inspire students to become change agents to bring about effective societal functioning.

6.2 Benefits of Leadership Programs

As mentioned, leadership programs in the university have different focuses. Therefore, different researchers have demonstrated the influence of these programs from various perspectives. Primarily, many scholars focus on the impact of cultivating fundamental skills that are needed to be a leader. Astin and Astin (2000) noted that formal leadership programs prepare students with essential skills required as future leaders. They further noted that involvement in student organizations, community service, and leadership education could enable students to achieve their personal goals. Equally important, some researchers emphasize the importance of ethical leadership and moral competence (Burns, 1978). If a student program is embedded with ethical leadership and can address the needs of organizations and society, the program is expected to influence both the students and the communities positively (Kiersch & Peters, 2017).

Many studies have utilized quantitative research to demonstrate that student leadership programs benefit students' personal development. According to one study on the effectiveness of 31 leadership programs, Zimmerman-Oster and Burkhardt (1999) found that students benefit from different aspects of personal and interpersonal development, including enhanced personal values and social engagement, more commitment to community services, developed communication skills, self-identity and self-worth, and integrity and ethics, which were consistent with the intended outcomes of the programs. More importantly, the programs not only positively impact student leadership skills but also influence the psychosocial aspects of students, such as personal growth and self-efficacy. In the follow-up study conducted by Cress et al. (2001), they applied grounded theory research and investigated student leadership programs in ten universities. The study showed that the programs positively influenced students' learning and personal development regarding civic engagement, leadership skills, cultural competence, leadership knowledge, and personal and organizational values. These studies show that leadership qualities can be taught and trained through leadership programs and activities.

Besides quantitative studies, researchers also utilized qualitative methods in the evaluation process. For instance, DiPaolo (2002) conducted a case study and found that students developed more positive values after participating in a 5-day leadership program. Furthermore, Hobbs and Spencer (2002) evaluated a 2-week leadership training program and reported that participants' communication and character-building skills were enhanced. Hoyt and Kennedy (2008) conducted interviews and focus groups in their assessment, and the participants reported that their initial understanding of leadership was insufficient and wrong before joining the program. Although they had hesitations in referring to themselves as leaders or spotting leadership qualities in themselves, the program broadened their horizons and built their confidence and self-awareness. Moreover, the interviewees stated that they had learned practical methods to tackle challenges, developed more confidence to manage their lives, and were inspired to be leaders in the future.

Generally speaking, many studies have shown that student leadership programs can cultivate student leaders with qualities and competencies for future leadership roles. In the study by Cohen et al. (2011), students revealed that apart from learning the skills, awareness, and knowledge acquired in the classroom setting, they learned how to apply them in their daily lives. Moreover, they agreed that the leadership program enhanced their confidence in job-hunting and helped them in the future. The students learned how to tackle challenges effectively and desired to act as change agents to bring about positive changes. The program conducted by Mukoza and Goodman (2013) also showed that the participants became more confident in performing leadership roles after joining leadership programs. Moreover, they became critical thinkers, being able to tackle challenges and resolve conflicts.

Research also showed that different leadership programs produce positive outcomes for the students. Notably, student leadership programs with elements of SL can help university students take up social responsibilities and react to social crises or global challenges. As Zimmerman-Oster and Burkhardt (1999) proposed, the forms of activities, such as SL, residential living, community service, and student organizations, can be diversified. Shek et al. (2021) demonstrated that SL programs can enhance students' interpersonal and intrapersonal competence. Many universities utilize practice-based learning, experiential learning, and SL to train students with effective communication skills, problem-solving abilities, and national and international perspectives (Shek et al., 2017). For instance, Shek and Cheung (2013) revealed that students taking SL courses experience holistic development and demonstrate positive changes in civic engagement, psychosocial competence, self-efficacy, social responsibility, as well as interpersonal and intrapersonal competence. Students have served as catalysts in leadership development programs. Schmalenbach et al. (2022) implemented elements of experiential learning, SL, and peer-assisted learning in their LIFE program, leading to students improving in leadership, teamwork, analytical thinking, and personal growth. In another study, Ferdiansyah et al. (2022) proved that SL programs can engage students in community service effectively and address the community's needs, especially during the pandemic. The students have developed more team-building skills and improved their interpersonal skills significantly.

Specifically, researchers have investigated the effectiveness of programs with different durations. Leadership programs are proven to have long-term effects on participants. In the follow-up study of a leadership development program after ten years, Garza (2000) ascertained that the program influenced the students' acquisition of leadership qualities and job-related competence in a positive way. Moreover, the program influenced the students' choice of further study. However, Dugan and Komives (2007) suggested that a short- or moderate-duration program produced more positive influence than programs with a longer duration. Possible reasons may be stagnation or students' self-doubt about their capacity or value of leadership. They highlighted that clarification of program outcomes and carefully designed program durations are needed. Posner (2009) examined the effect of a leadership program over time on students, tracking them from freshman to senior years. He reported that the participants showed significant changes in their leadership behaviors after three years. The studies show that leadership programs could positively impact students' leadership qualities in the long run. A similar conclusion was reached by Rosch and Caza (2012) that short-term leadership training programs cultivate a more integrated understanding of leadership among students, and this effect lasts over time.

6.3 Essential Qualities of Leadership

Exploring the theoretical foundation of leadership can help investigate why leadership programs positively influence students and what elements should be emphasized in leadership programs. Different scholars and practitioners have proposed various definitions of leadership, and the contents and forms of leadership training have also been diversified. Primarily, the Social Change Model of leadership development (SCM) was developed for university students who aspire to be socially responsible citizens and initiate social changes in their lives (Astin et al., 1996). SCM regards leadership as a "purposeful, collaborative, values-oriented process that generates positive social change" (Komives & Wagner, 2016). Therefore, leadership is inclusive and available for all people. Moreover, "community involvement and community service could be 'powerful vehicles' for the development of leadership qualities" (Astin, 1996). Notably, SCM was one of the most famous models in guiding student leadership development programs (Astin et al., 1996; Haber, 2006; Kezar et al., 2006). The model emphasizes the values of the "seven Cs," namely "consciousness of self," "congruence," "commitment," "collaboration," "common purpose," "controversy with civility," and "citizenship." All seven values work together in the process of initiating the transcendent "C" of "change" (Astin et al., 1996). Dugan (2006) agreed that the SCM model facilitates students' cultivation of self-awareness and competencies when working in a group. Haber and Komives (2009) suggested that higher education should offer diversified chances and sufficient resources for students on campus and in the community to experience leadership development. They demonstrated that multifaceted forms of formal and informal activities, such as involvement in student organizations' curricular or co-curricular programs, should be included in leadership programs.

Second, Conger (1992) suggested four strategies for developing student leaders: personal growth, conceptual knowledge, feedback, and skill building. In his view, effective leadership training should not be a one-week workshop but should integrate various approaches to facilitate learning and practice. Firstly, personal growth denotes reflection on behaviors, values, and aspirations, and it aims to increase students' self-awareness and facilitate self-exploration (Conger, 1992). Activities include group and individual reflection, SL, team building, and networking (Allen & Hartman, 2008). Moreover, the conceptual overview emphasizes enhancing one's knowledge base through various kinds of exposure, such as self-paced learning, class-based learning, or degree programs. Additionally, feedback provides participants with different tools and exercises to reveal their personalities, strengths, weaknesses, and values (Smith, 1993). Lastly, skill-building activities, such as games, personal development plans, or action learning, could develop participants' competence through actual mechanical processes (Conger, 1992). Nowadays, most leadership programs in universities have implemented some or all of the four methods.

Third, the transformational leadership theory proposed by Burns (1978) is gaining popularity nowadays. Burns (1978) stated that leadership can be relational, collective, and purposeful, and it aims to engage followers, cater to personal needs and group goals, and be socially responsible citizens. Tichy and Devanna (1986) highlighted seven qualities of transformational leaders, including being change agents, being courageous, having faith in people, being driven by values, being committed to lifelong learning, being able to address problems with uncertainty, and being a forward thinker. Ingleton (2013) argued that the transformational leadership theory can serve as a well-suited theoretical foundation for student development programs to equip students with skills and values needed in society and initiate positive changes.

Besides the above mainstream models, some scholars proposed other approaches. To name a few, Van Linden and Fertman (1998) listed three stages (having awareness, motivation interaction, and gaining mastery) and five dimensions (gaining knowledge, formulating positive values, facilitating communication, developing analytical skills, and emphasizing stress management skills) for youth leadership development. This model combines cognitive, emotional, and behavioral dimensions of youth development. Furthermore, Ricketts and Rudd (2002) proposed five elements of leadership education curriculum for youth, including (1) conceptual knowledge of leadership, (2) attitude, will, and desire, (3) analytical skills, (4) communication skills, and (5) interpersonal and intrapersonal relationships. Additionally, Straker (2008) emphasized that leadership qualities are influenced by the personal characteristics of leaders. Therefore, educators should focus on training students' personal qualities such as self-awareness of their strengths and weaknesses, trustworthiness, and cooperation.

The multifold theoretical basis of youth leadership programs suggests that the ingredients of these programs would be diversified. Nevertheless, leadership development programs are contextual, and the contents of such programs should be specifically designed to expose students to diverse learning opportunities (Allen & Hartman, 2008). In response to this call, various higher institutions have implemented multifaceted approaches in their programs to cultivate their student leaders. Therefore, choosing suitable approaches that cater to the school's characteristics, the students' development stage, and society's needs is necessary.

In terms of the learning outcomes, different programs emphasize diverse dimensions of leadership skills in their training. For instance, Robinson (2009) highlighted that leadership programs should embed the cultivation of ethical leadership and multicultural competence. Seemiller and Murray (2013) proposed eight categories of competencies, including "learning and reasoning," "self-awareness and development," "interpersonal interactions," "group dynamics," "civic responsibility," "communication," "strategic planning," and "personal behavior." Additionally, the leadership program implemented by Hendricks et al. (2010) aimed to develop six personal qualities of leadership, including "integrity," "dedication," "magnanimity," "humility," "openness," and "creativity," based on the philosophy of Bennis (2009).

6.4 Ways of Cultivating Leadership Skills

One powerful tool proposed by many scholars to cultivate leadership skills is reflection. The concept of "reflective leaders" has been identified and emphasized by many scholars and practitioners (Guthrie & Jones, 2012; Harvey & Jenkins, 2014; Hendricks et al., 2018; Lowe & Gardner, 2000). According to Roberts and Westville (2008), reflection is "critically thinking about one's behaviors, experiences, attitudes, beliefs, and values." They recommended that practitioners apply journal writing, group discussion in class, and dialogue through emails, websites, or discussion boards to facilitate students' reflective practice. Huber (2002) encouraged students to be involved in reflective practice to contemplate their behaviors and experiences and identify their values, attitudes, and beliefs, thus building the linkage between their inner self and the outside world. Morrison (1996) showed that students developed an enhanced level of self-awareness, self-efficacy, and self-value after conducting concrete reflection. Through reflection, students can build their value system and develop a concrete understanding of their strengths and weaknesses. They can also integrate their personal experiences and learning to gain a deeper understanding of themselves, personally, interpersonally, privately, or publicly (Roberts & Westville, 2008).

Another important vehicle for nurturing leadership is mentorship. Buckner and Williams (1995) highlighted that peer mentoring is effective when student leaders can act as mentors in a leadership program. Mentors can inspire students to develop self-awareness of leadership qualities and transfer and share information directly in that specific environment (Posner, 2009). The mentor–mentee relationship is a dynamic and mutually beneficial bonding, fostering personal growth, engagement, and acquisition of leadership skills (Hendricks et al., 2010). Chang et al. (2003) also implemented mentorship training and encouraged students to be role models, advisors, counselors, leaders, friends, and listeners. Besides theoretical knowledge, students practiced leadership skills through role-playing, public speaking, and team management activities. Moreover, they worked with local leaders in the program and participated in a community project to gain practical experience in leadership.

In order to meet the needs of the service economy and globalization, leaders are expected to lead an organization or group under different situations, which highlights the need to train future leaders' global outlook. Gregersen et al. (1998) proposed four approaches: traveling abroad, working with people from diverse backgrounds, participating in projects actively, and completing projects overseas. In this way, young people can be leaders in their lives and the outside world. Shek and Ng (2017) asserted that student leadership is related to building personal capacities, facilitating interpersonal communications, fostering teamwork, committing to community service, and inspiring a national and international outlook. Therefore, a global outlook is a crucial quality for future leaders.

Equally important, many scholars emphasize the importance of SL activities in leadership training programs. In SL, young people have opportunities to be involved in solving more comprehensive real-life problems. Moreover, they can act as change agents to address the real needs of the community. Des Marais and Farzanehkia (2000) proposed that young people can cultivate leadership in real-life contexts and that SL can effectively promote leadership development among youths. They argued that public policy-making, as well as analytical, communication, and management skills, could be trained through SL so that youths can learn about themselves and the outside world. Hoyt and Kennedy (2008) encouraged students to actively participate in community service and civic engagement to develop leadership qualities. Dugan et al. (2011) reinforced that experiential learning strategies, SL, mentoring relationships, and facilitating conversations across differences are critical factors in leadership program delivery. They urged universities and educators to incorporate these elements into their programs to train effective leaders. Similarly, Ngai et al. (2012) concluded that leadership training programs commonly use strategies such as experiential learning, SL, adventure-based training, international exposure, and project-based learning.

Interestingly, an increasing number of practitioners are proposing innovative approaches in student leadership programs. For instance, Jackson and Kelley (2002) asserted that the employment of technology, such as online learning, should be added to respond to the needs of globalization. Moreover, Shek and Chung (2018) believed that it is essential to cultivate youth leadership qualities through an alternative version of STEM education, which includes soft skills (e.g., interpersonal communication), trust (gaining trust from others), empathy (showing empathy toward others' feelings and experiences), and moral character (possessing sound moral reasoning). STEM education can prepare young students to be qualified leaders in service economies.

Apart from the co-curricular projects, some universities set up formal curricula in the form of credit-bearing subjects to nurture student leaders. For instance, the Global Youth Leadership Institute was established to train future leaders with essential skills, values, and characteristics (Shek et al., 2017, 2020). Firstly, the program invites prestigious leaders to share their vision and experience with the students. Moreover, it provides intensive training with lectures, field visits, and SL. Additionally, there is an experiential leadership training camp to consolidate the conceptual views of leadership and further cultivate leadership skills through experiential learning. Remarkably, both local and exchange students can enroll in this program to inspire cross-fertilization, mutual understanding, and multicultural competence among students.

Researchers investigated the effectiveness of various strategies and evaluated which activities should be included in student leadership programs. For instance, Zimmerman-Oster and Burkhardt (1999) reported that the most popular leadership program activities are conducting seminars and workshops, inviting mentors and guest speakers, and encouraging volunteer services. Moreover, strategies such as skill building, involvement in community, tackling intercultural issues, and public policy should be addressed in these programs. DiPaolo (2002) stated that outdoor activities, SL programs, and self-assessment and reflection are components of a successful leadership education program. Huber (2002) showed that encouraging students to participate in SL or volunteer activities in the community enriches students' experience, empowers them to be active and effective leaders, and better aligns with their aspirations. Micari et al. (2010) stated that one-day workshops, extracurricular activities, or credit-bearing courses were popular among the programs. Jenkins (2013) investigated 24 commonly used approaches in student leadership programs and concluded that educators preferred discussion-based methods and instructional approaches that could develop students' conceptual learning and personal growth. They also found that studying abroad and leadership retreats were often applied in most student leadership programs. However, traditional assessments such as tests or examinations and skill-building activities were seldom used in the programs. These studies have provided insight for higher education institutions and practitioners to implement effective and appropriate student leadership programs. With reference to Hong Kong, we have used Service-Learning as a vehicle to nurture the development of leadership qualities in university students (Li et al., 2023; Lin & Shek, 2021, 2023; Shek et al., 2022; Zhu et al., 2024).

In conclusion, students' leadership programs may be embedded with diversified content and objectives. Generally speaking, leadership programs should apply an integrated approach with action, reflection, learning, and practice to cultivate leaders' inward and outward qualities. No matter which elements of theories or models the programs have applied, most programs include four elements: leadership knowledge, skill building, reflection, and SL or community practice. Firstly, they taught leadership skills, including values, integrity, ethics, and morality in decision-making, as leadership knowledge and skills can be trained in the classroom (Bennis, 2009). Additionally, leadership skills require leaders to be aware of their talents and limitations and take effective action to address them (Lowe & Gardner, 2000). Effective leaders must have effective problem-solving skills, planning strategies, setting priorities, and making judgments (Gardner, 1990; Hart & Pounder, 1999; Jackson & Kelley, 2002). Besides teaching various leadership skills, reflecting on one's behaviors, attitudes, beliefs, and values is another powerful tool to prepare students with complex and multicultural competence (Hendricks et al., 2018; Roberts & Westville, 2008). Equally important, students should also be given the chance to work out to complete community development projects, preferably under the supervision of mentors (Dugan & Komives, 2007; Hendricks et al., 2010). Besides, SL is a vital vehicle to nurture youth leadership qualities, which will be discussed in the next chapter.

Acknowledgements The preparation of this chapter is financially supported by The Hong Kong Polytechnic University (ZZ4U and ZZUE), Li and Fung Endowed Professorship in Service Leadership Education, Wofoo Foundation, and the Matching Fund of Research Grants Council (ZECL and ZH4Q).

References

Allen, S. J., & Hartman, N. S. (2008). Leadership development: An exploration of sources of learning. *SAM Advanced Management Journal, 73*(1), 10–19.

Astin, A. W., & Astin, H. S. (2000). *Leadership reconsidered: Engaging higher education in social change.* W. K. Kellogg Foundation. https://files.eric.ed.gov/fulltext/ED444437.pdf

Astin, A. W., Astin, H. S., Boatsman, K., Bonous-Hammarth, M., Chambers, T., Goldberg, S., Johnson, C. S., Komives, S. R., Langdon, E. A., Leland, C., Lucas, N., Pope, R. L., Roberts, D., & Shellog, K. M. (1996). *A social change model of leadership development: Guidebook (version III).* Higher Education Research Institute.

Astin, H. S. (1996). Leadership for social change. *About Campus, 1*(3), 4–10. https://doi.org/10.1002/abc.6190010302

Bennis, W. (1999). The leadership advantage. *Leader to Leader, 12*(2), 18–23. https://doi.org/10.1002/ltl.40619991205

Bennis, W. (2009). *On becoming a leader.* Basic Books.

Bennis, W., & Nanus, B. (1985). *Leaders: The strategies for taking charge.* Harper & Row.

Buckner, J. K., & Williams, M. L. (1995, November 18–21). *Reconceptualizing university student leadership development programs: Applying the competing values model* [Conference presentation]. The 81st Annual Meeting of the Speech Communication Association, San Antonio, TX, United States.

Burns, J. (1978). *Leadership.* Harper & Row.

Carter, R. I., & Spotanski, D. R. (1989). Perceptions of leadership and personal development of selected high school students in Iowa. *Journal of Agricultural Education, 30*(4), 30–34. https://doi.org/10.5032/jae.1989.04030

Chang, P. P. W., Cohen, L., Pike, L. T., Pooley, J. A., & Breen, L. (2003). The Edith Cowan University School of Psychology mentoring programme: From reducing attrition to building learning communities. In F. Kochan & J. Pascarelle (Eds.), *Global perspectives of the reconstruction of contexts, learning communities and cultures through mentoring* (pp. 277–293). Information Age Publishing.

Chickering, A. W., & Reisser, L. (1993). *Education and identity* (2nd ed.). Jossey-Bass.

Cohen, L., Chang, P. P., Hendricks, J., Cope, V., & Harman, B. (2011). Enhancing psychology students' experiences: The development of an undergraduate leadership programme. *Psychology Learning & Teaching, 10*(2), 164–169. https://doi.org/10.2304/plat.2011.10.2.164

Conger, J. A. (1992). *Learning to lead: The art of transforming managers into leaders* (1st ed.). Jossey-Bass.

Cress, C. M., Astin, H. S., Zimmerman-Oster, K., & Burkhardt, J. C. (2001). Developmental outcomes of college students' involvement in leadership activities. *Journal of College Student Development, 42*, 15–27.

De Larrosa, L. L., & Butner, B. (2000, May 5). *Chickering's seven vectors of student development explained* [Paper presentation]. McNair Scholars Program, Texas Tech University, Lubbock, TX, United States. http://kvccdocs.com/KVCC/2013-Spring/FY125-OLA/content/L-17/Chickering-Vectors-Explained.pdf

Des Marais, J., & Farzanehkia, F. (2000). Service-learning leadership development for youths. *Phi Delta Kappan, 81*(9), 678–680. https://digitalcommons.unomaha.edu/cgi/viewcontent.cgi?article=1050&context=slcestgen

DiPaolo, D. G. (2002). Voices of leadership. *Journal of Leadership Education, 1*(2), 62–77. https://doi.org/10.12806/V1/I2/RF4

Dugan, J. P. (2006). Explorations using the social change model: Leadership development among college men and women. *Journal of College Student Development, 47*(2), 217–225. https://doi.org/10.1353/csd.2006.0015

Dugan, J. P., Bohle, C. W., Gebhardt, M., Hofert, M., Wilk, E., & Cooney, M. A. (2011). Influences of leadership program participation on students' capacities for socially responsible leadership.

Journal of Student Affairs Research and Practice, 48(1), 65–84. https://doi.org/10.2202/1949-6605.6206
Dugan, J. P., & Komives, S. R. (2007). *Developing leadership capacity in college students: Findings from a national study*. National Clearinghouse for Leadership Programs.
Ferdiansyah, S., Winarno, A., & Ardhita, Z. (2022). Service learning in Indonesia: Developing undergraduate students' leadership during COVID-19 pandemic. *Higher Education, Skills and Work-Based Learning, 12*(5), 884–899. https://doi.org/10.1108/HESWBL-06-2021-0123
Freeman, J. P., & Goldin, A. (2008). The increasing importance of student leadership development programs in higher education. *NASPA Net Results*, 1–5.
Gardner, J. W. (1990). Leadership and the future. *The Futurist, 24*(3), 8.
Garfield, N. J., & David, L. B. (1986). Arthur Chickering: Bridging theory and practice in student development. *Journal of Counseling & Development, 64*(8), 483–491. https://doi.org/10.1002/j.1556-6676.1986.tb01178.x
Garza, O. G. (2000). *A ten-year follow-up study of the completers' perceptions of the TAMU Community College and Technical Institute Leadership Development Program: Minority Leadership Development Project* (Publication No. 9980148) [Doctoral dissertation, Texas A&M University]. ProQuest Dissertations & Theses Global.
Goleman, D., Boyatzis, R., & McKee, A. (2001). Primal leadership: The hidden driver of great performance. *Harvard Business Review, 79*(11), 42–51.
Gregersen, H. B., Morrison, A. J., & Black, J. S. (1998). Developing leaders for the global frontier. *Sloan Management Review, 40*(1), 21–33. https://link.gale.com/apps/doc/A21276831/AONE?u=anon~e71ecd3d&sid=googleScholar&xid=609741f5
Guthrie, K. L., & Jones, T. B. (2012). Teaching and learning: Using experiential learning and reflection for leadership education. *New Directions for Student Services, 2012*(140), 53–63. https://doi.org/10.1002/ss.20031
Haber, P. (2006). Structure, design, and models of student leadership programs. In S. R. Komives, J. P. Dugan, J. E. Owen, C. Slack, & W. Wagner (Eds.), *Handbook for student leadership programs* (pp. 29–51). National Clearinghouse for Leadership Programs.
Haber, P., & Komives, S. R. (2009). Predicting the individual values of the social change model of leadership development: The role of college students' leadership and involvement experiences. *Journal of Leadership Education, 7*(3), 133–166. https://doi.org/10.12806/V7/I3/RF4
Hart, A. W., & Pounder, D. G. (1999). Reinventing preparation programs: A decade of activity. In J. Murphy & P. B. Forsyth (Eds.), *Educational administration: A decade of reform* (pp. 115–151). Corwin Press.
Harvey, M., & Jenkins, D. M. (2014). Knowledge, praxis, and reflection: The three critical elements of effective leadership studies programs. *Journal of Leadership Studies, 7*(4), 76–85. https://doi.org/10.1002/jls.21314
Heifetz, R. A. (1994). *Leadership without easy answers*. Harvard University Press. https://doi.org/10.4159/9780674038479
Hendricks, D. G., Yasuhara, K., & Taylor, A. C. (2018, June 24–27). *Enhancing student leadership competencies through reflection* [Conference presentation]. 2018 ASEE Annual Conference & Exposition, Salt Lake City, UT, United States. https://doi.org/10.18260/1-2--30428
Hendricks, J. M., Cope, V. C., & Harris, M. (2010). A leadership program in an undergraduate nursing course in Western Australia: Building leaders in our midst. *Nurse Education Today, 30*(3), 252–257. https://doi.org/10.1016/j.nedt.2009.12.007
Hobbs, E., & Spencer, S. (2002, February 7–9). *Perceived change in leadership skills as a result of the Wilderness Education Association wilderness stewardship course* [Paper presentation]. Wilderness Education Association 2002 National Conference, Bradford Woods, IN, United States.
Hoyt, M. A., & Kennedy, C. L. (2008). Leadership and adolescent girls: A qualitative study of leadership development. *American Journal of Community Psychology, 42*(3–4), 203–219. https://doi.org/10.1007/s10464-008-9206-8

Huber, N. S. (2002). Approaching leadership education in the new millennium. *Journal of Leadership Education, 1*(1), 25–34. https://doi.org/10.12806/V1/I1/C3

Ingleton, T. (2013). College student leadership development: Transformational leadership as a theoretical foundation. *International Journal of Academic Research in Business and Social Sciences, 3*(7), 219–229. https://doi.org/10.6007/IJARBSS/v3-i7/28

Jackson, B. L., & Kelley, C. (2002). Exceptional and innovative programs in educational leadership. *Educational Administration Quarterly, 38*(2), 192–212. https://doi.org/10.1177/0013161X0238 2005

Jenkins, D. M. (2013). Exploring instructional strategies in student leadership development programming. *Journal of Leadership Studies, 6*(4), 48–62. https://doi.org/10.1002/jls.21266

Karagianni, D., & Montgomery, A. J. (2018). Developing leadership skills among adolescents and young adults: A review of leadership programmes. *International Journal of Adolescence and Youth, 23*(1), 86–98. https://doi.org/10.1080/02673843.2017.1292928

Kezar, A., Carducci, R., & Contreras-McGavin, M. (2006). *Rethinking the "L" word in higher education: The revolution of research on leadership.* Wiley.

Kiersch, C., & Peters, J. (2017). Leadership from the inside out: Student leadership development within authentic leadership and servant leadership frameworks. *Journal of Leadership Education, 16*(1), 148–168. https://doi.org/10.12806/V16/I1/T4

Komives, S. R., Dugan, J. P., Owen, J. E., Slack, C., & Wagner, W. (2011). *The handbook for student leadership development* (2nd ed.). Jossey-Bass.

Komives, S. R., & Wagner, W. (2016). *Leadership for a better world: Understanding the social change model of leadership development* (2nd ed.). Wiley.

Li, X., Shek, D. T. L., Mok, B. P. W., Shek, E. Y. W., & Bai, Y. P. (2023). Effectiveness of electronic service-learning (e-SL) in primary school children in China during the COVID-19 pandemic. *Applied Research in Quality of Life, 19*(6), 3081–3108. https://doi.org/10.1007/s11482-023-102 44-2

Lin, L., & Shek, D. T. L. (2021). Serving children and adolescents in need during the COVID-19 pandemic: Evaluation of service-learning subjects with and without face-to-face interaction. *International Journal of Environmental Research and Public Health, 18*(4), Article 2114. https://doi.org/10.3390/ijerph18042114

Lin, L., Shek, D. T. L., & Li, X. (2023). Who benefits and appreciates more? An evaluation of online service-learning projects in mainland China during the COVID-19 pandemic. *Applied Research in Quality of Life, 18*(2), 625–646. https://doi.org/10.1007/s11482-022-10081-9

Lowe, K. B., & Gardner, W. L. (2000). Ten years of the leadership quarterly: Contributions and challenges for the future. *The Leadership Quarterly, 11*(4), 459–514. https://doi.org/10.1016/S1048-9843(00)00059-X

Micari, M., Gould, A. K., & Lainez, L. (2010). Becoming a leader along the way: Embedding leadership training into a large-scale peer-learning program in the STEM disciplines. *Journal of College Student Development, 51*(2), 218–230. https://doi.org/10.1353/csd.0.0125

Montgomery, A., & Kehoe, I. (Eds.). (2016). *Reimagining the purpose of schools and educational organisations: Developing critical thinking, agency, beliefs in schools and educational organisations.* Springer. https://doi.org/10.1007/978-3-319-24699-4

Morrison, K. (1996). Developing reflective practice in higher degree students through a learning journal. *Studies in Higher Education, 21*(3), 317–332. https://doi.org/10.1080/030750796123 31381241

Mukoza, S. K., & Goodman, S. (2013). Building leadership capacity: An evaluation of the University of Cape Town's Emerging Student Leaders Programme. *Industry and Higher Education, 27*(2), 129–137. https://doi.org/10.5367/ihe.2013.0147

National Association of Colleges and Employers. (2023, April 27). *The job market for the class of 2023: Key skills/competencies employers are seeking and the impact of career center use* [Press release]. https://www.naceweb.org/about-us/press/5bcffa5b-6fa6-4091-860e-c5ae5b103949

Ngai, N. P., Cheung, C. K., Ngai, S. S. Y., & To, S. M. (2012). Youth leadership training in Hong Kong: Current developments and the way ahead. *International Journal of Adolescence and Youth, 17*(2–3), 165–179. https://doi.org/10.1080/02673843.2012.656192

Posner, B. Z. (2009). A longitudinal study examining changes in students' leadership behavior. *Journal of College Student Development, 50*(5), 551–563. https://doi.org/10.1353/csd.0.0091

Ricketts, J. C., & Rudd, R. D. (2002). A comprehensive leadership education model to train, teach, and develop leadership in youth. *Journal of Career and Technical Education, 19*(1), 7–17. https://doi.org/10.21061/jcte.v19i1.655

Roberts, C., & Westville, I. (2008). Developing future leaders: The role of reflection in the classroom. *Journal of Leadership Education, 7*(1), 116–130. https://doi.org/10.12806/V7/I1/AB1

Roberts, D. C. (2007). *Deeper learning in leadership: Helping college students find the potential within.* Wiley.

Robinson, J. E. (2009). *Developing a student-centered leadership program at East Stroudsburg University* (Publication No. 3379866) [Doctoral dissertation, Rowan University]. ProQuest Dissertations & Theses Global.

Rosch, D. M., & Caza, A. (2012). The durable effects of short-term programs on student leadership development. *Journal of Leadership Education, 11*(1), 28–48. https://doi.org/10.12806/V11/I1/RF2

Schmalenbach, C., Monterrosa, H., Cabrera Larín, A. R., & Jurkowski, S. (2022). The LIFE programme—University students learning leadership and teamwork through service learning in El Salvador. *Intercultural Education, 33*(4), 470–483. https://doi.org/10.1080/14675986.2022.2090689

Seemiller, C., & Murray, T. (2013). The common language of leadership. *Journal of Leadership Studies, 7*(1), 33–45. https://doi.org/10.1002/jls.21277

Shankman, M. L., & Allen, S. J. (2009). *Emotionally intelligent leadership: A guide for college students.* Wiley.

Shek, D. T. L., & Cheung, B. P. (2013). Developmental issues of university students in Hong Kong. *International Journal of Adolescent Medicine and Health, 25*(4), 345–351. https://doi.org/10.1515/ijamh-2013-0032

Shek, D. T. L., & Chung, B. P. (2018). The quest for an alternative paradigm of STEM education for young people. *International Journal of Child and Adolescent Health, 11*(3), 259–270. https://ira.lib.polyu.edu.hk/bitstream/10397/93709/1/APSS-0395_Shek_Quest_Alternative_Paradigm.pdf

Shek, D. T. L., Li, X., Yu, L., Lin, L., & Chen, Y. (2022). Evaluation of electronic service-learning (e-service-learning) projects in mainland China under COVID-19. *Applied Research in Quality of Life, 17*(5), 3175–3198. https://doi.org/10.1007/s11482-022-10058-8

Shek, D. T. L., Ma, C., & Yang, Z. (2020). Transformation and development of university students through service-learning: A corporate-community-university partnership initiative in Hong Kong (Project WeCan). *Applied Research in Quality of Life, 15*(5), 1375–1393. https://doi.org/10.1007/s11482-019-09738-9

Shek, D. T. L., & Ng, E. C. (2017). Leadership training for university students in Hong Kong: A critical review. *International Journal of Child & Adolescent Health, 10*(1), 25–40. https://web-p-ebscohost-com.ezproxy.lb.polyu.edu.hk/ehost/pdfviewer/pdfviewer?vid=0&sid=497c2c2c-ce37-438c-8164-de49e148b4ad%40redis

Shek, D. T. L., Yang, Z., Ma, C. M. S., & Chai, C. W. Y. (2021). Subjective outcome evaluation of service-learning by the service recipients: Scale development, normative profiles and predictors. *Child Indicators Research, 14*(1), 411–434. https://doi.org/10.1007/s12187-020-09765-1

Shek, D. T. L., Yuen-Tsang, A. W. K, & Ng, E. C. W. (2017). Global Youth Leadership Institute: A platform to nurture leadership in university students. *International Journal of Child & Adolescent Health, 10*(1), 17–23. https://web-p-ebscohost-com.ezproxy.lb.polyu.edu.hk/ehost/pdfviewer/pdfviewer?vid=0&sid=703dea49-397c-44da-8af1-47e6ed4509f8%40redis

Sisk, D. (Ed.). (2022). *Gifted education, creativity and leadership development.* MDPI. https://doi.org/10.3390/books978-3-0365-5640-6

Smith, D. C. (1993). Learning to lead: The art of transforming managers into leaders. *Journal of Business Ethics, 12*(9), 676–688.
Straker, D. (2008). *Leadership vs. management*. ChangingMinds. http://changingminds.org/disciplines/leadership/articles/manager_leader.htm
Tichy, N. M., & Devanna, M. A. (1986). The transformational leader. *Training & Development Journal, 40*(7), 27–32.
Van Linden, J. A., & Fertman, C. I. (1998). *Youth leadership: A guide to understanding leadership development in adolescents*. Jossey-Bass.
Wise, S. M. (2017). Chickering's theory and the seven vectors of development. In W. K. Killam & S. Degges-White (Eds.), *College student development: Applying theory to practice on the diverse campus* (pp. 101–110). Springer. https://doi.org/10.1891/9780826118165.0010
Zhu, X., Wu, X., Zhang, S., & Shek, D. T. L. (2024). Evaluation of an electronic service-learning course utilizing regular and intensive delivery modes: The Hong Kong experience. *Research on Social Work Practice, 34*(8), 873–887. https://doi.org/10.1177/10497315231207054
Zimmerman-Oster, K., & Burkhardt, J. (1999). *Leadership in the making: Impact and insights from leadership development programs in US colleges and universities*. W. K. Kellogg Foundation. https://files.eric.ed.gov/fulltext/ED446577.pdf
Zubernis, L., Snyder, M., & McCoy, V. A. (2011). Counseling lesbian and gay college students through the lens of Cass's and Chickering's developmental models. *Journal of LGBT Issues in Counseling, 5*(2), 122–150. https://doi.org/10.1080/15538605.2011.578506

Chapter 7
Service-Learning as a Vehicle for Youth Holistic Development

Daniel T. L. Shek, Xiang Li, and Ginger C. C. Chau

Abstract This chapter introduces Service-Learning (SL) as an innovative pedagogical approach that fosters the holistic development of youth in higher education. Grounded in the classic educational theories of Dewey, Kolb, and Mezirow, SL emphasizes the importance of critical reflection on service experiences. Through a review of empirical evidence, this chapter further highlights the multifaceted impacts of SL on four principal stakeholders: students, service recipients, teachers, and communities. It demonstrates how SL facilitates mutually beneficial relationships among these parties. This chapter also discusses the implementation of SL in a global context, with a specific focus on The Hong Kong Polytechnic University (PolyU) as a notable example. Furthermore, the chapter addresses the successful adaptation of SL to electronic SL (e-SL) in response to the COVID-19 pandemic. In conclusion, the collective evidence supports the role of SL in bridging academic knowledge with real-world practice and community engagement. This underscores its significance as a valuable educational approach for the holistic development of youth.

Keywords Service-learning (SL) · Holistic development · SL theories · Impact · Global implementation · Hong Kong · Electronic service-learning (E-SL)

7.1 The Nature of Service-Learning

As a form of experiential learning, Service-Learning (SL) is gaining popularity in higher education. It has been recognized as an influential approach in promoting students' holistic learning, civic engagement, and personal development through providing community service and doing reflective practice. During the past few decades, a growing number of practitioners and universities have integrated SL subjects into their academic curricula (Giles & Eyler, 1994). As one of the pedagogies that emphasizes students' civic development, Kuh and Schneider (2008) pointed out that "SL is a high-impact educational practice and can prepare students for their work and life challenges and develop their citizenship effectively."

There have been two significant steps in the field of SL research. One milestone was the coining of the term "Service-Learning" in 1967 by Robert Sigmon, and another was Stanton's integration of SL into higher education in 1991 (Giles &

D. T. L. Shek, *Promoting Holistic Development in University Students*, Quality of Life in Asia 17, https://doi.org/10.1007/978-981-96-0251-3_7

Eyler, 1994). Nevertheless, different organizations, universities, and institutions have proposed diverse definitions of SL. Based on Kendall's (1990) review, there are 147 different terms and definitions related to SL. Two dimensions were derived from those definitions: SL as an educational pedagogy and SL as a philosophy. The two concepts share one similarity: "The equilibrium between service (to the community) and learning (from service) is meaningful and purposeful," which requires the students, faculty, and community partners to collaborate closely with each other (Flecky, 2010).

Perhaps the definition by Bringle and Hatcher (1995) is one of the most cited definitions: "SL is a course-based, credit-bearing educational experience, during which the students can take part in an organized service activity that meets community needs that have been identified, and the students reflect on the service activity to gain further understanding of course content, a broader appreciation of the discipline, and an enhanced sense of civic responsibility" (p. 112). Based on their definition, students and the community are in a reciprocal relationship, and both benefit from SL activities. SL is more than an "add-on" to a course or adding hours to meet the graduation requirement. Instead, while students serve, they benefit and learn, and communities collaborate and benefit (Lascell, 2014).

SL has widely been recognized as "a form of experiential learning that facilitates learning by doing or observing" (Sigmon, 1979). Sigmon's definition lays the foundation for developing standards for distinguishing SL from other types of experiential learning (Furco, 1996). Firstly, SL is unique as it aims to benefit the service providers and the community equally. Moreover, SL has been integrated into academic learning, and student learning outcomes are also embedded in SL courses (Kuh & Schneider, 2008). To establish a clear goal for SL, Sigmon (1994) broadened his definition of "reciprocal learning" and emphasized that "The balance between learning goals and service outcomes in SL is essential." Therefore, "service" and "learning" carry equally important goals and enhance each other (Jacoby, 2003).

Sigmon (1979) pointed out that there are 4Rs in a well-developed SL program: respect, reciprocity, relevance, and reflection. Essentially, the hyphen between "service" and "learning" is meaningful as it addresses the micro needs of meeting individual course objectives and the macro needs of engaging the community effectively. Jacoby (1996) highlighted that students involved in SL practice need to be sensitive, creative, and reflective in their service, as the community needs are often unique to that specific community. Therefore, there are no quick and prescribed ways to solve those deep-rooted community problems. Eyler and Giles (1999) denoted that there are several essential elements to define quality SL experiences, including sustainable curricula and projects, sound partnerships between students and the service recipients, meaningful activities for enhancing students' experiences and addressing community needs, solid and clear relevance between service activities that are addressing community problems and achieving the objective learning outcomes of the course, and well-designed challenges for students to learn effective ways to respond to diversity and diversified needs in the community. Likewise, Ehrlich (2000) stated that there are three essential components in SL: connection to course objectives, service activities to respond to community needs, and rich opportunities for reflection. According to Einfeld and Collins (2008), experience, reflection, and reciprocity are essential elements in SL programs. Jacoby (1996) believed that students learn through the integration of practice and reflection. Reflection integrates service as practice, inspiring the learners to reevaluate their perceptions of themselves and the learning experience and to think about how their activities are constructive and meaningful. Therefore, high-quality SL programs or courses can facilitate students' establishment of a concrete and strategic understanding of the course, enrich their learning experiences, enhance their skills, and deepen their civic responsibility while addressing real community needs.

7.2 Theories on Service-Learning

For decades, the theoretical foundation of SL practices has been mainly grounded in the work of Dewey, Kolb, and Mezirow (Cone & Harris, 1996). John Dewey's ideas have been particularly influential, who stated that "we reflect and utilize our prior knowledge from experiences to guide our future development" (Flecky, 2010). According to Dewey, integrating knowledge and skills with experience lays the foundation for learning. Therefore, the best way of learning does not come from reading brilliant books in a classroom but from going to the outside world to integrate real-world experience (Giles, 1987). Dewey believed in "learning by doing" (Salam et al., 2019a), and his work emphasizes that education is the bridge from academic knowledge to real-life experience by involving oneself in and reflecting on real-world problems (Noddings, 1998). Building on Dewey's idea, Ehrlich (2000) stated that learning begins with a problem and continues by developing comprehensive methods and practical skills to tackle the problem.

SL highlights the importance of reflection, emphasizing that SL practice should be sensitive, creative, and reflective to provide context and meaning through critical thinking (Giles & Eyler, 1994). Dewey (1938) defined reflective thinking as "active, persistent, and careful consideration of any belief or supposed form of knowledge in light of the grounds that support it and the further conclusions to which it tends" (pp. 19–20). Dewey highlighted two principles as the key to experiential learning, "continuity" and "interaction" (Mathieson, 2016). Regarding continuity, Dewey (1910) emphasized that experiences should build on previous ones and be directed toward growth and development. He also noted the teacher's role in inspiring students to shape their knowledge base and guide them in developing fitting experiences. In terms of interaction, learning is an outcome of communication and integration between the learner and the environment.

Specifically, Dewey (1986) stated that there are six steps in the process of inquiry, including "(1) encountering a problem; (2) formulating a problem or question to be resolved; (3) gathering information for effective solutions; (4) making hypotheses; (5) testing hypotheses; and (6) making warranted assertions." The critical elements in SL are experience, inquiry, and reflection. He added that there is no fixed sequence of the steps, so the six steps could be collapsed or expanded, but they are irreplaceable elements for practicing reflective thinking. The six steps guide the practitioners and researchers to explore "How does learning happen?" "What is learning?" and "What is the relationship between learning and action?" (Giles & Eyler, 1994). This argument lays the theoretical foundation of SL.

Based on Dewey's philosophy, the experiential model proposed by Kolb (1984) has long been regarded as the guidance for experiential education and for analyzing and designing SL programs. Kolb conceptualized "Dewey's six steps of inquiry" and formed the "four-stage experiential learning cycle" (Cone & Harris, 1996). The four steps involve moving from (1) concrete experiences—doing (e.g., having a direct and actual experience), through (2) reflective observation—observing (e.g., reflecting on the experience and thoughtful interpretation and comparison of experiences), to the development of (3) abstract conceptualization—thinking (e.g., conceptualizing theories or models from the experiences and reflection), and finally to the application of (4) active experimentation—planning (e.g., implementing effective ways for forthcoming experience). Effective learning takes place in cycles where a learner develops through each stage. Based on Kolb's framework, conducting written or oral reflection is critical for learners, and the learners have already been engaged in the learning cycle when they participate in community service. Reflective practice happens before, during, and after service. With the guidance of the teachers, students could form abstract concepts and hypotheses based on their critical reflection, which enables the reflection to cycle back into further and more profound concrete learning experiences (Morris, 2020). Going through the learning steps, students get the chance to exercise and develop their critical thinking skills.

Cone and Harris (1996) asserted that Kolb's philosophy is a student-centered model that facilitates students with diverse learning styles to establish personal skills and apply their learning from school in community service. Most researchers view Kolb's model as a guiding theory for how learners comprehend and transfer different academic learning and knowledge based on their experiences. Although Kolb's model is generally regarded as the most popular framework foundation for SL, there are criticisms regarding its neglect of the personal, social, and contextual dimensions of experiential learning (Fenwick, 2003; Jarvis, 2012; Miettinen, 2000).

The transformative learning model proposed by Mezirow (1978) emphasized how learners explore meaning from their experience and how the perception of social problems, critical events, and life events can contribute to significant learning and behavioral change. The model provides a theoretical foundation for an SL framework. Mezirow (2018) defined transformative learning as "a process where learners explore meaning in their experiences after critical and rational reflection" to achieve a meaningful mindset or reference for guiding individual and social action. There are ten non-sequential components in the model that describe the learning process, including: "(1) a disorienting dilemma, (2) self-examination with feelings of fear, anger, guilt, or shame, (3) a critical assessment of assumptions, (4) recognition that one's discontent and the process of transformation are shared, (5) exploration of options for new roles, relationships, and actions, (6) planning a course of action, (7) acquiring knowledge and skills for implementing one's plans, (8) provisionally trying new roles, (9) building competence and self-confidence in new roles and relationships, and (10) a reintegration into one's life based on conditions dictated." Although the degree of individual transformation is hard to predict, clarify, and examine, one must be empowered by this model to develop civic responsibility, self-directedness, and more critical thinking skills (Kiely, 2002).

The transformative learning theory proposed by Mezirow (2018) supports the idea that reflection is the most powerful driving force in SL programs, which can facilitate students' experiencing, comprehending, and reconstructing SL experiences to form meaningful and concrete knowledge. Based on this assertion, no learning takes place without reflection. According to Jones and Abes (2004), transformative SL enables students to engage in community services where the contexts and cultures are different from their own, and individual and social transformations will emerge from the experiences. Moreover, Naudé (2015) stated that transformative SL requires students to work collaboratively with the community and provides them with regular and structured spaces for reflection. Kiely (2002) demonstrated that transformative SL can foster students' critical consciousness, enhance analytical skills, and cultivate civic responsibility. Furthermore, it also empowers students to be more socially responsible and self-directed.

Researchers have also proposed different theories of SL. For instance, Schön (1987) emphasized reflection practice in experiential education, and his "reflection-in-action" model has been applied to cultivate reciprocal reflective activities in SL (Honnett & Poulsen, 1989). In his research, Schön (1987) proposed that the ability to learn by doing and build lifelong learning and problem-solving competence has influenced how reflection has been integrated into SL. Therefore, professional education should focus on cultivating the practitioners to be confident, skillful, and caring. Moreover, in his book, he described how to develop solid problem-solving skills: (1) practice facing real challenges; (2) test different solutions; (3) allow making mistakes; (4) seek assistance; and (5) refine approaches. Additionally, he emphasized that teachers have the responsibility to encourage and guide students to make meaningful reflections. He further urged professionals to utilize this model to prepare students for future challenges and complicated and unpredictable problems. Nevertheless, Schön's model has not been widely recognized as a popular theory of SL (Flecky, 2010).

7.3 Impact of Service-Learning on Different Stakeholders

Well-planned SL generates win–win benefits for every stakeholder, which is noteworthy (Lyday et al., 1998). SL can impact the service providers, departments or faculties, universities, service recipients, and the community. Indeed, higher education and the community share different motivations, perceived benefits, and objectives in the involvement of SL programs (Gray et al., 2000).

We can explore the benefits of SL to four groups of stakeholders. First, university students providing SL services will benefit from SL greatly. In fact, many studies have documented the influence of SL on various domains of development. Second, service recipients (e.g., primary and secondary school students served by university students) can also benefit from SL. For example, through STEM SL projects, students may acquire more STEM knowledge and develop more positive attitudes to STEM initiatives. Third, SL may also benefit the teachers of SL subjects such as sharpening their teaching skills and enhancing their understanding of community needs. Finally, SL may create a positive impact on the broader community, such as promoting community solidarity and identity.

7.3.1 Impacts on Service Providers

The effectiveness of SL for service providers has been widely studied and evaluated by many scholars. Various studies have demonstrated that SL programs not only address community needs but also enable students to integrate their learning into real-life situations and develop their personal, interpersonal, cognitive, and moral development (Eyler et al., 1997; Payne, 2000; Rhodes, 1999). SL courses usually specify student outcomes for community engagement, teaching students how to participate in public service and contribute to building a greater community as citizens (Gabelnick, 1997). Campus Compact (2016) showed that around 80% of the programs intended to enhance critical thinking, 77% addressed civic or democratic learning, and 77% tackled engagement across differences. Other outcomes included global learning (64%), social justice (62%), and policy knowledge (28%).

After reviewing 103 studies, Conway et al. (2009) found that SL could enhance students' academic outcomes, personal competence, and civic responsibility. Eyler et al. (2001) investigated and reviewed 135 studies from 1993 to 2000 that analyzed the impact of SL activities on students, departments, and universities, and 132 of the research suggested the positive or neutral influence of SL programs. Specifically, they found that SL positively influences students' personal development and interpersonal development, such as personal efficacy, self-identity, spiritual growth, moral development, leadership, and communication skills. Moreover, SL can generate positive social outcomes, such as reducing stereotypes, facilitating cultural competence, enhancing civic engagement, strengthening involvement in the community, or providing services to the community. Additionally, SL can influence learning outcomes, such as facilitating cognitive development and problem-solving skills, enhancing academic learning, and applying knowledge to the real world. In another study, Balčiūnienė and Mažeikienė (2008) categorized the benefits into several dimensions, including "emotional satisfaction, academic benefits, strengthening of cognitive thinking abilities, reinforcement of citizenship attitudes and competencies, and personal growth."

7.3.1.1 Impact on Social Behavior

Krug (1991) evaluated SL with at-risk youth in a program where the youth provided services for primary students. The study revealed that at-risk youth participating in the programs showed positive gains in potency, self-concept, and activity involvement in the community. Similarly, Luchs (1980) reported that students in SL programs exhibited more positive attitudes toward other people, and they developed a more substantial level of efficacy and self-esteem than the control groups. Calabrese and Schumer (1986) showed that students with disciplinary problems exhibited a lower degree of alienation and isolation and engaged in fewer risky behaviors after participating in SL programs. Conrad (1982) found that students began to view adults, other people, and their community more positively after participating in SL programs.

7.3.1.2 Impact on Self-identity

Apart from the changes in social behavior, the effectiveness of SL programs in students' psychological development has been evaluated by many scholars. Bontempo (1979) interviewed students and coordinators of SL programs in various schools and found that the students showed positive self-concepts and self-worth after joining the program. Sager (1973) investigated 22 students in a summer SL program providing hospital services. The study revealed that students showed significant improvement in self-esteem and self-confidence. Moreover, they demonstrated more self-acceptance, felt their services were worthwhile, and valued their interactions with peers. Similarly, Kelly (1973) found that students who were involved in SL programs exhibited more remarkable positive changes in self-image, self-consciousness, and other related variables than those who were not involved in SL activities. Using a case study approach, Martin (1977) also found positive changes in students' behaviors based on teacher interviews and self-reflection, indicating a gain in positive self-identity.

7.3.1.3 Impact on Moral Judgment

Alexander (1977) demonstrated significant changes in moral thinking, the development of ego, and the degree of prejudice among the students participating in SL courses. Edwards (1974) showed that students displayed a higher level of moral judgment, mutual trust, cooperation, and moral reasoning than those who were not involved in the programs. Similar results could be found in other studies (Mosher, 1977; Reck, 1978). Boss (1994) revealed that students in SL classes demonstrated higher gains in terms of moral reasoning relative to the control group. Similar findings could be seen in Gorman et al. (1994). Lies et al. (2012) demonstrated that students in the SL group notably exhibited a greater level of moral reasoning than those who were in the control group.

7.3.1.4 Impact on Cognitive Development

Hedin (1987) found that students showed significant gains in reading skills after the SL courses. Braza (1975) evaluated community-based SL programs and found that students significantly improved their knowledge, behavior, and attitudes after participating in the SL programs. Markus et al. (1993) evaluated the effectiveness of integrating SL into political science courses and revealed that students in the course had better academic performance and could apply their learning from the class to new situations more effectively. In their study utilizing the Measure of Epistemological Reflection, Wang and Rodgers (2006) showed that students revealed improved critical thinking skills and reasoning after taking SL courses, and their scores increased dramatically from the pretest to the posttest. The findings enriched the results of previous studies that SL programs benefit students' cognitive development (Eyler & Giles, 1999; Eyler et al., 1998; Osborne et al., 1998). Various studies have shown that SL courses can promote the cognitive development of students.

7.3.2 Impact on Service Recipients

Theoretically, reciprocity and mutual benefits are two characteristics that define SL. However, numerous studies have explored how SL influences service providers, while fewer studies evaluated the benefits of SL on service recipients (Shek et al., 2021). D'Arlach et al. (2009) have highlighted that the perceptions of service recipients can demonstrate a first-hand assessment of the influence of the SL programs. A reciprocal, assets-based partnership might enrich an SL course. Therefore, their voices are essential to show whether SL activities truly address their needs (Weah et al., 2000). For instance, Shek et al. (2021) used subjective outcome evaluation to investigate how SL programs benefit service recipients. The overwhelmingly positive responses revealed that the SL programs improved different Positive Youth Development (PYD) qualities of service recipients. They also validated a measure of client satisfaction based on the responses of the service recipients. The empirical evidence enhanced the idea that SL can have mutual benefits for both service providers and service recipients (Vogel & Seifer, 2011).

7.3.3 Impact on Teachers of Service-Learning Subjects

As one of the stakeholders in the partnership, teachers of SL subjects also benefit from SL. Vogel and Seifer (2011) asserted that SL programs create a context for teachers to develop skills and organizational infrastructure, enhance teachers' understanding of the value of partnership, and develop their competence and motivation to form partnerships with the community (Cashman & Seifer, 2008). In their review of the impact of SL on teachers, Eyler et al. (2001) drew four conclusions. First, SL reports could help teachers understand student satisfaction and their learning process (Berson & Younkin, 1998). Second, teachers could use SL reports for research purposes (Driscoll et al., 1996). Third, teachers could understand barriers in SL programs, such as resource insufficiency (Wade & Yarbrough, 1997) or lack of reward (Euster & Weinbach, 1994). Finally, teachers could integrate SL into academic subjects (Stanton, 1990).

Many studies have shown that SL can impact academic partners as well. Gelmon et al. (1998) conducted a multi-methods assessment to evaluate a three-year SL program in 17 schools. Their study showed that faculty member's benefit from the program from various perspectives, including strengthened relationships between students and communities, gained new insights into teaching, developed a high level of competence to integrate their personal lives with professional lives, and enhanced understanding of community needs. Other studies also showed that SL programs benefit academic institutions in increasing recruitment and retention rates among students (Astin & Sax, 1998; Roose et al., 1997). These studies demonstrated that institutional involvement in SL can cultivate a sustainable university-community partnership. Nevertheless, fewer studies have focused on the benefits of SL for teachers, particularly in the Chinese context, compared to those on students as service providers.

7.3.4 Impact on the Community

Lyday et al. (1998) summarized several benefits of SL to the community, including mobilizing youth as resources, tackling real-life community concerns, promoting a sense of community among students, cultivating future leaders, nurturing future workforce, generating good economic benefits, and establishing healthy communities. They highlighted that communities would become healthier places for people living there after the implementation of SL activities or programs. Similarly, Balčiūnienė and Mažeikienė (2008) categorized the community benefits into several dimensions, including enabling communities to receive help and better services, enhancing cooperation among communities and universities, gaining new insights and ideas to solve problems, providing emotional support and satisfaction for target groups, cultivating a deeper sense of community identity and belongingness, empowering the residents, and broadening their horizon.

Obviously, community partners are facilitators in students' learning and engagement process instead of passive service recipients. Studies have shown that SL allows communities to receive help and better satisfy their needs. According to Campus Compact (2016), 59% of SL programs have developed partnerships and shared outcome goals with their community partners. Additionally, community members integrate their experiences and knowledge and co-create activities to address their needs. Sandy and Holland (2006) revealed that "Community partners value their role as student educators and appreciate the resources and knowledge the program brings to the community." Lyday et al. (1998) also evaluated that SL activities enable communities to receive better services and assistance. Moreover, communities could launch new projects and receive fresh insights to address community problems. Additionally, Gelmon et al. (1998) reported that the community-university partnership was enhanced after the implementation of SL programs. Balčiūnienė and Mažeikienė (2008) found that students' participation enhanced the learning level of target groups and reinforced community members' involvement and self-esteem. Additionally, the positive emotions of the service recipients in the community improved after the SL activities, and their quality of life improved as well.

There is also enhanced cooperation between universities and the community as a result of SL. Gray et al. (2000) conducted interviews with the community representatives, and they reported that good cooperation enhanced the positive benefit of the SL activities. They also pointed out that the programs provided the community with accurate and essential assistance, enabled more access to diversified activities, and made it easier for community members to plan future activities. In their review, Balčiūnienė and Mažeikienė (2008) noted that students brought new ideas for solving existing problems in the community. Moreover, the community members also mentioned that their horizons had been broadened, and they became more open-minded to accept different ideas and attitudes.

Many researchers have also studied the social impact of SL. For instance, Trigos-Carrillo et al. (2020) investigated the effectiveness of SL projects regarding peace-building in Colombia. Results indicated that the students involved had developed cultural humility through affective understanding and the consolidation of community practice. While students gradually developed trust-based and co-constructed partnerships with the community members, the community was also initiated to create a relationship with the institution. Equally important, the students experienced positive social impact and intercultural competencies. Balčiūnienė and Mažeikienė (2008) also highlighted the impact of SL on emotional satisfaction. In their study, community members showed their appreciation toward SL programs and stressed that their feelings of belongingness to the communities were enhanced as well. Moreover, they stated that the students provided diligent and sincere help to them, which encouraged the community members to participate actively in the activities. One religious group indicated that SL activities enhanced their positive emotions and the feeling of being needed. Similarly, Driscoll et al. (1996) stressed that the communities appreciated the help of students in SL activities. They agreed that their involvement with the community was high, and they appreciated the capacity of students to provide service, enhance economic and social benefits to the community, and bring new insights about the operation to them.

Finally, the empowerment of the community to provide suggestions regarding SL activities and cooperation can also be regarded as a positive influence on the community. Balčiūnienė and Mažeikienė (2008) pointed out that community members felt empowered as their opinions were valued. The community members suggested ways to improve the programs in future, including cooperation with the university, forms of student activities, and adjustment of objectives. Interestingly, Sandy and Holland (2006) invited the community partners to give their recommendations for SL activities. By valuing and appreciating the role and impact of communities, community partners developed a more profound commitment to the objectives, values, and goals of SL activities. Miron and Moely (2006) revealed that community partners' positive views of SL activities could enhance their extent of involvement in the programs and activities. Communities value that SL activities bring additional resources and opportunities to cultivate future professionals and develop a deeper sense of community belongingness among community members (Basinger & Bartholomew, 2006). Community partners appreciated the opportunity to be involved in student recruitment, student reflection, faculty development, and curriculum improvement (Sandy & Holland, 2006).

In conclusion, several differences and similarities can be identified when comparing the effectiveness of SL activities on different stakeholders. First, students can gain academic benefits from participating in the programs, and their interpersonal and intrapersonal competence can be cultivated as well. Moreover, their civic responsibility and citizenship attitudes are enhanced. Regarding the benefits for the communities, they receive actual and concrete support and help. They also embrace new ideas to solve community challenges and develop more flexibility to adapt to changes. Additionally, the community members are empowered to join activities to strive for a better community. Furthermore, communities are able to strengthen cooperation with higher education. In addition, community members can build a deeper sense of belonging and a higher level of satisfaction with the community.

SL activities catalyze change, during which a diversity of attitudes, thinking styles, and beliefs are interchanged and reflected. Both students and the community can reflect on their values and rebuild new values based on their learning and participation. Balčiūnienė and Mažeikienė (2008) emphasized that SL contributes to the individual development of students and the formation of the personal identity of both students and communities. Moreover, both parties are becoming more aware of the importance of SL programs and striving to improve their implementation.

7.4 Development of Service-Learning in the Global Context

SL can be regarded as a relatively new pedagogy in universities and colleges in America and throughout the world (Kenny & Gallagher, 2002). According to Ehrlich (2000), the development of SL in the United States was closely tied to civic and political activism during the 1960s and 70s. SL enables students' active involvement in service projects, responding to the community's needs while achieving their academic goals. By the late 1980s, colleges and universities in America began putting more emphasis on community life and civic engagement (Hollander et al., 2002).

The concept of "Service-Learning" was first introduced by Sigmon and William in 1967 at the Regional Education Board (Sigmon, 1979). In the early 1960s, the National Society for Experiential Education (NSEE) supported SL as a principle of experiential learning. Additionally, the NSEE promoted research in the field of SL (Eyler & Giles, 1999). Lerner and Simon (2014) argued that higher education institutions at that time were under tremendous pressure to address real-world problems and contribute value to the community. As a result, universities began exploring ways to engage with the community through conducting research and teaching in a valuable and sustainable manner.

Notably, the philosophy of SL originated from social reform movements, especially after the "National and Community Service Act" passed in 1990. Throughout the 1980s, educational authorities and schools in the United States began to implement SL activities, with some even making community service a graduation requirement. However, these initiatives were limited to a small group of participants (Kenny et al., 2002). The movements laid the foundation for the blooming of SL programs (Kraft, 1996). By the late 1980s, SL had gained recognition as a distinct practice from community service and had been integrated with academic study (Hollander et al., 2002). When the 1990s began, the growing attention toward SL was regarded as a "vital force in educational change" (Kenny et al., 2002). Since then, the essence of SL has been embedded in higher education, with multiple attempts made to build the SL network and link this pedagogy to the higher education curriculum (Kenny & Gallagher, 2002). Boyer (1996) emphasized the importance of civic engagement and encouraged universities to support communities and integrate knowledge to address community needs by conducting research, implementing effective teaching, and providing services. From his perspective, learning is not merely for academic knowledge but also for the development of leadership qualities. Furthermore, active citizenship encompasses human rights, social responsibility, civic duty, and democratic participation.

Initially, SL courses were offered mainly by departments like social sciences, education, or humanities while being scarce in hard sciences. Moreover, these courses were often not credit-bearing or integrated with scholarship opportunities (Howard, 1993). Recognizing the value and impact on student development, an increasing number of educators and administrators worked toward incorporating SL into their curricula. In 1984, it was estimated that nearly 27% of high schools (5400 schools) had different kinds of SL programs involving approximately 900,000 students, which constituted 6.6% of the high school students (Newmann & Rutter, 1985). Nonetheless, the majority of these school-based programs focused on white students instead of at-risk and minority youth (Kraft, 1996). In the same year, the SL programs were enhanced by the Campus Out-Reach Opportunity League (COOL). Subsequently, this organization strived to facilitate more university students in serving their communities, expand SL across hundreds of universities in America, and enhance SL in the country (Kenny & Gallagher, 2002). In 1985, Campus Compact was established to promote democratic, civic, and community engagement movements and to cultivate citizenship values and skills by serving the public and communities (Heffernan, 2001). By the year 2000, SL had received increasing attention and become a significant educational movement in the United States. Currently, Campus Compact provides resources to help faculty and members build their SL programs. It now has over 1100 presidential members, representing over 6 million students dedicated to enhancing civic engagement (University of Hawaii at Manoa, 2022).

Today, there are diverse SL and civic engagement programs offered by various universities in America. Campus Compact (2007) revealed that each university had an average of 77 community partners from different natures, such as NGOs, community-based organizations, schools, and government organizations. Notably, Campus Compact (2016) reported that for each university, the SL programs cooperated with a variety of community partners, including "community-based organizations (99%), business partners (67%), faith-based organizations (82%), and K-12 schools (95%)." Moreover, many students already had experience in providing SL before entering the university, as SL programs were embedded in K-12 learning environments. Thus, the partnership among students, universities, and communities continues to thrive and develop, and SL programs and courses become more integrated into higher education in America.

Apart from the US, the United Kingdom has a longstanding tradition of encouraging active participation in citizenship, which stresses citizens' responsibilities (Birdwell et al., 2013). In the UK, based on the *Dearing Report* (1997), one primary goal of higher education is to "build a democratic, civilized, and inclusive society," which addresses the necessity of reforming higher education curricula to cultivate students to be active and responsible citizens and developing essential skills and competencies. The Council for Citizenship and Learning in the Community (CSV/CCLC) has been building a platform to promote and encourage SL in higher education. This platform aims to link national, multidisciplinary, and community-linked networks in SL through university and community partnerships. In 2002, the British government initiated the Higher Education Active Community Fund to provide financial support for developing community and SL programs in all English universities. These initiatives laid the foundation for integrating SL and citizenship education into higher education in the United Kingdom (Annette, 2002).

In contrast to Western societies, the research and practice of SL are relatively new in Asia. In recent years, higher education in the Asia-Pacific region has taken the initiative to embed SL in their curricula or education philosophies, leading to the flourishing of diverse forms of programs (Permaul, 2009). In 1999, "the International Partnership for SL and Leadership (IPSL)" and "the United Board for Christian Higher Education in Asia (UBCHEA)" supported the development of SL in Asian institutions by providing training, offering funding, and facilitating program development. Realizing the importance of SL, "the United Board for Christian Higher Education (UB)" aimed to promote SL programs in higher education and assist Asian universities in SL research and practice within the Asian community (Ma et al., 2019). After its establishment, UB facilitated the founding of the SL Asia Network (SLAN). SLAN has connected more than 55 institutions in 11 Asian countries to expand SL research and practice (Shumer et al., 2021). In 1999, SLAN held the first SL faculty workshop, which facilitated the development of local and international SL cooperation. SLAN members emphasized that academic SL should integrate service, encourage reflection, and fulfill requirements of learning outcomes (McCarthy, 2009). Over the past decade, research and study of SL have been conducted in Japan (Lim, 2019) and Taiwan (Lin et al., 2014). As more institutions and universities apply for SL courses, others in Asia, such as Singapore, Indonesia, mainland China, and Hong Kong SAR, are increasingly conducting SL research.

In Hong Kong, SL was first adopted at Chung Chi College of The Chinese University of Hong Kong in 1995 as a volunteering concept. In 2006, Lingnan University set up the first Office of SL. In 2011, The Hong Kong Polytechnic University (PolyU) implemented SL as a credit-bearing course for undergraduates. Now, more universities have established SL offices to promote the motto "Serving to learn" and "Learning to serve" (Ma et al., 2019; Xing & Ma, 2010). With the increasing popularity of SL both internationally and in the Asian context, the Higher Education SL Network was formed in Hong Kong in 2009, which provides a platform for local universities to share their SL experiences and resources. In 2017, the first Asia-Pacific Regional Conference on SL was conducted in Hong Kong, and more universities in Asia explored different forms of SL engagement (Ma, 2018; Ma et al., 2019).

The philosophical foundation for SL in Asia is enriching and diverse. Moreover, Asian countries have embraced SL as a critical learning model (Ma & Chan, 2013). For instance, Ma (2021) at Singapore University integrated Confucius's five ethical principles into the SL course for the moral and ethical education of students. This theoretical framework served as a guiding principle for the SL course. Her research revealed that integrating Eastern and Western philosophies could facilitate a dynamic whole-person development for students. By encouraging youth to adhere to moral standards, SL courses not only engage the community and provide real-life practice for students' critical reflection but also cultivate their social responsibility. This study proved the influence of Asian culture in the development of SL, especially in Chinese contexts.

In Hong Kong, Law (2021) from Lingnan University applied cross-disciplinary theories and qualitative research to investigate an innovative practice of one SL course. In this course, she utilized art as a visual language to facilitate SL practice in improving the community's sense of well-being. In India, Nayagam et al. (2021) from Union Christian College used the SL Efficiency Predictor Index to analyze the qualitative data gathered over five years to examine the overall success of SL courses. This study revealed a unique perspective on the overall impact of SL programs, suggesting that integrating art as an innovative idea with SL principles could improve community well-being (Shumer, 2021).

Although an increasing number of institutions and universities in Asia are embedding SL courses, Asian countries still have a long way to go. More tremendous joint efforts should be made to ensure the sustainability of SL practice, maintaining the impact on students, agencies, schools, and communities. Expanding and sustaining the benefits of SL necessitates meticulous planning of SL courses and programs. Moreover, it is essential to go beyond merely providing service, to engage the community actively, and to ensure a lasting impact (Permaul, 2009).

7.5 Service-Learning at PolyU

Although SL is recognized as an effective pedagogy in the West, it remains relatively new in many Asian communities, including Hong Kong (Ma, 2018). In these communities, teachers and faculty members are not adequately prepared for planning, designing, and teaching SL. Moreover, there are some misunderstandings about SL among academic staff. For instance, SL is marginalized as not being "academic enough" or a "waste of time." Some staff also consider it informal or similar to volunteerism. In Chinese societies, despite the expansion of different community service projects, SL programs are often regarded as mere volunteerism without clear intended learning outcomes.

In the past, PolyU students mainly provided voluntary services through the Community SL Program (CSLP). Since the learning elements embedded in this program were weak, the effectiveness of the community service was limited. Additionally, it was challenging to make the projects sustainable because the turnover rate in voluntary services was high. Therefore, there was a strong demand for providing systematic training, purposeful teaching, and structured reflections of SL instead of merely focusing on volunteer activities (Chan et al., 2019).

Before making the bold move to mandate a three-credit SL subject, PolyU faced three significant challenges, which termed "three zeroes": no credit-bearing subject of similar orientation, no teacher has experience in teaching SL subjects, and no recognition for SL in existing ranking systems. Therefore, there were many obstacles and doubts in making SL mandatory at PolyU at the beginning. Despite these challenges, PolyU took the first initiative among universities in Hong Kong to introduce SL as a graduation requirement. In the summer of 2011, PolyU decided to pilot SL subjects. In particular, we paid special attention to overcome the above three challenges. First, we built up credit-bearing SL subjects. Second, we trained SL teachers. Third, although there is still no ranking in terms of SL, we have influenced the government to pay more attention to the importance of SL. For example, in the University Accountability Agreement (UAA) for each Government funded universities, SL is one of the metric in the assessment. Furthermore, we also made reference to the international best practice in SL and to benchmark our SL subjects with reference to such standards. In particular, we emphasize that SL is "academic service learning" instead of community service.

The overall goal of the new program is to cultivate holistic development in undergraduate students. Shek et al. (2015) identified six major qualities for the students, namely professional competence, critical thinking abilities, effective communication skills, problem-solving abilities, lifelong learning attributes, and ethical leadership qualities. To achieve the above goals, PolyU designed and implemented General University Requirements (GUR) in the 2012/13 academic year as a new element in the undergraduate courses at PolyU. The 3-credit SL is one of the components of the GUR. Up to now, PolyU has formed collaborative relationships with over 150 community partners, including NGOs, universities and institutions, K12 schools, and different organizations from Hong Kong, mainland China, and several countries worldwide (Shek et al., 2018).

Specifically, the various SL subjects aim to cater to the well-being of both students undertaking the courses and the communities receiving the services, which can be revealed in the intended learning outcomes (Shek et al., 2018). Based on the Subject Proposal Form, upon completing the subject, students will be able to:

- Apply the knowledge and skills they have acquired to deal with complex issues in the service setting.
- Reflect on their role and responsibilities both as professionals in their chosen discipline and as responsible citizens.
- Demonstrate empathy for people in need and a strong sense of civic responsibility.
- Demonstrate an understanding of the linkage between SL and the academic content of the subject.

Besides, all SL subjects incorporate three key components: (1) purpose-designed academic teaching, (2) challenging, meaningful, and demanding services, and (3) structured reflection and assessment (Office of Service Learning, 2016). Students enrolled in SL subjects are expected to provide services for the community or participate in civic engagement activities, addressing the specific needs of the service sites. Furthermore, to provide the students with more room to apply their abilities and interests, the subject teachers only design outlines and clear the boundaries of the programs. This approach allows students to investigate the needs of the community and apply their learning to design tailored services. Moreover, this flexibility allows students to exercise their adaptability, creativity, teamwork, and leadership.

Although PolyU emphasizes "hard" sciences, such as engineering, construction, mathematics, and physics, it also puts great efforts into "promoting civic engagement among undergraduate students" and "enhancing their commitment to serving society," which is clearly shown in the motto of PolyU, "To learn and to apply, for the benefit of mankind" (Ngai & Shek, 2022). For instance, engineers need to be equipped with both technical and soft skills like social responsibility, intercultural competence, communication skills, and leadership qualities (Galloway, 2007). To respond to this call, PolyU has implemented a long tradition of organizing engineering-related SL projects.

Maurrasse (2002) stressed that a good relationship between the university and the community is one of the essential elements that contribute to the success of academic SL. For instance, PolyU initiated an innovative project, the Project WeCan, which involved collaboration between the business sector, the university, and the community. Project WeCan was launched in 2011 with the support of Wharf, aiming to provide more learning opportunities and enhance the well-being of underprivileged secondary school students (Shek & Ho, 2018). This partnership connected and mobilized the resources available, enhancing the project's impact.

The impact of SL on the staff members is remarkable as well. Shek et al. (2015) found that staff from various disciplines involved in SL subjects realized their ability to contribute to the community and society. Additionally, teachers had the autonomy to add additional learning outcomes to address community needs. The findings in the longitudinal evaluation study indicated that SL requirements effectively cultivated students' holistic development. Firstly, the results from the Student Feedback Questionnaire (SFQ) data, students' focus groups, qualitative evaluations, and longitudinal case studies indicated that students evaluated SL subjects positively. Moreover, most students agreed that SL was the most engaging subject among all the GUR subjects, and their understanding of their majors and future careers was enhanced after taking the SL subjects in their departments. Equally important, students specified that SL subjects had cultivated their psychosocial skills and social responsibility.

Apart from the views of service providers, the perceptions of service recipients and other stakeholders are essential to be noted. Yu et al. (2019) analyzed the views of different stakeholders and found that 99.2% of the service recipients evaluated the tutors positively, and 99.4% had a positive assessment of the program. Overall, 98.9% of service recipients were satisfied with the program. The quantitative ratings provided by the observers and the evaluation data from service collaborators revealed similar findings. All the results indicated that the program benefited both service providers and service recipients, and different stakeholders evaluated the services and programs positively.

Developing SL subjects at PolyU represents a cultural breakthrough for the university. Although taking SL is a mandatory requirement, PolyU students can choose different subjects offered by various disciplines, providing diverse services to different communities. There are nearly 70 subjects in PolyU provided by over 95% of academic departments, which motivate the students to be familiar with the community, develop empathy for people in need, and solve real-life challenges by themselves. Approximately 170 staff members teach or assist in these subjects. The SL subject comprises lectures, workshops, community service for 40 hours, reflection, and continuous assessment. Remarkably, the subjects are designed to serve different groups in need, such as children, adolescents, older adults, people with disability, ethnic groups, and immigrants (Chan et al., 2019).

Nevertheless, major challenges are ahead, such as ensuring a competitive edge, maintaining the quality of SL initiatives, and integration across multi-disciplines. To tackle the challenges, Shek et al. (2018) highlighted that several valuable experiences can be drawn from SL initiatives in PolyU, including (1) the flexibility of providing a variety of SL subjects in most disciplines, (2) the provision of systematic training for teachers to equip them with essential knowledge and skills, (3) the offering of comprehensive training and blended learning materials of both students and teachers, (4) comprehensive support from the senior management such as the establishment of the Office of SL, and multi-sectoral collaboration with NGOs, schools, government departments, and business sectors, and (5) the recognition of evaluation and research in a scholarly model in the implementation of SL.

7.6 Electronic SL Under the Pandemic

Electronic SL (E-SL) is a kind of SL course in which the instructions or service activities are conducted online (Marcus et al., 2020). This shift in SL from high-touch to high-tech caters to the increasing needs of digital learners worldwide (Waldner et al., 2012). As an experiential learning pedagogy, SL effectively promotes students' personal development and civic engagement. The nature of SL activities mainly relies on the interpersonal interaction between service providers and recipients. However, due to the social distancing measures implemented during the COVID-19 pandemic, close physical interaction was restricted, promoting the adaptation of online SL as an alternative approach. Waldner et al. (2012) described how online learning facilitated SL by eliminating geographical barriers. Therefore, e-SL holds the key to the future of SL, offering opportunities to adapt and evolve in response to changing circumstances and needs.

Waldner et al. (2012) identified four types of e-SL: Hybrid Type 1, Hybrid Type 2, Hybrid Type 3, and Hybrid Type 4, e.g., the Extreme SL. Hybrid Type 1 refers to students providing service on-site while studying course contents or instructions entirely online. Hybrid Type 2 involves students providing service entirely online while studying course contents or instructions fully on-site. Hybrid Type 3 represents a mixed learning mode where service and learning happen partially online and partially on-site. Hybrid Type 4 depicts that learning and service are carried out entirely online. Waldner et al. (2012) also reminded educators to carefully employ different e-SL methods as each type has its strengths and limitations. A single type of e-SL cannot adequately meet the diverse needs of students and community service recipients.

When framing the guidelines for developing e-SL, Salam et al., (2019b) suggested that educators should revise and customize suitable technologies that align with the nature and objectives of SL projects at all stages of the SL-teaching process. Lawler (2011) emphasized the critical role of "project management, strategy and technology, and organization collaboration" in successful e-SL projects. Instead of simply applying technology to replace face-to-face instruction, effective e-SL should make full use of technology to engage students, innovate learning activities, and create new learning opportunities to fill the gap in traditional face-to-face SL contexts. E-SL also ensures that instructors and students enjoy flexibility (Griffin et al., 2011). Moreover, e-SL can involve more partners regionally, nationally, or even globally, intensifying the impact of the SL projects (Malvey et al., 2006). Nevertheless, as Bringle and Clayton (2020) pointed out, "E-SL is not merely using a virtual format to deliver an SL course or implanting a virtual community service component to an existing SL course." Innovative methods and tools could be applied to facilitate engagement. Moreover, teachers should be cautious, as body language, along with verbal and nonverbal communication, could also greatly influence communication (Ngai et al., 2023).

Many scholars have identified the benefits of e-SL. Yusof et al. (2019) proved that the hybrid mode that combines traditional SL and e-SL enables students to gain skills such as online team building, global citizenship, scholarship, and adaptability with online SL. Nielsen (2016) demonstrated that online SL can cultivate the professional skills of students and train them to be responsible for their learning. Guthrie and McCracken (2014) proposed that instructors can utilize reflective journals to facilitate students' learning in their online SL courses. Lehman and Conceição (2010) had a similar conclusion that self-reflection is critical to successful e-SL courses. They further suggested that e-SL courses enabled students to develop a deeper sense of learning. E-SL can engage a variety of populations unable to join in traditional SL activities, such as those with disabilities (Malvey et al., 2006), travel limitations (Waldner et al., 2012), scheduling conflicts (Waldner et al., 2012), and those who are shy or have introvert personalities (Seifer & Mihalynuk, 2005).

During the COVID-19 pandemic, because of school and city lockdown (Shek, 2021), e-SL has developed even more rapidly. The pandemic's restrictions on social interaction and the impossibility of continuing traditional classroom-based teaching and learning activities have compelled educators to explore alternative methods to carry out SL activities and engage students, such as distance teaching or online teaching. The transition from a physical classroom to virtual teaching has become the norm. Schmidt (2021) stated that online SL has emerged as the preferred choice for engaging students during the pandemic. Burton and Winter (2021) proposed that e-SL can address the limitations of social distancing. Educators worldwide need to be prepared to respond to challenges swiftly, continue to develop education, and reduce the negative influence on teaching and learning.

For example, the Johns Hopkins School of Nursing (JHUSON) collaborated with local community leaders and established a phone-based support network for older adults in the community. In the project, faculty members and students provided rapid support and trained their competence during the crisis (Tian & Noel, 2020). At DePaul University, students participated in virtual SL activities to help the community, such as writing personalized letters and cards for healthcare professionals, making face masks, conducting online research work with community partners, producing exercise and fitness videos, and making small donations. During their virtual SL activities, the participants also utilized creative means, such as art, painting, and drawing (Gresh et al., 2021). The University of Alabama at Birmingham (UAB) integrated an e-SL module into their traditional SL course. This module included online lectures, digital infographics, and post-reflection assignments to help students better understand the pandemic and its influence on the community (Adkins-Jablonsky et al., 2021). Similarly, at Iona College New York, Veyvoda and Van Cleave (2020) organized students to conduct teleconferences with the service users and prepared "Zoom Trivia" and FaceTime on a weekly basis to have one-to-one conversations and made memoirs for the residents and their families. The COVID-19 pandemic has necessitated rapid and creative responses from educators and students alike. In this time of uncertainty, e-SL has become indispensable. Moreover, the quarantine measures have shown the advantages of e-SL.

Physical distancing does not mean disconnection between human beings. Instead of responding passively to suspend, postpone, or cancel SL courses during the pandemic, PolyU adopted fully online teaching and hybrid teaching in response to the social distancing measures under COVID-19. When the pandemic hit Hong Kong, all lectures and workshops in the course titled "Promotion of Children and Adolescent Development" were conducted online, and most on-site activities were replaced with online services and educational video production. To engage service recipients, students made videos covering various topics based on their needs. Although physical interaction was limited, virtual materials and online classrooms provided support and encouragement for primary students during the pandemic. Another example is the subject "Service Leadership through Serving Children and Families with Special Needs." In this subject, service recipients could join in online career talks, English workshops, and mock interviews where they learned experiences from students from PolyU. Moreover, PolyU students created videos to introduce different skills (Shek et al., 2022a).

In terms of offshore service, the two subjects, "Service Leadership through Serving Children and Families with Special Needs" and "Promotion of Children and Adolescent Development," provided outbound SL programs to mainland China. Due to the outbreak of the pandemic, all summer camps were transformed into online formats. Specifically, students attended online lectures and workshops to acquire knowledge and service skills. They worked in groups to composite their service plans and completed individual reflective journals. During the service, students utilized a web platform to engage primary students from mainland China. These subjects also formed collaborations with local universities and schools, which served as independent assessors to evaluate the quality and process of the programs. Shek et al. (2022b) analyzed the subjective and objective outcome evaluation data, as well as process evaluation data, gathered from three sites in China during the summer of 2020 and 2021. The results showed that both PolyU students and other stakeholders had positive evaluations of their experiences. More importantly, PolyU students, as service providers, demonstrated positive changes in PYD attributes, including leadership qualities and life satisfaction. Additionally, the data collected over time in multiple sites during the pandemic revealed similar findings, which increased the reliability of the conclusions. The study also supported the effectiveness of e-SL in teaching, learning, and services in a Chinese context.

Apart from addressing immediate public health emergencies, PolyU has a long-term vision of establishing an online platform. This platform offers online learning courses for mixed-mode teacher training programs and online sessions for teachers and students. Moreover, two specific components have been developed: "SL Pedagogy & Practice" to assist teachers in comprehending and implementing SL, and "Learn to Serve, Serve to Learn: Introduction to SL" designed for students. The online resource platform is an effective and practical way to respond to the challenges of the pandemic. Despite the suspension of on-site SL activities at PolyU due to social distancing, students and teachers can access online resources to develop a basic understanding of SL theories and practices (Leung et al., 2021; Lin & Shek, 2021).

Many people may question the effectiveness of virtual SL. To assess the concern, educators at PolyU conducted several studies to evaluate the impact of e-SL on student learning outcomes. Lin and Shek (2021) applied objective outcome evaluation to examine the effects of e-SL on students' learning and life satisfaction, while subjective outcome evaluation was adopted to investigate students' perceptions of the subjects. The findings revealed that non-face-to-face SL significantly promoted college students' positive growth and quality of life. Moreover, students in the e-SL subjects also experienced improvements in different domains of PYD compared with those in traditional SL courses. Leung et al. (2021) compared the learning outcomes and perceptions of students from two traditional SL classes and e-SL classes and reported that both modes of classes were effective in achieving their objectives. The scholars further concluded that e-SL effectively promoted PYD competencies, service leadership qualities, and life satisfaction among students. In a large-scale study conducted by Ngai et al. (2023) from the Service-Learning and Leadership Office at PolyU, the learning outcomes of students enrolled in e-SL subjects were examined and compared with pre-pandemic data. The study showed that e-SL was beneficial in promoting student learning. Nevertheless, e-SL subjects were less effective in facilitating civic learning outcomes. More importantly, the research demonstrated that the quality of reflection and interaction with the community were critical factors influencing the effectiveness of e-SL subjects. The study implied that e-SL was not merely transforming teaching content online (Bringle & Clayton, 2020).

The initiatives and efforts undertaken by PolyU have demonstrated that e-SL can be an effective approach, challenging the notion that SL is limited to traditional face-to-face modes. The integration of e-SL elements has shown developments in PYD competencies among students. More importantly, e-SL is flexible and sustainable in reacting to public health emergencies in future and addressing the needs of more needy groups with physical, mental, and geographical limits (Leung et al., 2021; Li et al., 2023; Lin et al., 2023; Zhu et al., 2023).

As pointed out by Waldner et al. (2012), "E-SL can cater to the increasing needs of digital learners around the globe." Engaging students online is indeed challenging in e-SL. Educators, students, and communities should be well prepared to interact with each other online. As a form of teaching emphasizing intensive interpersonal interaction, the transition from high-touch to high-tech is promising. Future e-SL should make great efforts to address reflection, verbal and nonverbal communication, and interaction.

7.7 Conclusion

This chapter begins by introducing the definition and nature of SL and explores innovative ways to integrate it into higher education courses. Furthermore, it analyzes and discusses the impact of SL classes or programs on various stakeholders, including students, teachers, institutions, community stakeholders, and schools. Specifically, the chapter highlights the implementation of SL at PolyU, where the university strives to enhance the quality of SL subjects, strengthen the effectiveness of SL programs, and develop innovative approaches to engage students. The chapter also delves into an innovative practice known as e-SL, which has gained prominence during the pandemic. More importantly, future e-SL initiatives should focus on addressing key aspects such as reflection, verbal and nonverbal communication, and interaction. These elements are crucial to ensure the meaningful cultivation of social responsibility and psychosocial competence among university students through SL.

Acknowledgements The preparation of this chapter is financially supported by The Hong Kong Polytechnic University (ZZ4U and ZZUE), Li and Fung Endowed Professorship in Service Leadership Education, Wofoo Foundation, and the Matching Fund of Research Grants Council (ZECL and ZH4Q).

References

Adkins-Jablonsky, S., Fleming, R., Esteban, M., Bucio, D., Morris, J. J., & Raut, S. (2021). Impacts of a COVID-19 E-service-learning module in a non-major biology course. *Journal of Microbiology & Biology Education, 22*(1), 1–10. https://doi.org/10.1128/jmbe.v22i1.2489

Alexander, R. C. (1977). *A moral education curriculum on prejudice* (Publication No. 7711349) [Doctoral dissertation, Boston University]. ProQuest Dissertations & Theses Global. https://www.proquest.com/openview/72a23cbea17834ba7a41c5bfa178aa98/1?pq-origsite=gscholar&cbl=18750&diss=y

Annette, J. (2002). Service learning in an international context. *Frontiers: The Interdisciplinary Journal of Study Abroad, 8*(1), 83–93. https://doi.org/10.36366/frontiers.v8i1.95

Astin, A. W., & Sax, L. J. (1998). How undergraduates are affected by service participation. *Journal of College Student Development, 39*(3), 251–263.

Balčiūnienė, I., & Mažeikienė, N. (2008). Benefits of service-learning: Evaluations from students and communities. *Social Research, 1*(11), 53–66. https://etalpykla.lituanistika.lt/object/LT-LDB-0001:J.04~2008~1367164310738/J.04~2008~1367164310738.pdf

Basinger, N., & Bartholomew, K. (2006). Service-learning in nonprofit organizations: Motivations, expectations, and outcomes. *Michigan Journal of Community Service Learning, 12*(2), 15–26. https://files.eric.ed.gov/fulltext/EJ843837.pdf

Berson, J. S., & Younkin, W. F. (1998). Doing well by doing good: A study of the effects of a service-learning experience on student success. *Higher Education, 184*. https://digitalcommons.unomaha.edu/slcehighered/184

Birdwell, J., Scott, R., & Horley, E. (2013). Active citizenship, education and service learning. *Education, Citizenship and Social Justice, 8*(2), 185–199. https://doi.org/10.1177/1746197913483683

Bontempo, B. T. (1979). *A study of experience-based learning in alternative public high schools: Implications for a new role for educators*. [Unpublished doctoral dissertation]. Indiana University.

Boss, J. A. (1994). The effect of community service work on the moral development of college ethics students. *Journal of Moral Education, 23*(2), 183–198. https://doi.org/10.1080/0305724940230206

Boyer, E. L. (1996). The scholarship of engagement. *Bulletin of the American Academy of Arts and Sciences, 49*(7), 18–33. https://doi.org/10.2307/3824459

Braza, G. F. (1975). A comparison of experiential and classroom learning models in teaching health problems of the poor. *The Journal of School Health, 45*(6), 353–355. https://doi.org/10.1111/j.1746-1561.1975.tb01975.x

Bringle, R. G., & Clayton, P. H. (2020). Integrating service learning and digital technologies: Examining the challenge and the promise. *Revista Iberoamericana de Educación a Distancia, 23*(1), 43–65. https://doi.org/10.5944/ried.23.1.25386

Bringle, R. G., & Hatcher, J. A. (1995). A service-learning curriculum for faculty. *Michigan Journal of Community Service Learning, 2,* 112–122. http://hdl.handle.net/2027/spo.3239521.0002.111

Burton, C., & Winter, M. A. (2021). Benefits of service-learning for students during the COVID-19 crisis: Two case studies. *Scholarship of Teaching and Learning in Psychology, 10*(4), 370–378. https://doi.org/10.1037/stl0000292

Calabrese, R. L., & Schumer, H. (1986). The effects of service activities on adolescent alienation. *Adolescence, 21*(83), 675–687. https://digitalcommons.unomaha.edu/slcek12/43

Campus Compact. (2007). *2007 service statistics: Highlights and trends of Campus Compact's annual membership survey.* https://compact.org/sites/default/files/2022-04/2007-Statistics-Layout-1.pdf

Campus Compact. (2016). *Revitalizing our democracy: Building on our assets: 2016 annual member survey executive summary.* https://compact.org/sites/default/files/2022-04/2016-campus_compact_executive_summary_2016_final3-2-1-2-1.pdf

Cashman, S. B., & Seifer, S. D. (2008). Service-learning: An integral part of undergraduate public health. *American Journal of Preventive Medicine, 35*(3), 273–278. https://doi.org/10.1016/j.amepre.2008.06.012

Chan, S. C., Ngai, G., Yau, J., Yuen, W. W., Shek, D. T. L., & Au, H. S. (2019). Service-learning as a vehicle for youth leadership: The case of The Hong Kong Polytechnic University. In D. T. L. Shek, G. Ngai, & S. C. Chan (Eds.), *Service-learning for youth leadership: The case of Hong Kong* (Vol.12, pp. 19–31). Springer. https://doi.org/10.1007/978-981-13-0448-4_2

Cone, D., & Harris, S. (1996). Service-learning practice: Developing a theoretical framework. *Michigan Journal of Community Service Learning, 3,* 31–43. https://digitalcommons.unomaha.edu/cgi/viewcontent.cgi?article=1192&context=slceslgen

Conrad, D. (1982). *Youth participation and experiential education.* Psychology Press.

Conway, J. M., Amel, E. L., & Gerwien, D. P. (2009). Teaching and learning in the social context: A meta-analysis of service learning's effects on academic, personal, social, and citizenship outcomes. *Teaching of Psychology, 36*(4), 233–245. https://doi.org/10.1080/00986280903172969

D'Arlach, L., Sánchez, B., & Feuer, R. (2009). Voices from the community: A case for reciprocity in service-learning. *Michigan Journal of Community Service Learning, 16*(1), 5–16. https://quod.lib.umich.edu/cgi/p/pod/dod-idx/voices-from-the-community-a-case-for-reciprocity-in-service.pdf?c=mjcsl;idno=3239521.0016.101;format=pdf

Dewey, J. (1910). What is thought? In J. Dewey (Ed.), *How we think* (pp. 1–13). D.C. Heath and Company.

Dewey, J. (1938). *Experiential learning.* Pentice Hall.

Dewey, J. (1986). Experience and education. *The Educational Forum, 50*(3), 241–252. https://doi.org/10.1080/00131728609335764

Driscoll, A., Holland, B., Gelmon, S., & Kerrigan, S. (1996). An assessment model for service-learning: Comprehensive case studies of impact on faculty, students, community, and institution. *Michigan Journal of Community Service Learning, 3*(1), 66–71. https://digitalcommons.unomaha.edu/cgi/viewcontent.cgi?article=1174&context=slceslgen

Education in the UK. (1997). *Dearing report: Higher education in the learning society.* https://education-uk.org/documents/dearing1997/dearing1997.html

Edwards, C. P. (1974). *The effect of experience on moral development: Results from Kenya* (Publication No. 7516860) [Doctoral dissertation, Harvard University]. ProQuest Dissertations and Theses Global. https://www.proquest.com/openview/f3774ed69ef29a966137e9af07464ba4/1?pq-origsite=gscholar&cbl=18750&diss=y

Ehrlich, T. (2000). *Civic responsibility and higher education.* Oryx Press.

Einfeld, A., & Collins, D. (2008). The relationships between service-learning, social justice, multicultural competence, and civic engagement. *Journal of College Student Development, 49*, 95–109. https://doi.org/10.1353/csd.2008.0017

Euster, G. L., & Weinbach, R. W. (1994). Faculty rewards for community service activities: An update. *Journal of Social Work Education, 30*(3), 317–324. https://doi.org/10.1080/10437797.1994.10672242

Eyler, J., & Giles Jr., D. E. (1999). *Where's the learning in service-learning?* Jossey-Bass.

Eyler, J., Giles Jr, D. E., & Braxton, J. (1997). The impact of service-learning on college students. *Michigan Journal of Community Service Learning, 4*, 5–15. https://quod.lib.umich.edu/m/mjcsl/3239521.0004.101/1/--impact-of-service-learning-on-college-students?size=100;view=text

Eyler, J., Giles Jr, D. E., Stenson, C. M., & Gray, C. J. (2001). *At a glance: What we know about the effects of service-learning on college students, faculty, institutions and communities, 1993–2000: Third edition.* https://digitalcommons.unomaha.edu/slcehighered/139

Eyler, J. S., Root, S., & Giles, D. E. (1998). Service-learning and the development of expert citizens: Service-learning and cognitive science. In R. G. Bringle & D. K. Duffy (Eds.), *With service in mind: Concepts and models for service-learning in psychology* (pp. 85–100). Routledge. https://doi.org/10.4324/9781003448754

Fenwick, T. J. (2003). *Learning through experience: Troubling orthodoxies and intersecting questions.* Krieger. http://hdl.voced.edu.au/10707/42954

Flecky, K. (2010). Foundations of service-learning. In K. Flecky & L. Gitlow (Eds.), *Service-learning in occupational therapy education: Philosophy and practice* (pp. 1–12). Jones and Bartlett Learning. https://samples.jbpub.com/9780763759582/59582_CH01_FINAL.pdf

Furco, A. (1996). Service-learning: A balanced approach to experiential education. *Service Learning, General, 128*. https://digitalcommons.unomaha.edu/slceslgen/128

Gabelnick, F. (1997). Educating a committed citizenry. *Change: The Magazine of Higher Learning, 29*(1), 30–35. https://doi.org/10.1080/00091389709603111

Galloway, P. D. (2007). The 21st-century engineer: A proposal for engineering education reform. *Civil Engineering Magazine Archive, 77*(11), 46–104. https://doi.org/10.1061/ciegag.0000147

Gelmon, S. B., Holland, B. A., Seifer, S. D., Shinnamon, A., & Connors, K. (1998). Community-university partnerships for mutual learning. *Michigan Journal of Community Service Learning, 5*, 97–107. https://quod.lib.umich.edu/m/mjcsl/3239521.0005.110?rgn=main;view=fulltext

Giles Jr., D. E. (1987). Dewey's theory of experience: Implications for service-learning. *Journal of Cooperative Education, 27*(2), 87–90. https://digitalcommons.unomaha.edu/slceslgen/151

Giles Jr., D. E., & Eyler, J. (1994). The theoretical roots of service-learning in John Dewey: Toward a theory of service-learning. *Michigan Journal of Community Service Learning, 1*(1), 7–85. https://digitalcommons.unomaha.edu/slceslgen/150

Gorman, M., Duffy, J., & Heffernan, M. (1994). Service experience and the moral development of college students. *Religious Education, 89*(3), 422–431. https://doi.org/10.1080/0034408940890308

Gray, M. J., Ondaatje, E. H., Fricker Jr, R. D., & Geschwind, S. A. (2000). Assessing service-learning: The benefits of community service for students. *Change: The Magazine of Higher Learning, 32*(2), 30–39. https://doi.org/10.1080/00091380009601721

Gresh, A., LaFave, S., Thamilselvan, V., Batchelder, A., Mermer, J., Jacques, K., Greensfelder, A., Buckley, M., Cohen, Z., Coy, A., & Warren, N. (2021). Service learning in public health nursing education: How COVID-19 accelerated community-academic partnership. *Public Health Nursing, 38*(2), 248–257. https://doi.org/10.1111/phn.12796

Griffin, M., Saitta, E., Bowdon, M., & Walters, L. J. (2011). Engaging stem: Service-learning, technology, science education and community partnerships. In M. Bowdon & R. G. Carpenter (Eds.), *Higher education, emerging technologies, and community partnerships: Concepts, models and practices* (pp. 51–56). IGI Global. https://doi.org/10.4018/978-1-60960-623-7.ch005

Guthrie, K. L., & McCracken, H. (2014). Reflection: The importance of making meaning in e-service-learning courses. *Journal of Computing in Higher Education, 26*, 238–252. https://doi.org/10.1007/s12528-014-9087-9

Hedin, D. (1987). Students as teachers: A tool for improving school climate and productivity. *Social Policy, 17*(3), 42–47.

Heffernan, K. (2001). Campus compact: Developing partnerships for community service. *Community & Junior College Libraries, 10*(2), 55–59. https://doi.org/10.1300/J107v10n02_07

Hollander, E. L., Saltmarsh, J., & Zlotkowski, E. (2002). Indicators of engagement. In M. E. Kenny, L. A. K. Simon, K. Kiley-Brabeck, & R. M. Lerner (Eds.), *Learning to serve: Promoting civil society through service learning* (pp. 31–49). Springer. https://doi.org/10.1007/978-1-4615-0885-4_3

Honnett, E. P., & Poulsen, S. J. (1989). *Principals of good practice for combining service and learning: A wingspread special report*. https://digitalcommons.unomaha.edu/slceguides/27

Howard, J. (1993). *Praxis I: A faculty casebook on community service learning*. OCSL Press.

Jacoby, B. (1996). *Service-learning in higher education: Concepts and practices*. Jossey-Bass.

Jacoby, B. (2003). *Building partnerships for service-learning*. Jossey-Bass.

Jarvis, P. (2012). *Adult learning in the social context* (Vol. 78). Routledge.

Jones, S. R., & Abes, E. S. (2004). Enduring influences of service-learning on college students' identity development. *Journal of College Student Development, 45*(2), 149–166. https://doi.org/10.1353/csd.2004.0023

Kelly, H. J. (1973). *The effect of the helping experience upon the self-concept of the helper* [Doctroal dissertation, Seattle University]. Dr. C.C. & Mabel L. Criss Library. https://digitalcommons.unomaha.edu/slcedt/4

Kendall, J. C. (1990). *Combining service and learning: A resource book for community and public service* (Vol. 2). National Society for Internships and Experiential.

Kenny, M. E., & Gallagher, L. A. (2002). Service-learning: A history of systems. In M. E. Kenny, L. A. K. Simon, K. Kiley-Brabeck, & R. M. Lerner (Eds.), *Learning to serve: Promoting civil society through service learning* (pp. 15–29). Springer. https://doi.org/10.1007/978-1-4615-0885-4_2

Kenny, M., Simon, L. A. K., Kiley-Brabeck, K., & Lerner, R. M. (Eds.). (2002). Promoting civil society through service learning: A view of the issues. In M. E. Kenny, L. A. K. Simon, K. Kiley-Brabeck, & R. M. Lerner (Eds.), *Learning to serve: Promoting civil society through service learning* (pp. 1–14). Springer. https://doi.org/10.1007/978-1-4615-0885-4_1

Kiely, R. (2002). *Toward an expanded conceptualization of transformational learning: A case study of international service-learning in Nicaragua* [Doctroal dissertation, Cornell University]. Dr. C.C. & Mabel L. Criss Library. https://digitalcommons.unomaha.edu/slcedt/23

Kolb, D. (1984). *Experiential learning: Experience as the source of learning and development*. Prentice Hall.

Kraft, R. J. (1996). Service learning: An introduction to its theory, practice, and effects. *Education and Urban Society, 28*(2), 131–159. https://doi.org/10.1177/0013124596028002001

Krug, J. L. (1991). *Select changes in high school students' self-esteem and attitudes toward their school and community by their participation in service learning activities at a Rocky Mountain high school* (Publication No. 9318063) [Doctoral dissertation, University of Colorado Boulder]. Russian Science Citation Index.

Kuh, G. D., & Schneider, C. G. (2008). *High-impact educational practices: What they are, who has access to them, and why they matter.* Association of American Colleges and Universities.

Lascell, W. A. (2014). *Academic service-learning faculty handbook.* SUNY Oneonta. https://www.oneonta.edu/academics/csrc/documents/PDFs/SL_Handbook_Lascell_2014.pdf

Law, S. S. (2021). Sharing and realization of the vision and practice of art facilitation through service-learning. In R. Shumer, C. H. K. MA, & C. W. Y. Chan (Eds.), *Food for thought: Service-learning research in Asia* (pp. 21–32). Information Age Publishing.

Lawler, J. (2011). Critical success factors for partnering with nonprofit organizations on digital technology service-learning projects: A case study. In M. Bowdon & R. G. Carpenter (Eds.), *Higher education, emerging technologies, and community partnerships: Concepts, models and practices* (pp. 106–123). IGI Global.

Lehman, R. M., & Conceição, S. C. (2010). *Creating a sense of presence in online teaching: How to "be there" for distance learners*. Jossey-Bass.

Lerner, R. M., & Simon, L. A. K. (2014). *University-community collaborations for the twenty-first century: Outreach scholarship for youth and families*. Routledge. https://doi.org/10.4324/9781315790046

Leung, H., Shek, D. T. L., & Dou, D. (2021). Evaluation of service-learning in project WeCan under COVID-19 in a Chinese context. *International Journal of Environmental Research and Public Health, 18*(7), 3596. https://doi.org/10.3390/ijerph18073596

Li, X., Shek, D. T. L., Mok, B. P. W., Shek, E. Y. W., & Bai, Y. P. (2023). Effectiveness of electronic service-learning (e-sl) in primary school children in China during the COVID-19 pandemic. *Applied Research in Quality of Life. 19*, 3081–3108. https://doi.org/10.1007/s11482-023-10244-2

Lies, J. M., Bock, T., Brandenberger, J., & Trozzolo, T. A. (2012). The effects of off-campus service learning on the moral reasoning of college students. *Journal of Moral Education, 41*(2), 189–199. https://doi.org/10.1080/03057240.2012.669925

Lim, T. W. (2019). Case study 2: Service learning. In *Industrial revolution 4.0, tech giants, and digitized societies* (pp. 105–120). Palgrave Macmillan. https://doi.org/10.1007/978-981-13-7470-8_7

Lin, L., & Shek, D. T. L. (2021). Serving children and adolescents in need during the COVID-19 pandemic: Evaluation of service-learning subjects with and without face-to-face interaction. *International Journal of Environmental Research and Public Health, 18*(4), 2114. https://doi.org/10.3390/ijerph18042114

Lin, L., Shek, D. T. L., & Li, X. (2023). Who benefits and appreciates more? An evaluation of Online Service-Learning Projects in mainland China during the COVID-19 pandemic. *Applied Research in Quality of Life, 18*(2), 625–646. https://doi.org/10.1007/s11482-022-10081-9

Lin, C. Y., Wu, S. W., Wu, S. F., Pan, B. S., & Liao, H. C. (2014). Effects of service-learning in a University in Taiwan. *Procedia-Social and Behavioral Sciences, 116*, 902–906. https://doi.org/10.1016/j.sbspro.2014.01.317

Luchs, K. P. (1980). *Selected changes in urban high school students after participation in community based learning and service activities* [Doctoral dissertation, The University of Maryland]. Dr. C.C. & Mabel L. Criss Library. https://digitalcommons.unomaha.edu/slcedt/51

Lyday, W. J., Winecoff, H. L., & Hiott, B. C. (1998). *Connecting communities through service-learning* (ED430128). ERIC. https://files.eric.ed.gov/fulltext/ED430128.pdf

Ma, H. K. C. (2018). Service-learning development in higher education in Hong Kong. In T. W. Lim & T. Y. Kong (Eds.), *Studying Hong Kong: 20 years of political, economic and social developments* (pp. 43–61). World Scientific. https://doi.org/10.1142/9789813223554_0004

Ma, H. K. C. (2021). The implication of confucianism for service learning. In R. Shumer, C. M. H. Ka, & C. C. W. Yee (Eds.) *Food for thought: Service-learning research in Asia* (pp. 7–19). Information Age Publishing.

Ma, H. K. C., & Chan, M. A. C. (2013). A Hong Kong university first: Establishing service-learning as an academic credit-bearing subject. *Gateways: International Journal of Community Research and Engagement, 6(1)*, 178–198. https://doi.org/10.5130/ijcre.v6i1.3286

Ma, H. K. C., Fung, C. C. W., & Hoi, I. T. P. (2019). A common outcome measurement for service-learning in Hong Kong. *Journal of Higher Education Outreach and Engagement, 23*(3), 3–20. https://ojs01.galib.uga.edu/jheoe/article/view/1517/1454

Malvey, D. M., Hamby, E. F., & Fottler, M. D. (2006). E-service learning: A pedagogic innovation for healthcare management education. *The Journal of Health Administration Education, 23*(2), 181–198. http://dx.doi.org/10.13140/2.1.1613.3760

Marcus, V. B., Atan, N. A., Yusof, S. M., & Tahir, L. (2020). A systematic review of e-service learning in higher education. *International Journal of Interactive Mobile Technologies, 14*(6), 4–14. https://doi.org/10.3991/ijim.v14i06.13395

Markus, G. B., Howard, J. P., & King, D. C. (1993). Integrating community service and classroom instruction enhances learning: Results from an experiment. *Educational Evaluation and Policy Analysis, 15*(4), 410–419. https://doi.org/10.3102/01623737015004410

Martin, W. (1977). *A participant observation study of an outdoor education experiential curriculum experiment in a public secondary school* [Doctoral dissertation, Michigan State University]. MSU Libraries Digital Repository. https://d.lib.msu.edu/etd/43716

Mathieson, L. (2016). Synergies in critical reflective practice and science: Science as reflection and reflection as science. *Journal of University Teaching & Learning Practice, 13*(2). https://doi.org/10.53761/1.13.2.4

Maurrasse, D. J. (2002). Higher education-community partnerships: Assessing progress in the field. *Nonprofit and Voluntary Sector Quarterly, 31*(1), 131–139. https://doi.org/10.1177/0899764002311006

McCarthy, F. E. (2009). Where we are now: A review of service-learning among SLAN Colleges and universities in Asia. *New Horizons in Education, 57*(3), 8–19. https://files.eric.ed.gov/fulltext/EJ893700.pdf

Mezirow, J. (1978). Perspective transformation. *Adult Education, 28*(2), 100–110. https://doi.org/10.1177/074171367802800202

Mezirow, J. (2018). Transformative learning theory. In K. Illeris (Ed.), *Contemporary theories of learning* (2nd ed., pp. 114–128). Routledge. https://doi.org/10.4324/9781315147277

Miettinen, R. (2000). The concept of experiential learning and John Dewey's theory of reflective thought and action. *International Journal of Lifelong Education, 19*(1), 54–72. https://doi.org/10.1080/026013700293458

Miron, D., & Moely, B. E. (2006). Community agency voice and benefit in service-learning. *Michigan Journal of Community Service Learning, 12*(2), 27–37. https://files.eric.ed.gov/fulltext/EJ843838.pdf

Morris, T. H. (2020). Experiential learning–a systematic review and revision of Kolb's model. *Interactive Learning Environments, 28*(8), 1064–1077. https://doi.org/10.1080/10494820.2019.1570279

Mosher, R. (1977). Theory and practice: A new E.R.A? *Theory into Practice, 16*(2), 81–88. https://doi.org/10.1080/00405847709542679

Naudé, L. (2015). On (un) common ground: Transforming from dissonance to commitment in a service learning class. *Journal of College Student Development, 56*(1), 84–102. https://doi.org/10.1353/csd.2015.0002

Nayagam, J. R., Simon, T. K., & Nair, M. R. (2021). Evoking eco consciousness through service learning. In R. Shumer, C. M. H. Ka, & C. C. W. Yee (Eds.), *Food for thought: Service-learning research in Asia* (pp. 57–73). Information Age Publishing.

Newmann, F. M., & Rutter, R. A. (1985). A profile of high school community service programs. *Educational Leadership, 43*(4), 65–71.

Ngai, G., Lau, K.-H., & Kwan, K.-P. (2023). A large-scale study of students' e-service-learning experiences and outcomes during the pandemic. *Journal of Experiential Education, 47*(1), 29–52. https://doi.org/10.1177/10538259231171852

Ngai, G., & Shek, D. T. L. (2022). *Service-learning capacity enhancement in Hong Kong higher education* (1st ed., Vol. 14). Springer. https://doi.org/10.1007/978-981-19-2437-8

Nielsen, D. (2016). Facilitating service learning in the online technical communication classroom. *Journal of Technical Writing and Communication, 46*(2), 236–256. https://doi.org/10.1177/0047281616633600

Noddings, N. (1998). Perspectives from feminist philosophy. *Educational Researcher, 27*(5), 17–18. https://doi.org/10.3102/0013189X027005017

Office of Service Learning. (2016). *Learn to serve, serve to learn: The Hong Kong Polytechnic University's experience of mandatory service-learning*. The Hong Kong Polytechnic University. https://www.polyu.edu.hk/osl/files/publications/TheHKPolyUsExperienceOfMandatorySL.pdf

Osborne, R. E., Hammerich, S., & Hensley, C. (1998). Student effects of service-learning: Tracking change across a semester. *Michigan Journal of Community Service Learning, 5*(1), 5–13. https://quod.lib.umich.edu/m/mjcsl/3239521.0005.101/1

Payne, C. A. (2000). Changes in involvement preferences as measured by the community service involvement preference inventory. *Michigan Journal of Community Service Learning, 7*(1), 41–53. http://hdl.handle.net/2027/spo.3239521.0007.105

Permaul, J. S. (2009). Theoretical bases for service-learning: Implications for program design and effectiveness. *New Horizons in Education, 57*(3), 1–7. https://files.eric.ed.gov/fulltext/EJ893699.pdf

Reck, C. J. (1978). *A study of the relationship between participation in school service programs and moral development* [Doctorcal dissertation, St. Louis University]. Russian Science Citation Index.

Rhodes, C. P. (1999). *Psychosocial changes in student development of college sophomore women along Chickering's seven vectors with service-learning as an institutional effect* (Publication No. 9929120) [Doctoral dissertation, Vanderbilt University]. ProQuest Dissertations & Theses Global. https://www.proquest.com/docview/304517181?parentSessionId=FX07OHEVUtEVDkIlGvJNVHy6xFti%2BdfyewqxVJYuwX0%3D&pq-origsite=primo&accountid=16210&sourcetype=Dissertations%20&%20Theses

Roose, D., Daphne, J., Miller, A. G., Norris, W., Peacock, R., White, C., & White, G. (1997). *Black student retention study: Oberlin College.* Oberlin College.

Sager, W. G. (1973). *A study of changes in attitudes, values, and self-concepts of senior high school youth while working as full-time volunteers with institutionally mentally retarded people* [Unpublished doctoral dissertation]. University of South Dakota.

Salam, M., Iskandar, D. N. A., Ibrahim, D. H. A., & Farooq, M. S. (2019a). Service learning in higher education: A systematic literature review. *Asia Pacific Education Review, 20*, 573–593.https://doi.org/10.1007/s12564-019-09580-6

Salam, M., Iskandar, D. N. A., Ibrahim, D. H. A., & Farooq, M. S. (2019b). Technology integration in service-learning pedagogy: A holistic framework. *Telematics and Informatics, 38*, 257–273.https://doi.org/10.1016/j.tele.2019.02.002

Sandy, M., & Holland, B. A. (2006). Different worlds and common ground: Community partner perspectives on campus-community partnerships. *Michigan Journal of Community Service Learning, 13*(1), 30–43. https://files.eric.ed.gov/fulltext/EJ843845.pdf

Schmidt, M. E. (2021). Embracing e-service learning in the age of COVID and beyond. *Scholarship of Teaching and Learning in Psychology, 10*(3), 337–341. https://doi.org/10.1037/stl0000283

Schön, D. A. (1987). *Educating the reflective practitioner: Toward a new design for teaching and learning in the professions.* Jossey-Bass.

Seifer, S. D., & Mihalynuk, T. V. (2005). The use of technology in higher education service-learning. In A. Seidman (Ed.), *College student retention: Formula for student success* (pp. 360–362). National Service-Learning Clearinghouse. https://searchworks.stanford.edu/view/9612004

Shek, D. T. L. (2021). COVID-19 and quality of life: Twelve reflections. *Applied Research in Quality of Life, 16*(1), 1–11. https://doi.org/10.1007/s11482-020-09898-z

Shek, D. T. L., & Ho, W. W. (2018). Serving clients in a drug rehabilitation agency as a vehicle to promote service leadership in university students. In D. T. L. Shek, G. Ngai, & S. C. Chan (Eds.), *Service-learning for youth leadership: The case of Hong Kong* (Vol. 12, pp. 65–82). Springer. https://doi.org/10.1007/978-981-13-0448-4_5

Shek, D. T. L., Li, X., Chak, Y. L., & Lin, L. (2022a). Service-learning in the context of business-community-university partnership: The Project WeCan in Hong Kong. In G. Ngai, & D. T. L. Shek (Eds.), *Service-learning capacity enhancement in Hong Kong higher education* (Vol. 14, pp. 181–201). Springer. https://doi.org/10.1007/978-981-19-2437-8_10

Shek, D. T. L., Li, X., Yu, L., Lin, L., & Chen, Y. (2022b). Evaluation of electronic service-learning (e-service-learning) projects in mainland China under COVID-19. *Applied Research in Quality of Life, 17*, 3175–3198. https://doi.org/10.1007/s11482-022-10058-8

Shek, D. T. L., Ngai, G., & Chan, S. C. (2018). *Service-learning for youth leadership: The case of Hong Kong* (Vol. 12). Springer. https://doi.org/10.1007/978-981-13-0448-4

Shek, D. T. L., Yang, Z., Ma, C., & Chai, C. (2021). Subjective outcome evaluation of service-learning by the service recipients: Scale development, normative profiles and predictors. *Child Indicators Research, 14*(1), 411–434. https://doi.org/10.1007/s12187-020-09765-1

Shek, D. T. L., Yu, L., & Ngai, J. (2015). Evaluation of a general education program in Hong Kong: Secondary data analyses based on student feedback questionnaires. *International Journal on Disability and Human Development, 14*(4), 401–406. https://doi.org/10.1515/ijdhd-2015-0462

Shumer, R., Ma, C. H. K., & Chan, C. W. Y. (2021). *Food for thought: Service-learning research in Asia*. Information Age Publishing.

Sigmon, R. (1979). Service-learning: Three principles. *Synergist, 8*(1), 9–11.

Sigmon, R. (1994). *Linking service with learning: A report from CIC*. Council of Independent Colleges.

Stanton, T. (1990). Service learning: Groping toward a definition. In J. C Kendall, & Associates (Eds.). *Combining service and learning: A resource book for community and public service* (Vol. 1, pp. 65–67). National Society for Internships and Experiential Education.

Tian, Q., & Noel, T. Jr. (2020). Service-learning in Catholic higher education and alternative approaches facing the COVID-19 pandemic. *Journal of Catholic Education, 23*(1), 184–196. https://doi.org/10.15365/joce.2301142020

Trigos-Carrillo, L., Fonseca, L., & Reinoso, N. (2020). Social impact of a transformative service-learning experience in a post-conflict setting. *Frontiers in Psychology, 11*, 47. https://doi.org/10.3389/fpsyg.2020.00047

University of Hawaii at Manoa. (2022). *Campus Compact*. https://manoa.hawaii.edu/undergrad/civic-engage/campus-compact/

Veyvoda, M. A., & Van Cleave, T. J. (2020). Re-imagining community-engaged learning: Service-learning in communication sciences and disorders courses during and after COVID-19. *Perspectives of the ASHA Special Interest Groups, 5*(6), 1542–1551. https://doi.org/10.1044/2020_PERSP-20-00146

Vogel, A. L., & Seifer, S. D. (2011). Impacts of sustained institutional participation in service-learning: Perspectives from faculty, staff and administrators. *Gateways: International Journal of Community Research and Engagement, 4*, 186–202. https://doi.org/10.5130/IJCRE.V4I0.1789

Wade, R. C., & Yarbrough, D. B. (1997). Community service learning in student teaching: Toward the development of an active citizenry. *Michigan Journal of Community Service Learning, 4*, 42–55. https://quod.lib.umich.edu/m/mjcsl/3239521.0004.105?rgn=main;view=fulltext

Waldner, L. S., Widener, M. C., & McGorry, S. Y. (2012). E-service learning: The evolution of service-learning to engage a growing online student population. *Journal of Higher Education Outreach and Engagement, 16*(2), 123–150. https://openjournals.libs.uga.edu/jheoe/article/view/936/935

Wang, Y., & Rodgers, R. (2006). Impact of service-learning and social justice education on college students' cognitive development. *NASPA Journal, 43*(2), 316–337. https://doi.org/10.2202/1949-6605.1642

Weah, W., Simmons, V. C., & Hall, M. (2000). Service-learning and multicultural/multiethnic perspectives: From diversity to equity. *Phi Delta Kappan*, 673. https://digitalcommons.unomaha.edu/slcediversity/3

Xing, J., & Ma, C. H. K. (2010). *Service-learning in Asia: Curricular models and practices* (Vol. 1). Hong Kong University Press.

Yu, L., Shek, D. T. L., & Xing, K. Y. (2019). Impact of a service-learning programme in mainland China: Views of different stakeholders. In D. T. L. Shek, G. Ngai, & S. C. Chan (Eds.), *Service-learning for youth leadership: The case of Hong Kong* (Vol 12, pp. 49–63). Springer. https://doi.org/10.1007/978-981-13-0448-4_4

Yusof, A., Atan, N. A., Harun, J., & Doulatabadi, M. (2019). Developing students graduate attributes in service learning project through online platform. *Proceedings of the International Conference on Industrial Engineering and Operations Management, Thailand*, 3524–3537. https://ieomsociety.org/ieom2019/papers/815.pdf

Zhu, X., Wu, X., Zhang, S., & Shek, D. T. L. (2023). Evaluation of an electronic service-learning course utilizing regular and intensive delivery modes: The Hong Kong experience. *Research on Social Work Practice, 34*(8), 873–887. https://doi.org/10.1177/10497315231207054

Chapter 8
General Education Program as a Vehicle to Promote Holistic Student Development

Daniel T. L. Shek and Lu Yu

Abstract In the rapidly changing global landscape, university students confront numerous uncertainties and challenges. The provision of General Education (GE) has become crucial in equipping students with interdisciplinary knowledge, 21st-century skills, and psychosocial competences, enabling them to cope with the challenges. GE offers exposure to multiple disciplines, laying the groundwork for the development of intellectual, psychosocial, and civic capacities. To broaden students' knowledge base, foster positive values, and develop essential generic skills for navigating a swiftly evolving world and contributing to a prosperous society, The Hong Kong Polytechnic University (PolyU) has developed a GE program known as the General University Requirements (GUR). This program encompasses various components, including Leadership Education and Development and Service Learning. Both qualitative and quantitative evaluations have demonstrated the effectiveness of the GUR in promoting students' holistic development and well-being. This highlights the importance of integrating GE programs into university curricula and provides insightful perspectives on the ongoing development and innovation of GE programs in higher education.

Keywords General education · University students · General university requirements (GUR) · Evaluation · Leadership education and development

8.1 Introduction

With reference to the fast-changing world and the intensification of globalization, university students face many uncertainties and challenges, and they need to acquire interdisciplinary competences and a flexible mindset to tackle these challenges. Most importantly, they should possess 21st-century skills and psychosocial competences, such as effective communication, cognitive competence, troubleshooting mindset, critical thinking, relationship building, and cross-cultural competence (Gersten, 2011; Lundberg, 2012). Leaders and practitioners in colleges and universities, as well as the public, are exploring effective ways to equip students with cognitive competence and effective communication skills (Jones, 1996). In response to such

D. T. L. Shek, *Promoting Holistic Development in University Students*, Quality of Life in Asia 17, https://doi.org/10.1007/978-981-96-0251-3_8

challenges, providing General Education (GE) courses for students is becoming more and more critical.

One heuristic definition of GE is provided by the American Association of Colleges and Universities (2009): "General Education is part of a liberal education curriculum shared by all students. It provides broad exposure to multiple disciplines and forms the basis for developing important intellectual and civic capacities." Based on this definition, GE is commonly regarded as a standard educational component of undergraduate education, helping students explore rich experiences of academic disciplines and promote their intellectual and civic development. Besides, GE is also seen as a vehicle to motivate learners to consolidate their knowledge and develop life skills such as cognitive competence, interpersonal and intrapersonal communication, integration ability, and team-building skills. These skills equip students with lifelong learning ability and a sense of responsibility in a rapidly changing and increasingly uncertain world (Nelson Laird & Garver, 2010). Furthermore, considering the well-being issues faced by university students outlined in the previous chapters, GE is an active agent that can enhance their well-being.

Aloi et al. (2003) estimated that around 95% of higher education institutions in America provide GE courses for students. Historically, the forms of GE were usually lecture-oriented courses with large enrollments and provided a limited range of disciplines for students to select, such as science or humanities (Glynn et al., 2005). The curriculum was fragmented and lacked coherence. As time went by, an increasing number of higher education institutions in America have evaluated, debated, and modified their GE programs (Gaff, 1994). With this development, GE programs have reformed from lecture-oriented foundational courses to embrace an interdisciplinary instructional goal (Glynn et al., 2005).

8.2 The Roles and Importance of General Education Programs

The importance of GE in engaging students in their learning process has been increasingly emphasized in higher education. In the era of digitalization, acquiring technical competence is far from enough for students to thrive and flourish in the ever-changing world. There is an increasing call to prepare students as competent individuals who can meet the demands of a complex world beyond their specific area of disciplines. Wehlburg (2010) highlighted that GE is essential and critical, and that universities should utilize GE and develop related programs to promote the well-being of students. As interactive settings and collaborative environments are always applied in GE programs, stakeholders in higher education attempt to integrate GE courses to enhance students' learning and engagement (Glynn et al., 2005; Jones, 1996). Attributes such as cognitive competence, writing and reading skills, as well as methods to evaluate the skills, should be addressed in GE courses. More importantly, these competences can enable students to thrive, succeed, and maintain a high level of well-being throughout their lives (Chernyshenko et al., 2018). Therefore, educational institutions should make more efforts to nurture the "knowledge, skills, and attitudes" of students through the GE curriculum (Aloi et al., 2003).

More importantly, scholars and practitioners are exploring effective ways to integrate GE courses into their curricula. Gaff and Ratcliff (1997) emphasized the principles of cohesion, integration, and interdisciplinary connections in designing and implementing GE. Schneider and Schoenberg (1998) stated that "GE should equip students with intellectual capacities and perceive the ability to engage in inquiry, civic knowledge, and values" (p. 7). Bastedo (2002) argued that GE in the contemporary world should help students understand critical issues and develop interdisciplinary capacities in independent learning and acting. Glynn et al. (2005) stressed that GE should cultivate skills like communication, surveying, and cognitive competence and prepare students for intense studies in their discipline. Moreover, GE should develop students' global sensitivity in social, political, economic, technological, and cultural areas. In this way, students can develop better cultural competence and assess real-life issues objectively and comprehensively. Therefore, it is not surprising that GE programs are widely discussed and implemented by more and more colleges and universities.

Besides, the roles and functions of GE have been discussed from different perspectives. GE programs enhance the success and well-being of students, the community and society, and higher education (Li & Li, 2023). In terms of facilitating students' learning outcomes, Gaff (1994) pointed out that GE programs should "continuously strive for educational coherence" and "start with diversity but aim at coherence." Therefore, GE should embrace a wide breadth of knowledge, enable students to undertake meaningful lifelong projects, and create coherence from the varieties (p. 14). Moreover, developing a high level of critical thinking skills in students should be emphasized. Wehlburg (2010) emphasized that students can learn critical approaches, theories, methodologies, and concepts across different professions. Students can gather and filter information, utilize adequate resources, and apply academic learning in their daily lives. Li and Li (2023) stated that GE plays a critical part in nurturing students' intellectual competence, promoting ethical competence, and achieving whole-person development.

In addition, GE implementation can enhance the well-being of the community and society. Firstly, GE can enhance students' social responsibility as educated citizens, which can contribute to building a better community and society (Bok, 2013). It can also empower students to be actively involved in society to improve the well-being of the community. Specifically, by nurturing the concept and awareness of social justice and the global community, GE empowers students to be actively involved in actions that can enhance the well-being of the whole world (Li & Li, 2023). Gaff (1994) argued that GE programs are "self-consciously value-based and teach social responsibility," and he proposed that faculty should provide opportunities for students to be involved in critical, active, and reflective processes (p. 17). For example, as stated in the core curriculum handbook of Susquehanna University, one mission of university education is "educating citizens of the world." Susquehanna University offers a core curriculum called "Futures Seminar," which includes components "Managing

Tomorrow's Crises," "The Future of the World Oceans," and "World Order Models" in their GE courses. Students learn to view their current behaviors and choices critically and think about the future and the world from a futuristic perspective (Gaff, 1994). Moreover, components of multicultural education and Service-Learning (SL) are always adopted in GE programs (Wehlburg, 2010). By participating in these courses, students develop multicultural competence, provide service to the community, and develop a strong sense of citizen participation, civic responsibility, and social understanding, ultimately enabling substantial societal contributions in future.

Equally important, GE promotes the development of institutions by enhancing integrative learning, which enables students to integrate their learning and knowledge effectively, enriches their learning experiences, and nurtures a comprehensive and multidisciplinary knowledge base (Wehlburg, 2010). In discussing "12 principles for effective GE programs," Gaff (1994) emphasized that GE programs should "embody institutional mission" and "be grounded in the sense of public purpose, its history and tradition, the character of its students, and its geographical setting ..." (p. 11). As Lewis (2006) noted, GE can have a significant impact on the design and implementation of education programs in institutions. Faculties and institutions can reflect on and reconsider their mission and identity and innovate their programs. Equally important, GE can help frame and fulfill the overall educational philosophy, values, goals, and mission of higher education institutions (Menand, 2010). Therefore, promoting GE is beneficial for the development of educational programs that are consistent with the institution's mission.

8.3 General Education Program at PolyU

Many countries and regions have recognized the significance of the above GE and have introduced different GE curriculum models into their courses to enhance students' learning experiences at university. Among the various models adopted by different universities, the most widely used and referenced model is the GE model implemented by American colleges and universities. Students usually take a series of GE courses in the first two years of their university study, followed by courses related to their major in the third and fourth years. Today, many countries and regions, including mainland China, Hong Kong, Taiwan, and others, have incorporated this model into their curriculum (Xing et al., 2013; Weiland, 1989).

In the context of Hong Kong, the undergraduate study structure has gone through changes over the past decade. When Hong Kong was still under British colonial rule (i.e., until June 30, 1997), the university structure was modeled after that of the United Kingdom, where students took seven years of high school education followed by three years of undergraduate study. With the education reform carried out after 1997, starting in the 2012/2013 academic year, the duration of high school was reduced to six years, and university education was extended from three to four years. An additional year of university education allowed for the incorporation of GE to broaden students' worldviews. Past studies suggest that this approach would help broaden students' knowledge base and vision, cultivate positive values, and nurture basic generic skills, ultimately strengthening Hong Kong's human resources pool. These changes would also facilitate Hong Kong's response to the rapidly changing financial and social environment, enable the transformation into a high-value-added services economy in the twenty-first century (Jaffee, 2013; Sutherland, 2002), and contribute to the development of Hong Kong as a civilized society (Curry, 2012).

In the 2012–2013 academic year, The Hong Kong Polytechnic University (PolyU) launched a new GE program in the undergraduate program. Known as the General University Requirements (GUR), the university core curriculum consists of six main sections, each described in the following paragraphs. Through this six-part framework, the core curriculum aims to nurture PolyU students with five desirable graduation qualities: critical thinking, effective communication, innovative problem-solving, lifelong learning, and ethical leadership, thereby cultivating them to be competitive professionals and global citizens. The GUR components include:

- "Freshman Seminar": The Freshman Seminar, the first part of the University's core curriculum, is a three-credit course offered by PolyU faculties to all first-year students in each faculty.
- "Leadership and Intrapersonal Development (LIPD).": This component is designed to help students develop the intrapersonal and interpersonal skills required of a virtuous leader. It comprises two subjects (each with three credits), one is "Tomorrow's Leaders," which is compulsory for all first-year students (except students majoring in business administration). The other, "Tango! Managing Yourself and Leading Others," is primarily for first-year students in the Faculty of Business.
- "Language and Communication Requirements": This component aims to enhance students' language proficiency. Students are required to take one Chinese subject (3 credits) and two English subjects (6 credits) based on their linguistic competence.
- "Cluster-Area Requirements": The general studies course covers four major areas: (1) "Human Nature, Relations and Development," (2) "Cultures, Organisations, Societies and Globalisation," (3) "Chinese History and Culture" and (4) "Science, Technology and Environment." At the same time, the content design of each category includes at least one of the following two additional requirements: Chinese Reading and Writing Requirements and English Reading and Writing Requirements. Students need to take one course (3 credits each, totaling 12 credits) in each of the above four areas, and the selected subjects must also meet the above two additional study requirements. The general studies course is intended to nurture students' "intellectual capacity, global outlook, communication and critical thinking skills from a multidisciplinary perspective."
- "Service Learning": Students are required to take a subject (3 credits) that contains social service elements. This course aims to "develop students' sense of social responsibility, empathy and ability to apply professional knowledge."
- "Healthy Lifestyle": This course does not award any credits, and students need to complete a series of different projects, such as "introductory classes,"

"physical training," "e-learning," and "wrap-up classes." This section aims to "develop students' understanding of healthy living patterns and to acquire relevant knowledge and skills."

Over the years, the desired graduate attributes and the GUR curriculum have undergone some changes. In the recent revamp of the GUR, the Freshman Seminar was removed, and two new graduation requirements ("Artificial Intelligence and Data Analytics" and "Innovation and Entrepreneurship") were added. Besides, the "Leadership and Intrapersonal Development" has been renamed "Leadership Education and Development".

8.3.1 Leadership and Intrapersonal Development: "Tomorrow's Leaders"

University students are the leaders of tomorrow. Hence, there is a need to nurture their leadership qualities. Unfortunately, few credit-bearing leadership subjects are offered at universities, and most leadership programs are non-credit-bearing and extracurricular. Besides, leadership programs in the university context are commonly designed for "elite students," leaving behind students who are late starters. Embracing the beliefs that "every student can shine" and "students can lead (at least leading themselves)," we aim to develop the intrapersonal and interpersonal skills of university students via a leadership subject entitled "Tomorrow's Leaders." Specifically, this subject is based on the Positive Youth Development (PYD) approach, which was modeled after Project P.A.T.H.S. in Hong Kong. Project P.A.T.H.S. was developed to promote the holistic development of junior secondary school students in Hong Kong. As a university version of P.A.T.H.S., in this subject, we focus on several PYD attributes, including "self-understanding," "self-leadership," "cognitive competence," "emotional competence," "moral competence," "resilience," "social competence," "team building," and "conflict resolution."

Due to the implementation of the Hong Kong National Security Law in 2020, universities are now responsible for providing education on national security. As such, we have incorporated national security education into "Tomorrow's Leaders," renaming the area "Leadership Education and Development (LEAD)." We devote a 3-hour lecture to law abidance leadership (plus 7 hours of self-study) to nurture students' law abidance leadership. We will discuss this issue in Chap. 13, which can capture the attention of scholars in the local and international contexts.

This subject has received several teaching awards, including the "Silver Award (Ethical Leadership)" and "Gold Award (Nurturing Well-Being and Purpose)" in "QS Reimagine Education Awards" and the "University Grants Committee Teaching Award," the highest teaching award in the higher education sector in Hong Kong.

8.3.2 Cluster Area Requirement (Area A): Service Leadership

Besides taking the compulsory subject of leadership under LIPD, students can also take another elective subject on Service Leadership under "Cluster Area Requirement (Area A)." This cluster, entitled "Human Nature, Relations and Development," includes subjects from social sciences and interdisciplinary perspectives, which enables students to understand and appreciate human nature and explore its development from diverse theoretical perspectives.

The subject "Service Leadership" was developed against the backdrop of the global economy's shift from manufacturing-oriented to service-oriented. With the support of the Fung Education Initiative and the seminal ideas from Dr. Po Chung, Service Leadership highlights the qualities of "leadership competence," "character," and "care." Adopting the PYD approach, we emphasize the importance of intelligence (IQ), emotional intelligence (EQ), and spirituality (SQ) in leadership competence, character traits emphasized in Western and Chinese cultural contexts, and caring dispositions. Besides, we highlight the quality of self-leadership, which states that "one needs to lead oneself before leading others." Moreover, we stress the differences between the Service Leadership Theory and contemporary leadership models.

This subject has received many teaching awards, including the "Bronze Award (Ethical Leadership)" and "Gold Award (Nurturing Well-Being and Purpose)" in "QS Reimagine Education Awards" and the "University Grants Committee Teaching Award," the highest teaching award in the higher education sector in Hong Kong.

8.3.3 Service-Learning: Promotion of Child and Adolescent Development

As mentioned in the previous chapter, SL is a pedagogy that can strengthen students' learning and promote their sense of social responsibility and civic engagement. Besides, SL helps to promote a sense of empathy and understanding of community needs, which are essential qualities for leadership. In the subject titled "Promotion of Child and Adolescent Development," we help students understand the theories and research on child and adolescent development and to integrate their academic learning into SL projects. The program has several project sites in Hong Kong, including schools admitting students with low academic achievements, organizations providing service for families and children with special needs, and organizations helping students with emotional and behavioral problems. Students taking this subject also implement the SL project in mainland China in the form of summer camps. During these camps, university students develop programs for primary school students in subjects such as English, Health Education, Personal Development, and Science. In Hangzhou, we conducted summer camps for a primary school that admitted children of migrant workers. During the COVID-19 pandemic, we conducted online SL from 2019 to 2022.

This subject has received several teaching awards, including the "Silver Award (Ethical Leadership)" and "Gold Award (Nurturing Well-Being and Purpose)" in "QS Reimagine Education Awards" and the "University Grants Committee Teaching Award," the highest teaching award in the higher education sector in Hong Kong.

8.3.4 Service-Learning: Service Leadership Through Serving Children and Families with Special Needs

We have also developed another SL subject titled "Service Leadership through Serving Children and Families with Special Needs" to enable students to gain a comprehensive understanding of the Service Leadership Theory and to highlight the essential qualities of service leaders. Besides, students are expected to develop leadership qualities of "competence, character, and care" and to integrate this knowledge into their SL projects. In Hong Kong, university students implement SL projects in ordinary high schools to help students with poor academic achievement, in special schools to support students with emotional and behavioral problems, and in an organization to assist young people with behavioral and substance abuse problems. Outside Hong Kong, students taking this subject also implement related SL projects in Chengdu and Xi'an in the form of summer camps. At these sites, we organize summer camps for primary school students from families of migrant workers or low-income households. To enrich the development of these students, SL implementers provide different programs in English Language, Health Education, Science Education, and Personal Development. During the pandemic, we also provided online SL projects for primary school students in Chengdu and Xi'an.

This subject has received several teaching awards, including the "Bronze Award (Social Enterprise)" and "Gold Award (Nurturing Well-Being and Purpose)" in "QS Reimagine Education Awards" and the "University Grants Committee Teaching Award," the highest teaching award in the higher education sector in Hong Kong.

8.4 Evaluation of the General University Requirements

In order to explore the impact and effectiveness of GUR at PolyU, we have conducted a variety of evaluation strategies after its implementation. These evaluation methods include "objective outcome evaluations," "subjective outcome evaluations," and "qualitative evaluations." These studies supported the conclusion that the GUR has a positive impact on the holistic development and well-being of PolyU students.

Manifold types of evaluation studies on the impact of GUR have been conducted. Specifically, quantitative methods such as online surveys and the Collegiate Learning

Assessment Plus (CLA+) were adopted to investigate student-level developmental indicators. In the 2013/2014 academic year, Shek et al. (2016a) investigated the students' learning gains in attributes of cognitive competence and intrapersonal and interpersonal communication based on their results in the CLA+ scale and other subscales from both freshmen ($N = 150$) and sophomores ($N = 150$). The objective outcome evaluation data displayed that sophomores performed better than first-year students on the attributes of problem-solving, effective communication, and critical thinking, which showed that GUR has a positive impact on promoting the desired development attributes and whole-person development. Remarkably, the researchers noted that multiple components of the GUR curriculum enabled students to apply their academic learning to their daily lives. Moreover, a variety of experiential learning and collaborative learning activities were utilized in GUR subjects to train students' cognitive competence and interpersonal and intrapersonal communication skills. Additionally, students developed a sense of responsibility and citizenship after participating in a wide range of community services in SL courses provided by GUR. It is not surprising to discover that the GUR curriculum is beneficial for students in developing desired graduate attributes defined by PolyU.

Regarding subjective outcome evaluation, the researchers utilized the standard student feedback questionnaire (SFQ) to examine students' feedback. In the first semester of the 2012/2013 academic year, Shek and Yu (2016) applied a tailor-made SFQ to understand students' perceptions of a subject under GUR. The questionnaire included universal items for all subjects and "refined" items for this targeted subject. Despite considering the students' evaluation of teachers and the subjects, the study also regarded students' final grades as one of the outcome measures and as an objective indicator of students' learning attainment. Altogether, 748 students completed SFQ. The overall data supported the hypothesis that the subject nurtured five desirable graduate attributes of PolyU students ("critical thinking, effective communication, ethical leadership, lifelong learning, and innovative problem-solving"). Qualitative data also showed that students gained different levels of interpersonal and intrapersonal competence. Interestingly, the ratings displayed faculty-based differences, which highlighted the need for in-depth qualitative studies to explore these variations in the future.

To replicate the findings, Shek et al. (2017f) conducted a similar study on the same subject in the second semester. SFQ data from 674 students were analyzed, which were consistent with the first semester in that students generally appreciated the subject design, the teacher quality, and the perceived learning outcomes and benefits. The two studies proved that this subject was implemented effectively in its first year and further suggested that providing leadership and intrapersonal development subjects under GUR is necessary. More importantly, the successful implementation of this subject provides guidelines for other universities to incorporate similar subjects in their curriculum.

Another replication quantitative research was conducted by Shek et al. (2016b). They assessed the SFQ and students' final grades in one subject under the GUR framework to assess its impact on students over two years. Altogether, 1,406 students from the 2012/2013 academic year and 1,283 students from the 2013/2014 academic year completed the SFQ. Students agreed that the subject, teacher's performance, and perceived benefits were beneficial for them. The results also displayed that the GUR subject has a favorable effect on students' positive development, such as reflection skills and self-understanding. More importantly, the study revealed that the evaluation data were related to students' academic performance. These results were consistent with previous subjective evaluations conducted by Shek (2013a), who found that this subject under the GUR framework was effective in enhancing the positive development of university students.

Despite focusing on one subject, Shek et al. (2015a) analyzed longitudinal SFQ data of all GUR subjects during the 2012/2013 and 2013/2014 academic years. The study involved a large sample size of 15,810 students and 17,463 students from these two academic years, respectively. The study proved that the students generally agreed with the effectiveness of the GUR subjects, including the learning experiences and the teaching quality of teachers. In terms of different GUR components, some subjects, such as Language and Communication Requirement, displayed an increase in satisfaction over time, while some subjects, such as SL, showed a slight decline in satisfaction. Therefore, differences regarding various GUR subjects were examined. The findings were consistent with the qualitative study conducted by Shek et al. (2015b), which found that GUR was successful at PolyU. Equally important, this study suggested considering variations across different domains and over time in further studies.

Qualitatively, to understand students' experiences of all GUR subjects, Shek et al. (2017d) recruited 163 students from different faculties to collect their qualitative data during the 2012–2013 academic year. Students were invited to describe their experiences using descriptors and metaphors. Most students reported unforgettable experiences gained from the GUR subjects. To cite some examples, "having opportunities to make new friends," "new learning methods," "experiential learning stimulated interest," and "enriched learning experiences" were reported by students. The frequently adopted positive descriptors include "interesting," "practical," "useful," "helpful to development," and "have increased knowledge." In terms of unforgettable experiences, over 76% of students reported remarkable and positive experiences. Around 8% gave neutral responses, and less than 16% provided negative feedback. Students appreciated the forms of experiential learning and collaborative learning. Many GUR subjects in PolyU adopted experiential learning and collaborative learning to enhance students' learning experiences. Remarkably, many scholars have identified the impact of experiential learning. For instance, Eyler (2009) emphasized that experiential learning develops students' competence and helps students' link academic study to real-life learning. It enables students to be well-prepared for future work and to be responsible citizens after their graduation. The study also discussed obstacles or challenges encountered by students, including language barriers, poor time management, and heavy workloads. Equally important, from the narratives, over 95% of students reported that they have benefited from subjects such as "communication skills," "critical thinking skills," "enhanced physical and mental health," and "ethical leadership skills." Moreover, students agreed that the GUR subjects expanded their worldviews. This study is meaningful as it involved a large number of participants from various disciplines. As the first qualitative study to examine the 4-year curriculum in Hong Kong, this study also filled the knowledge gap in the qualitative evaluation of students. Remarkably, GUR programs need to integrate the element of experiential learning to support the planning and implementation of experiential learning.

Notably, focus groups for students and teachers were carried out to understand the perceptions of different stakeholders. Shek et al. (2017a) conducted 18 student focus groups in the 2013/2014 academic year. Altogether, 74 participants joined the study. Most students appreciated the well-designed subject contents, good quality of teachers, devoted and caring way of teaching, and experiential teaching and learning methods. Moreover, they agreed that the subject was beneficial for broadening their learning experience, enhancing their holistic development and well-being, and training their reading and writing skills. For example, one student commented, "My most impressive experience was to visit and talk with people who lived in the 'rippled room.' This experience really let me know more." Another student responded, "I think I had developed more confidence through doing a variety of tasks such as group work and individual projects. In my first several group projects, I often felt that I had less contribution to the project and did not dare to express my views. Then, after experiencing so many group projects, I feel that the group project is not so scary, and I am able to express what I am thinking now." Notably, the challenges encountered by students were discussed, which provided practical suggestions for improving the quality of the GUR curriculum. The findings displayed that the GUR curriculum equips students with indispensable competences and promotes their all-round development.

Equally important, students' reflections and sharing were recognized as valuable feedback. In the 2011/2012 academic year, Shek and Law (2014) invited students to illustrate their experiences using three descriptors and one metaphor after taking one GUR subject. The subject was in the second pilot stage. Altogether, 143 students provided their responses. Regarding the descriptors, over 94% of them were positive, and around 2% were negative. To cite some examples, positive descriptors such as "helpful to development," "useful/helpful," "reflective," "interactive," "interesting," "inspiring," "impressive," "self-enhancement," and "skills development" were identified. Likewise, in terms of metaphor descriptions, more than 92% of students gave positive feedback, and less than 5% of the metaphors were negative. Positive metaphors, such as "compass," "GPS," "map," and "an enjoyable, nice, exploring, exciting, and unforgettable journey," were provided by students. The results were consistent with the previous study conducted by Shek (2013b) when this GUR subject was in the first pilot stage. The findings suggested that this GUR subject is effective in promoting leadership and intrapersonal development of PolyU students.

Apart from the reflection on the subject, students' perceptions of teachers were also evaluated. In the 2012/2013 academic year, Shek and Wu (2014) invited students to write personal reflective journals to share their views. A framework analysis methodology was adopted for this study. In total, 66 pieces of personal reflections were received. The qualitative data displayed that students appreciated the subject and teachers' performance. Firstly, students reflected that the professional arrangement and personal engagement of teachers were adequate, including various methods of teaching, professional delivery of content, rich forms of activities, and in-depth reflection. Additionally, students recognized the caring, warm, and supportive attitude of teachers. For instance, one student reflected, "Our lecturer has done her best to make it interesting and easy to understand with direct explanations." Another student wrote, "Our lecturer and tutor gave us full and valuable support, helping us to find out our mistakes and improving our presentation." Moreover, the respondents appreciated the rich personal engagement and effective communication with teachers. This study revealed that teachers take up an inspiring role in promoting students' psychosocial well-being in GUR subjects.

In addition to the perceptions of students, qualitative evaluation was applied to explore teachers' feedback. Teachers are regarded as significant stakeholders, and their feedback and suggestions regarding program design, objectives, and rationales are critical for the positive development of the program (Fuchs et al., 2001). To understand the impact of the subjects from the teachers' perspectives, in the 2013/2014 academic year, Shek et al. (2017b) invited 40 teachers who had taught the GUR subjects to join a focus group. The teachers reported that they were satisfied with the arrangement and implementation of GUR subjects. Remarkably, teachers appreciated the integration of interactive learning and teaching methods, including fieldwork, group projects, and debates, in GUR subjects, which could strengthen students' self-learning skills, involve students actively in their studies, and inspire them to understand the contents. Moreover, the respondents recognized its beneficial effect of enhancing students' academic and psychosocial well-being. One teacher reported, "I think the design of the course is not only for text examination but also for promoting students' capability for dealing with difficulties in life." Another teacher added, "Many students treat the course very positively because they think the course really broadens their horizons and attracts them. Science students think the content talking about culture in the course is very interesting." In addition to the benefits, the respondents also reported challenges encountered during their teaching, such as heavy workload, low learning motivation of some students, and English learning difficulties encountered by some students. The challenges mentioned by teachers indicated that improvements were needed to enhance the quality of the GUR subjects. Despite the limitations and challenges, this qualitative study was consistent with the previous findings that the GUR subjects are beneficial for students (Shek & Sun, 2013; Shek et al., 2015c, 2017c).

To explore "whether students in the 4-year undergraduate program were better than those in the 3-year program," Shek and Yu (2017b) applied a static group comparison design with an experimental group (Year 3 students of the 4-year program) and control group (Year 3 students of the 3-year program) from the 2014/2015 student cohort. It was the first study to validate the effectiveness of the educational reforms in higher education in Hong Kong. In this study, students in the comparison group showed better performance on various developmental outcome indicators, such as "intrapersonal competence," "interpersonal competence," and "PYD attributes." Moreover, by utilizing methods such as "experiential learning," "reflective learning," and "collaborative learning," students who took GUR subjects displayed an enhanced level of engagement compared to students who were not involved in the GUR curriculum. The findings showed that GUR at PolyU is beneficial for students, which was consistent with the previous research (Shek & Ma, 2014; Shek & Yu, 2014; Shek et al., 2015b, 2015c, 2017e).

Interestingly, the researchers utilized the data obtained from the same experimental group to explore whether and how GUR is beneficial. Shek and Yu (2017a) utilized another static group comparison design, where the same experimental group (Year 3 students of the 4-year program) in Shek and Yu (2017b) was compared with the control group (Year 3 students of the 3-year program) from another university in Hong Kong. Notably, students from PolyU (the experimental group) performed better than students in the control group at a comparable university. For instance, students in the treatment group scored higher in terms of psychosocial competence, cognitive competence, emotional management, and moral competence. Moreover, the life satisfaction of PolyU students was higher than that of the comparable group, which suggested that the GUR has a positive impact on enhancing the all-round development of students.

After the GUR was implemented for five years, Shek et al. (2015c) conducted a 5-year longitudinal study. This study is the first longitudinal study in the local context to examine the impact of GUR. With the principle of triangulation, they collected objective and subjective data as well as qualitative and quantitative data. Moreover, the perceptions of students and teachers were valued and recognized, which presented a comprehensive picture of the implementation process and the effectiveness of GUR programs. The study suggested that GUR is effective in enhancing five desirable graduate attributes of PolyU, including "problem-solving skills," "critical thinking competence," "effective communication," "ethical leadership," and "lifelong learning." All of the above studies and findings strengthened the conclusion that GUR is beneficial for promoting the holistic development of students.

8.5 Conclusion

The roles and importance of GE programs in university education are unequivocally presented. GE courses enable students to explore and establish a diverse knowledge base and develop multidisciplinary competences. Essential competences, such as cognitive competence, effective communication, critical thinking, and creative thinking, help students thrive and flourish in the rapidly changing world. More importantly, GE courses cultivate a sense of social responsibility and civic engagement as responsible citizens and future leaders. With a commitment to lifelong learning and enhanced psychosocial well-being, students will benefit throughout their lives. Furthermore, this chapter discusses the implementation and structure of GUR at PolyU. There are multifaceted components in its curriculum, thereby facilitating students to embrace a holistic educational experience. Many subjects under the GUR curriculum at PolyU have received many awards, which is inspiring. Additionally, evaluations and studies on the effectiveness of GUR at PolyU were carried out after its implementation. Both qualitative and quantitative evaluation methods have reinforced the hypothesis that the GUR is effective in enriching students' learning experiences and fostering holistic development. These findings provide meaningful insights for the reflection, implementation, ongoing refinement, and innovation of the GUR curriculum in the higher education sector.

Acknowledgements The preparation of this chapter is financially supported by The Hong Kong Polytechnic University (ZZ4U and ZZUE), Li and Fung Endowed Professorship in Service Leadership Education, Wofoo Foundation, and the Matching Fund of Research Grants Council (ZECL and ZH4Q).

References

Aloi, S. L., Gardner, W. S., & Lusher, A. L. (2003). A framework for assessing general education outcomes within the majors. *The Journal of General Education, 52*(4), 237–252. http://www.jstor.org/stable/27797962

American Association of Colleges and Universities. (2009). *What is liberal education?* https://www.aacu.org/trending-topics/what-is-liberal-education

Bastedo, M. (2002). General education. In J. Forest & K. Kinser (Eds.), *Higher education in the United States: An encyclopedia* (pp. 273–276). ABC-CLIO.

Bok, D. (2013). *Higher education in America* (Rev. ed.). Princeton University Press. https://doi.org/10.1515/9781400866120

Chernyshenko, O. S., Kankaraš, M., & Drasgow, F. (2018). *Social and emotional skills for student success and well-being: Conceptual framework for the OECD study on social and emotional skills.* (OECD Education Working Papers No. 173). OECD Publishing. https://doi.org/10.1787/db1d8e59-en

Curry, J. M. (2012). Cultural challenges in Hong Kong to the implementation of effective general education. *Teaching in Higher Education, 17*(2), 223–230. https://doi.org/10.1080/13562517.2012.658565

Eyler, J. (2009). The power of experiential education. *Liberal Education, 95*(4), 24–31. https://files.eric.ed.gov/fulltext/EJ871318.pdf

Fuchs, D., Fuchs, L. S., Thompson, A., Otaiba, S. A., Yen, L., Yang, N. J., Braun, M., & O'Connor, R. E. (2001). Is reading important in reading-readiness programs? A randomized field trial with teachers as program implementers. *Journal of Educational Psychology, 93*(2), 251–267. https://doi.org/10.1037/0022-0663.93.2.251

Gaff, J. G. (1994). *Strong foundations: Twelve principles for effective general education programs. American Association of Colleges and Universities.*

Gaff, J. G., & Ratcliff, J. L. (1997). *Handbook of the undergraduate curriculum: A comprehensive guide to purposes, structures, practices, and change.* Jossey-Bass.

Gersten, K. (2011). General education: Learning from the past, preparing for the future. *Higher Learning Research Communications, 2*(2), 8–17. https://doi.org/10.18870/hlrc.v2i2.67

Glynn, S. M., Aultman, L. P., & Owens, A. M. (2005). Motivation to learn in general education programs. *The Journal of General Education, 54*(2), 150–170. https://doi.org/10.2307/27798014

Jaffee, D. (2013). Building general education with Hong Kong characteristics. *International Education, 42*(2), 41–59. https://trace.tennessee.edu/internationaleducation/vol42/iss2/4

Jones, E. A. (1996). National and state policies affecting learning expectations. *New Directions for Higher Education, 1996*(96), 7–18.https://doi.org/10.1002/he.36919969603

Lewis, H. R. (2006). *Excellence without a soul: How a great university forgot education.* Public Affairs.

Li, X., & Li, Y. (2023). Individualized and innovation-centered general education in a Chinese STEM University. *Education Sciences, 13*(8), Article 846. https://doi.org/10.3390/educsci13080846

Lundberg, T. C. (2012). Learning to innovate in twenty-first-century community colleges: Searching for the general education niche in two-year colleges. *New Directions for Community Colleges, 2012*(157), 83–95. https://doi.org/10.1002/cc.20008

Menand, L. (2010). *The marketplace of ideas: Reform and resistance in the American university.* W. W. Norton & Company.

Nelson Laird, T. F., & Garver, A. K. (2010). The effect of teaching general education courses on deep approaches to learning: How disciplinary context matters. *Research in Higher Education, 51*(3), 248–265. https://doi.org/10.1007/s11162-009-9154-7

Schneider, C., & Schoenberg, R. (1998). *The academy in transition: Contemporary understandings of liberal education.* American Association of Colleges and Universities.

Shek, D. T. L. (2013a). Promotion of holistic development in university students. *Best Practices in Mental Health, 9*(1), 47–61. https://doi.org/10.70256/428239ofjkeh

Shek, D. T. L. (2013b). Reflections of Chinese students on a university subject on leadership and intrapersonal development. *International Journal on Disability and Human Development, 12*(2), 213–219. https://doi.org/10.1515/ijdhd-2013-0019

Shek, D. T. L., & Law, M. Y. M. (2014). Evaluation of a subject on leadership and intrapersonal development: Views of the students based on qualitative evaluation. *International Journal on Disability and Human Development, 13*(4), 435–441. https://doi.org/10.1515/ijdhd-2014-0339

Shek, D. T. L., & Ma, C. M. S. (2014). Do university students change after taking a subject on leadership and intrapersonal development? *International Journal on Disability and Human Development, 13*(4), 451–456. https://doi.org/10.1515/ijdhd-2014-0341

Shek, D. T. L., & Sun, R. C. F. (2013). Process evaluation of a leadership and intrapersonal development subject for university students. *International Journal on Disability and Human Development, 12*(2), 203–211. https://doi.org/10.1515/ijdhd-2013-0018

Shek, D. T. L., & Wu, F. K. Y. (2014). The role of teachers in youth development: Reflections of students. *International Journal on Disability and Human Development, 13*(4), 473–480. https://doi.org/10.1515/ijdhd-2014-0344

Shek, D. T. L., & Yu, L. (2014). Post-course subjective outcome evaluation of a subject on leadership and intrapersonal development for university students in Hong Kong. *International Journal on Disability and Human Development, 13*(4), 457–464. https://doi.org/10.1515/ijdhd-2014-0342

Shek, D. T. L., & Yu, L. (2016). Student feedback on a subject on leadership and intrapersonal development for university students in Hong Kong. *International Journal on Disability and Human Development, 15*(3), 339–346. https://doi.org/10.1515/ijdhd-2015-6002

Shek, D. T. L., & Yu, L. (2017a). General university requirements and holistic development in university students in Hong Kong. *International Journal of Adolescent Medicine and Health, 29*(1), 41–48. https://doi.org/10.1515/ijamh-2017-3006

Shek, D. T. L., & Yu, L. (2017b). The impact of 3-year and 4-year undergraduate programs on university students: The case of Hong Kong. *International Journal of Adolescent Medicine and Health, 29*(1), 49–55. https://doi.org/10.1515/ijamh-2017-3007

Shek, D. T. L., Yu, L., & Chai, W. Y. (2017a). Evaluation of the general university requirements: What did students say? *International Journal of Adolescent Medicine and Health, 29*(1), 75–82. https://doi.org/10.1515/ijamh-2017-3010

Shek, D. T. L., Yu, L., Chan, K. H. W., & Ho, W. W. L. (2016a). Assessing learning gains of university students in Hong Kong adopting the Collegiate Learning Assessment Plus (CLA+). *International Journal on Disability and Human Development, 15*(3), 331–337. https://doi.org/10.1515/ijdhd-2015-6001

Shek, D. T. L., Yu, L., & Chi, X. (2017b). Focus group evaluation of teachers' views on a new general education program in Hong Kong. *International Journal of Adolescent Medicine and Health, 29*(1), 67–74. https://doi.org/10.1515/IJAMH-2017-3009

Shek, D. T. L., Yu, L., & Ngai, J. (2015a). Evaluation of a general education program in Hong Kong: Secondary data analyses based on student feedback questionnaires. *International Journal on Disability and Human Development, 14*(4), 401–406. https://doi.org/10.1515/ijdhd-2015-0462

Shek, D. T. L., Yu, L., Wu, F. K. Y., & Chai, W. Y. (2015b). General university requirements at Hong Kong Polytechnic University: Evaluation findings based on student focus groups. *Assessment and Evaluation in Higher Education, 40*(8), 1017–1031. https://doi.org/10.1080/02602938.2014.960362

Shek, D. T. L., Yu, L., Wu, F. K. Y., & Chai, W. Y. (2017c). Teachers' views of a new general education program in Hong Kong: A qualitative study. *International Journal of Adolescent Medicine and Health, 29*(1), 57–65. https://doi.org/10.1515/ijamh-2017-3008

Shek, D. T. L., Yu, L., Wu, F. K. Y., & Ng, C. S. M. (2015c). General education program in a new 4-year university curriculum in Hong Kong: Findings based on multiple evaluation strategies. *International Journal on Disability and Human Development, 14*(4), 377–384. https://doi.org/10.1515/ijdhd-2015-0459

Shek, D. T. L., Yu, L., Wu, F. K. Y., Ng, C. S. M., & Chai, W. Y. (2017d). Qualitative evaluation of general university requirements in a new 4-year university curriculum: Findings based on experiences of students. *International Journal of Adolescent Medicine and Health, 29*(1), 91–102. https://doi.org/10.1515/ijamh-2017-3012

Shek, D. T. L., Yu, L., Wu, F. K. Y., Zhu, X. Q., & Chai, W. Y. (2017e). Teachers' views on a new general education program in Hong Kong: Qualitative data collected over two years. *International Journal of Child & Adolescent Health, 10*(2), 233–243.

Shek, D. T. L., Yu, L., & Xie, Q. Z. (2017f). Student feedback on a pioneer subject on leadership and intrapersonal development in Hong Kong. *International Journal of Adolescent Medicine and Health, 29*(1), 83–89. https://doi.org/10.1515/ijamh-2017-3011

Shek, D. T. L., Yu, L., & Zhu, X. Q. (2016b). Evaluation of a leadership and intrapersonal development subject for university students in Hong Kong: Findings based on 2 years. *International Journal on Disability and Human Development, 15*(1), 101–109. https://doi.org/10.1515/ijdhd-2015-0028

Sutherland, S. R. (2002). *Higher education in Hong Kong: Report of the University Grants Committee.* University Grants Committee. https://www.ugc.edu.hk/doc/eng/ugc/publication/report/her/hereport.pdf

Wehlburg, C. M. (2010). Integrated general education: A brief look back. *New Directions for Teaching and Learning, 2010*(121), 3–11. https://doi.org/10.1002/tl.383

Weiland, J. S. (1989). General education in the universities after 1992. *European Journal of Education, 24*(4), 371–380. https://doi.org/10.2307/1503305

Xing, J., Ng, P., & Cheng, C. (eds.). (2013). *General education and the development of global citizenship in Hong Kong.* Routledge.

Chapter 9
Development, Implementation, and Evaluation of a Leadership Subject for University Students—"Tomorrow's Leaders"

Daniel T. L. Shek and Xiang Li

Abstract The prevalence of developmental issues among university students is on the rise. To promote students' holistic development, The Hong Kong Polytechnic University (PolyU) has developed a 3-credit leadership course titled "Tomorrow's Leaders." This course aims to cultivate students' positive youth development (PYD) attributes, focusing on intrapersonal and interpersonal qualities essential for effective leadership, thereby enhancing their developmental assets. Its teaching philosophy is rooted in the belief that every student has the potential to be a leader. The curriculum is designed to integrate academic knowledge with personal growth, fostering intense interactions between teachers and students, as well as among students themselves. It encourages experiential, collaborative, and reflective learning. Engagement methods include group discussions, reflective activities, sharing exercises, and post-lecture evaluations. The impact of the course has been rigorously evaluated through objective outcome evaluation, subjective outcome evaluation, process evaluation, and qualitative evaluation. Findings consistently show improvements in students' PYD attributes, their positive views on the course and instructors, and the perceived benefits they gained from the course. In addition to positive feedback from students, this subject has also received external recognition. The chapter further discusses teacher training and future direction.

Keywords Leadership · Positive youth development (PYD) · Tomorrow's Leaders · University · Impact and evaluation · Student learning experience

9.1 Introduction

The developmental issues among university students, such as mental health problems and rising egocentrism, are growing (Li et al., 2021; Shek & Wong, 2011; Twenge, 2014). To address the developmental issues, Lewis (2006) highlighted that "Over the decades, I have heard many academic discussions about teaching, about the curriculum, about grading, about athletics, and about responding to student misdeeds. I have almost never heard discussions among professors about making students better

D. T. L. Shek, *Promoting Holistic Development in University Students*, Quality of Life in Asia 17, https://doi.org/10.1007/978-981-96-0251-3_9

people" (p. xiii). Similarly, Dalton and Crosby (2006) claimed that universities should provide resources and support for students to "make internal connections to the defining beliefs and purposes in their lives … since they do not reach that part of students' lives where things really matter" (p. 1). Nevertheless, universities have been criticized for failing to shoulder the responsibility of helping students develop holistically (Shek, 2013).

Based on the PYD approach, we argue that cultivating PYD attributes among adolescents can help strengthen developmental assets in students, which would eventually protect them from developmental problems and help them thrive (Shek, 2010; Shek & Wong, 2011). In this regard, the subject "Tomorrow's Leaders," which applied a leadership framework to integrate theories and research on PYD, was developed. Students are expected to learn, reflect on, and practice their intrapersonal and leadership competencies by participating in a range of experiential learning activities provided by this leadership subject. Notably, many credit-bearing leadership subjects do not focus on attributes of youth development, or many subjects do not carry any credit. Moreover, most youth leadership programs usually adopt an "elitist" approach without a well-articulated conceptual framework. Therefore, implementing this leadership subject is unique and creative among universities, particularly in universities in Hong Kong. Besides, systematic evaluative works to assess leadership and intrapersonal development in university students are lacking (Shek & Ng, 2017; Shek & Yuen, 2019).

The subject "Tomorrow's Leaders," which aimed to promote holistic development in university students, was implemented at The Hong Kong Polytechnic University (PolyU). The subject was developed under a leadership framework to facilitate students' learning and integration of theories, research, and concepts of the basic personal qualities of effective leaders, particularly intrapersonal and interpersonal qualities highlighted in the PYD framework (Shek et al., 2015). Moreover, students will be able to develop and reflect on their intrapersonal and interpersonal competencies and train their ability to apply their learning to their daily lives (Shek & Yuen, 2019). Equally important, the subject highlights the importance of intrapersonal and interpersonal qualities in developing effective leadership, particularly ethical leadership. In the 2010/11 and 2011/12 academic years, we piloted a 2-credit subject based on PYD concepts and theories. When it comes to the 2012/13 academic year, with the university implementing the new four-year undergraduate curriculum, we initiated a 3-credit subject on leadership. Initially, the subject was implemented in a face-to-face format (Shek et al., 2015). With the occurrence of the pandemic in 2020, we have also taught this subject via online and hybrid modes (Shek et al., 2023c; Shek et al., 2023d).

According to the intended learning outcomes of Tomorrow's Leaders, "Upon completion of the subject, students will be able to:

(1) Understand and integrate theories, research, and concepts on the basic qualities (particularly intrapersonal and interpersonal qualities) of effective leaders.
(2) Develop self-awareness and self-understanding.
(3) Demonstrate self-leadership in pursuit of continual self-improvement.

(4) Apply intrapersonal and interpersonal skills in daily lives.
(5) Appreciate the importance of intrapersonal and interpersonal qualities in effective leadership, particularly the connection of learning in the subject to one's professional development and personal growth.
(6) Recognize and accept their responsibility as professionals and citizens to the society and the world."

9.2 Core Beliefs About Students as Leaders

The PYD approach attempts to cultivate the talents, strengths, and potential of adolescents (Li et al., 2022). Consistent with the PYD framework, we firmly believe that cultivating developmental assets (particularly psychosocial competencies) is crucial for strengthening the holistic youth development of university students (Shek et al., 2020). Therefore, "Tomorrow's Leaders" embeds themes of different PYD qualities, including self-leadership, positive and healthy identity, resilience, emotional competence, critical thinking, interpersonal competence, morality, spirituality, team building, interpersonal communication, and mental health. As stated in Shek and Yuen (2019), "Our teaching philosophy underlying this subject includes:

(1) *Every student is (and can be) a leader*, although most students may not be aware of their potential and abilities.
(2) *Self-understanding and intrapersonal competence* are critical to effective leadership. Through the structured and systematic curriculum, self-understanding, interpersonal communication, and ethical leadership in students will be enhanced.
(3) *Experiential learning* is an important vehicle to help students understand themselves. As such, individual, group, and class experiential learning activities with high interaction with the students are developed.
(4) *Individual reflection* is the key to student development and learning.
(5) *Collaborative learning* can help students develop intrapersonal and interpersonal competence. Learning through group sharing, discussion, evaluation, and presentation is essential.
(6) There is an *equal emphasis on the academic knowledge* of PYD and leadership and on applying *that knowledge in real life.* Students are encouraged to apply what they have learned to their lives consciously.
(7) *Systematic evaluation* utilizing different evaluation mechanisms is crucial to understanding the effectiveness of the subject developed."

9.3 Curriculum Design and Student Engagement

The subject is genuinely innovative and integrative in terms of curriculum design, incorporating several principles. First, we emphasize the importance of both academic knowledge and personal development in the subject. Students taking this subject are expected to develop their intrapersonal and interpersonal sensitivity and competencies (Shek et al., 2013b). Second, we expect teacher-student and student–student interactions in the subject to be intense, particularly in a classroom setting (Shek & Yuen, 2019). This subject has gradually evolved to use "flipped classroom" and "blended learning" approaches in some teaching units. With the increased use of online teaching and learning, we have also developed and piloted virtual teaching and learning videos (Li et al., 2022; Shek et al., 2022b). Third, approaches such as intellectual thinking, experiential learning, collaborative learning, and reflective learning are emphasized in the subject (e.g., students learn through experience in activities). Fourth, we uphold the importance of reflection in teaching and learning. Fifth, we encourage students to learn together through collaborative learning activities. Sixth, we strive to create enjoyable learning experiences for the students. Finally, students are involved in assessments, in-class participation, and group presentations. Students are required to do the preparatory work before the class and are encouraged to deepen their understanding through peer-led discussions and debates.

The above principles are upheld in the subject through several strategies. First, we promote an interactive atmosphere in class that forms the cornerstones of experiential learning. Second, various forms of teaching practices, including integration of multimedia, in-class discussions and sharing, group presentations, case studies and role-plays, interactive games, creative arts, and debates, are applied. Third, we constantly encourage students to reflect and self-evaluate to facilitate deep learning. The above methods are effective in encouraging students to be attentively involved in class and in facilitating students' learning, participation, and reflection. In particular, learner-centered approaches are adopted to meet the needs of the students. First, experiential learning activities engage students through active participation. Second, collaborative learning is another approach that can empower and motivate students to learn. More importantly, students are enabled to reflect on their learning and integrate the knowledge and experiences to solve their real-life problems (e.g., application in real-life settings) (Shek & Yuen, 2019). Through such applications, students can learn how to use abstract theoretical concepts in the real world. Finally, through reflective learning, students can understand their thinking, feelings, and behavior on a deeper level.

In this subject, engaging and inspiring the students is essential. First, small group discussions give students a sense of belonging and ownership. Second, students are engaged through reflection activities and related sharing exercises. We believe the reflection and discussion processes can deepen the students' learning. Third, routine post-lecture evaluations help to engage students. We give feedback on students' comments so that they know that we care about their learning experiences. Fourth, instructors are expected to share their personal experiences (e.g., self-disclosure) to engage students. Fifth, the basic philosophy that "everyone is (and can be) a leader" strengthens students' confidence and capability, which is a powerful tool of empowerment. Sixth, students are guided to understand the nature and importance of their holistic development, including ethical leadership in their career and chosen profession. The creation of personal relevance of the subject to students' lives can also engage the students. Finally, student engagement is involved in the assessment.

Students are assessed based on their preparation for class and class participation, such as completion of worksheets and taking the initiative to join Q&A sessions and class discussions. Peer assessment is also adopted, where students are invited to evaluate the performance of other group members honestly and authentically regarding group participation and group projects.

9.4 Impact and Evaluation

The subject was piloted in the 2010/11 and 2011/12 school years, with 463 students enrolled in this subject. Since the 2012/13 academic year, the subject was formally implemented, with over 2000 students taking it annually. Until now, the subject has been taken by 22,576 students (Shek & Yuen, 2019). A wide range of evaluative tools have been applied to evaluate the impact of the subject, including objective outcome evaluation, subjective outcome evaluation, process evaluation, and qualitative evaluation (Shek et al., 2015). Shek and Sun (2012a) highlighted that "this subject also disseminates the evaluation findings based on the spirit of 'scholarship of teaching and learning' (SOTL)."

9.4.1 Objective Outcome Evaluation

Two objective outcome evaluation strategies have been applied to examine changes in students after taking the subject. First, to evaluate the effectiveness of the subject, a "one-group pretest–posttest" design was utilized, using an instrument modeled after the Chinese Positive Youth Development Scale (Shek & Ma, 2010; Shek et al., 2007), which includes measures of PYD outcomes.

For the pilot subjects, Shek and Yuen (2019) revealed that the students improved in various domains, such as emotional competence and positive competence. Utilizing a pretest–posttest pre-experimental design, Shek and Sun (2012a) revealed that students ($N = 50$) changed in a positive direction on different measures of PYD, including resilience, psychosocial competencies (social, emotional, cognitive, behavioral, and moral competence), self-determination, self-efficacy, optimism, positive identity, spirituality, bonding, and prosocial norms. Furthermore, students' scores on the composite measures of PYD also increased after taking the subject.

After the inception of the new 4-year undergraduate curriculum in the 2012/13 academic year, there are also findings suggesting that students showed positive changes based on various outcome measures after taking this subject (Shek et al., 2020). Utilizing a pre-experimental design, Shek and Ma (2014a) collected data from 1029 students on measures of PYD and life satisfaction. Results showed that students had higher ratings on several outcome measures (self-determination, thriving, and life satisfaction), although there were some odd findings. Similarly, utilizing a single-group pre-experimental design with pretest and posttest data (N

= 2876 undergraduate students) to understand student changes on measures of PYD, psychological well-being, and desired graduate attributes, Li and Shek (2019) found that students improved in most of the measures of PYD attributes, such as psychosocial competence, spirituality, and clear and positive identity. Moreover, students showed higher scores on satisfaction with life and institutional learning outcomes, including the ability to solve problems, critical thinking, leadership with ethics, and lifelong learning. During the COVID-19 pandemic, we taught this subject via online and hybrid teaching methods. Based on the responses of 630 students, Chai et al. (2022) revealed that students improved on individual measures of PYD (e.g., resilience, moral competence, spirituality), higher-order PYD measures (e.g., cognitive-behavioral competence, positive identity), well-being (thriving and life satisfaction), and desired graduate attributes (e.g., ethical leadership).

Besides the one-group pretest–posttest design, we have also used a quasi-experimental design, which included a control group (Shek et al., 2013a). Compared with the control group participants, students taking this subject revealed more positive changes indexed by eight measures, including resilience, psychosocial competence, self-efficacy, and optimism.

9.4.2 Subjective Outcome Evaluation

To assess students' views of the subject, the instructor teaching the subject, and the perceived benefits of the subject, we used a validated measure based on validated measures in previous projects, such as the Project P.A.T.H.S. (Shek & Ma, 2014b; Shek & Sun, 2014). In the pilot stage, subjective outcome evaluation findings were very positive. For example, students had very positive views of the subject, the teacher, and the value of the subject (Shek & Sun, 2013a). In the full implementation stage, after the inception of the new 4-year program in the 2012/13 academic year, findings also consistently showed that students appreciated the subject, the teacher, and the benefits of the subject (Li et al., 2023). In particular, most participants reflected that the subject was effective in promoting their development in different domains. For instance, Shek et al. (2016) showed that 92% of the students agreed that the subject promoted their ethical decision-making; around 94% of the students also reported that the subject promoted their self-reflection. In a recent study based on a subjective outcome evaluation strategy (Yu et al., 2022), a positive evaluation of the findings was replicated. For example, 93% of the students agreed that they positively evaluated the subject. There are also findings demonstrating that students had positive evaluations of the subject during the pandemic (Chai et al., 2022), with 78% agreeing that the subject could promote their ability in ethical leadership. Additionally, 93% of the students showed overall satisfaction with the subject.

In addition to post-course subjective outcome evaluation, we conducted post-lecture evaluation studies using a subjective outcome evaluation strategy (Shek & Li, 2023). The purpose of the post-lecture evaluation is to collect immediate feedback from the students after a lecture so that the teachers can reflect on their teaching and identify areas for improvement. For example, Leung et al. (2016) conducted a post-lecture evaluation and found that a very high proportion of students were satisfied with the lecture, particularly in their evaluation of the lecture and the teacher. Yu et al. (2016) similarly reported that most students were satisfied with the lectures, including the classroom interaction and the benefits of the lectures to their development, such as awareness of the importance of personal development.

9.4.3 Process Evaluation

In the early days of subject development, as several teachers were involved in teaching, there was a need to understand the degree of adherence to the developed curriculum and the quality of the subject's implementation. Hence, in the pilot stage, we conducted two process evaluations to assess the quality of the implementation process using a process evaluation instrument.

After the subject was piloted in the second term of the 2010/11 school year, a process evaluation was conducted in 14 lectures. The findings showed that teachers followed the developed curriculum closely (although they might customize some PowerPoint slides), with a mean adherence rate of 86%. This process evaluation applied a 7-point rating scale, with a higher score suggesting better implementation quality. Specifically, in this study, the overall mean score of other items rated by the two evaluators was generally high. For instance, high scores were observed in the areas of student interest (5.25/7), classroom management (5.43/7), application of the interactive delivery method (5.5/7), use of strategies to enhance student motivation (5.51/7), and the opportunity for reflection (5.5/7). Overall, the subject was identified to be able to promote the students' psychosocial competence (Shek & Sun, 2012b).

To replicate the findings, Shek and Sun (2013b) conducted another process evaluation for 19 lectures in the first term of the 2011/2012 academic year. A 7-point rating scale was applied, and the findings supported that inter-rater reliability was generally high. For example, the average level of program adherence was high (95%). Besides, the high quality and success of the program were enhanced by many factors, such as student participation and involvement (6.03/7), interactive delivery method (5.84/7), enhancement of student motivation (5.76/7), and achievement of the lecture objectives (5.92/7). The study replicated and extended the findings of the first piloting exercise and proved the high implementation quality of this subject (Shek & Sun, 2013b).

9.4.4 Qualitative Evaluation

Besides the quantitative evaluation findings, we also conducted qualitative evaluation through two strategies, namely reflective comments made by the students and focus groups. Studies in the pilot and full implementation stages revealed that students' views of the subjects, the teachers, and the perceived benefits are overwhelmingly positive. For example, Shek and Sun (2012c) invited students ($N = 189$) to use "descriptors" and "metaphors" to describe the subject. In terms of descriptors, students used positive descriptors, including "self-understanding," "interesting," "informative," "funny," "cooperation," "motivating," "reflective," "useful," "relaxing," "happy," "meaningful," "good," "enlightening," "understand leadership," "communication skills improvement," and "enjoyable." For metaphors, students generally used positive metaphors to describe the subject. Some examples included "smiley/happy face," "buffet," "light," "an interesting/enjoyable/meaningful/lovely tour," "a guide/cookbook," "faith," "compass," "gift," "ice-cream," "relaxing course," "a mirror and a telescope," "journey," "fun with interaction and friends," and "star."

Besides qualitative evaluation, we conducted focus groups to understand the subjects' subjective experience and perceived impact (Shek & Law, 2014). From the students' narratives, we noted that they had positive learning experiences and found the subject helpful. Some examples are shown below:

- "There was one unique feature of this subject. It was not purely theoretical. The use of activities could help us understand the meaning of the theory, which made the whole thing not so abstract."
- "I had a deep impression of the group activities, games, and sharing. I liked this course because it was not rigid, and it was enjoyable. It was like an interest group where you could chat and play with the classmates."
- "I appreciated students coming from Mainland China. I appreciated their courage to speak in public."
- "Before taking the course, I did not know how to stand in others' positions and think about other people. In other words, I looked at things from my perspective. I thought about myself first—it was your fault, but not my fault. I am a perfectionist. I do not like other people intruding in my life, and I am very stubborn. In particular, I always have quarrels with my mum, and I do not understand her feelings. For example, I always go out at night until very late, and my mum worries about me. In the past, I simply ignored her and thought it was her business if she worried about me … But now I will stand in my mum's position to look at things. I think our relationship has improved. My mum said that our relationship had improved. She also said that I had a better temper and became more easygoing. In the past, we would stop talking when we were unhappy. Now, we would communicate, and I would understand her feelings."

Besides the specific evaluation of "Tomorrow's Leaders," we also conducted several studies to evaluate the effectiveness of General University Requirements curricula (e.g., General Education), where the leadership requirement is an integral component of the 4-year curriculum (Shek & Yuen, 2019). Findings revealed that this subject was implemented successfully and well-received by the students, as the students' feedback was generally positive (Shek & Yu, 2017; Shek et al., 2017).

9.5 Student Learning Experience

In recent years, we have used different ways to encourage students to share their learning experiences and perceptions of the subject. Besides asking students to reflect on the subject, we also invited the scholarship recipients to write reflections about the subject (Shek & Wu, 2012). In the following section, we present some of the students' salient views on this subject.

9.5.1 Initial Views and Subsequent Learning Experience

Some students shared that they initially held the view that the subject was easy or not meaningful. However, their subsequent experiences have changed their views. Some examples are presented below:

- "To be honest, in the beginning, I thought this subject should be easy to pass … Therefore, I had viewed the subject as 'relaxing hours' at the beginning. After attending a few classes, I found that it was enjoyable and relaxing. Compared with my initial attitude, such efforts were definitely out of my expectations … After struggling for several days, I was fortunate to have performed excellently in the presentation."
- "Frankly speaking, I never thought that this subject could be so meaningful and reflective. At the very beginning, I thought this subject would be theory-based again and boring. However, it turns out that it is a subject that promoted my personal growth and provided me with the valuable opportunity to reflect on my life. The leadership skills I have learned can also be applied in daily life and my future career. I have to say that the experience of taking 'Tomorrow's Leader' is absolutely unforgettable and wonderful."
- "At the first lesson, I defended strongly as I had to share my understanding with five unfamiliar faces; I felt strange at that time. However, now, I feel very happy having lessons with my dearest group mates. During the lessons, we can be involved in a natural and genuine discussion and sharing. Even though the physical environment is not favorable for sharing, I am still positively influenced by the encouraging atmosphere of the lessons."
- "In the beginning, I did not think there was a strong correlation between leadership and my future career as a physiotherapist … Therefore, I initially thought that being a leader was a doctor's job. It was not important for me to learn how to be a good leader. However, I found that this concept was wrong after attending the lectures. In the class, our lecturer told us that everybody would have a chance to become a leader in everyday life … This actually impressed me a lot as the teacher can encourage us to understand things from others' points of view, which I did not think about before."
- "To be frank, I thought I was already a successful leader before I studied this subject. I believe that as long as we can produce something together, we are

already a successful team. Nevertheless, I found how wrong I was after realizing the true meaning of team building. I genuinely appreciate the content of this course, as it was helpful to my personal development. The skills I learned in this course are suitable for group presentations and useful for my future development. It is because working in a team is inevitable in society."

9.5.2 Design and Pedagogy of the Subject

Students generally appreciated the design and arrangement of the subject, particularly its interactive nature, good organization, and a high degree of student engagement in the subject. Some comments are presented below:

- "Incorporated with many meaningful class activities, the lectures were well-organized, and the learning materials were very well-prepared. Each lecture had a lecture outline, providing an overview of the content. The outlines are good materials for preview and review. The lecture content was presented on PowerPoint slides, which were also well-structured and informative, offering concise explanations for various aspects and vivid examples for the explanation."
- "Instead of holding lectures in a boring and dull manner, where students sit in the lecture hall and simply listen to what the lecturer says, 'Tomorrow's Leaders' gave us an interesting and unforgettable learning experience. Well-organized lectures were given to facilitate our understanding of various useful leadership theories. These theories included the basic personal qualities of effective leaders and were integrated into different in-class activities. Various in-class activities were held to give practical experiences. With in-class interactions, the frame of the classroom disappeared."
- "It is good for the subject to use many activities to facilitate our learning. This is a unique aspect of the subject, as it uses an experiential learning approach. We could learn the qualities of a leader through participating in the activities."
- "Unlike regular lectures offered by my home department, the atmosphere is relaxed, and interaction between the students and lecturers is highly promoted. The mode of learning is no longer a dull listening and notes-jotting process but rather an active thinking and sharing process. The lecturers appreciated their students' participation, and the students found it fruitful to express their thoughts. The subject demonstrates an enjoyable yet insightful way of learning. I am sure I cannot find this environment elsewhere in other lectures or tutorials."
- "I like attending this lecture because of its relaxing atmosphere and the chit-chat with my group mates. I did learn a lot from this subject."
- "When I first saw the name of this subject, 'Tomorrow's Leaders,' I thought it would be a theories-based subject with a boring lecturer explaining complex concepts in leadership in depth. However, I knew I was wrong from the first lesson. Instead of spoon-fed teaching, the lecturer emphasized teaching through interactive games, movie watching, and personal sharing. This kind of two-way

learning helped me think, analyze, and reflect during the class, making the complex theories easier to understand and remember."

- "My first big impression of this subject is that there are many group discussions and games during each lecture. It is my first time taking a subject with so many interactions during each lesson. I find it very necessary and beneficial. The discussions allow me to communicate more with my group mates and better understand others' views on the same issue. By interacting with others, I have also improved my interpersonal skills. I try to be more open rather than keeping quiet."
- "Another stimulating thing in this course is the reflective activities. One unforgettable activity is about self-understanding and personality, which was held during the lecture."
- "Reflecting on the days when I was studying this course, they were more than significant! I genuinely learned many things that will never be covered in other courses I studied."

9.5.3 Nurturing Leadership Qualities

Generally, students agreed that the subject was effective in cultivating their knowledge, attitudes, and skills about leadership. Some narratives of the students are presented below:

- "Through attending the lectures and reading the lecture notes, our understanding of each leadership competence deepened."
- "The subject helped me to be more confident in taking on a leader's role in my social work profession. The course introduced thirteen elements that a successful leader should possess. Some of them I have heard of before, but some are new to me. One new element has inspired me a lot and provided me with insight into being a leader. That is spirituality. A spiritual leadership style should include spiritual values such as integrity, honesty, and humility."
- "Concerning how this subject assisted my personal development, it changed my belief in leadership. I used to think that leadership was innate. The idea consolidated during my secondary school life when only the best students were nominated to join leadership camps and workshops. They had excelled academically in primary school. Later, they tended to become the student union president or other important student posts in the school. Nevertheless, the subject proved me otherwise. The topics covered suggest that leadership attributes can be developed. Everyone can be a leader. It grants me a new hope."
- "Through these lectures, we could understand the theories and concepts of leadership. Also, we can learn to develop our own leadership. Actually, I believe that leadership is very important to us. In the course of schooling, effective leadership can help us accomplish different tasks. Furthermore, effective leadership is essential for our future life."
- "After finishing this course, I realized that leadership is not as simple as I used to think. It relates to many other social skills, such as emotions, resilience, and even

ethics. This course covered a wide range of qualities of effective leaders and gave me a deeper understanding of myself. Recognizing my weaknesses and strengths through class activities made me know what areas I need to improve in order to be an effective leader."

9.5.4 Contribution to Personal Development

Many students shared that the subject enables them to promote their overall personal development.

- "No matter whether it is for my study or personal development, the subject is definitely beneficial to me … For me, the completion of this subject has given me a fresh perspective and altered my mind on my sense of being, everyday life, and my future career plan. For example, my system of thinking has changed, and my approaches to processing data have changed. I have learned how to control my emotional intelligence when facing pressure, and I have developed a better approach to pleasing others and forming teamwork. These changes will all be valuable for reshaping my mind, rewarding my study, strengthening my leadership skills, and probably sharpening my future life."
- "I think the most important point is that I started to think more after attending this subject. Since I am a Year-1 student, there are lots of things I have to adapt to in this university, including the busy learning schedule and heavy workloads; it is easy for us to forget to think about our life meaning. This subject talks a lot about morality, resilience, and spirituality. Those things might not have any direct benefits or linkages to getting good grades or making money in the future. However, it is very important for whole well-being."
- "After finishing the course, I find that it provided a good introduction to various leadership traits and allowed us to reflect on ourselves. I think this is paramount for our personal development."
- "Personally, this module is very useful and inspiring to me in my life experience. I know that being a successful leader or improving my weaknesses is a lifelong process, but I will try my best on it."

9.5.5 Promotion of Psychosocial Competence

As the subject focuses on PYD attributes, students generally shared that the subject was effective in cultivating their psychosocial competence. Some comments are presented below:

- *Ability to Apply*: "These life skills are very useful, especially in the last few weeks of the semester when all the assignments and presentation deadlines are compacted together."
- *Teamwork*: "The knowledge helped us to be a leader during teamwork."

- *Coping with Stress*: "It also taught us how to lead our own life—coping with life stress instead of coping by stresses."
- *Optimism*: "It helped us to keep an optimistic attitude toward life."
- *Accepting One's Limitation and Initiating Change*: "I am relatively weak in English, especially in oral English. Every time I feel stressed when speaking English. However, after realizing my limitations and being encouraged by the teacher, I decided to take the initiative to express my opinion in English in class. This course gives me a chance to improve my attitude toward challenges, and I think it will be very useful in my future career."
- *Resilience*: "A week before I learned this topic, the results of all mid-terms were released. Although the results were fair, I was so disappointed since my family and I had high expectations for me. What was more disappointing was that I worked really hard, but I could not get satisfactory results. I could not accept this truth and felt extremely frustrated. I even thought of giving up my dream and stopped expecting myself to improve. However, after attending the lecture titled 'Resilience,' all the negative thoughts disappeared … I further discovered that I should not magnify my failures blindly! It was not as bad as I had imagined. Then, I worked harder and tried new ways of studying to find one that suited me the most. Therefore, I attained satisfactory results in the final examinations."
- *Emotional Control*: "I have also learned emotional control. Recognizing my own emotions is the first step in emotional control. No matter whether I feel upset or joyful, I have to admit the feeling. Then, managing emotions and expressing them in an appropriate manner is the second step."
- *Communication Skills*: "For communication skills, I learned that 'listen' is as important as 'speak.' In the past, I sometimes ignored the feelings of my friends and only focused on my sharing. Though I was not doing that on purpose, they might feel uncomfortable and not being respected. In the pursuit of preventing misinterpretation, I ought to listen when others are ready to share and give an appropriate response to show my love and care."
- *Empathy*: "Empathy is another topic that has had a positive effect on me. In real life, I think I always play the role of a leader. I used to put many pressures on my teammates and asked them to submit assignments within 2–3 days after our meeting. Because I think only stress can motivate them to work harder. However, I seldom considered their workload, which made them feel upset and too stressed. Luckily, I learned how important 'empathy' is, and I am becoming more flexible and caring about my group mates' feelings more."
- *Self-understanding*: "This course also enables me to know more about myself. It helps me to know myself and think about what areas of qualities I lack. It made me realize that I am not good at social cognition. I used to respect others' wants and needs without thinking about myself. Yet, this realization makes me feel stressed afterward."
- *Self-awareness*: "Another benefit I have gained from this subject is a better self-understanding. While learning about the concept of the personal qualities of effective leaders, the lecturer also encouraged us to think about ourselves. Therefore, I have learned to do self-reflection. I think it helped me improve my self-awareness."

- *Self-expression*: "Besides, I learned to express myself more as this course gave us many chances to discuss leadership traits with our group mates. In daily life, we seldom evaluate our emotions or relationships with other people."
- *Ethics*: "Ethical issues was another topic covered in 'Tomorrow's Leaders.' This topic was important but was frequently ignored by people. Ethics determines the proper way of action for an individual. It was the method for us to categorize our values and pursue them."

9.5.6 Reflection

"Tomorrow's Leaders" strongly emphasizes the importance of reflection. Students also underscored the value of reflection in this subject.

- "The teacher asked us, 'If you had a living funeral like Morrie did, what comments about yourself would you expect to hear from your parents, siblings, or good friends?' This question inspired me to think about how others view me. I reflected on what I have done since I came to this world and what I expect myself to achieve in the future. My answer is, 'Dear, I am proud of you, and you leave with no regrets.' It showed my personality and aspiration thoroughly."
- "During my self-reflection, I thought deeply about my strengths and weaknesses, my opportunities and threats, my past, present and future, my turning points … just everything happened in my life. I discovered that opportunities are always there for me, but the point is whether I am fully prepared to grasp those chances tightly or not. I must say, self-reflection helps me to identify my goals and further determine my dreams."
- "My whole journey of taking Tomorrow's Leaders is incredible and unforgettable. Unlike other subjects that I have taken, Tomorrow's Leaders not only aims at giving students the related theories or knowledge but also provides a chance to reflect on ourselves to promote personal growth in such a short period of time, only fourteen weeks, and to me, it does work. I am able to gain those leadership skills in a very relaxing way because the lessons are all in an interactive way."
- "Tomorrow's Leaders was also useful to our daily lives."
- "This subject also highlights the learning of lifelong skills. Positive self-talk, time management, and emotion control are just some examples of life skills that were taught during the lectures. Without exaggeration, all of them are very useful skills that can be applied throughout my university life and even in my future work."

9.5.7 Group Presentation

- "This job was not easy; we had to plan what content to include, what format to use, and how much time for each section … During the process, it gave me a feeling of being a teacher. The fact is that preparing a class activity that can articulate your theory is not easy … At that time, I suddenly realized how mighty our lecturer was. On the day of the presentation, our group wore full suits to present. In my opinion, we looked very smart and united. During the presentation, we used many different formats to facilitate classmates' understanding and increase their level of participation."

- "At the same time, interpersonal skills were trained during the discussion. It lets us practice theories in daily life experiences. Since there were many members in one group, we learned to listen to and accept different opinions."
- "Therefore, I reflected on whether we built a successful team or not after the presentation. I ultimately found that as a team leader, there were two things I needed to improve, including adjusting the speed of work and believing in my group members."

9.5.8 Individual Term Paper

Students appreciated the value of the individual term paper, although they also experienced challenges and difficulties. However, they regarded it as an excellent opportunity to consolidate their learning.

- "The Individual Term Paper was a great challenge to all of us … We think it was not easy because we are science students. It is unusual for us to discuss conceptual stuff, let alone to critically analyze the concept … However, writing the Individual Term Paper gives me a valuable opportunity to have a very deep understanding of the specific competence."
- "As a science student, it is a challenge for me to write an article about social science. The term paper was not easy to do, but it provided me with a good chance to learn and search for something new. Through the article searching and reading process, I had a deeper understanding of my topic and its relevance to my future career. Actually, this is the first time I'm writing something about social science in English, and the positive feedback from my lecturers about my work has given me great fulfillment."
- "One thing that should be noted is our final written assignment. It is a personal reflection journal that requires us to evaluate ourselves in terms of leadership qualities. When doing this assignment, I found that I had a better understanding of myself. I really evaluate myself with the leadership qualities taught in the lectures."

9.6 Training for Teachers of "Tomorrow's Leaders"

As 10–12 colleagues are typically involved in teaching Tomorrow's Leaders, there is a need for coordination and coaching involving several training strategies. First, we conduct monthly meetings to exchange views on issues of common concerns (e.g., how to deal with challenging students). Second, we hold mock teaching sessions before the start of each semester. Third, we conduct training for colleagues based on unique teaching and learning needs. For example, under COVID-19, we conducted several training workshops to facilitate colleagues to adopt online teaching (Shek et al., 2021; Shek et al., 2022b; Shek et al., 2022c). Another example is that we include law abidance leadership in the updated curriculum (Shek et al., 2023a; Shek et al., 2023b; Shek et al., 2022a). To empower colleagues to teach this politically sensitive topic, we regularly conduct training, which is regarded as very helpful by the teachers. Finally, we encourage colleagues to share their teaching experiences in the form of publications. Besides contributing to the scholarship of teaching and learning, we also empower teachers in their professional development. Some narratives are presented below:

- "For me, the experience of teaching 'Tomorrow's Leaders' was very precious, not only in my pursuit to be a teacher but also in my understanding of the needs and ideas of the students. This subject opened the door for me to share the aspirations and despair, ups and downs, and strengths and weaknesses of the students, which required mutual trust, acceptance, and recognition. Engagement of the students, self-disclosure, high but reasonable expectations of the students' performance, encouragement, and acknowledgment of students' potential are essential keys to breaking the ice and building trust with the students. Though I had been a social worker who needed to engage well with my clients in the helping process, engaging the students in the classroom and accompanying them in their learning was a refreshing and treasurable experience for me. Another reflection of teaching 'Tomorrow's Leaders' is the personal growth that I have experienced." (Leung, 2016b, p. 226).
- "Tomorrow's Leaders has helped me develop professionally in that it has changed my perception of what a teacher should aim to achieve … I came into teaching Tomorrow's Leaders with a high degree of openness accompanied by a sense of curiosity about the extent to which Tomorrow's Leaders would impact my students. I started teaching Tomorrow's Leaders with the feeling that it is like driving on a highway with no streetlights at night; you can only see what is in front of you and know that you are getting closer and closer to where you want to be, but exactly how far you are away from your destination is not always clear … My belief now is that the value of Tomorrow's Leaders (or teaching Tomorrow's Leaders) is more of a means to an end than an end itself. Leadership is a lifelong journey and not a destination in my students that I should 'drive' towards." (Leung, 2016a, p. 218).
- "The experience of teaching 'Tomorrow's Leaders' has also changed me both as a teacher and a person. First and foremost, my views about teaching have been transformed. Trained in the traditional teacher-centered educational environment, I used to believe that a good teacher's job is to disseminate knowledge clearly and that students have the responsibility to absorb the knowledge if I have done my job. I was able to deliver a lecture with clarity, explain a concept/theory with many examples, and answer students' questions effectively. However, I did not

have much know-how in terms of students' active learning and teacher-student interaction. By shifting the focus from teacher's teaching to learner's learning and taking into account each student's interests and individual style, the teacher can actively involve students in the learning process and desirable learning outcomes can be then achieved." (Yu, 2016, p. 200).

- "Through reflective teaching, I continuously recalled and evaluated my teaching experiences in order to improve my performance in the future ... Little is known about its beneficial effects on teachers. The present study provides a case study to demonstrate how a teacher can utilize reflective capabilities (e.g., identifying problems, gathering information, searching, and experimenting with solutions) when teaching a holistic leadership program. It highlights the role of reflective practice on a teacher's professional development." (Ma, 2016, p. 192).
- "In delivering the lectures of 'Tomorrow's Leaders,' I do not see myself only as a 'fixed entity' of achieving the goals and outcomes set in times of preparation. Instead, I intend to accept a more satisfying realization of entering 'the process of becoming' ... to let myself be in the class. Besides investigating the inwardness, that is, the teacher's self towards teaching, it is equally important to examine how the beliefs and rationale are delivered to the students; that is the 'process' that Rogers emphasized." (Wu, 2016, p. 207).

9.7 External Recognition

To date, we have generated many refereed journal articles, book chapters, and books based on the development and implementation of the subject (see Appendix). This subject was shortlisted for the 2015 Reimagine Education Awards (Ethical Leadership), and it was awarded the Silver Award (Ethical Leadership) in the 2017 Reimagine Education Awards, and the Gold Award (Nurturing Student Well-Being and Purpose) in the 2021 Reimagine Education Awards. We also won the University Grants Committee Award 2018 in Hong Kong.

9.8 Directions for Future Development

There are several directions for the development of this subject. First, to develop a comprehensive understanding of the effectiveness of the subject, evaluation work should continue. In addition to the collection of routine data, including pretest–posttest objective outcome evaluation, post-course subjective outcome evaluation, and qualitative evaluation, it will be helpful if we plan to conduct a study that adopts a quasi-experimental design that includes control groups. This strategy can give more definitive findings regarding the effectiveness of the subject over time. Moreover, a long-term follow-up study can be considered. As the first cohort of students under the new 4-year undergraduate program graduated in 2016, it would be exciting to collect their views on how the subject benefits them in the work context. Through the gradual accumulation of evaluation data, a credible scientific database will be constructed in leadership education for university students in both Chinese and international contexts.

As teachers are one of the key factors in contributing to the success of teaching this subject, systematic and adequate training should be given to the teachers involved. In the future, we may consider developing a training manual and an e-learning package for the teachers, which would ensure that new teachers would have adequate training before teaching this subject. This strategy is an important quality assurance mechanism. Finally, apart from PolyU, the subject can benefit other universities within and outside Hong Kong. To help colleagues understand the philosophy and curriculum of this subject, we conducted a symposium in February 2020 and produced a DVD documenting the curriculum. Equally important, a dedicated website can be considered in the future to consolidate the impact.

Acknowledgements The preparation of this chapter is financially supported by The Hong Kong Polytechnic University (ZZ4U and ZZUE), Li and Fung Endowed Professorship in Service Leadership Education, Wofoo Foundation, and the Matching Fund of Research Grants Council (ZECL and ZH4Q).

Appendix

Tomorrow's Leaders Publication List

A. **Books and special issues**

1 Shek, D. T. L., Sun, R. C. F., & Merrick, J. (Eds.). (2012). Positive youth development constructs: Conceptual review and application [Special issue]. *The Scientific World Journal, 2012*, Article ID 152923, 3 pages. https://doi.org/10.1100/2012/152923

2 Shek, D. T. L., Sun, R. C. F., & Merrick, J. (Eds.). (2012). Positive youth development: Theory, research and application [Special issue]. *Journal of Alternative Medicine Research, 4*(4), 343–421.

3 Shek, D. T. L., Sun, R. C. F., & Merrick, J. (Eds.). (2013). Developmental issues in Chinese adolescents [Special issue]. *International Journal of Child Health and Human Development, 6*(1), 1–166.

4 Shek, D. T. L., Sun, R. C. F., & Merrick, J. (Eds.). (2013). *University and college students: Health and development issues for the leaders of tomorrow* [Reprint]. New York, NY: Nova Science Publishers.

5 Shek, D. T. L., Siu, A. M. H., & Merrick, J. (2015). *Tomorrow's leaders: Service leadership and holistic development in Chinese university students* [Reprint]. New York, NY: Nova Science Publishers.

6 Shek, D. T. L., Wu, F. K. Y., & Merrick, J. (Eds.). (2015). *Leadership and service learning education: Holistic development for Chinese university students* [Reprint]. New York, NY: Nova Science Publishers.
7 Shek, D. T. L., Ma, C. M. S., & Merrick, J. (Eds.) (2016). Promoting leadership and intrapersonal development in university students [Special issue]. *International Journal on Disability and Human Development, 15*(2), 125–239.
8 Shek, D. T. L., Ma, C. M. S., & Merrick, J. (Eds.). (2017). *Leadership: Promoting leadership and intrapersonal development in university students* [Reprint]. New York, NY: Nova Science Publishers.
9 Shek, D. T. L., Yu, L., Wu, F. K. Y., & Merrick, J. (Eds.) (2017). Evaluation of positive youth development and leadership programs in Hong Kong [Special issue]. *International Journal of Adolescent Medicine and Health, 29*(1), 1–109.
10 Shek, D. T. L., Yu, L., & Merrick, J. (Eds). (2017). *University students: Promotion of holistic development in Hong Kong* [Reprint]. New York, NY: Nova Science Publishers.

B. **Book Chapters**

1 Shek, D. T. L. (2012). Post-lecture evaluation of a positive youth development subject for university students in Hong Kong [Reprint]. In D. T. L. Shek, R. C. F. Sun, & J. Merrick (Eds.), *Developmental issues in Chinese adolescents* (pp. 81–94). New York, NY: Nova Science Publishers.
2 Shek, D. T. L., & Wu, F. K. Y. (2012). Reflective journals of student taking a positive youth development course in a university context in Hong Kong [Reprint]. In D. T. L. Shek, R. C. F. Sun, & J. Merrick (Eds.), *Developmental issues in Chinese adolescents* (pp. 1–12). New York, NY: Nova Science Publishers.
3 Shek, D. T. L., & Sun, R. C. F. (2013). Post-course subjective outcome evaluation of a course promoting leadership and intrapersonal development in university students in Hong Kong [Reprint]. In D. T. L. Shek, R. C. F. Sun, & J. Merrick (Eds.), *Chinese adolescent development: Economic disadvantages, parents and intrapersonal development* (pp. 137–152). New York, NY: Nova Science Publishers.
4 Shek, D. T. L., & Sun, R. C. F. (2013). Post-lecture evaluation of a university course on leadership and intrapersonal development [Reprint]. In D. T. L. Shek, R. C. F. Sun, & J. Merrick (Eds.), *Chinese adolescent development: Economic disadvantages, parents and intrapersonal development* (pp. 125–136). New York, NY: Nova Science Publishers.
5 Shek, D. T. L., & Sun, R. C. F. (2013). Process evaluation of a leadership and intrapersonal development subject for university students [Reprint]. In D. T. L. Shek, R. C. F. Sun, & J. Merrick (Eds.), *Chinese adolescent development: Economic disadvantages, parents and intrapersonal development* (pp. 153–166). New York, NY: Nova Science Publishers.

6 Shek, D. T. L., & Tung, L. Y. K., (2013). Reflections of Chinese students on a university subject on leadership and intrapersonal development [Reprint]. In D. T. L. Shek, R. C. F. Sun, & J. Merrick (Eds.), *Chinese adolescent development: Economic disadvantages, parents and intrapersonal development* (pp. 167–178). New York, NY: Nova Science Publishers.

7 Shek, D. T. L., Sun, R. C. F. Tsien-Wong, T. B. K., Cheng, C. T., & Yan, H. R. (2013). Objective outcome evaluation of a leadership and intrapersonal development subject for university students [Reprint]. In D. T. L. Shek, R. C. F. Sun, & J. Merrick (Eds.), *Chinese adolescent development: Economic disadvantages, parents and intrapersonal development* (pp. 179–190). New York, NY: Nova Science Publishers.

8 Shek, D. T. L., Sun, R. C. F., Yuen, W. W. H., Chui, Y. H., Dorcas, A., Ma C. M. S., Tsui, P. F. (2013). Second piloting of a leadership and intrapersonal development subject at The Hong Kong Polytechnic University [Reprint]. In D. T. L. Shek, R. C. F. Sun, & J. Merrick (Eds.), *Chinese adolescent development: Economic disadvantages, parents and intrapersonal development* (pp. 111–124). New York, NY: Nova Science Publishers.

9 Shek, D. T. L., Sun, R. C. F., & Merrick, J. (2013). Introduction: neglected research on Chinese adolescent development [Reprint]. In D. T. L. Shek, R. C. F. Sun, & J. Merrick (Eds.), *Chinese adolescent development: Economic disadvantages, parents and intrapersonal development* (pp. i–xii). New York, NY: Nova Science Publishers. (70%; Refereed book.)

10 Shek, D. T. L. (2013). Development of a positive youth development subject in a university context. In D. T. L. Shek & R. C. F. Sun (Eds.), *Development and evaluation of positive adolescent training through holistic social programs (P.A.T.H.S.)* (pp. 279–289). Heidelberg, Germany: Springer.

11 Shek, D. T. L. (2013). Development of a positive youth development subject in a university context in Hong Kong [Reprint]. In D. T. L. Shek, R. C. F. Sun, & J. Merrick (Eds.), *University and college students: Health and development issues for the leaders of tomorrow* (pp. 179–191). New York, NY: Nova Science Publishers.

12 Shek, D. T. L. (2013). Post-lecture evaluation of a positive youth development subject for university students in Hong Kong [Reprint]. In D. T. L. Shek, R. C. F. Sun, & J. Merrick (Eds.), *Positive youth development: Theory, research and application* (pp. 81–94). New York, NY: Nova Science Publishers.

13 Shek, D. T. L., & Sun, R. C. F. (2013). Focus group evaluation of a positive youth development course in a university in Hong Kong [Reprint]. In D. T. L. Shek, R. C. F. Sun, & J. Merrick (Eds.), *University and college students: Health and development issues for the leaders of tomorrow* (pp. 245–255). New York, NY: Nova Science Publishers.

14 Shek, D. T. L., & Sun, R. C. F. (2013). Process evaluation of a positive youth development course in a university setting in Hong Kong [Reprint]. In D. T. L. Shek, R. C. F. Sun, & J. Merrick (Eds.), *University and college students:*

Health and development issues for the leaders of tomorrow (pp. 221–231). New York, NY: Nova Science Publishers.

15 Shek, D. T. L., & Sun, R. C. F. (2013). Promoting leadership and intrapersonal competence in university students: What can we learn from Hong Kong [Reprint]? In D. T. L. Shek, R.C.F. Sun, & J. Merrick (Eds.), *University and college students: Health and development issues for the leaders of tomorrow* (pp. 193–207). New York, NY: Nova Science Publishers.

16 Shek, D. T. L., & Sun, R. C. F. (2013). Promoting psychosocial competencies in university students: Evaluation based on a one group pretest–posttest design [Reprint]. In D. T. L. Shek, R. C. F. Sun, & J. Merrick (Eds.), *University and college students: Health and development issues for the leaders of tomorrow* (pp. 209–219). New York, NY: Nova Science Publishers.

17 Shek, D. T. L., & Sun, R. C. F. (2013). Qualitative evaluation of a positive youth development course in a university setting in Hong Kong [Reprint]. In D. T. L. Shek, R. C. F. Sun, & J. Merrick (Eds.), *University and college students: Health and development issues for the leaders of tomorrow* (pp. 233–243). New York, NY: Nova Science Publishers.

18 Shek, D. T. L., Sun, R. C. F., & Merrick, J. (2013). Introduction: How to promote holistic development in university students? [Reprint]. In D. T. L. Shek, R. C. F. Sun, & J. Merrick (Eds.), *University and college students: Health and development issues for the leaders of tomorrow* (pp. xi–xiv). New York, NY: Nova Science Publishers.

19 Shek, D. T. L. (2014). Post-lecture evaluation of a positive youth development subject for university students in Hong Kong [Reprint]. In J. Merrick (Ed.), *Child health and human development yearbook 2013* (pp. 83–94). New York, NY: Nova Science Publishers.

20 Shek, D. T. L., & Wu, F. K. Y. (2014). Reflective journals of students taking a positive youth development course in a university context in Hong Kong [Reprint]. In J. Merrick (Ed.), *Child health and human development yearbook 2013* (pp. 3–14). New York, NY: Nova Science Publishers.

21 Shek, D. T. L., & Yu, L. (2015). Post-course subjective outcome evaluation of a subject on leadership and intrapersonal development for university students in Hong Kong [Reprint]. In D. T. L. Shek, A. M. H. Siu, & J. Merrick. (Eds), *Tomorrow's leaders: Service leadership and holistic development in Chinese university students* (pp. 77–90). New York, NY: Nova Science Publishers.

22 Shek, D. T. L., Siu, A. M. H., & Merrick, J. (2015). A tale of innovative leadership program in Hong Kong [Reprint]. In D. T. L. Shek, A. M. H. Siu, & J. Merrick. (Eds), *Tomorrow's leaders: Service leadership and holistic development in Chinese university students* (pp. 3–6). New York, NY: Nova Science Publishers.

23 Shek, D. T. L., & Law, M. Y. M. (2015). Evaluation of a subject on leadership and intrapersonal development: Views of the students based on qualitative evaluation [Reprint]. In D. T. L. Shek, A. M. H. Siu, & J. Merrick. (Eds), *Tomorrow's leaders: Service leadership and holistic development*

in Chinese university students (pp. 43–54). New York, NY: Nova Science Publishers.

24 Shek, D. T. L., & Leung, H. (2015). Post-lecture subjective outcome evaluation of a university subject on leadership and positive youth development in Hong Kong [Reprint]. In D. T. L. Shek, A. M. H. Siu, & J. Merrick. (Eds), *Tomorrow's leaders: Service leadership and holistic development in Chinese university students* (pp. 91–104). New York, NY: Nova Science Publishers.

25 Shek, D. T. L., & Leung, J. T. Y. (2015). Perceived benefits of a university subject on leadership and intrapersonal development [Reprint]. In D. T. L. Shek, A. M. H. Siu, & J. Merrick. (Eds), *Tomorrow's leaders: Service leadership and holistic development in Chinese university students* (pp. 117–130). New York, NY: Nova Science Publishers.

26 Shek, D. T. L., & Ma, C. M. S. (2015). Do university students change after taking a subject on leadership and intrapersonal development? [Reprint]. In D. T. L. Shek, A. M. H. Siu, & J. Merrick. (Eds), *Tomorrow's leaders: Service leadership and holistic development in Chinese university students* (pp. 67–76). New York, NY: Nova Science Publishers.

27 Shek, D. T. L., & Wu, F. K. Y. (2015). The role of teachers in youth development: Reflections of students [Reprint]. In D. T. L. Shek, A. M. H. Siu, & J. Merrick. (Eds), *Tomorrow's leaders: Service leadership and holistic development in Chinese university students* (pp. 105–116). New York, NY: Nova Science Publishers.

28 Shek, D. T. L., Wu, F. K. Y., & Law, M. Y. M. (2015). Perceptions of a university subject on leadership and intra-personal development: Reflections of the scholarship recipients [Reprint]. In D. T. L. Shek, A. M. H. Siu, & J. Merrick. (Eds), *Tomorrow's leaders: Service leadership and holistic development in Chinese university students* (pp. 55–66). New York, NY: Nova Science Publishers.

29 Yu, L., Shek, D. T. L., & Leung, E. Y. K. (2015). Leadership and Intrapersonal Development: Post-Lecture Evaluation [Reprint]. In D. T. L. Shek, F. K. Y. Wu, & J. Merrick (Eds.), *Leadership and service-learning education: Holistic development for Chinese university students* (pp. 9–22). New York, NY: Nova Science Publishers.

30 Leung, H., Shek, D. T. L., & Mok, B. P. W. (2015). Student evaluation of "Tomorrow's Leaders" course [Reprint]. In D. T. L. Shek, F. K. Y. Wu, & J. Merrick (Eds.), *Leadership and service-learning education: Holistic development for Chinese university students* (pp.75–94). New York, NY: Nova Science Publishers.

31 Yu, L., Shek, D. T. L., & Leung, E. Y. K. (2017). Post-lecture evaluation of a university subject on leadership and intrapersonal development [Reprint]. In J. Merrick (Ed), *Child and adolescent health yearbook 2016* (pp. 20–29). New York, NY: Nova Science Publishers.

32 Leung, H., Shek, D. T. L., & Mok, B. P. W. (2017). Post-lecture subjective outcome evaluation of a university subject on leadership and intrapersonal development [Reprint]. In J. Merrick (Ed), *Child and adolescent health yearbook 2016* (pp. 105–118). New York, NY: Nova Science Publishers.
33 Shek, D. T. L., Yuen-Tsang, A. W. K., & Ng, E. C. W. (2016). Global Youth Leadership Institute [Reprint]. In D. T. L. Shek, C. M. S. Ma, L. Lin & J. Merrick (Eds.), *Education in Hong Kong: Service leadership for university students* (pp. 147–155). New York, NY: Nova Science Publishers.
34 Shek, D. T. L., Ma, C. M. S., & Merrick, J. (2017). Can we nurture university students to become the leaders of tomorrow? [Reprint]. In D. T. L. Shek, C. M. S. Ma, & J. Merrick (Eds.), *Leadership: Promoting leadership and intrapersonal development in university students* (pp. 3–8). New York, NY: Nova Science Publishers.
35 Shek, D. T. L. & Ma, C. M. S. (2017). Emotional competence [Reprint]. In D. T. L. Shek, C. M. S. Ma, & J. Merrick (Eds.), *Leadership: Promoting leadership and intrapersonal development in university students* (pp. 11–22). New York, NY: Nova Science Publishers.
36 Shek, D. T. L. & Yu, L. (2017). Cognitive competence [Reprint]. In D. T. L. Shek, C. M. S. Ma, & J. Merrick (Eds.), *Leadership: Promoting leadership and intrapersonal development in university students* (pp. 23–38). New York, NY: Nova Science Publishers.
37 Shek, D. T. L. & Wu, F. K. Y. (2017). Development of a clear and positive identity [Reprint]. In D. T. L. Shek, C. M. S. Ma, & J. Merrick (Eds.), *Leadership: Promoting leadership and intrapersonal development in university students* (pp. 39–48). New York, NY: Nova Science Publishers.
38 Shek, D. T. L. & Leung, H. (2017). Resilience, Leadership and Intrapersonal Development [Reprint]. In D. T. L. Shek, C. M. S. Ma, & J. Merrick (Eds.), *Leadership: Promoting leadership and intrapersonal development in university students* (pp. 49–60). New York, NY: Nova Science Publishers.
39 Shek, D. T. L. & Leung, H. (2017). Developing self-leadership and responsibility [Reprint]. In D. T. L. Shek, C. M. S. Ma, & J. Merrick (Eds.), *Leadership: Promoting leadership and intrapersonal development in university students* (pp. 61–74). New York, NY: Nova Science Publishers.
40 Shek, D. T. L. & Leung, J. Y. T. (2017). Developing social competence [Reprint]. In D. T. L. Shek, C. M. S. Ma, & J. Merrick (Eds.), *Leadership: Promoting leadership and intrapersonal development in university students* (pp. 61–74). New York, NY: Nova Science Publishers.
41 Shek, D. T. L. & Ho, W. W. L. (2017). Spirituality [Reprint]. In D. T. L. Shek, C. M. S. Ma, & J. Merrick (Eds.), *Leadership: Promoting leadership and intrapersonal development in university students* (pp. 75–90). New York, NY: Nova Science Publishers.
42 Shek, D. T. L. & Ho, W. W. L. (2017). Moral Competence [Reprint]. In D. T. L. Shek, C. M. S. Ma, & J. Merrick (Eds.), *Leadership: Promoting leadership and intrapersonal development in university students* (pp. 91–102). New York, NY: Nova Science Publishers.

43 Shek, D. T. L., Wu, F. K. Y., Leung, C. T. L., Fok, H. K., Li, P. P. K., & Law, M. Y. M. (2017). Focus group evaluation [Reprint]. In D. T. L. Shek, C. M. S. Ma, & J. Merrick (Eds.), *Leadership: Promoting leadership and intrapersonal development in university students* (pp. 219–233). New York, NY: Nova Science Publishers.
44 Ma, C. M. S., Shek, D. T. L., Li, P. P. K., & Leung, E. Y. K. (2017). Evaluation of a leadership and intrapersonal development program [Reprint]. In D. T. L. Shek, C. M. S. Ma, & J. Merrick (Eds.), *Leadership: Promoting leadership and intrapersonal development in university students* (pp. 235–246). New York, NY: Nova Science Publishers.
45 Shek, D. T. L., Fok, H. K., Leung, C. T. L., Li, P. P. K., & Law, M. Y. M. (2017). Qualitative evaluation of leadership [Reprint]. In D. T. L. Shek, C. M. S. Ma, & J. Merrick (Eds.), *Leadership: Promoting leadership and intrapersonal development in university students* (pp. 201–217). New York, NY: Nova Science Publishers.
46 Chan, S. C. F., Ngai, G., & Shek, D. T. L. (2017). Leadership qualities as a foundation of service learning [Reprint]. In D. T. L. Shek, L. Yu, & J. Merrick (Eds.), *University students: Promotion of holistic development in Hong Kong* (pp. 9–22). New York, NY: Nova Science Publishers.
47 Shek, D. T. L., & Yuen, A. (2017). What should be the desired attributes of youth leaders? [Reprint] In D. T. L. Shek, L. Yu, & J. Merrick (Eds.), *University students: Promotion of holistic development in Hong Kong* (pp. 59–88). New York, NY: Nova Science Publishers.
48 Shek, D. T. L., & Yu, L. (2017). Student feedback on a pioneer subject on leadership and intrapersonal development [Reprint]. In D. T. L. Shek, L. Yu, & J. Merrick (Eds.), *University students: promotion of holistic development in Hong Kong* (pp. 251–261). New York, NY: Nova Science Publishers.
49 Shek, D. T. L., & Yu, L. (2017). An evaluation study on a university general education subject in Hong Kong [Reprint]. In D. T. L. Shek, L. Yu, & J. Merrick (Eds.), *University students: Promotion of holistic development in Hong Kong* (pp. 283–295). New York, NY: Nova Science Publishers.
50 Shek, D. T. L., Fok, H. K., Leung, C. T. L., & Li, P. P. K. (2017). Qualitative evaluation of a credit-bearing leadership subject in Hong Kong [Reprint]. In J. Merrick (Ed.), *Child health and human development yearbook 2016* (pp. 209–222). New York, NY: Nova Science Publishers.
51 Shek, D. T. L., Wu, F. K. Y., Leung, C. T. L., Fok, H. K., & Li, P. P. K. (2017). Focus group evaluation of a subject on leadership and intrapersonal development in Hong Kong [Reprint]. In J. Merrick (Ed.), *Child health and human development yearbook 2016* (pp. 223–235). New York, NY: Nova Science Publishers.
52 Ma, C. M. S., Shek, D. T. L., Li, P. P. K., Mok, B. P. W., & Leung, E. Y. K. (2017). Qualitative evaluation of a leadership and intrapersonal development subject for university students in Hong Kong [Reprint]. In J. Merrick (Ed.),

Child health and human development yearbook 2016 (pp. 263–272). New York, NY: Nova Science Publishers.
53 Shek, D. T. L., Yuen-Tsang, A. W. K., & Ng, E. C. W. (2018). Global youth leadership institute: A platform to nurture leadership in university students [Reprint]. In J. Merrick (Ed.), *Child and adolescent health yearbook 2017* (pp. 15–23). New York, NY: Nova Science Publishers.
54 Ma, C. M. S., Shek, D. T. L., & Li, P. P. K. (2018). Evaluation of a leadership and intrapersonal development subject for university students: Experience in Hong Kong [Reprint]. In J. Merrick (Ed.), *Child and adolescent health yearbook 2017* (pp. 395–408). New York, NY: Nova Science Publishers.
55 Shek, D. T. L., Yu, L., & Chai, W. Y. (2018). Qualitative evaluation of a new general education program at a university in Hong Kong: Teachers' experience [Reprint]. In J. Merrick (Ed.), *Child and adolescent health yearbook 2017* (pp. 87–107). New York, NY: Nova Science Publishers.
56 Shek, D. T. L., Yu, L., Wu, F. K. Y., Zhu, X., & Chai, W. (2018). Teachers' views on a new general education program in Hong Kong: Qualitative data collection over two years [Reprint]. In J. Merrick (Ed.), *Child and adolescent health yearbook 2017* (pp. 271–284). New York, NY: Nova Science Publishers.
57 Shek, D. T. L., Yu, L, Wu, F. K. Y., & Zhu, X. (2018). Implementation of the general university requirements in a university in Hong Kong: Experience based on the third year [Reprint]. In J. Merrick (Ed.), *Child and adolescent health yearbook 2017* (pp. 285–296). New York, NY: Nova Science Publishers.
58 Shek, D. T. L., Wu, F. K. Y., Lu, H. C., Leung, J. T. Y., Ho, W., …Law, M. Y. M. (2018). Views of Chinese students on general education based on individual interviews [Reprint]. In J. Merrick (Ed.), *Child and adolescent health yearbook 2017* (pp. 379–393). New York, NY: Nova Science Publishers.
59 Shek, D. T. L., Yu, L., & Zhu, X. (2018). Qualitative evaluation of a new general education program in Hong Kong: Findings based on students [Reprint]. In J. Merrick (Ed.), *Child and adolescent health yearbook 2017* (pp. 409–420). New York, NY: Nova Science Publishers.
60 Shek, D. T. L., Wu, F. K. Y., & Chai, W. Y. (2018). How do teachers view and experience a new general education program in Hong Kong? A study based on descriptors and open-ended questions [Reprint]. In J. Merrick (Ed.), *Public health yearbook 2017* (pp. 347–364). New York, NY: Nova Science Publishers.
61 Shek, D. T. L., Wu, F. K. Y., & Chai, W. Y. (2018). Chinese students in Hong Kong and their view on general education [Reprint]. In D. T. L. Shek, J. T. Y. Leung, & J. Merrick (Eds.), *Soft skills and aspirations in Chinese children and youth* (pp. 243–262). New York, NY: Nova Science Publishers.
62 石丹理,柴文玉, &于璐. (2018). 香港理工大學 「大學核心課程」的綜合評估研究.載於甘陽&孫向晨(主編),通識教育評論(頁14–36). 上海:復旦大學出版社.

63 Shek, D. T. L. (2019). Development of the new 4-year undergraduate program in Hong Kong. In D. T. L. Shek, G. Ngai, & S. C. F. Chan (Eds.), *Service-learning for youth leadership: The case of Hong Kong* (pp. 01–18). Singapore: Springer.

64 Shek, D. T. L., Yu, L., & Zhu, X. (2020). Student development under a new general education program in Hong Kong: A 3-year longitudinal assessment [Reprint]. In A. Tenenbaum, D. T. L. Shek, M. Y. M. Law, & J. Merrick (Eds.), *Advances in Chinese children, adolescent and family research* (pp. 289–312). New York, NY: Nova Science Publishers.

65 Yu, L., Shek, D. T. L., & Zhu, X. (2020). The influence of personal well-being on learning achievement in university students over time: Mediating or moderating effects of internal and external university engagement [Reprint]. In W. Duan, & S. M. Y. Ho (Eds.), *Positive Education: Theory, Practice, and Evidence* (pp.53–68). Lausanne: Frontiers Media SA.

C. **Journal Articles**

1 Shek, D. T. L. (2010). Nurturing holistic development of university students in Hong Kong: Where are we and where should we go? *The Scientific World Journal: TSW Child Health & Human Development, 10*, 563–575.

2 Shek, D. T. L. (2012). Development of a positive youth development subject in a university context in Hong Kong. *International Journal on Disability and Human Development, 11*(3), 173–179.

3 Shek, D. T. L. (2012). Post-lecture evaluation of a positive youth development subject for university students in Hong Kong. *The Scientific World Journal, 2012*, Article ID 934679, 8 pages. https://doi.org/10.1100/2012/934679

4 Shek, D. T. L., & Sun, R. C. F. (2012). Focus group evaluation of a positive youth development course in a university in Hong Kong. *International Journal on Disability and Human Development, 11*(3), 249–254.

5 Shek, D. T. L., & Sun, R. C. F. (2012). Promoting leadership and intrapersonal competence in university students: What can we learn from Hong Kong? *International Journal on Disability and Human Development, 11*(3), 221–228.

6 Shek, D. T. L., & Sun, R. C. F. (2012). Promoting psychosocial competencies in university students: Evaluation based on a one group pre-test/post-test design. *International Journal on Disability and Human Development, 11*(3), 229–234.

7 Shek, D. T. L., & Sun, R. C. F. (2012). Qualitative evaluation of a positive youth development course in a university setting in Hong Kong. *International Journal on Disability and Human Development, 11*(3), 243–248.

8 Shek, D. T. L., Sun, R. C. F., & Merrick, J. (2012). Editorial: How to promote holistic development in university students? *International Journal on Disability and Human Development, 11*(3), 171–172.

9 Shek, D. T. L., Sun, R. C. F., Chui, Y. H., Lit, S. W., Yuen, W. W., Chung, Y. Y. H., & Ngai, S. W. (2012). Development and evaluation of a positive youth development course for university students in Hong Kong. *The Scientific World Journal, 2012*, Article 263731, 8 pages. https://doi.org/10.1100/2012/263731
10 Shek, D. T. L., & Wu, F. K. Y. (2012). Reflective journals of students taking a positive youth development course in a university context in Hong Kong. *The Scientific World Journal, 2012*, Article ID 131560, 8 pages. https://doi.org/10.1100/2012/131560
11 Shek, D. T. L. (2013). Post-lecture evaluation of a positive youth development subject for university students in Hong Kong. *International Journal of Child Health and Human Development, 6*(1), 69–79.
12 Shek, D. T. L. (2013). Promotion of holistic development in university students: A credit-bearing subject on leadership and intrapersonal development. *Best Practices in Mental Health, 9*(1), 47–61.
13 Shek, D. T. L. (2013). Reflections of Chinese students on a university subject on leadership and intrapersonal development. *International Journal on Disability and Human Development, 12*(2), 213–219.
14 Shek, D. T. L., & Sun, R. C. F. (2013). Post-course subjective outcome evaluation of a course promoting leadership and intrapersonal development in university students in Hong Kong. *International Journal on Disability and Human Development, 12*(2), 193–201.
15 Shek, D. T. L., & Sun, R. C. F. (2013). Post-lecture evaluation of a university course on leadership and intrapersonal development. *International Journal on Disability and Human Development, 12*(2), 185–191.
16 Shek, D. T. L., & Sun, R. C. F. (2013). Process evaluation of a leadership and intrapersonal development subject for university students. *International Journal on Disability and Human Development, 12*(2), 203–211.
17 Shek, D. T. L., & Wu, F. K. Y. (2013). Reflective journals of students taking a positive youth development course in a university context in Hong Kong. *International Journal of Child Health and Human Development, 6*(1), 7–15.
18 Shek, D. T. L., Sun, R. C. F., Tsien-Wong, T. B. K., Cheng, C. T., & Yan, H. R. (2013). Objective outcome evaluation of a leadership and intrapersonal development subject for university students. *International Journal on Disability and Human Development, 12*(2), 221–227.
19 Shek, D. T. L., Sun, R. C. F., Yuen, W. W. H., Chui, Y. H., Dorcas A., Ma, C. M. S., Yu L., Chak, Y. L. Y., Law M. Y. M., Chung Y. Y. H., & Tsui, P. F. (2013). Second piloting of a leadership and intrapersonal development subject at The Hong Kong Polytechnic University. *International Journal on Disability and Human Development, 12*(2), 107–114.
20 Shek, D. T. L., & Law, M. Y. M. (2014). Evaluation of a subject on leadership and intrapersonal development: Views of the students based on qualitative evaluation. *International Journal on Disability and Human Development, 13*(4), 435–441.

21 Shek, D. T. L., & Leung, H. (2014). Post-lecture subjective outcome evaluation of a university subject on leadership and positive youth development in Hong Kong. *International Journal on Disability and Human Development, 13*(4), 465–472.
22 Shek, D. T. L., & Leung, J. T. Y. (2014). Perceived benefits of a university subject on leadership and intrapersonal development. *International Journal on Disability and Human Development, 13*(4), 481–488.
23 Shek, D. T. L., & Ma, C. M. S. (2014). Do university students change after taking a subject on leadership and intrapersonal development? *International Journal on Disability and Human Development, 13*(4), 451–456.
24 Shek, D. T. L., & Wu, F. K. Y. (2014). The role of teachers in youth development: Reflections of students. *International Journal on Disability and Human Development, 13*(4), 473–480.
25 Shek, D. T. L., & Yu, L. (2014). Post-course subjective outcome evaluation of a subject on leadership and intrapersonal development for university students in Hong Kong. *International Journal on Disability and Human Development, 13*(4), 457–464.
26 Shek, D. T. L., Siu, A. M. H. & Merrick J. (2014). Editorial: A tale of two innovative leadership subjects in Hong Kong, People's Republic of China. *International Journal on Disability and Human Development, 13*(4), 409–411.
27 Shek, D. T. L., Wu, F. K. Y. & Law, M. Y. M. (2014). Perceptions of a university subject on leadership and intrapersonal development: Reflections of the scholarship recipients. *International Journal on Disability and Human Development, 13*(4), 443–450.
28 Shek, D. T. L., Yu, L., & Zhu, X. (2016). Evaluation of a leadership and intrapersonal development subject for university students in Hong Kong: Findings based on 2 years. *International Journal on Disability and Human Development, 15*(1), 101–109.
29 Leung, H., Shek, D. T. L., Mok, B. P. W. (2016). Post-lecture subjective outcome evaluation of a university subject on leadership and intrapersonal development. *International Journal of Child and Adolescent Health, 9*(2), 223–233.
30 Yu, L., Shek, D. T. L., & Leung, E. Y. K. (2016). Post-lecture evaluation of a university subject on leadership and intrapersonal development. *International Journal of Child and Adolescent Health, 9*(2), 155–163.
31 Shek, D. T. L., Ma, C. M. S., & Merrick, J. (2016). Editorial: Nurturing university students to be Tomorrow's Leaders [Special issue]. *International Journal on Disability and Human Development, 15*(2), 125–126.
32 Shek, D. T. L., & Ma, C. M. S. (2016). Emotional competence: A key leadership competence for university students [Special issue]. *International Journal on Disability and Human Development, 15*(2), 127–134.
33 Shek, D. T. L., & Yu, L. (2016). Cognitive competence: A key positive youth development construct for university students [Special issue]. *International Journal on Disability and Human Development, 15*(2), 135–142.

34 Shek, D. T. L., & Wu, F. K. Y. (2016). Clear and positive identity as an attribute of an effective leader [Special issue]. *International Journal on Disability and Human Development, 15*(2), 143–148.
35 Shek, D. T. L., & Leung, H. (2016). Resilience as a focus of a subject on leadership and intrapersonal development [Special issue]. *International Journal on Disability and Human Development, 15*(2), 149–155.
36 Shek, D. T. L., & Leung, H. (2016). Developing self-leadership and responsibility and moving away from egocentrism [Special issue]. *International Journal on Disability and Human Development, 15*(2), 157–164.
37 Shek, D. T. L., & Leung, J. T. Y. (2016). Developing social competence in a subject on leadership and intrapersonal development [Special issue]. *International Journal on Disability and Human Development, 15*(2), 165–173.
38 Shek, D. T. L., & Ho, W. (2016). Spirituality as a key positive youth development construct for university students [Special issue]. *International Journal on Disability and Human Development, 15*(2), 175–180.
39 Shek, D. T. L., & Ho, W. (2016). Nurturing moral competence in university students via a credit-bearing subject [Special issue]. *International Journal on Disability and Human Development, 15*(2), 181–186.
40 Shek, D. T. L., Liang, J., & Law, M. Y. M. (2016). Subjective outcome evaluation of a university subject on leadership and intrapersonal development [Special issue]. *International Journal on Disability and Human Development, 15*(2), 231–239.
41 Shek, D. T. L., Fok, H. K., Leung, C. T. L., & Li, P. P. K. (2016). Qualitative evaluation of a credit-bearing leadership subject in Hong Kong. *International Journal of Child Health and Human Development, 9*(2), 173–183.
42 Shek, D. T. L., Wu, F. K. Y., Leung, C. T. L., Fok, H. K., & Li, P. P. K. (2016). Focus group evaluation of a subject on leadership and intrapersonal development in Hong Kong. *International Journal of Child Health and Human Development, 9*(2), 185–194.
43 Ma, C. M. S., Shek, D. T. L., Li, P. P. K., Mok, B. P. W., & Leung, E. Y. K. (2016). Qualitative evaluation of a leadership and intrapersonal development subject for university students in Hong Kong. *International Journal of Child Health and Human Development, 9*(2), 217–224.
44 Shek, D. T. L., & Yu, L. (2016). Student feedback on a subject on leadership and intrapersonal development for university students in Hong Kong. *International Journal on Disability and Human Development, 15*(3), 339–346.
45 Shek, D. T. L., Yu, L., & Xie, Q. Z. (2017). Student feedback on a pioneer subject on leadership and intrapersonal development in Hong Kong. *International Journal of Adolescent Medicine and Health, 29*(1), 83–89.
46 Shek, D. T. L., Yuen-Tsang, A.W.K., & Ng, E. C. W. (2017). Global Youth Leadership Institute: A platform to nurture leadership in university students. *International Journal of Child and Adolescent Health, 10*(1), 17–23.

47 Shek, D. T. L., & Ng, E. C. W. (2017). Leadership training for university students in Hong Kong: A critical review. *International Journal of Child and Adolescent Health, 10*(1), 25–40.
48 Ma, C. M. S., Shek, D. T. L., & Li, P. P. K. (2017). Evaluation of a leadership and intrapersonal development subject for university students: Experience in Hong Kong. *International Journal of Child and Adolescent Health, 10*(3), 337–346.
49 Shek, D. T. L. (2019). Leadership qualities as a foundation of service learning: The Hong Kong experience. *International Journal of Child and Adolescent Health, 12*(1), 9–18.
50 Li, X. & Shek, D. T. L. (2019). Objective outcome evaluation of a leadership course utilizing the positive youth development approach in Hong Kong. *Assessment & Evaluation in Higher Education, 45*(5), 741–757. https://doi.org/10.1080/02602938.2019.1696944
51 Shek, D. T. L., & Yuen, A. (2019). The quest for holistic youth leadership development: What should be the desired attributes of youth leaders? *International Journal of Child and Adolescent Health, 12*(1), 43–61.
52 Shek, D. T. L., Yu, L., Lin, L., Li, X., Zhu, X., Dou, D., Chai, W. Y., Chak, Y., Ho, W., Leung, E., Li, P., Mok, B., Shek, V., Shek, E., & Jin, T. Y. (2021). Nurturing leadership qualities under COVID-19: Student perceptions of the qualities and effectiveness of online teaching and learning on leadership development. *International Journal of Child and Adolescent Health, 14*(1), 89–100.
53 Li, X., Shek, D. T. L., & Shek, E. Y. (2021). Psychological morbidity among university students in Hong Kong (2014–2018): Psychometric properties of the Depression Anxiety Stress Scales (DASS) and related correlates. *International Journal of Environmental Research and Public Health, 18*(16), 8305. https://doi.org/10.3390/ijerph18168305
54 Shek, D. T. L., Zhu, X., Li, X., & Dou, D. (2022). Satisfaction with HyFlex teaching and law-abiding leadership education in Hong Kong university students under COVID-19. *Applied Research in Quality of Life, 17*(5), 2833–2858. https://doi.org/10.1007/s11482-022-10040-4
55 Shek, D. T., Yu, L., Li, X., Zhu, X., Dou. D., Chan, C. H. M., Zhu, L. Z., & Shek, E. Y. W. (2022). Online teaching of a leadership course under COVID-19: Evidence based on two semesters. *International Journal of Child and Adolescent Health, 15*(1), 29–40.
56 Chai, W., Li, X., & Shek, D. T. L. (2022). The effectiveness of a leadership subject using a hybrid teaching mode during the pandemic: Objective outcome and subjective outcome evaluation. *International Journal of Environmental Research and Public Health, 19*(16), 9809. https://doi.org/10.3390/ijerph19169809
57 Shek, D.T.L., Dou, D., Zhu, X., Li, X. (2022). Law abidance leadership education for university students in Hong Kong: Post-lecture evaluation. *Frontiers in Psychology, 13*, Article 994448. https://doi.org/10.3389/fpsyg.2022.994448

58 Yu, L., Lin, L., Shek, T. L. D., & Chai, W. (2022). Students' perceived attributes and benefits of a leadership course: Subjective outcome evaluation. *Research on Social Work Practice, 32*(2), 199–214. https://doi.org/10.1177/10497315211042823
59 Shek, D. T. L., Li, X., Wong, T. Y., Yu, L., Chai, W. Y., Cheng, N. S., Mok, P. W., Chiu, T. Y., Dou, D. Y., Chak, L. Y., Shek, K. F., Ho, W. L., Zhu, X. Q., & Chau, C. C. (2022). Development of virtual teaching and learning videos for leadership education for university students in Hong Kong. *International Journal of Public Health, 14*(4), 377–389.
60 Li, X., Shek, D. T., Wong, T., & Yu, L. (2022). Subjective outcome evaluation of instructional videos in leadership education. *International Journal of Environmental Research and Public Health, 20*(1), 367. https://doi.org/10.3390/ijerph20010367
61 Shek, D. T., & Li, X. (2023). Video teaching materials for leadership education: Subjective outcome evaluation based on university students in Hong Kong. *International Journal of Child Health & Human Development, 16*(1), 73–87.
62 Shek, D. T., Zhu, X., Dou, D., & Li, X. (2023). National security law education in Hong Kong: Qualitative evaluation based on the perspective of the students. *International Journal of Environmental Research and Public Health, 20*(1), 553. https://doi.org/10.3390/ijerph20010553
63 Shek, D. T. L., Chau, C., Mok, B., Chai, W., Cheng, N., Shek, V., Ho, W., Chiu, T., & Chak, Y. (2023). Teachers' experience in law-abiding leadership education: Replication across time. *International Journal of Child Health and Human Development 16*(1), 27–39.
64 Shek, D. T. L., Chau, C., Mok, B., Chak, Y., Cheng, N., Shek, V., Li, P., & Xiao, Z. (2023). Education on law-abidance leadership: Does face-to-face teaching matter? *International Journal of Child Health and Human Development, 16*(1), 89–102.
65 Shek, D. T. L., Wong, T., Li, X., & Yu, L. (2023). Use of instructional videos in leadership education in higher education under COVID-19: A qualitative study. *PLoS ONE, 18*(9): Article e0291861. https://doi.org/10.1371/journal.pone.0291861
66 Li, X., Shek, D. T. L., Dou, D., Zhu, X., & Wu, X. (2023). Law abidance leadership education for university students in Hong Kong: Subjective outcome evaluation. *Applied Research in Quality of Life*, 19, 683–708. https://doi.org/10.1007/s11482-023-10260-2

D. **Conference Presentations**

1 Shek, D. T. L., Chui, Y.H., Yuen W., Chung Y., & Ngai S. (2011, July). *Preparing university students for adulthood and the labor force: Role of positive youth development.* Paper presented at International Conference on Transitioning to Adulthood in Asia: Courtship, Marriage, and Work organized by University Hall Auditorium, National University of Singapore.

2 Shek, D. T. L., & Sun, R. C. F. (2012, May). *Nurturing university students to be Tomorrow's Leaders: The role of positive youth development*. Paper presented at the International Conference on "Youth Development in the Global Context: Emergent Issues and Responses" organized by the Project P.A.T.H.S., Hong Kong.
3 Shek, D. T. L. (2012, June). *Promotion of holistic development of university students* via *the formal curriculum.* Paper presented at the "General Education and University Curriculum Reform: An International Conference in Hong Kong" organized by City University of Hong Kong and the Hong Kong America Centre.
4 Shek, D. T. L. (2012, November). *Nurturing social responsibility in university students: The Hong Kong experience*. Paper presented at the "Summit on University Social Responsibility in an Era of Globalization" organized by The Hong Kong Polytechnic University and China Institute of Education Policy.
5 Wu, F. K. Y., Shek, D. T. L., Yu, L., Chai, C., & Zhu, X. (2016, August). *Well-being of university students in Hong Kong: A longitudinal case study*. Paper presented at the 14th International Society for Quality-of-Life Studies Annual Conference: Bridging Quality-of life Experiences from East to West, Seoul, South Korea.
6 Leung, H., Yu, L., Shek, D. T. L., & Cheung, R. (2017, September). *A holistic approach to the promotion of a healthy lifestyle among university students*. Paper presented at the 15th International Society for Quality-of-Life Studies Annual Conference—"Quality of Life: Towards a Better Society", Innsbruck, Austria.
7 Yuen, C., Yu, L., & Shek, D. T. L. (2018, June). *The role of emotional competence in the relationship between self-leadership and life satisfaction.* Paper presented at the 16th International Society for Quality-of-Life Studies Annual Conference—"Promotion of Quality of Life in the Changing World", The Hong Kong Polytechnic University, Hong Kong.
8 Leung, E. Y. K., Yu, L., & Shek, D. T. L. (2018, June). *Mental health status of first-year university students in Hong Kong*. Paper presented at the 16th International Society for Quality-of-Life Studies Annual Conference—"Promotion of Quality of Life in the Changing World", The Hong Kong Polytechnic University, Hong Kong.
9 Mok, B. P. W., Yu, L., & Shek, D. T. L. (2018, June). *Students' perceived learning gains from a general education subject: A case study in Hong Kong*. Paper presented at the 16th International Society for Quality-of-Life Studies Annual Conference—"Promotion of Quality of Life in the Changing World", The Hong Kong Polytechnic University, Hong Kong.
10 Zhu, A. Y. F., Yu, L., & Shek, D. T. L. (2018, June). *Evaluation of a general education programme amongst university students in Hong Kong*. Paper presented at the 16th International Society for Quality-of-Life Studies Annual Conference—"Promotion of Quality of Life in the Changing World", The Hong Kong Polytechnic University, Hong Kong.

Summary of publications	No
A. Books and special issues	10
B. Book chapters	65
C. Journal articles	66
D. Conference presentations	10
Total	**151**

References

Chai, W. Y., Li, X., & Shek, D. T. L. (2022). The effectiveness of a leadership subject using a hybrid teaching mode during the pandemic: Objective outcome and subjective outcome evaluation. *International Journal of Environmental Research and Public Health, 19*(16), Article 9809. https://doi.org/10.3390/ijerph19169809

Dalton, J., & Crosby, P. (2006). The neglected inner lives of college students. *Journal of College and Character, 7*(8), 1–2. https://doi.org/10.2202/1940-1639.1237

Leung, H. (2016a). Levels of reflection on teaching a leadership and positive youth development subject. *International Journal on Disability and Human Development, 15*(2), 211–220. https://doi.org/10.1515/ijdhd-2016-0712

Leung, H., Shek, D. T. L., & Mok, B. P. W. (2016). Post-lecture subjective outcome evaluation of a university subject on leadership and intrapersonal development. *International Journal of Child and Adolescent Health, 9*(2), 223–233.

Leung, J. (2016b). Riding on a roller coaster: Personal reflections of teaching a subject on leadership and intrapersonal development. *International Journal on Disability and Human Development, 15*(2), 221–229. https://doi.org/10.1515/ijdhd-2016-0713

Lewis, H. R. (2006). *Excellence without a soul: How a great university forgot education.* Citeseer.

Li, X., & Shek, D. T. L. (2020). Objective outcome evaluation of a leadership course utilising the positive youth development approach in Hong Kong. *Assessment & Evaluation in Higher Education, 45*(5), 741–757. https://doi.org/10.1080/02602938.2019.1696944

Li, X., Shek, D. T. L., Dou, D. Y., Zhu, X. Q., & Wu, X. (2024). Law abidance leadership education for university students in Hong Kong: Subjective outcome evaluation. *Applied Research in Quality of Life, 19*(2), 683–708. https://doi.org/10.1007/s11482-023-10260-2

Li, X., Shek, D. T. L., & Shek, E. Y. (2021). Psychological morbidity among university students in Hong Kong (2014–2018): Psychometric properties of the Depression Anxiety Stress Scales (DASS) and related correlates. *International Journal of Environmental Research and Public Health, 18*(16), Article 8305 https://doi.org/10.3390/ijerph18168305

Li, X., Shek, D. T. L., Wong, T., & Yu, L. (2022). Subjective outcome evaluation of instructional videos in leadership education. *International Journal of Environmental Research and Public Health, 20*(1), 367. https://doi.org/10.3390/ijerph20010367

Ma, C. M. (2016). Reflective teaching in a holistic personal development course for Chinese university students: A case study. *International Journal on Disability and Human Development, 15*(2), 187–193. https://doi.org/10.1515/ijdhd-2016-0709

Shek, D. T. L. (2010). Positive youth development and behavioral intention to gamble among Chinese adolescents in Hong Kong. *International Journal of Adolescent Medicine and Health, 22*(1), 163–172. https://doi.org/10.1515/IJAMH.2010.22.1.163

Shek, D. T. L. (2013). Promotion of holistic development in university students. *Best Practices in Mental Health, 9*(1), 47–61. https://doi.org/10.70256/428239ofjkeh

Shek, D. T. L., Chau, C. C., Mok, B., Chai, W., Cheng, N. S., Shek, V., Ho, W., Chiu, T. Y., & Chak, Y. (2023a). Teachers' experience in law-abiding leadership education: Replication across time. *International Journal of Child Health and Human Development, 16*(1), 27–39.

Shek, D. T. L., Chau, C. C., Mok, B. P., Chak, L. Y., Cheng, N. S., Shek, K. F., Li, P. K., & Xiao, Z. (2023b). Education on law-abidance leadership: Does face-to-face teaching matter? *International Journal of Child and Adolescent Health, 16*(1), 89–102.

Shek, D. T. L., Dou, D., Zhu, X., & Li, X. (2022a). Law abidance leadership education for university students in Hong Kong: Post-lecture evaluation. *Frontiers in Psychology, 13*, Article 994448. https://doi.org/10.3389/fpsyg.2022.994448

Shek, D. T. L., & Law, Y. M. (2014). Evaluation of a subject on leadership and intrapersonal development: Views of the students based on qualitative evaluation. *International Journal on Disability and Human Development, 13*(4), 435–441. https://doi.org/10.1515/ijdhd-2014-0339

Shek, D. T. L., & Li, X. (2023). Video teaching materials for leadership education: Subjective outcome evaluation based on university students in Hong Kong. *International Journal of Child Health & Human Development, 16*(1), 73–87.

Shek, D. T. L., Li, X., Wong, T. Y., Yu, L., Chai, W. Y., Cheng, N. S., Mok, B. P., Chiu, T. Y., Dou, D. Y., Chak, L. Y., Shek, K. F., Ho, W. L., Zhu, X. Q., & Chau, C. C. (2022b). Development of virtual teaching and learning videos for leadership education for university students in Hong Kong. *International Public Health Journal, 14*(4), 377–389.

Shek, D. T. L., Liang, J. Q., & Law, Y. M. (2016). Subjective outcome evaluation of a university subject on leadership and intrapersonal development. *International Journal on Disability and Human Development, 15*(2), 231–239. https://doi.org/10.1515/ijdhd-2016-0714

Shek, D. T. L., & Ma, M. S. (2010). Dimensionality of the Chinese Positive Youth Development Scale: Confirmatory factor analyses. *Social Indicators Research, 98*(1), 41–59. https://doi.org/10.1007/s11205-009-9515-9

Shek, D. T. L., & Ma, M. S. (2014a). Do university students change after taking a subject on leadership and intrapersonal development? *International Journal on Disability and Human Development, 13*(4), 451–456. https://doi.org/10.1515/ijdhd-2014-0341

Shek, D. T. L., & Ma, M. S. (2014b). Validation of a subjective outcome evaluation tool for participants in a positive youth development program in Hong Kong. *Journal of Pediatric and Adolescent Gynecology, 27*, S43–S49. https://doi.org/10.1016/j.jpag.2014.02.011

Shek, D. T. L., & Ng, E. C. W. (2017). Leadership training for university students in Hong Kong: A critical review. *International Journal of Child and Adolescent Health, 10*(1), 25–40.

Shek, D. T. L., Siu, A. M. H., & Lee, T. Y. (2007). The Chinese Positive Youth Development Scale: A validation study. *Research on Social Work Practice, 17*(3), 380–391. https://doi.org/10.1177/1049731506296196

Shek, D. T. L., Siu, M. H. A., & Merrick, J. (2015). *Tomorrow's leaders: Service leadership and holistic development in Chinese university students*. Nova Science Publishers, Inc.

Shek, D. T. L., & Sun, C. F. (2012a). Promoting psychosocial competencies in university students: Evaluation based on a one-group pre-test/post-test design. *International Journal on Disability and Human Development, 11*(3), 229–234. https://doi.org/10.1515/ijdhd-2012-0039

Shek, D. T. L., & Sun, C. F. (2012b). Process evaluation of a positive youth development course in a university setting in Hong Kong. *International Journal on Disability and Human Development, 11*(3), 235–241. https://doi.org/10.1515/ijdhd-2012-0038

Shek, D. T. L., & Sun, C. F. (2012c). Qualitative evaluation of a positive youth development course in a university setting in Hong Kong. *International Journal on Disability and Human Development, 11*(3), 243–248. https://doi.org/10.1515/ijdhd-2012-0040

Shek, D. T. L., & Sun, C. F. (2013a). Post-course subjective outcome evaluation of a course promoting leadership and intrapersonal development in university students in Hong Kong. *International Journal on Disability and Human Development, 12*(2), 193–201. https://doi.org/10.1515/ijdhd-2012-0136

Shek, D. T. L., & Sun, C. F. (2013b). Process evaluation of a leadership and intrapersonal development subject for university students. *International Journal on Disability and Human Development, 12*(2), 203–211. https://doi.org/10.1515/ijdhd-2013-0018

Shek, D. T. L., & Sun, C. F. (2014). Positive youth development programs for adolescents with greater psychosocial needs: Subjective outcome evaluation over 3 years. *Journal of Pediatric and Adolescent Gynecology, 27*, S17–S25. https://doi.org/10.1016/j.jpag.2014.02.008

Shek, D. T. L., Sun, C. F., Yuen, W. H., Chui, Y. H., Dorcas, A., Ma, M. S., Yu, L., Chak, L. Y., Law, Y. M., Chung, Y. H., & Tsui, P. F. (2013a). Second piloting of a leadership and intrapersonal development subject at The Hong Kong Polytechnic University. *International Journal on Disability and Human Development, 12*(2), 107–114. https://doi.org/10.1515/ijdhd-2013-0007

Shek, D. T. L., & Wong, K. K. (2011). Do adolescent developmental issues disappear overnight? Reflections about holistic development in university students. *The Scientific World Journal, 11*(1), 353–361. https://doi.org/10.1100/tsw.2011.5

Shek, D. T. L., Wong, T., Li, X., & Yu, L. (2023c). Use of instructional videos in leadership education in higher education under COVID-19: A qualitative study. *PLOS One, 18*(9), Article e0291861. https://doi.org/10.1371/journal.pone.0291861

Shek, D. T. L., & Wu, F. K. (2012). Reflective journals of students taking a positive youth-development course in a university context in Hong Kong. *The Scientific World Journal, 2012*, Article 131560. https://doi.org/10.1100/2012/131560

Shek, D. T. L., & Yu, L. (2017). An evaluation study on a university general education subject in Hong Kong. *The International Journal of Adolescent Medicine and Health, 29*(1), 103–109. https://doi.org/10.1515/ijamh-2017-3013

Shek, D. T. L., Yu, L., & Chai, W. Y. (2017). Evaluation of the general university requirements: What did students say? *The International Journal of Adolescent Medicine and Health, 29*(1), 75–82. https://doi.org/10.1515/ijamh-2017-3010

Shek, D. T. L., Yu, L., Li, X., Zhu, X. Q., Dou, D. Y., Chan, H. M., Zhu, L. Z., & Shek, Y. W. (2022c). Online teaching of a leadership course under COVID-19: Evidence based on two semesters. *International Journal of Child and Adolescent Health, 15*(1), 29–40.

Shek, D. T. L., Yu, L., Lin, L., Li, X., Zhu, X. Q., Dou, D. Y., Chai, W. Y., Chak, L. Y., Ho, W. L., Leung, E., Li, P., Mok, B., Shek, V., Shek, E., & Jin, T. Y. (2021). Nurturing leadership qualities under COVID-19: Student perceptions of the qualities and effectiveness of online teaching and learning on leadership development. *International Journal of Child and Adolescent Health, 14*(1), 89–100. https://ira.lib.polyu.edu.hk/bitstream/10397/93770/1/Shek_Nurturing_Leadership_Qualities.pdf

Shek, D. T. L., Yu, L., Ma, C. M., Sun, R. C., & Liu, T. T. (2013b). Development of a credit-bearing service leadership subject for university students in Hong Kong. *International Journal of Adolescent Medicine and Health, 25*(4), 353–361. https://doi.org/10.1515/ijamh-2013-0033

Shek, D. T. L., & Yuen, A. (2019). The quest for holistic youth leadership development: What should be the desired attributes of youth leaders? *International Journal of Child and Adolescent Health, 12*(1), 43–61. https://ira.lib.polyu.edu.hk/bitstream/10397/93756/1/APSS-0282_Shek_Quest_Holistic_Youth.pdf

Shek, D. T. L., Zhu, X. Q., Dou, D. Y., Law, M. Y. M., Yu, L., Ma, C. M. S., & Lin, L. (2020). Nurturing holistic development in university students through leadership courses: The Hong Kong experience. In G. Tonon (Ed.), *Teaching quality of life in different fields* (Vol. 79, pp. 61–80). Springer. https://doi.org/10.1007/978-3-030-21551-4_4

Shek, D. T. L., Zhu, X. Q., Dou, D. Y., & Li, X. (2023d). National security law education in Hong Kong: Qualitative evaluation based on the perspective of the students. *International Journal of Environmental Research and Public Health, 20*(1), 553. https://doi.org/10.3390/ijerph20010553

Twenge, J. M. (2014). *Generation me-revised and updated: Why today's young Americans are more confident, assertive, entitled and more miserable than ever before.* Simon and Schuster.

Wu, K. Y. (2016). "Know thyself": Some personal reflections in teaching a subject on leadership and intrapersonal development. *International Journal on Disability and Human Development, 15*(2), 203–209. https://doi.org/10.1515/ijdhd-2016-0711

Yu, L. (2016). A teacher's reflection on teaching "Tomorrow's Leaders" in university students in Hong Kong. *International Journal on Disability and Human Development, 15*(2), 195–202. https://doi.org/10.1515/ijdhd-2016-0710

Yu, L., Lin, L., Shek, D. T. L., & Chai, W. Y. (2022). Students' perceived attributes and benefits of a leadership course: Subjective outcome evaluation. *Research on Social Work Practice, 32*(2), 199–214. https://doi.org/10.1177/10497315211042823

Yu, L., Shek, D. T. L., & Leung, E. Y. K. (2016). Post-lecture evaluation of a university subject on leadership and intrapersonal development. *International Journal of Child and Adolescent Health, 9*(2), 155–163. https://ira.lib.polyu.edu.hk/bitstream/10397/93766/1/APSS-0592_Yu_Post-Lecture_Evaluation_University.pdf

Chapter 10
Development, Implementation, and Evaluation of a Service Leadership Subject for University Students

Daniel T. L. Shek and Xiaoqin Zhu

Abstract Because of the changing requirements in the service economy, there is a great need to nurture university students into effective service leaders who possess not only leadership competencies in different aspects but also caring and character attributes. Grounded on the Service Leadership Theory proposed by Po Chung, Co-Founder of DHL International, a credit-bearing subject entitled "Service Leadership" and non-credit-bearing training programs were developed at The Hong Kong Polytechnic University (PolyU). Such Service Leadership education cultivates the belief that "Everyone is (can be) a leader" in students and emphasizes the importance of leadership qualities in the service economy, including competence, character, and care. Findings from different evaluation approaches have shown that the Service Leadership education has been well received by students, who rated the program content, teacher(s), and the gains from participation positively and exhibited significant positive changes in Service Leadership qualities and well-being. To document the development and achievement of Service Leadership education and to further promote it in and out of Hong Kong, journal articles, book chapters, and special issues on theoretical understanding, curriculum development, and evaluation findings have been published. In addition, two international conferences have been organized to exchange experiences and insights. Future directions include more effects in conducting comprehensive evaluations, teacher training, and project extension.

Keywords Service leadership subject · Evaluation findings · Student sharing · Benefit · Teacher training

10.1 Introduction

Under the influence of industrial transformation and globalization, the service sector has dominated Hong Kong's economy (Nations Encyclopedia, 2023). Around 84.7% of the GDP in Hong Kong was contributed by all service sectors in 1998, and this figure rose to 93.7% in 2021 (Census & Statistics Department, 2023). The success of a service-oriented economy highlights the need for developing a new theory of leadership. Different from the emphasis on authority, ranking, and concern about

D. T. L. Shek, *Promoting Holistic Development in University Students*, Quality of Life in Asia 17, https://doi.org/10.1007/978-981-96-0251-3_10

oneself in a manufacturing economy, the postindustrial economy values attributes such as relationship, empowerment, integrity, trust, and service (Grönfeldt & Strother, 2006; Kezar et al., 2006; Rost, 1993). With the service sector contributing to the pillar of Hong Kong's economy, many researchers urge universities to cultivate effective leaders who can respond to the needs of the service economy. Nevertheless, the higher education sector in Hong Kong fails to provide holistic training and education programs or courses to address this need (Shek et al., 2013, 2021), and the value of some leadership qualities, such as care and moral character, have always been ignored (Shek & Chung 2015b; Shek & Yuen, 2019).

In this regard, a credit-bearing subject entitled "Service Leadership" was developed at The Hong Kong Polytechnic University (PolyU) (Shek et al., 2015d). Theoretically, its curriculum framework was built on the Service Leadership and Management (SLAM) initiated by Po Chung, the co-founder of DHL International (Asia Pacific) (Shek & Yuen, 2019). Chung (2012) defined Service Leadership as "Satisfying needs by consistently providing quality personal service to everyone that one comes into contact with, including one's self, others, groups, communities, systems, and environments." Using an equation of $E = MC^2$, SLAM proposes that the effectiveness of leadership (E) is influenced by the competencies (C), the caring disposition (C), and moral character (M) of the leaders perceived by superiors, subordinates, and peers. Later, the three essential determinants of effective service leadership are further referred to as "three Cs" or 3Cs (e.g., competence, care, and character) (Shek et al., 2022). Within this framework, this subject focuses on developing students' competencies, caring disposition, and character (Shek & Yuen, 2019).

10.2 Course Objectives and Intended Learning Outcomes

Against the above background, universities should provide enough support, resources, and training to cultivate competent, caring, and moral service leaders of tomorrow (Shek & Yuen, 2019). However, few credit-bearing leadership subjects adopt a holistic manner to nurture students in these three aspects. In addition, many leadership programs in the local and international contexts hold the belief that only elite students can serve as leaders.

To respond to this call, a 3-credit subject entitled "Service Leadership" was developed at PolyU. This subject aims to cultivate effective service leaders, and all university students at PolyU are eligible to take this subject (Shek et al., 2013). Firstly, this subject intends to facilitate students to reflect on their initial understanding of leadership and the basic qualities of service leaders. In addition, this subject strives to enable students to explore and develop their intrapersonal and interpersonal competencies, caring disposition (such as active listening, being empathetic, and showing love and care), and moral character (building character strengths and valuing Chinese virtues). Finally, this subject expects students to appreciate the importance of Service Leadership to their development and wellness as well as that of other people and society.

Specifically, as stated in the course outline, "Upon completion of the course, students will be able to:

(1) Understand the contemporary models of leadership with reference to the service sector, including their assertions, strengths, and weaknesses;
(2) Demonstrate understanding of the basic leadership attributes intrinsic to effective service leaders, including leadership competencies, moral character, and caring disposition;
(3) Reflect upon the need for developing the qualities of effective service leaders and their own leadership qualities, particularly ethical leadership; and
(4) Appreciate the potential application of knowledge on effective Service Leadership gained in this subject to oneself."

While service industries are gradually replacing or complementing traditional manufacturing industries worldwide, the framework of Service Leadership is suitable for Hong Kong society and in contexts outside Hong Kong.

10.3 Pedagogical Approach

The SLAM framework highlights that several factors, including the competencies, moral character, and caring disposition of the leader, determine effective Service Leadership. Therefore, the subject covers topics on the basic Service Leadership Theory (SLT) (e.g., seven core beliefs and three realms of Service Leadership) and three essential leadership qualities (e.g., competencies, caring disposition, and moral character). Moreover, the teaching/learning methods of this subject are diversified, including lectures, experiential classroom activities, reflective exercises, a group project presentation, and an individual paper (Shek & Yuen, 2019; Shek et al., 2013). As stated in the proposal of this subject, "This subject embeds the teaching philosophy that:

(1) *Every student is (and can be) a leader*. Teachers should encourage every student to develop his/her leadership and appreciate the merits of every student.
(2) *Self-understanding and self-reflection* are very important for effective Service Leadership. Individual self-reflection exercises should be conducted to allow students to enhance their self-understanding.
(3) *Experiential learning* is an effective approach to enhance student learning. Individual, group, and class experiential learning activities should be conducted, in which students can work individually or collaboratively to experience the knowledge learned.
(4) *Collaborative learning* can help students develop competencies, caring disposition, and moral character. Learning will be facilitated through group sharing, discussion, evaluation, and presentation.
(5) *Critical thinking* is encouraged in learning. As such, debates and critical appraisals of the SLAM framework can be conducted, which allows students to think from multiple perspectives.

(6) *Equal emphasis is placed on the theoretical knowledge* of Service Leadership and on the *application of that knowledge in real life*. Teachers should highlight the link between theoretical knowledge and students' lives and future careers. Students are encouraged to apply the knowledge to their lives consciously.
(7) *Systematic evaluation* utilizing different evaluation approaches is critical to understanding the effectiveness of the course developed."

10.4 Engagement of Students

Specifically, this subject adopts a student-centered approach and applies various methods to facilitate students' engagement, including:

(1) Small groups are formed at the beginning of the class. The interaction among students enhances their willingness to share and facilitates students' active participation in group activities (e.g., collaborative learning).
(2) Reflection exercises are conducted by completing worksheets. The written task facilitates active reflection of students (e.g., reflective learning).
(3) In addition to lectures, this subject utilizes manifold experiential teaching/learning strategies to engage students, facilitate their participation, enhance their learning, and stimulate their reflection, including multimedia stimulation, in-class discussion, sharing, role-plays, debates, and expressive arts.
(4) Teachers are encouraged to do attentive self-disclosure. The sharing of their personal experiences helps to build a trustful relationship between teachers and students and motivates the students to share their personal feelings and thoughts (e.g., learning through trust).
(5) The interaction between teachers and students is intense through in-class discussions and other experiential learning activities. This subject strives to establish an enjoyable and encouraging atmosphere in the classroom to encourage students' engagement.
(6) Teachers always bear the basic philosophy that "everyone is (and can be) a leader" in mind and through actions, which boosts students' confidence and helps explore individual capacity. The sharing and performance of every student is appreciated.
(7) Students are inspired to explore how they can apply the philosophy of Service Leadership to help their personal development. After building such awareness and learning with real-life applications, students can be motivated to participate actively in class.

Additionally, the assessment also helps engage the students. First, students will be assessed in terms of their preparation for and participation in class, such as completion of worksheets, volunteering to answer questions, and participation in class activities. Moreover, the arrangement of group presentations motivates students to develop collaborative learning and team-building competence. Finally, students are invited to evaluate the performance and contribution of other group mates in the group presentation.

10.5 Special Issues on the Service Leadership Curriculum

To document the curriculum material for Service Leadership, we have published two special issues on the theory and teaching materials on Service Leadership (Shek et al., 2015c, 2015e). In the editorial of Shek et al. (2015e), the editors highlighted several characteristics of the Service Leadership model. First, the service aims to meet the ethical demands of different stakeholders. According to this view, we lead not simply because of self-interest motives such as seeking personal fame. Second, a systems orientation is adopted, with the understanding that leadership influences oneself, the followers, and the habitat. Within the person, there are different dimensions, such as the physical, emotional, interpersonal, and spiritual dimensions. Third, three Cs are emphasized in the SLT (Shek et al., 2022). The first "C" is competencies that refer to the skills relevant to task requirements, such as analytical skills and interpersonal communication skills. The second "C" is the character, which refers to qualities such as integrity, responsibility, and honesty. The third "C" is care, which is closely linked with care and consideration for others. In fact, the emphasis on the personal qualities of leadership can be revealed in the principle of "the server is the service." Fourth, in contrast to the elitist view of leadership, Service Leadership advocates the idea that "Everybody is (and can be) a leader." The key issue is how to unleash the potential of an individual. For example, a teacher may play a leader's role when there is a fire outbreak by leading the students to evacuate safely. Fifth, to provide the best service, leaders need to upgrade and improve themselves constantly. Sixth, among the different modes of training leaders, it is argued that the mentor-apprentice model is the best training strategy. Finally, the Service Leadership model maintains that besides Western theories and research, it is crucial to consider Chinese philosophies in understanding successful leadership as well as its dark side.

In the paper by Shek et al. (2015b), differences between the manufacturing economy and the service economy were highlighted (e.g., tangible raw materials and products under the manufacturing economy versus intangible knowledge and skills as well as service under the service economy). Because of these fundamental differences, the "desired" leadership qualities also differ for manufacturing and service economies (e.g., minimal empowerment under the manufacturing economy versus nurturance of empowerment under the service economy). They also introduced the 25 principles of Service Leadership proposed by Po Chung (Chung & Bell 2015). These include the principles of "15 minutes of leadership, self-leadership, people leadership, the server, three Cs, co-creation, who you are, personal ethics, who you hire, authoritarian versus distributed leadership, virtues (e.g., trust and fairness), personal operating system, personal brand, relationship, service, mentor–mentee, historical service development, non-tradable service, service mindset, transformation and inspiration, global extension of relationships, habitat management, maritime mindset, Anna Karenina and constructive criticism." In another paper comparing the Service Leadership model and other models, Shek et al. (2015a) highlighted the unique characteristics of the Service Leadership model, such as service and systems orientation and the focus on character and care.

Regarding the curriculum of the subject, there are several parts. In the first part, the focus is on the intrapersonal competencies of successful service leaders (Shek & Lin, 2015). In this topic, we focus on several fundamental competencies in service leaders. These include the adversity quotient (successful adaptation and responses to adversity) and emotional quotient (understanding one's emotions and those of others; management of emotions, particularly negative ones). In the second part, the focus is on interpersonal competencies, including assertiveness and conflict management (Shek et al., 2015g). Besides, ways to promote interpersonal competencies are also touched upon. In the next part (Shek et al., 2015f), we introduce the importance of developmental assets in Service Leadership. Based on the positive youth development (PYD) approach, we highlight that the attributes of self-esteem, self-efficacy, meaning in life, and optimism about the future are essential in Service Leadership. The leadership ramifications of these positive developmental assets are also discussed. In another paper (Shek & Lin, 2015), how Service Leadership plays an essential role in social entrepreneurship is introduced.

In another special issue, we also cover several topics in the curriculum. Based on the positive psychology perspective, we talk about the importance of character strengths in Service Leadership (Shek et al., 2015g). In particular, we focus on the Values in Action framework proposed by Peterson and Seligman (2004), which includes 24 character strengths that can be subsumed under six dimensions: "wisdom and knowledge, courage, humanity, justice, temperance, and transcendence." Besides the Values in Action model that was developed in the Western context, we also cover the notion of character with reference to Chinese philosophies, particularly Confucian virtues. Students are facilitated to reflect on the importance and relevance of Confucian virtues in contemporary Hong Kong.

As the third C in the 3Cs model, we cover the topic of caring disposition in Service Leadership, including its antecedents and consequences, as well as the ways to promote caring disposition. In a related topic, we cover the issue of how to nurture a sense of care in service leaders. In addition to the three basic components of care (love, listening, and empathy) and related skills, we discuss the linkage between care in service leaders and outcomes in different systems, including leaders themselves, followers, and organizations. As Service Leadership involves the relationship between service providers and service recipients, another topic concerns the origin, development, maintenance, and importance of social relationships. Moreover, we cover self-leadership with the belief that "Before leading others, one has to lead oneself." Through this topic, we encourage the students to examine the origin and consequences of self-leadership, as well as the strategies that could be used to promote self-leadership. Finally, as Service Leadership emphasizes the mentor-apprenticeship training model, we also cover the topic of mentorship as a role of service leaders. Mentoring does not only contribute to the development of mentees but also to the personal and professional growth of service leaders as mentors. Besides the determinants and benefits of mentorship, we also explore ways to nurture mentorship as an attribute of effective Service Leadership.

10.6 Evaluation of the Impact of the Subject

In the 2012/13 academic year, this subject was developed as one of the General Education subjects and offered to students under the 3-year undergraduate program. Initially, it carried two credits, and a total of 190 students took this subject. When it turned to the 2014/15 academic year, this subject was modified and enriched to be a 3-credit subject and offered to students under the 4-year undergraduate program. To date, a total of 1817 students took this subject. Various evaluation approaches have been utilized to investigate the effectiveness of the subject (Shek & Yuen, 2019).

(1) Objective outcome evaluation: One group pretest–posttest design was applied to investigate the outcome of the subject. The data gathered from all classes showed that students exhibited significant increases in the scores of PYD, Service Leadership qualities and beliefs, and life satisfaction, no matter whether they came from the 3-year program or the 4-year program. The questionnaire can be seen in Appendix 1.
(2) Subjective outcome evaluation: Students were invited to complete the subjective outcome evaluation questionnaire after completion of the course. The data proved that students evaluated the subject, instructor(s), and the gains from this subject positively. The subjective outcome evaluation questionnaire can be seen in Appendix 2.
(3) Process evaluation: In the first two semesters, two independent raters were invited to observe and assess the program implementation quality and program adherence. The data from the process evaluation revealed that the program adherence and implementation quality were high.
(4) Qualitative evaluation: After the completion of the subject, students were encouraged to write reflective feedback and participate in focus groups to express their feelings and views toward this subject. The findings revealed that students generally had positive feelings toward the subject and regarded learning experiences and achievement in this subject as favorable.

Up until now, the evaluation results have been published in refereed journals, a book series entitled "Quality of Life in Asia," and two special issues in the "International Journal on Disability and Human Development." The achievement of the Service Leadership project has also been documented in a recent special issue, "International Journal of Child and Adolescent Health," edited by Shek et al. (2020c). Appendix 3 outlines the publications arising from this subject and the related evaluation.

10.7 Special Issue on the Origin of the Service Leadership Theory

Based on his successful experience at DHL, Po Chung formulated the SLT. Fundamentally, he believed that everybody has to play a leader's role. For example, if there is a traffic problem, a courier has to decide (thus "lead") how to deliver the package to the customer efficiently and safely. Hence, Chung (2012) proposed that "An effective service leader must possess three attributes: competence, character, and care." Besides, a service leader must continuously improve and be self-led. In terms of the nurture of Service Leadership, the best model is a mentor-apprentice model, which is in sharp contrast to mass training programs involving many trainees.

To document the origin of the SLT, we conducted a study based on interviews with Po Chung and his former colleagues on the different aspects of Service Leadership (Shek et al., 2021). Based on the study, we published a special issue covering the different aspects of the SLT. Based on the written work and personal interviews with Po Chung, Shek and Yang (2021) described the timeline for the development of SLT, including his original intention, major milestones, and major propositions of the theory. His basic view on leadership in the service economy can be shown in his saying, "I clearly showed how management was designed for industrial manufacturing and making sure things are done well. This is crucial when a production line must produce millions of identical objects. High-level services, on the other hand, are complex exchanges between people that help one another thrive, be more fulfilled, and reach their whole self-actualization" (p. 376). At the same time, Po Chung pointed out the gaps in contemporary higher education as follows: "We have found a gross lack of training, discussion or investigation in the leader's character. We have noted how universities skimp on character education, and this oversight has created many problems for leaders that we would describe as 'toxic.' To put it using our 3Cs of Service Leadership, other models are great for covering Competence and even Care, but Character has gone ignored for too long. There are many examples of leaders who did very well or got far ahead with only one strong C. More importantly, there are many examples of bad or toxic leaders in history who led followers on the wrong track or used corrupt practices for advancement and achievement" (p. 377).

In the other papers in the special issue, we highlighted several other major attributes of the SLT, including its emphases on humanistic leadership, moral character, care, trust, and self-leadership. In particular, SLT alerts us to the "dark side" of leadership, which can have detrimental effects on leaders, followers, organizations, and the community (Dou & Shek, 2021). The humanistic orientation of the SLT can be seen in Po Chung's statements: "We are in the post-industrial age because the making of things is over, because AI is coming, and we have to be more human to lead other humans. So, we are changing from making things to motivating humans to do better so that humans can become better. And what we are organizing in our, we would have to call it, our set of knowledge, is to become better humans and make humans work better … We realize that we have to lead the staff instead of managing them. We have to let them work happily and feel pleasant when they come back to the workplace. We also have to take care of their needs if we want them to feel joyful and work diligently … DHL has bottom-up leadership. What we are doing is the delivery of service with people orientation instead of managing production lines … They (couriers) keep making decisions and making improvements. We also let them know that their contributions are key to the success of the company, to the success of customers, and also to the success of themselves … Therefore, these are psychic income and joyfulness of carrying the job" (Zhu et al., 2021, p. 385).

One special emphasis of the SLT is its focus on moral character (Dou et al., 2021). As pointed out by Po Chung, "One of the aims of Service Leadership training is to highlight the crucial role that a leader's character plays for success in a service organization. Service is not necessarily customer service, by the way, but across a network of people who are united by a vision and positive energy. Therefore, a person's character is of the kind that is free from the toxic behaviors and qualities that erode trust across those in the group" (p. 396). Besides, he contrasts leadership under the manufacturing economy and service economy as follows: "Management is all about operational efficiency, stability, and excellence, in short, doing things 'right' or well. In our view, leadership is more about doing the right things with the right heart and about ensuring that what a company does is aligned with human values and needs, resulting in the greatest good for communities and stakeholders … The Service Leadership model I designed, on the other hand, is most interested in helping a leader improve their character through careful self-knowledge, self-governance, and commitment to continuous learning and development. To put it another way, a leader's greatest self-actualization comes by helping everyone in his or her network meet all their needs, including each person's self-actualization" (p. 397).

According to Po Chung, "trust" is an indispensable part of the three facets of Service Leadership (Chai & Shek, 2021). As he argued, "We can link trust to the 3Cs [Competence, Character, and Care]. The first one is competence-based trust: whether a person is reliable or not [in doing things]; whether a person has a high standard of doing things or not. The second one is morality-based trust or character-based trust: whether a person will cheat others, does he lie, does he steal things? The third one is that trusting a person based on whether he would put his heart into doing things; if you are doing work together with him, whether he cares about you and cares about the work to be done will also influence your judgment of whether he is trustworthy or not" (p. 429).

In addition, one can build trust by staying away from behavior that should not be done. "[Among] the Ten Commandments, the first three are talking about God; the fourth to the tenth regulate how people have to behave or not behave if they want to live together as a community, for example, 'do not steal, do not lie, and do not cheat' … And now, we compare it with Confucianism. We can see Confucian moral principles as positive ones: *xiao, ti, zhong, xin, li, yi, lian, chi, zhi, ren, yong, shu*' ('filial piety, brotherly love, loyalty, truthfulness, propriety, righteousness, integrity, shamefulness, wisdom, benevolence, courage, forgiveness'). I talk about the Ten Commandments when I talk about ethics and character, saying that you should not do these. These are the things that, if you do, people will move away from you. And if people hear enough about these behaviors and there is a pattern, then you have a bad reputation. People don't trust you, they don't do business with you, and you stop being a leader … The key ingredients behind a great service leader are his or her 3Cs of Competence, Character, and Care. By making each one as strong as possible, the intersection of the 3Cs is our leadership potential. This is also the building block for establishing and maintaining our level of trustworthiness" (pp. 430–431).

In the final paper on this special issue (Shek & Yang, 2021), we introduced the Fung Service Leadership Initiative, which was initiated by the Victor and William Fung Foundation, with the Hong Kong Institute of Service Leadership and Management (HKI-SLAM) and all public universities funded by the University Grants Committee. While the Victor and William Fung Foundation proposed the SLI with funding support, HKI-SLAM served as the Secretariat, coordinating the universities and helping to organize activities such as international conferences. The eight public universities were invited to develop credit-bearing subjects, non-credit-bearing programs, and curriculum materials. Each university had its free hand to develop the programs with respect to its circumstances, including student needs and institutional progress.

Some information on HKI-SLAM is also in order. In 2011, Po Chung founded and funded HKI-SLAM to promote Service Leadership education, which is an innovative paradigm shift in conceiving service, leadership, and their combination. The HKI-SLAM embraces several principles, including (a) "leadership is a service," which involves meeting the needs of oneself and other stakeholders in different ecological systems in an ethical manner; (b) "every day, people experience service and leadership opportunities," including the potential to promote leadership and service satisfaction; and (c) "the server is the service"—evaluation of effectiveness and satisfaction in terms of competency, character, and caring.

Finally, HKI-SLAM upholds the belief that "Service Leadership is about creating new personal service propositions and consistently striving to provide high-quality, caring service to everyone whom one comes into contact with, including oneself." HKI-SLAM works together with the Victor and William Fung Foundation on the Fung Service Leadership Initiative. At the end of the three-year initiative, many valuable achievements had been made. Because HKI-SLAM has completed and over-achieved its historical mission, it was winded up after the completion of SLI. As Po Chung pointed out, "We went to (the) eight universities, and we faced a lot of skepticism in the beginning, but now it is mostly accepted by all eight universities. Why did we go to (the) eight universities? Why did we go to universities? Because those are the gatekeepers of values or gatekeepers of knowledge … But now, nobody resists it anymore. EdU [The Education University of Hong Kong] does it. PolyU is teaching it, BU [Hong Kong Baptist University] is teaching it, and Lingnan (Lingnan University) is; all of them are doing it" (Shek & Yang, 2021, p. 375).

10.8 International Conferences on Service Leadership

With the funding of the Victor and William Foundation, the Fung Service Leadership Education Initiative was launched in 2012 with the involvement of eight public universities in Hong Kong (e.g., universities receiving funding from the University Grants Committee). These universities included: the City University of Hong Kong, Hong Kong Baptist University, Hong Kong University of Science and Technology, Lingnan University, The Chinese University of Hong Kong, The Education University of Hong Kong, The Hong Kong Polytechnic University, and The University of Hong Kong. In each university, different education initiatives, including credit-bearing Service Leadership subjects and non-credit-bearing Service Leadership programs, were developed (Shek & Chung, 2015a).

The first international conference was held on May 14–15, 2014. As described in the conference brochure, the Fung Service Leadership Initiative (SLI) is "a collaborative partnership of the Victor and William Fung Foundation, HKI-SLAM, and the eight UGC-funded universities in Hong Kong. HKI-SLAM provides its SLAM curriculum framework and serves as the secretariat of the Fung Service Leadership Initiative. The Victor and William Fung Foundation provides catalyst funding and intellectual support. Each university provides a principal investigator and other supporting colleagues who participate in the regular exchange of research findings about Service Leadership and share ideas about how university education might help sustain Hong Kong's reputation as a global service leader. This collaboration provides a unique curriculum development research platform for the universities. Each participating university is empowered to autonomously develop its own research-supported curriculum that is reasonably aligned with the SLAM framework and the unique needs of its students, the institution, and the communities the university serves. UGC provides additional funding through its matching grant scheme" (p. 3).

There were two main parts in this conference. In the first part, several keynote speeches underscored the importance of Service Leadership and Service Leadership education (Shek and Chung 2015a). In the welcome address, the President of PolyU remarked that "since the inception of the Initiative, the eight institutions have successfully incorporated the Service Leadership framework in their curriculum or have included a wide variety of co-curricular activities such as service-learning, student leadership, and civic engagement programs. Research on Service Leadership is also growing. At PolyU, for example, several credit-bearing Service Leadership subjects and non-credit-bearing Service Leadership training workshops have been conducted with positive evaluation results" (pp. v–vi).

Similarly, the importance of Service Leadership was highlighted by Edward Cheng, Chairman of the University Grants Committee: "As the Chairman of the University Grants Committee (UGC), I am pleased to see the successful collaborative efforts of the eight UGC-funded institutions on the Fung Service Leadership Initiative. I understand that the major objective of the Initiative is to benefit a prosperous and vibrant Hong Kong by nurturing the younger generation to meet the demands of the growing service economy and promoting service values. It is an objective that the UGC shares. To the same end, I have focused the work of the UGC on two initiatives that also aim to better prepare students for the exciting future lying ahead, especially against the background of the new 4-year academic program and the rise of Asia, particularly in China. As I briefly outline them here, you will see how the aims and values of the Li & Fung Service Leadership Initiative sit well with them" (p. vii).

In the opening address, John Tsang, the Financial Secretary of the Hong Kong Special Administrative Region, emphasized the importance of leadership training for university students: "The theme of this conference is closely related to the prospects for Hong Kong's economic development and aligns with the Government's effort to enhance our city's overall competitiveness. Economies globally have experienced great transformation in recent decades, with service industries becoming more prominent in the overall picture. Hong Kong is a good example. Our economy is highly oriented around the provision of services delivered domestically and exported to other places. More than 90% of our GDP is derived from services … The answer lies in developing our human capital, which is our city's greatest natural resource. We must nurture service leaders who respond effectively to the needs of this service era. Our prosperity depends on the quality of the next generation of service leaders. The Fung Service Leadership Initiative is a valuable platform for nurturing self-leadership, continuous self-improvement, interpersonal trust, and respect, which are important attributes for successful service leaders" (pp. ix–x).

The importance of Service Leadership was also highlighted in the speech by Victor Fung, Chairman of the Fung Group: "I think the future of Hong Kong's competitiveness lies in services and the development of services. All of you know that 94% of Hong Kong's GDP comes from services. Beyond Hong Kong's own borders, I think one has to look to China. If you look at the Chinese 12th Five-Year Plan, there is a huge emphasis on services. 43% of the Chinese economy is in services. That must be raised over time. We all know that any developed economy would have over 60% of its GDP from services. So, China has a long way to go. Moreover, even in the 12th Five-Year Plan that we see today, the plan is only to move services from 43 to 47% in 5 years. There is a huge role that Hong Kong can play if we get our service sector right. And in terms of our positioning, vis-a-vis the Mainland, to be able to assist the Mainland to achieve the development of the service sector faster than it would otherwise, I think, would be a huge contribution … That is why I am so interested and excited to see that the Service Leadership Initiative is now in its second year and that it involves all eight institutions of higher learning in Hong Kong to develop a whole new curriculum and teaching in Service Leadership. Because unless we do that, we will not be a service leader" (pp. xi–xii).

Finally, in his keynote address, Po Chung highlighted the emphasis on the importance of Service Leadership education: "So that is the vision. Strengthening our Service Leadership is how we can differentiate and thrive … Our invisible pillars are our values DNA. On the one hand, it is our regional and global respectability and trustworthiness, and on the other hand, it is our ability to think critically and independently. The first set is on being, and the second is on doing. We benefit from our traditional Chinese values and thrive when an organization needs bottom-up and top-down management. We are also comfortable with trusting our frontline service people to improvise on the spot and make decisions ... Because of our values, DNA, and thinking ability, and we are the home base of the world's best global bank, the best international airline, the best courier network, the best supply chain company, and one of the best professional services communities of lawyers, auditors, and arbitrators. We house the regional head office base of top-tier advertising agencies, trading companies, HR and PR companies, as well as the headquarters of several top-tier hotels ... As I said when we began, where there is no vision, the people will perish. We now have the vision, and it is simply about staying on track and committing to what we have been doing as global service leaders. We must explain all of these so that parents, students, teachers, and the broader community understand what we need to succeed and that our ability to deliver superior service through trustworthiness and improvisation is something very hard to copy. Even after several generations, the competition may never catch up!" (pp. xvi–xviii).

To wrap up the three-year Fung Service Leadership Initiative, we conducted another international conference on January 6–7, 2016 (Shek et al., 2018). Once again, the importance of Service Leadership and Service Leadership education in the global service economy was highlighted. In her keynote address entitled "Embrace Innovation and Technology to Strengthen Leadership," the Chief Secretary for Administration of the Hong Kong Special Administrative Region (and Chief Executive of Hong Kong from 2017 to 2022) noted, "Human capital is Hong Kong's most important asset. It is no exaggeration for me to say that Hong Kong's prosperity depends on its Government, businesses, and individuals delivering high-quality services. Allow me to share a few observations from my over three decades of government service ... As compared with Hong Kong, the service industries only accounted for 48.1% of China's GDP in 2014, marginally higher than the contribution of the manufacturing industries (47.1%). With the manufacturing processes gradually moving from Mainland China to lower-cost manufacturing bases in Southeast Asia and South Asia, China has to diversify its economy to the service sector to sustain its economic growth. With the so-called 'twin engines of growth,' namely 'increasing the supply of public products and services' and 'promoting mass entrepreneurship and innovation (大眾創業、萬眾創新)' in place, there is huge potential for growth in the service industries. The Mainland will open up at a higher level, promoting technologies, standards, and services around the world. Hong Kong, which has evolved as a mature service economy over the years, certainly could have a great role to play in the process" (p. 13).

In his key address entitled "Service Leadership and the Second Education Revolution," Victor Fung said, "There is a huge potential in the Chinese Mainland's service economy, especially in light of the emphasis placed on services in the 12th Five-Year Plan, which concluded at the end of 2015. Under that plan, the target was for China's economy to move services from 43 to 47% of GDP in five years. Given the size of the Chinese economy, this represents a huge shift. According to the latest data, services now account for about 51.4% of Mainland GDP. So, we can see that China is moving full steam ahead with services development ... The quality of the services that are embedded in production is, in fact, what differentiates one product from another. This has significant implications for the producers and providers of goods and highlights the need to study, understand, and teach services management. Support for the 'Service Leadership Initiative' is a contribution by the Fung Foundation to the important area of training our next generation of leaders in services. Our approach from the outset has been to encourage each of the eight universities to implement the principles of Service Leadership in their own way. Each university will present its own achievements and experiences. Our hope, ultimately, is that the 'Service Leadership Initiative' provides rewarding and life-changing curricula and experiences for our young people and promising new horizons of research for our professors and scholars" (pp. 15–16).

In his keynote address entitled "Almost All Human Social Activity is Service Leadership," Po Chung highlighted "The idea of a 'second education revolution' that had sometimes been mentioned in academic circles. The 'first education revolution' was when Prussia created the first public education system hundreds of years ago, which was an effort to turn farmers into factory workers. Our effort now is to develop training yet again, no longer churning out competent factory workers but nurturing excellent service providers … What I learned over the years was that in order to inspire and bring out the best engagement and quality from our people, we must do things the right way and do the right things with care and compassion. Doing things right is competence. Doing the right things is character. Then, doing the right things with compassion is care. Competence, character, and care are the fundamental needs to bring out the best in people. People trust ethical leaders, no matter where they come from. People will not trust unethical leaders, no matter where they are from, be it from Alaska, Chile, Greenland, or Cape Town … Last but not least, I will wrap up by suggesting a theory. This theory states that everything that falls under human activity can be better understood through Service Leadership. This includes self-leadership, family leadership, tribal leadership, organization leadership, community leadership, professional leadership, and political leadership. This also includes the products that come to us wrapped in service. The Asia Pacific Business Advisory Council defines service as: 'If you are not in growing or catching, if you are not in digging or mining, and if you are not repeatedly making or building, then everything else is service.' In other words, and this is at the root of our call for a 'second education revolution,' '*almost all human social activity is Service Leadership*'" (pp. 17–19).

In another keynote speech (pp. 29–36), Po Keung Ip described the leadership lessons learned from the Zhen Guan period in the Tang Dynasty in China. These include the emphasis on the proper behavior of the Emperor, interdependence of the ruler and the ruled, governing by virtues and care, heightened awareness of possible risk, staying away from extravagance, and learning from history. Besides, other leadership lessons include identifying and recruiting talents, identifying able officials, encouraging expressions of different views, accepting advice, collaborating well with the ministers, being willing to give credit to others, establishing a central institutional decision body, and enforcing fair laws.

In addition to the above keynote speeches, colleagues from different universities shared their Service Leadership initiatives (Shek et al., 2018). At the City University of Hong Kong, Service Leadership initiatives that include education, social innovation incubation, research, knowledge transfer, and student Service Leadership were put under Project Flame, with a focus on inter-disciplinary collaboration and community involvement. For Hong Kong Baptist University, colleagues developed 10 Service Leadership subjects under the General Education program. At The Chinese University of Hong Kong, the SLI included a General Education subject, video cases for flipped classroom teaching, service-learning modules, and a social website. The Education University of Hong Kong developed non-credit-bearing leadership programs through the "Achiever" project. For PolyU, there were both credit-bearing subjects and non-credit-bearing Service Leadership programs outside Hong Kong. At the Hong Kong University of Science and Technology, colleagues collaborated with several faculties to include engineering and Service Leadership knowledge in leadership programs. At The University of Hong Kong, Service Leadership education was conducted through community service projects in the Faculty of Social Sciences.

10.9 Special Issues on Evaluation Research

To illustrate our work on evaluation work, we referred to a special issue entitled "Service Leadership Education in an Era of Service Economy" in 2020 (Shek et al., 2020b). In the editorial, we recapped our work surrounding Service Leadership (Shek et al., 2020b). These include the development of the 2-credit and 3-credit subjects on "Service Leadership." While the 2-credit subject was offered for students in the 3-year program (old university structure before the 2012/13 academic year), the 3-credit subject was offered to students studying in the new 4-year program. The 3-credit subject was also conducted in Xi'an in mainland China and Cambodia in the form of an intensive summer course, with local students in these two places also joining the subjects. Second, besides the classroom-based "Service Leadership," we also developed a Service-Learning (SL) subject called "Service Leadership through Serving Children and Families with Special Needs." Third, Service Leadership education was included in non-credit-bearing leadership programs, with students from Hong Kong and Mainland China (Peking University and Xi'an Jiaotong University) joining the programs. Finally, intensive Service Leadership components were also developed for the Wofoo Leaders' Network.

In the paper, Chai et al. (2020) reported the evaluation findings based on a pre-experimental design (e.g., one group pretest–posttest research design). Based on the strategy of objective outcome evaluation, we assessed students' outcomes, including "PYD attributes, life satisfaction, and Service Leadership qualities" at the beginning as well as the end of the subject using validated measures. Based on the questionnaires collected from 148 students taking the subject in two semesters, we found that there were positive changes in the PYD attributes, satisfaction with life, and Service Leadership qualities. Similar positive changes were observed for another cohort of students ($N = 88$), where students showed positive changes in several indicators, including Service Leadership qualities (self-leadership, character strengths, care, and beliefs about Service Leadership), satisfaction with life, and PYD attributes (Zhu et al., 2020). Moreover, there were significant correlations among changes in Service Leadership qualities, life satisfaction, and PYD attributes.

Additionally, subjective outcome evaluation was implemented to assess the perceptions of the students on the subject by using a validated measure (Shek et al., 2020a). The subject was offered in the 2015/16 academic year, and it involved 106 university students. Results indicated that the students generally evaluated the subject, teachers, and perceived the benefits of the subjects positively. For example, over 90% of the students denoted that the subject was well-designed, the classroom atmosphere was very good, and interaction among students was very good during class. The participants had positive views of the teacher. An overwhelmingly high proportion of the students agreed that the teachers had very good skills and attitudes, cared about students, and were ready to help the students. Furthermore, students generally perceived that the subject benefitted them, including their psychosocial competence, ethical decision-making, and optimism. They also felt that the subject promoted their Service Leadership qualities. It was found that program and instructor qualities predicted perceived benefits.

In another paper on subjective outcome evaluation based on an intensive leadership program in the SOAR Youth Leadership Program 2017/2018 in Beijing (Law et al., 2020), 41 completed questionnaires were collected. Results showed that students had positive evaluations of the program (e.g., program design, classroom atmosphere, and student interaction) and the trainers (e.g., teachers cared about the students and encouraged the students to reflect). Most importantly, the majority of the students perceived that the subject was beneficial in promoting their holistic development, particularly their Service Leadership qualities. For example, most students agreed that the program promoted their social competence (90%), self-leadership (93%), compassion and care (98%), and attributes of successful leaders (100%). In addition to the rating scales, we also invited students to give some descriptors and metaphors that can represent the program. Some examples of the descriptors included "inspiring," "enlightening," "meaningful," "enjoyable," "practical," and "touching and warm." For the metaphors, some examples included "buffet," "melting pot," "light bulb," "lighthouse," and "butterfly." For the metaphor of "melting pot," some students shared that "the people attendants are from different backgrounds, all the diverse thinking patterns, languages, and cultures come together, melt with each other, forming an unbelievably perfect class. Everyone learns something about who they are, what other cultures are like, and most importantly, how to be a service leader" (p. 147).

Utilizing a qualitative methodology, Yang et al. (2020a) asked students in three cohorts (the 2016/17 academic year) to use descriptors and metaphors to examine their learning experience. Results showed that most students used positive descriptors and metaphors to describe their experiences. For example, students used "helpful to personal growth, useful subjects, useful to my development," "interesting, fun," "caring, warm, full of love, supportive, love, empathy," "impressive, unforgettable," "informative, knowledgeable, fruitful, comprehensive, gaining lots of knowledge," and "practical, able to apply daily, real-life experience" to describe their experiences.

For metaphors, students used positive metaphors, including “road signs” (“Service Leadership stresses not only personal growth but also others’ growth. It guides you the right way and sense of achievement!”), “light” (“It guides me to understand what a leader should be equipped with and gives me the tips and clues of how to become a successful leader …”), “compass in life” (“My program [Hotel Management] is something related to service leadership, which is knowledgeable for my career path”), and “wonderful journey” (“In our daily life, we seldom try to study about how we control our emotion, how we care others. In fact, it is a good way for me to review how we treat others appropriately. It is a matter of caring about others’ feelings. Try not to only care about own feelings and interests, which is selfish and not a good manner”).

Similarly, we conducted evaluations for three cohorts of students in the 2017/18 academic year, including local students in the regular terms and summer school in Cambodia (Yang et al., 2020b). Based on descriptors, results showed that students positively described their learning experiences using positive words, such as “useful,” “inspiring,” “meaningful,” “joyful,” “helpful,” “reflective,” and “memorable and unique.” Students also used positive metaphors to represent the subject. Some examples include “light” (“It leads us into the right way, and it lights up my career path”), “compass” (“It gives me different ideas of Service Leadership, and it helps me to develop. Also, it shows the way to become a successful service leader”), “map” (“It provides guidance to Service Leadership. It shows a clear path for my future leadership execution”), and “an inspiring journey” (“It would be like a journey to extremely new things, and concepts are really interesting and inspiring for me. I would be able to grow and learn through the journey”).

10.10 Sharing of the Students

To understand the views and feelings of the students toward Service Leadership, we have invited students to write reflections. Based on the data collected, several themes could be extracted from the narratives.

10.10.1 Unique Features of the Subject

Many students agreed that the subject was exceptional, including its design and pedagogy. In particular, the subject was engaging and encouraging from the students’ point of view.

- *Special Subject*: “Service Leadership is the most special subject that I have taken in the past two years. Through interactive lessons, helpful guidelines from lecturers, and extended readings, I have gained more than what I expected. This subject cultivated my critical thinking skills, self-reflecting habit, and communication technique in general, which has changed my mindset when encountering different situations."

- *Classroom Atmosphere*: "My first impression of this subject was the vivid atmosphere in the lessons."
- *Promotion of Thinking*: "We presented our group name with reasons and listened to others' interpretations of their group names. I was surprised by their interpretations, and [it] broadened my understanding of Service Leadership. Service Leadership is not only a theory-based subject, but also a subject that requires our own comprehensive interpretations on different concepts achieved by sharing our own opinion and consequently applying these theories in diverse circumstances."
- *Promotion of Creative Learning*: "I like the approach that our tutors used to deliver their messages in lessons. We always had a relaxing atmosphere during lessons. With creative learning ways, my interest in the subject has been greatly enhanced. I enjoyed the lessons, and it was fun to learn many new ideas that we could not easily come into contact with in other lessons."
- *Interacting Learning Style*: "The interacting learning style of this subject helps me to have a better understanding and deeper impression of the learning materials and theories. The lecturers gave us a lot of time to have discussions with my group mates. Through discussions, I could check whether I understand the concept just taught or not. If I found anything that was not clear enough, my group would try to clarify the concept together, and I could make self-corrections when listening to the conversation."
- *Sharing Orientation*: "During the lessons, we were encouraged to share our feelings on each topic. Also, there were many class activities. [For example,] we were asked to prepare role plays among groups. Apart from speaking out our feelings, we could act out it. Some of us were too shy to express our feelings in public. But if we changed it into dramas, it became more interesting and easier to speak out. This kind of sharing made me understand that 'share' is a key to showing kindness and care to the people we love."
- *Real-Life Examples*: "This subject uses numerous real-life examples to demonstrate how to be a successful service leader."

10.10.2 Personal Transformation and Future Development

Many students highlighted that the subject enhanced their personal development and motivated them to be better people in future. Some examples are presented below.

- *Subject as a Transit Point in Life*: "This subject is meaningful and useful for our future development. When [I was] asked to create a metonymy for this subject, I chose to describe it as a transit point in the stations. Every lesson, we have time to sit in the lecture [hall] and take a rest and think of ourselves and our journey so far. We learned from the lectures, discovered what could be improved, and had a self-reflection. We walked out of the lecture hall with a more determined mind on what we should do and what we should change to face our lives and become a better person. It gave us a point to stop and think, and I thought I had gained more, which was beyond my expectations."

- *Handle Challenges in Future*: "I sincerely appreciate the syllabus incorporated in the course based on the belief that it will greatly benefit my ability to handle challenges in future. My conviction is that we all have various unique purposes in our existence, and those purposes may somehow require different applications in different situations. An individual could be a team leader at the workplace, a family head at home, or a consultant at the local community committee, etc."
- *Gaining Strength to Face the Future*: "To be a qualified service leader is definitely not a walk in the park. However, the challenges ahead won't defeat me easily, as I have a strong desire to shine brighter, as well as brighten up the lives of others."
- *Impact on Future Life*: "Service Leadership is a unique subject, and studying this subject was an unforgettable experience. The knowledge that I have learned during the lessons may not directly contribute to my future career, but it has changed my point of view toward things that happened around me and improved my attitude when facing problems and challenges in future. More importantly, it taught me how to be an effective service leader for my own life, my career, and the whole society."
- *New Page in Life*: "The end of the semester marked a new page for my journey. To me, Service Leadership suits my personality and values to those of different stakeholders. A good service leader is not determined by the quantity but by the quality of the service. APSS1A21 Service Leadership gave me a new direction on the concept of 'service' and 'leadership,' which can work hand in hand to serve myself, others, and the community comprehensively. I promise I will be a good service leader. Thank you."
- *Learning New Things and Reflection*: "For me, this subject is like a short trip during the summer holidays. I learned new things every lesson and made new friends in the class. Time is short, but I felt satisfied and pleased. This learning experience must become one of the most unforgettable memories of my university life. Beyond my expectations, this subject was really helpful, and I began to reflect on myself and apply it to real life."
- *Preparation for Future Career*: "Apart from boosting my personal growth, the course helps me a lot in preparing for my career, as leadership is a prominent quality that employers wish their employees to have. Service Leadership is even more crucial to us, future workers, due to the fast-changing economy around the globe."
- *Contribution to Future Career Development*: "I have benefited a great deal from this subject. After taking this subject, I have also changed some of my thoughts and behaviors. This supported and enhanced my current development. I believe these changes would also contribute to my future career development."
- *Encouragement to Face the Future*: "Before attending this course, I lacked self-confidence and thought that being a leader was a position that I could not bear. When I was chosen to be a leader, I usually refused and gave opportunities to others. Nonetheless, the core belief of Service Leadership inspires me that I can also become a leader, even if it is just a tiny event. I will keep this statement in

my mind and be brave to try. With this encouragement, I believe that I can be more confident in shouldering any responsibilities and grasping the opportunities to hold an important position in my future."

- *Enhanced Self-understanding*: "This subject has, more importantly, allowed me to have a deeper self-understanding and self-reflection on the potential leader that I would like to become. I was becoming more aware of the different attributes that impact the characteristics of a leader. In the past, while I generally believed that skills and understanding of the company and industry were among the major attributes of a leader, I realized that while these attributes are essential, they do not necessarily make you a good leader."
- *Enhanced Personal Development*: "This subject has greatly enhanced [my] personal development … I have become more aware of the things that make one colleague stand out from the others or why a particular staff is chosen for promotion and not the other … By putting yourself in other people's shoes rather than letting emotion control you, you will have a better understanding in realizing that the mistake was not purposely made."

10.10.3 Leadership Qualities

As a subject on Service Leadership, students reflected that the subject helped them enhance their understanding of Service Leadership and acquire positive leadership attitudes and leadership skills. Some of the students' sharing is presented below.

- *Understanding of Service Leadership*: "Before taking Service Leadership, leadership was an abstract concept to me … There was no clear definition in my mind, and it was simply interpreted as the way to lead a team efficiently. However, after taking this subject, I understand that leadership is a complicated process … In the past, leaders may only focus on how to lead followers, and we may usually think that the most important criteria for leaders are the skills and knowledge they possess to lead a team. But now, I understand that there are three significant elements that are equally important to perform effective Service Leadership—competences, moral character, and care."
- *Clarification of Leadership Concepts*: "I used to think that Service Leadership equals servant leadership. However, I discovered that I was wrong after having the first lesson on this subject. Service Leadership not only focuses on serving others and satisfying their needs but also on achieving your own goals at the same time. It took me some time to adapt to this new viewpoint of leadership."
- *The Uniqueness of Service Leadership*: "Theory-wise, not only do I know more about the Service Leadership model, in the process of comparing it to other leadership models, I learned the difference of the Service Leadership models [in comparison] to some other leadership models as well. To my understanding, I would agree that Service Leadership is a suitable and effective leadership model for the economy of Hong Kong, which consists of a high percentage of service industries."

- *Change in Conception of Leadership*: "This inspires me to believe that a leader does not only need to be autocratic, but he should build up good relationships with subordinates so as to increase the spirit of teamwork."
- *Caring*: "I discovered that successful leaders should take care of their followers. In the beginning, I suspected this argument and believed that caring is pointless. However, after the lecture, I found out that caring is positively associated with followers' performance, profits of the firm, and social stability. Consequently, I realized that caring is one of the vital elements in leadership, and we should show our care to our followers in a daily setting."
- *Holistic Conception of Leadership*: "This course inspires me to satisfy followers' needs. It is a common belief that a leader should make the final decision and control their followers in an autocratic way. In contrast, Service Leadership defines leadership as providing high-quality service to satisfy the needs of everyone one comes into contact with, including self, others, and the system."
- *Deeper Understanding of Leadership*: "One of the best things about this subject is that it motivates me to think out of the box and look at leadership from multiple perspectives. My previous perception of leaders is superficial, simply focusing on the positive things enjoyed by leaders, such as giving orders and enjoying the services provided by others."
- *New Conception of Leadership*: "'Service Leadership drew a new picture of leadership and broke my inherent views towards leadership. Leadership is not only about leaders themselves but also underlines how to use self-capacity to influence others. If a leader cannot accurately utilize his abilities to serve others, even if he has a high level of leadership competence, he is still not a good leader. This reminds me to take care of others and listen to others' feedback when being a leader."
- *Enhanced Understanding of Leadership*: "During the lectures, what inspired me the most was the explanation of different leadership styles. Not until then did I realize that there is a wide variety of leadership styles, and each of them has its own edge. It reminds me that my leadership style was too authoritarian before, and I planned to improve myself in the coming years."
- *Everyone Can be a Leader*: "As mentioned, I have always been a follower. I did not believe I could be a leader, so I did not become a leader. Service Leadership states that everyone, no matter what position, can serve and lead someone. Leadership can be nurtured … I am convinced that every person, no matter how decent he is, can develop himself to practice Service Leadership to some extent by leading himself, getting prepared to lead close people by ethically leading the close people, making contributions to those beyond them."
- *Comprehensive Understanding of Leadership*: "From my point of view, this is definitely a successful leadership training course. Before signing up for this course, I actually didn't have many leadership skills. In my understanding of leadership, I was trying my best to ask others to listen to me. However, I found that it is completely wrong, and I now have a comprehensive understanding, and my belief has been further strengthened after taking this course."

- *The Subject as a Lighthouse*: "Due to my lack of understanding of the term 'leadership,' I had no confidence in myself when it came to taking leading positions. I thought I was not talented enough to be a leader and did not have the capability or the charm to lead others. However, the first lecture of the course illuminated me as it pointed out that one of the main theories of Service Leadership is that 'everyone could be a leader.' It was like a lighthouse that showed me the way to accomplish something that I regarded as impossible in the past, motivating me to study harder in the subject."
- *Developing a Spiritual Health of Service*: "The subject of 'Service Leadership' is surely inspiring in two ways, not only providing me with a solid knowledge ground of this concept but also preparing me a spiritual heart of service to be a service leader in future. This course provides me with an invaluable opportunity to reflect and review what I have been doing in my university life and what should be improved before I graduate, especially when I am a final-year student. It enables me to increase my self-understanding of my strengths, weaknesses, and competence and rethink the meaning of my life. Generally, this course has turned me into a more proactive and energetic person with a more positive attitude and optimistic future projection through picturing my future success."

10.10.4 Benefits to the Students

In addition to leadership knowledge, attitude, and skills, students also mentioned that this subject promoted their psychosocial competencies in different areas:

- *Building up Arguments*: "I learned how to collect objective evidence, including data and empirical studies to support my arguments."
- *Interpersonal Relationship*: "In the past, I only focused on my interests without considering others' positions and thus failed to create a strong bond with my colleagues. After I recognize the importance of followers' feelings, I try to provide some mental and physical support to my followers."
- *Friendship*: "Sometimes, the curriculum and the system of the university make me feel that we are competitors between my classmates and me. However, except in this class, there are strong connections between the lecturers and students. We care about others, such as studies, emotions, and human relationships. I am glad that I have decided to join this class and built up a close relationship among my groupmates. I hope we can keep a life-long contact and support each other even after we graduate from PolyU."
- *Utilization of Leadership Skills*: "I started to utilize some of the self-leadership skills I heard in the lecture. Service Leadership considers self-control as an important element in leadership and provides some methods such as self-goal setting and self-reward to regulate our behaviors. These skills are really useful, and I can manage myself better after this course."

- *Communication Capacity*: "Apart from the above inspiration, my communication capacity has improved after the course. As a group coordinator, it is my responsibility to book a consultation with the lecturers. This action involves coordination with different parties such as my teammates and professors."
- *Admit One's Shortcomings and Cheer Up*: "Apart from the lecturers' sharing, they also threw challenges to us to let us realize our shortcomings. In one lesson, the lecturer invited one student to share one miserable incident and asked the class to cheer him up. Before this practice, I did not realize how hard it is to cheer a person up. However, in the real practice, I became speechless. It is hard to provide constructive advice or cheering words to help the student. Luckily, this course provided us chances to listen to others and learn from them."
- *Understanding Strengths and Weaknesses*: "The thorough class discussion in the realms of competencies, particularly the intrapersonal and interpersonal, with deep appreciation allows self-reflection by utilizing the provided scale to identify areas of improvement. The stated topics provided the needed opportunity to examine myself as I tried to focus more on my weaknesses and how best I could mold them to be my strengths over time."
- *Learning by Doing*: "I really enjoy studying APSS1A21 Service Leadership because the knowledge of effective Service Leadership taught is meaningful and practical in real life. I realize the importance of learning by doing that studying the contents written in books is definitely inadequate, and we should also work it out."
- *Team Building Skills*: "Apart from learning abstract concepts of leadership, I was also granted many opportunities to practice my leadership competences via group work, especially my team building skills. In the first lecture, all students were randomly divided into ten groups, and I did not have any group mates who were familiar with me."
- *Active Learning*: "I am used to receiving answers from the tutor instead of finding the solutions by myself. Nevertheless, after taking this subject, I knew the advantages and necessity of active learning."
- *Ethics and Morality*: "I was particularly impressed by the emphasis on ethics and morality in Service Leadership … This course revealed the true nature of leadership and led me to reflect on how effective leadership should be. Leadership should not be limited to making the most profits for the company. Instead, leadership should be a tool to promote the growth of self and others."
- *Self-Understanding*: "In the lecture, I had a really deep impression of the discussion on how important it is to know ourselves. I said, 'Feel your own feelings so that you can feel others' feelings.' It means that you need to always do reflection so you can know yourself and your goal better. Then, you can help others and listen to others' feelings."
- *Opportunity to Grow*: "I remember I was a bit surprised and scared when our group was told to role-play in front of the whole class during the second lesson. However, after performing on the stage, I felt quite enjoyable. Also, I have found that the knowledge I have learned becomes more understandable and rooted in my mind."

- *Development of Multiple Perspectives*: "One of the best things about this subject is that it motivates me to think out of the box and look at leadership from multiple perspectives. My previous perception of leaders was superficial, simply focusing on the positive things enjoyed by leaders, such as giving orders and enjoying the services provided by others. However, Service Leadership tells us that leaders are those who provide services and support. At the same time, although leaders are the service providers, it does not mean that good leaders should only care about others. Their own needs should also be considered."
- *Reflection*: "Due to the program, I can reflect more on my own life."
- *Self-Improvement*: "Interpersonal competencies, intrapersonal competencies, character strength and so on are the 'fruits' I got in the course, which has increased my awareness of myself and the impact of oneself on the whole organization. This learning experience changed my thoughts on how to improve myself before leading others. This course will become one of the most important courses I take in the PolyU."
- *Personal Transformation*: "It is very important that Service Leadership can strengthen my personality, attitude, and values. Honestly, it is easy for university students to lose themselves when they only focus on their academic results."

10.11 The Way Forward

Future directions are noted regarding evaluation, teacher training, and program extension.

10.11.1 Evaluation

Evaluation tools will be strengthened to assess the effectiveness of this subject. First, a quasi-experimental design with a control group can be applied to investigate whether this subject influences students in positive ways. Second, a long-term follow-up study will be helpful to examine whether the effectiveness of this subject can be sustained. In addition to the three qualities of Service Leadership, more attributes (e.g., leadership knowledge, attitude, and behavior) will be assessed during the learning.

10.11.2 Teacher Training

Since the philosophy of Service Leadership is relatively new, and as this subject applies an interactive approach instead of a traditional didactic approach, enriching teachers' knowledge and qualities is a crucial factor. To establish comprehensive knowledge of Service Leadership, teachers can participate in a training program offered by Po Chung. Moreover, to strengthen teacher training, our research team is developing an e-learning package to introduce interactive teaching methodology.

10.11.3 Program Extension

Another subject using Service Leadership pedagogy ("Service Leadership through Serving Children and Families with Special Needs") has been organized. Besides PolyU, the subject can also benefit students from other higher education sectors in Hong Kong. For instance, we plan to carry out a range of workshops with condensed versions for students from other tertiary education institutions. In addition, although the SLAM framework was developed in the service economy of Hong Kong, the philosophy of Service Leadership applies to places suitable for a postindustrial paradigm of leadership, such as Mainland China and other societies. There are some successful endeavors, such as the "Global Youth Leadership Program" co-organized by PolyU and Peking University, the "Silk Road Youth Leadership Program" by PolyU, Peking University, and Xi'an Jiaotong University. In particular, Peking University and PolyU co-organized a summer school for Service Leadership in 2016, and around 60 students participated in the camp at that time. We plan to deliver more comprehensive Service Leadership education that will benefit more students from universities outside Hong Kong.

Acknowledgements The preparation of this chapter is financially supported by The Hong Kong Polytechnic University (ZZ4U and ZZUE), Li and Fung Endowed Professorship in Service Leadership Education, Wofoo Foundation, and the Matching Fund of Research Grants Council (ZECL and ZH4Q).

Appendix 1: Objective Outcome Evaluation Form

學生問卷調查 I
Student Questionnaire I

Dear Student,

As part of the assessment of APSS1A21/M, you are expected to complete two sets of student questionnaires by Lecture 3 (e.g., Student Questionnaire I) and Lecture 12 (i.e., Student Questionnaire II). Successful completion of Student Questionnaires I and II would entitle you to **2 and 3 marks for Class Participation/ Preparation**, respectively. In the coming lectures, we will share with you some main findings and response profiles gathered from the Student Questionnaire I. Results regarding Student Questionnaire II will be uploaded to the Blackboard following the completion of the course. Failing to submit this in-class assignment means that **you will receive no marks**. Please rest assured that **all information collected will be kept confidential,** and **your identity will NOT be disclosed** at any point in time.

Meanwhile, we wish to seek your permission to use the data gathered from this questionnaire for *research and education purposes*, including submissions for publications in the forms of reports, book chapters, and academic journal articles. Any relevant data analyses of the data generated from this questionnaire will be conducted anonymously. We sincerely pledge your help **by checking "YES" below** and **signing at the bottom of this page**.

□ **YES.** I am granting my permission to use the data collected strictly for research and education purposes. I understand that all my information would be kept confidential, and all the analyses would be conducted in an anonymous fashion.

□ **NO.** I do not allow any data gathered from this questionnaire to be used.

Should you be inclined to learn more about this questionnaire, please do not hesitate to email Dr. Julie ZHU (xiaoqin.zhu@polyu.edu.hk) and Dr. Diya Dou (diya.dou@polyu.edu.hk) from the research team for more information. Thank you!

________________________ ________________________

Signature of student Date

第一部份 Part 1

請小心閱讀下列各句子,然後在下表圈出一個您認為最能夠代表您的想法的數字。答案沒有對錯之分,請憑自己的感覺和認識誠實作答。

Please read each sentence carefully and ***circle the number*** that best describes your thoughts. There is no right or wrong answer. Please answer the questions honestly based on your knowledge and impression of yourself.

		非常不同意**Strongly disagree**	不同意**Disagree**	有點不同意**Slightly disagree**	有點同意**Slightly agree**	同意**Agree**	非常同意**Strongly agree**	**CODE**
1	我懂得怎樣與人溝通。 I know how to communicate with others	1	2	3	4	5	6	**SC_01**
2	我了解人與人相處的規則和要求。 I understand the rules and expectations in interacting with others	1	2	3	4	5	6	**SC_02**
3	我能夠與其他人融洽相處。 I can get along well with others	1	2	3	4	5	6	**SC_03**
4	當我不開心時,我能夠適當地表達我的情緒。 When I am unhappy, I can appropriately express my emotions	1	2	3	4	5	6	**EC_01**
5	在與人發生衝突時,我通常能夠處理我的情緒。 When I have conflicts with others, I can usually manage my emotions	1	2	3	4	5	6	**EC_02**
6	我能夠站在別人的角度看問題和了解他們的感受。 I can stand in the shoes of others	1	2	3	4	5	6	**EC_03**

(continued)

(continued)

		非常不同意**Strongly disagree**	不同意**Disagree**	有點不同意**Slightly disagree**	有點同意**Slightly agree**	同意**Agree**	非常同意**Strongly agree**	**CODE**
7	我懂得從不同角度去看事物。 I know how to see things from different angles	1	2	3	4	5	6	**CC_01**
8	我會嘗試用創新的方法去解決我面對的問題。 I try new ways to solve my problems	1	2	3	4	5	6	**CC_02**
9	我懂得分析問題的成因和尋找解決的方法。 I know how to find the causes of and solutions to a problem	1	2	3	4	5	6	**CC_03**
10	我能夠分辨事情的好與壞。 I can differentiate between the good and the bad aspects of things	1	2	3	4	5	6	**CC_04**
11	我能夠以開放的態度面對批評。 I can face criticisms with an open mind	1	2	3	4	5	6	**BC_01**
12	我能夠表達與其他人不同的意見。 I can express views that are different from others'	1	2	3	4	5	6	**BC_02**

(continued)

(continued)

		非常不同意Strongly disagree	不同意Disagree	有點不同意Slightly disagree	有點同意Slightly agree	同意Agree	非常同意Strongly agree	CODE
13	對於自己的行為,我有較高的道德要求。 I have high moral standards about my behavior	1	2	3	4	5	6	**MC_01**
14	我向他人承諾了會做的事,我會把它完成。 I fulfill my promises	1	2	3	4	5	6	**MC_02**
15	為了賺錢而放棄一些道德原則,並沒有太大問題。(reversely coded) It is no big deal to give up some of our moral principles in exchange for money	1	2	3	4	5	6	**MC_03**
16	我有自我檢討的習慣。 I have a habit of self-reflection	1	2	3	4	5	6	**MC_04**
17	我有能力作出明智的抉擇。 I am capable of making wise choices	1	2	3	4	5	6	**SD_01**
18	我對自己所作的決定有信心。 I am confident about my decisions	1	2	3	4	5	6	**SD_02**

(continued)

(continued)

		非常不同意**Strongly disagree**	不同意**Disagree**	有點不同意**Slightly disagree**	有點同意**Slightly agree**	同意**Agree**	非常同意**Strongly agree**	**CODE**
19	我相信將來發生在我身上的事情, 大部分取決於我自己。 I believe that the things that will happen in my life are mostly determined by myself	1	2	3	4	5	6	**SD_03**
20	我是一個有自信的人。 I am a person with self-confidence	1	2	3	4	5	6	**CPI_01**
21	我相信自己有領袖的特質及能力。 I believe I have the qualities and abilities of a leader	1	2	3	4	5	6	**CPI_02**
22	我有信心解決我將來會面對的問題。 I have the confidence to solve my future problems	1	2	3	4	5	6	**BF_01**
23	我有信心能夠大學畢業。 I have the confidence to graduate from university	1	2	3	4	5	6	**BF_02**
24	我有信心畢業後能夠成為一個有用的人。 I have confidence that I will be a useful person after I graduate	1	2	3	4	5	6	**BF_03**

(continued)

(continued)

		非常不同意Strongly disagree	不同意Disagree	有點不同意Slightly disagree	有點同意Slightly agree	同意Agree	非常同意Strongly agree	CODE
25	在很多方面，我的生活接近我理想中的狀態。In most ways, my life is close to my ideal	1	2	3	4	5	6	**LS_01**
26	我的生活狀況是極好的。The conditions of my life are excellent	1	2	3	4	5	6	**LS_02**
27	我對自己的人生感到滿意。I am satisfied with my life	1	2	3	4	5	6	**LS_03**
28	到目前為止，我已經取得生命中我想得到的重要東西。So far, I have gotten the important things I want in life	1	2	3	4	5	6	**LS_04**
29	如果我能夠再活一次，我依然會選擇現有的生活。If I could live my life over, I would still choose the life I have now	1	2	3	4	5	6	**LS_05**
30	我的生命很有意義。My life is meaningful	1	2	3	4	5	6	**SP_01**
31	我已經找到人生的目標。I have found my purpose in life	1	2	3	4	5	6	**SP_02**

(continued)

(continued)

		非常不同意**Strongly disagree**	不同意**Disagree**	有點不同意**Slightly disagree**	有點同意**Slightly agree**	同意**Agree**	非常同意**Strongly agree**	**CODE**
32	我考慮過自殺。I have considered committing suicide before. (reversely coded)	1	2	3	4	5	6	**SP_03**
33	我相信心靈上的富有比物質上的富有更為重要。I believe spiritual riches are more important than material prosperity	1	2	3	4	5	6	**SP_04**
34	面對困難時,我不會輕易放棄。When I face difficulties, I do not give up easily	1	2	3	4	5	6	**RE_01**
35	我的信念是:「就算明天變得更差,我仍會好好地生活下去。」I believe that even though tomorrow becomes worse, I will still live in a good manner	1	2	3	4	5	6	**RE_02**
36	我相信人生中的困難是可以解決的。I believe problems in life can be solved	1	2	3	4	5	6	**RE_03**

第二部份 **Part 2**

Please read each sentence carefully and ***circle the number*** that best describes your views toward the role of leader or leadership process. There is no right or wrong answer. Please answer the questions honestly based on your knowledge and impression of yourself.

		Strongly disagree	**Disagree**	**Slightly disagree**	**Slightly agree**	**Agree**	**Strongly agree**	**CODE**
1	A good leader calmly deals with stressful situations	1	2	3	4	5	6	**SLA_01**
2	A good leader leads the team with an inspiring and strategic vision	1	2	3	4	5	6	**SLA_02**
3	A good leader is able to articulate his/her vision of the organization	1	2	3	4	5	6	**SLA_03**
4	Good leadership requires that a leader copes effectively with adversity	1	2	3	4	5	6	**SLA_04**
5	A good leader is open to challenge or criticism	1	2	3	4	5	6	**SLA_05**
6	A good leader encourages his/her followers to take responsibility for what they do	1	2	3	4	5	6	**SLA_06**
7	A good leader listens to his/her subordinates' views	1	2	3	4	5	6	**SLA_07**

(continued)

(continued)

		Strongly disagree	Disagree	Slightly disagree	Slightly agree	Agree	Strongly agree	CODE
8	When providing service, a leader should consider the characteristics of the service recipient	1	2	3	4	5	6	**SLA_08**
9	A good leader has sympathy for people who suffer	1	2	3	4	5	6	**SLA_09**
10	The ability and willingness to love followers is one of the most important leadership qualities	1	2	3	4	5	6	**SLA_10**
11	A good leader provides physical and psychological support for followers to accomplish their work assignments	1	2	3	4	5	6	**SLA_11**
12	A good leader uses himself/herself as an example to influence the behavior of followers	1	2	3	4	5	6	**SLA_12**
13	A good leader acts as an ethical model for the followers	1	2	3	4	5	6	**SLA_13**
14	A good leader sets an example for others to follow	1	2	3	4	5	6	**SLA_14**

(continued)

(continued)

		Strongly disagree	Disagree	Slightly disagree	Slightly agree	Agree	Strongly agree	CODE
15	Effective leaders appreciate and respect different opinions and viewpoints	1	2	3	4	5	6	**SLA_15**
16	Effective leadership largely involves good communication with followers	1	2	3	4	5	6	**SLA_16**
17	A good leader has good self-reflection ability	1	2	3	4	5	6	**SLA_17**
18	A leader should closely examine his/her own thoughts and behavior	1	2	3	4	5	6	**SLA_18**
19	A true leader knows his/her own strengths and weaknesses	1	2	3	4	5	6	**SLA_19**
20	Everyone can be a leader regardless of his/her current role and position	1	2	3	4	5	6	**SLA_20**
21	Everyone has the potential to be a leader	1	2	3	4	5	6	**SLA_21**
22	Whether or not a person can become a leader is fundamentally shaped by one's personality and not much can be changed	1	2	3	4	5	6	**SLA_22**

(continued)

(continued)

		Strongly disagree	Disagree	Slightly disagree	Slightly agree	Agree	Strongly agree	CODE
23	One's leadership competences are inborn and cannot be changed very much	1	2	3	4	5	6	**SLA_23**

第三部份 Part 3

The following statements describe some leaders' behaviors. Please read each statement carefully and indicate how similar it is to your own situation if you were a leader ***by circling the number***. There is no right or wrong answer. Please answer the questions honestly based on your knowledge and impression of yourself.

		Very dissimilar to me	Moderately dissimilar to me	Slightly dissimilar to me	Slightly similar to me	Moderately similar to me	Very similar to me	CODE
1	I learn through reflecting on my experiences	1	2	3	4	5	6	**SLB_01**
2	I often reflect on my work and life	1	2	3	4	5	6	**SLB_02**
3	I often reflect on my own strengths and weaknesses	1	2	3	4	5	6	**SLB_03**
4	I keep learning new knowledge	1	2	3	4	5	6	**SLB_04**
5	I am committed to continually improving myself	1	2	3	4	5	6	**SLB_05**
6	When there is a conflict between morality and self-interest, I would do things that are morally right	1	2	3	4	5	6	**SLB_06**

(continued)

(continued)

		Very dissimilar to me	Moderately dissimilar to me	Slightly dissimilar to me	Slightly similar to me	Moderately similar to me	Very similar to me	CODE
7	When I talk to someone who is upset, I try to understand his/her situation	1	2	3	4	5	6	**SLB_07**
8	I often try my best to help other people to overcome difficulties	1	2	3	4	5	6	**SLB_08**
9	Adversity, such as failures and setbacks, usually makes me stronger rather than weaker	1	2	3	4	5	6	**SLB_09**
10	When difficulties or setbacks appear in my life, I do not give up easily	1	2	3	4	5	6	**SLB_10**
11	I have faith to deal with challenges in my life	1	2	3	4	5	6	**SLB_11**
12	I have a sense of purpose in my life, which helps me cope with stressful situations	1	2	3	4	5	6	**SLB_12**
13	I am able to maintain positive relationships with other people	1	2	3	4	5	6	**SLB_13**

(continued)

(continued)

		Very dissimilar to me	Moderately dissimilar to me	Slightly dissimilar to me	Slightly similar to me	Moderately similar to me	Very similar to me	CODE
14	I am able to develop harmonious relationships with other people	1	2	3	4	5	6	**SLB_14**
15	I am able to think independently	1	2	3	4	5	6	**SLB_15**
16	I am able to think critically	1	2	3	4	5	6	**SLB_16**
17	I am able to argue in a logical way	1	2	3	4	5	6	**SLB_17**
18	I grab every opportunity to help other people grow	1	2	3	4	5	6	**SLB_18**
19	I invest time and put my energy into helping people to realize their potential	1	2	3	4	5	6	**SLB_19**

第四部份 **Part 4**

Please read each question carefully and ***circle the answer*** that you think is most appropriate according to your current knowledge.

	Note: Correct answer	CODE
1.	According to the Service Leadership and Management (SLAM) Model, competence, _______ and ______ influence the loyalty and commitment of the employees. A. fame; character B. intelligence; care C. intelligence; character D. character; care	SLK_01
2.	Which of the following statements are consistent with the Service Leadership and Management (SLAM) Model? (1) Service Leadership is about leading by trust and respect (2) Service Leadership is about leading by issuing orders. (3) Service Leadership is about leading by education and inspiration. (4) Service Leadership is about punishing mistakes. A. (1) and (2) B. (1) and (3) C. (2) and (4) D. (3) and (4)	SLK_02
3.	Which of the following statements is consistent with the Service Leadership and Management (SLAM) Model? A. Service Leadership is about giving commands. B. Service Leadership is about correcting others' mistakes. C. Service Leadership is about inspiring and empowering others. D. Service Leadership is about manipulating followers and others.	SLK_03
4.	Which of the following statements about Service Leadership is correct? A. Service Leaders do not need to consider the responses of actual people at work. B. Service Leaders do not need to satisfy actual people's needs at work. C. Service Leaders' work is tied inextricably to the needs of actual people. D. Service Leaders are elites	SLK_04
5.	According to the Service Leadership and Management (SLAM) Model, leadership is a service aimed at _________satisfying the needs of self, others, groups, communities, systems, and environments. A. ethically B. intuitively C. conditionally D. ideally	SLK_05
6.	A manager in the service economy wants to hire an employee. Based on the Service Leadership model, which of the following advice would you give him/her: A. Hire for skills, train for character. B. Hire for character, train for skills. C. Hire for attractiveness, train for character. D. Hire for efficiency, train for attitude.	SLK_06
7.	A good Service Leader often engages in self-reflection exercises in order to improve his/her own self. Which situational context would this be? A. Individual B. Habitat C. Community D. None of the above	SLK_07
8.	Jason performs good Service Leadership in the habitat. This indicates that he operates well in ___________. A. his own mind B. his own spirit C. his own body D. his own team	SLK_08

	Note: Correct answer	CODE
9.	Which of the following statements is consistent with the Core Beliefs of Service Leadership? A. A Service Leader should serve the needs of others only. **B. A Service Leader can ethically serve the needs of the self.** C. Making self-improvement is not related to leadership. D. Serving the needs of the self is not ethical for a Service Leader.	SLK_09
10.	The self-serving effort includes improving one's _______ to help in satisfying the needs of others. A. fame B. wealth C. authority and power D. **competences, abilities, and willingness**	SLK_10
11.	According to Manz's (1980) theory, which of the following strategies is a typical self-management strategy? A. **Setting a personal goal to achieve.** B. Hiding one's emotions. C. Asking for help from others. D. Holding one's opinions if they are different from others'.	SLK_11
12.	The Service Leadership and Management (SLAM) Model asserts that everyone can be a leader. Which of the following statements is NOT the rationale underlying this proposition? A. Self-development can be regarded as one sort of leadership. B. Every day, there are many service transactions in which one can take a leading role. C. Leadership quality is malleable and improvable. D. **Leadership is an inborn quality.**	SLK_12
13.	Which of the following individuals can become Service Leaders? (1) A dustman cleaning the offices. (2) A student who has not taken any leading position. (3) A frontline worker working at an assembly line for smartphone production. (4) A lawyer defending his clients' rights. A. (1) and (2) B. (2) and (3) C. (1) and (4) D. **All of them**	SLK_13
14.	The Service Leadership and Management (SLAM) Model maintains that ________. A. **everyone is a leader** B. only some people are leaders C. only competent people are leaders D. low educated people are not leaders	SLK_14
15.	According to the Service Leadership and Management (SLAM) Model, if Kate wants to become an effective Service Leader, she needs to: (1) develop her leadership, intrapersonal, and interpersonal competencies. (2) have excellent scholastic achievement. (3) enhance her moral character. (4) consider the needs of others and provide care to others when they are in need. A. (1) and (2) B. (1) and (3) C. (1), (2), and (3) D. **(1), (3), and (4)**	SLK_15
16.	Which statement is in line with the Service Leadership and Management (SLAM) Model? A. Improving one's competencies is more important than developing one's character strengths and caring disposition. B. Improving one's caring disposition is the only way to become a successful Service Leader. C. **Developing one's character strengths and developing caring disposition are equally important as improving one's competencies.** D. Improving one's competences is the only way to become a successful Service Leader.	SLK_16
17.	Quality Service Leadership is a(n) ___________ process that requires service leaders to _______ bring about improvement in each domain of E = MC2.	SLK_17

	Note: Correct answer	CODE
	A. one-time qualification; remarkably B. one-time qualification; continuously C. ongoing development; remarkably D. ongoing development; continuously	
18.	Leadership competency refers to leading in the most appropriate and satisfying way in order to ________. A. achieve a personal goal only B. solve all social problems C. satisfy needs given the current situation and context D. establish authority and power in the organization	**SLK_18**
19.	Of the four options below, which one is the attribute of intelligence quotient (IQ)? A. Emotional management B. Religious beliefs C. Physical strength D. Problem-solving skills	**SLK_19**
20.	According to the definition from Goleman (1998), which of the following capacities is considered as an aspect of emotional intelligence (EQ)? A. Recognizing the reasons for failure B. Questing about the meaning of life C. Suppressing others' emotions D. Managing our negative and positive emotions	**SLK_20**
21.	According to Goleman's (2001) model of emotional intelligence (EQ), which of the following domains was proposed? A. Self-awareness B. Self-sacrifice C. Self-achievement D. Self-reliance	**SLK_21**
22.	The ability to cope with adversity and bounce back is ______________. A. *assertiveness* quotient (AQ) B. *aspiration* quotient (AQ) C. *adventure* quotient (AQ) D. *adversity* quotient (AQ)	**SLK_22**
23.	Andy's student association failed to get a fund to support their project. Andy realized that failure also has meaning, felt motivated again, and tried to motivate his teammates. Andy showed a high A. intelligence quotient (IQ) B. physical quotient (PQ) C. cultural quotient (CQ) D. spiritual quotient (SQ)	**SLK_23**
24.	A leader with moral character can win _____ and _____ of their followers in the workplace. A. power; authority B. power; obedience C. authority; obedience D. trust; respect	**SLK_24**
25.	Jenny devoted herself to her career in helping people who suffered from hunger, isolation, and poverty. Which dimension of character strengths was demonstrated by her dedication? A. Wisdom B. Curiosity C. Humanity D. Knowledge	**SLK_25**
26.	The caring disposition of a service leader could be illuminated by the following level(s) of concern: (1) The wellbeing of one's own mind, body, and spirit. (2) The wellbeing of others' mind, body, and spirit. (3) The wellbeing of groups affected by one's actions and leadership. (4) The wellbeing of the environment. A. (1) only	**SLK_26**

	Note: Correct answer	CODE
	B. (1) and (2) C. (1), (2), and (3) D. All of the above	
27.	Caring disposition involves caring for others and society (Radke-Yarrow & Zahn-Waxler, 1986). A. a sense of obligation and support B. a sense of empathy and responsibility C. providing qualified products and good services D. providing excellent leadership and management	SLK_27
28.	Which of the following attributes is one of the three major components of caring disposition covered in the Service Leadership and Management (SLAM) Model? A. Warmth B. Support C. Responsibility D. Empathy	SLK_28
29.	In the Service Leadership and Management (SLAM) Model, "empathy" is an important aspect of caring disposition, and it refers to _______. A. understanding the position and circumstances of others B. making judgments in terms of others' background and occupation C. making an effort to convince others to accept one's viewpoints D. providing generous suggestions to others with mercy	SLK_29
30.	Being a "caring" leader in a positive social relationship, he/she needs to build up ____________ with followers and _______________. A. a secure affective bonding; to actively respond to their needs B. a relaxing working environment; to actively respond to their needs C. a secure affective bonding; to actively encourage them to have fun D. a relaxing working environment; to actively encourage them to have fun	SLK_30
31.	Manufacturing economy has a (an) _________ production process with _________ allowance for deviations. A. standardized; small B. standardized; large C. unstandardized; small D. unstandardized; large	SLK_31
32.	The desirable organizational structure under the service economy should be _________ and _________. A. decentralized; less formalized B. decentralized; formalized C. centralized; less formalized D. centralized; formalized	SLK_32
33.	Leaders in the service economy should primarily possess the following attributes: A. Showing respect toward the followers B. High intelligence C. Good academic achievement D. Good political sensitivity	SLK_33
34.	Leaders in the service economy should possess the following attributes EXCEPT: A. directive B. high in openness C. collaborative D. flexible	SLK_34
35.	According to Chung (2014), in order for Hong Kong to maintain its service-industry edge, we must leverage our competitive edge, which includes the following EXCEPT: A. ability to think critically B. ability to think independently C. trustworthiness D. courage	SLK_35

	Note: Correct answer	CODE
36.	Service Leadership is multidisciplinary in nature as it bridges and encompasses theoretical concepts and research from disciplines, including: (1) Psychology (2) Sociology (3) Anthropology (4) Behavioral Ecology (5) Economics A. (1), (2), and (3) B. (2), (3), and (4) C. (1), (2), (3) and (5) D. All of the above	**SLK_36**
37.	According to the Service Leadership and Management (SLAM) paradigm of leadership, leadership is: A. A means of improving one's own fame. B. A means of improving one's own fortune. C. Service aimed at ethically satisfying the needs of self and others. D. Service aimed to benefit others.	**SLK_37**
38.	According to the Service Leadership and Management (SLAM) Model, which of the following statements is most appropriate? A. Service is delivering one-size-fits-all service to customers. B. Service is delivering personal service to everyone one comes into contact with. C. Service is delivering prompt and timely service. D. Service is serving customers.	**SLK_38**
39.	According to the 25 principles of Service Leadership, which statement is the most appropriate? A. Service Leaders must try to predict and avoid errors that are costly to one's service reputation. B. It is not the duty of service leaders to predict and avoid errors that are costly to one's service reputation. C. Service leaders should hide errors that are costly to their service reputation. D. Service Leaders can easily compensate for the errors that are costly to one's service reputation.	**SLK_39**
40.	The crux (i.e., the most important point at issue) of an excellent service is _______. A. A healthy/mutually sustained relationship between the server and the person being served. B. The ability to promote affordable services. C. The ability to maximize profits in the process. D. The protection of the interest of the service provider.	**SLK_40**

第五部份 Part 5

This part will ask about your personal information. The information you provide will be kept strictly confidential. Please ***choose or fill in your answer*** in the space provided.

	CODE
Gender: 1. Male 2. Female	**Gender**
Date of birth: yyyy/mm/dd //	**DOB**
Age:	**Age**

(continued)

(continued)

	CODE
In which year did you begin your study at PolyU (Undergraduate Program)? 1. 2020 2. 2019 3. 2018 4. 2017 5. 2016 or before	**Entry**
Faculty/School: 1. Faculty of Applied Science and Textiles 2. Faculty of Business 3. Faculty of Construction and Environment 4. Faculty of Engineering 5. Faculty of Health and Social Sciences 6. Faculty of Humanities 7. School of Design 8. School of Hotel and Tourism Management 9. Other, please specify:___________________	**Faculty**
Have you ever taken the CAR subject "Service Leadership" (APSS1A21)? 1. Yes, I have taken the subject before 2. No, I have never taken the subject	**CAR**
Have you ever taken the service-learning subject "Service Leadership through Serving Children and Families with Special Needs" (APSS2S09)? 1. Yes 2. No	**SL_SCF**
Have you ever taken the Silk Road Youth Leadership Program? 1. Yes 2. No	**SRY**
Have you ever taken the following GUR leadership subjects? 1. Tomorrow's Leaders (APSS1L01) 2. Tango! Managing Self and Leading Others (MM1051) 3. Neither	**GUR**
Have you ever taken any other leadership course or workshop besides GUR leadership subjects? 1. Yes 2. No	**GUR_E**
How much do you think you know about Service Leadership (please circle your choice)? 1. I have NO knowledge about Service Leadership 2. I have LITTLE knowledge about Service Leadership 3. I have SOME knowledge about Service Leadership 4. I have A LOT of knowledge about Service Leadership 5. I have ALL the knowledge about Service Leadership	**SLKnow**

(continued)

(continued)

	CODE
Have you ever served in any leadership position in an organization (e.g., student association)? 1. Yes 2. No	**Lpost**
Have you had any work experience? *(You can pick more than one answer.)* 1. No work experience *(single choice only)* 2. Full-time work experience 3. Part-time work experience 4. Internship experience	**Wexp**
Which one of the results below did you use in your current undergraduate application? 1. Hong Kong Diploma of Secondary Education Examination (HKDSEE) (香港中學文憑考試) 2. Hong Kong Advanced Level Examination (HKALE) (香港高級程度會考) 3. National College Entrance Examination (NCEE)—in Mainland China (大陸高考) 4. Associate Degree/ Higher Diploma in Hong Kong (在香港取得的副學士學位/高級文憑) 5. Other, please specify: ___________________	**Result**
Your current GPA: _______________	**GPA**

Appendix 2: Subjective Outcome Evaluation

課程檢討問卷調查

Course Evaluation Form

親愛的同學:

為了幫助我們瞭解APSS1A21/M (Service Leadership) 科目的成效, 現懇請您完成此問卷。問卷內的問題沒有對或錯的答案, 所以請您憑著您的觀感誠實作答。當您完成這份問卷後, 請將問卷直接交給在場的工作人員。您無需在問卷寫下您的名字, 您所提供的一切意見及資料, 均絕對保密。有關講師在日後絕對不會知道個別同學的答案, 所有的資料只會供研究人員作整體分析之用。如有任何疑問, 請詢問在場的工作人員。謝謝您的幫忙!

Dear Students:

In order to better understand the impacts of APSS1A21/M (Service Leadership), we sincerely invite you to complete this questionnaire. The questions in the questionnaire **do not have correct or incorrect answers.** Please **honestly answer them based on your views**. After completing the questionnaire, please give it back to our staff directly. You do not need to provide your name on the questionnaire, and the information you provide will be **kept strictly confidential**. The lecturer(s) concerned will not know the responses of individual students, and the data will be used for overall analyses only. Should you have any questions, please contact the staff conducting this survey. Thank you for your help!

第一部分 **Part 1**

請回想一下您對APSS1A21/M (Service Leadership) 科目內容的觀感, 然後在下表圈出一個您認為最能夠代表您觀感的數字。

Please think about your impression concerning the curriculum contents of APSS1A21/M (Service Leadership), and then ***circle the number*** that best describes your views.

您對**APSS1A21/M (Service Leadership)** 課程內容的觀感: **Your views towards the course contents:**		非常不同意 **Strongly disagree**	不同意 **Disagree**	中立 **Neutral**	同意 **Agree**	非常同意 **Strongly agree**	**CODE**
1.1	科目的目標很清楚。 The objectives of the curriculum are very clear	1	2	3	4	5	**C1**
1.2	科目內容設計得很好。 The curriculum's content design is very good	1	2	3	4	5	**C2**
1.3	教學活動安排得很有條理。 The activities were carefully arranged	1	2	3	4	5	**C3**
1.4	科目進行時的氣氛很好。 The classroom atmosphere was very pleasant	1	2	3	4	5	**C4**
1.5	在課堂中, 同學間有很多交流。 There was much peer interaction among the students	1	2	3	4	5	**C5**

(continued)

(continued)

您對**APSS1A21/M (Service Leadership)** 課程內容的觀感: **Your views towards the course contents:**		非常不同意 **Strongly disagree**	不同意 **Disagree**	中立 **Neutral**	同意 **Agree**	非常同意 **Strongly agree**	**CODE**
1.6	我積極參與科目內的活動 (包括: 討論、分享、遊戲等)。 I participated actively in the class activities (including discussions, sharing, games, etc.)	1	2	3	4	5	**C6**
1.7	在課堂中, 我獲得鼓勵去做到最好。 I was encouraged to do my best	1	2	3	4	5	**C7**
1.8	課堂中的學習經驗, 增加我對這個科目的興趣。 The learning experience enhanced my interest in the course	1	2	3	4	5	**C8**
1.9	整體而言, 我對這個科目有非常正面的評價。 Overall speaking, I have a very positive evaluation of the course	1	2	3	4	5	**C9**
1.10	整體而言, 我很喜歡這個科目。 On the whole, I like this course very much	1	2	3	4	5	**C10**

第二部分 **Part 2**

請回想一下您對APSS1A21/M (Service Leadership) 科目講師的觀感, 然後在下表圈出一個您認為最能夠代表您觀感的數字。

Please think about your impression concerning the lecturer(s) of APSS1A21/M (Service Leadership), and then ***circle the number*** that best describes your views.

您對**APSS1A21/M (Service Leadership)** 講師的觀感: **Your views toward the lecturer(s):**		非常不同意 **Strongly disagree**	不同意 **Disagree**	中立 **Neutral**	同意 **Agree**	非常同意 **Strongly agree**	**CODE**
2.1	講師對這個科目有充分的掌握。 The lecturer(s) had a good mastery of the course	1	2	3	4	5	**L1**
2.2	講師的準備功夫充足。 The lecturer(s) was (were) well prepared for the lessons	1	2	3	4	5	**L2**
2.3	講師的教學技巧良好。 The teaching skills of the lecturer(s) were good	1	2	3	4	5	**L3**
2.4	講師的專業態度很好。 The lecturer(s) showed good professional attitude	1	2	3	4	5	**L4**
2.5	講師表現很投入。 The lecturer(s) was (were) very involved	1	2	3	4	5	**L5**
2.6	講師鼓勵同學參與課堂活動。 The lecturer(s) encouraged students to participate in the activities	1	2	3	4	5	**L6**

(continued)

(continued)

您對**APSS1A21/M (Service Leadership)** 講師的觀感: **Your views toward the lecturer(s):**		非常不同意 **Strongly disagree**	不同意 **Disagree**	中立 **Neutral**	同意 **Agree**	非常同意 **Strongly agree**	**CODE**
2.7	講師關心同學。 The lecturer(s) cared for the students	1	2	3	4	5	**L7**
2.8	同學有需要時, 講師樂意提供協助。 The lecturer(s) was (were) ready to offer help to students when needed	1	2	3	4	5	**L8**
2.9	導師與同學有很多交流。 The lecturer(s) had much interaction with the students	1	2	3	4	5	**L9**
2.10	我對講師的整體表現有非常正面的評價。 Overall speaking, I have a very positive evaluation of the lecturer(s)	1	2	3	4	5	**L10**

第三部分 **Part 3**

請評估APSS1A21/M (Service Leadership) 科目對您的幫助有多大, 然後在下表圈出一個您認為最能夠代表您觀感的數字。

Please evaluate to what extent you have benefited from APSS1A21/M (Service Leadership), and then ***circle the number*** that best describes your views.

APSS1A21/M (Service Leadership) 對您的幫助: The extent to which the course has helped you:		沒有幫助 Unhelpful	幫助不大 Not very helpful	不確定 Not sure	頗有幫助 Helpful	有很大幫助 Very helpful	CODE
3.1	促進我與人相處的能力。 It has enhanced my social competence	1	2	3	4	5	**H1**
3.2	增強我表達及處理情緒的能力。 It has improved my ability to express and handle my emotions	1	2	3	4	5	**H2**
3.3	加強我批判思考的能力。 It has enhanced my critical thinking	1	2	3	4	5	**H3**
3.4	加強我作出明智抉擇的能力。 It has increased my competence in making sensible and wise choices	1	2	3	4	5	**H4**
3.5	幫助我作出合符道德標準的決定。 It has helped me make ethical decisions	1	2	3	4	5	**H5**
3.6	加強我面對逆境的能力。 It has strengthened my resilience in adverse conditions	1	2	3	4	5	**H6**
3.7	加強我的自信。 It has strengthened my self-confidence	1	2	3	4	5	**H7**

(continued)

(continued)

APSS1A21/M (Service Leadership) 對您的幫助: The extent to which the course has helped you:		沒有幫助 **Unhelpful**	幫助不大 **Not very helpful**	不確定 **Not sure**	頗有幫助 **Helpful**	有很大幫助 **Very helpful**	**CODE**
3.8	幫助我更積極面對將來。 It has helped me face the future with a positive attitude	1	2	3	4	5	**H8**
3.9	提升我對生活的熱愛。 It has enhanced my love for life	1	2	3	4	5	**H9**
3.10	幫助我探索人生的意義。 It has helped me explore the meaning of life	1	2	3	4	5	**H10**
3.11	增強我領導自我的能力。 It has enhanced my ability of self-leadership	1	2	3	4	5	**H11**
3.12	培養我對他人的憐憫和愛護。 It has helped me cultivate compassion and care for others	1	2	3	4	5	**H12**
3.13	有助於全面地提升我的品質。 It has helped me enhance my character strengths comprehensively	1	2	3	4	5	**H13**

(continued)

(continued)

APSS1A21/M (Service Leadership) 對您的幫助: The extent to which the course has helped you:		沒有幫助 Unhelpful	幫助不大 Not very helpful	不確定 Not sure	頗有幫助 Helpful	有很大幫助 Very helpful	CODE
3.14	使我明白專業能力、個人品質和關愛他人對於成功領袖的重要性。 It has enabled me to understand the importance of situational task competencies, character strength, and caring disposition in successful leadership	1	2	3	4	5	**H14**
3.15	培養我貢獻社會的責任感。 It has promoted my sense of responsibility to serve society	1	2	3	4	5	**H15**
3.16	促進我的整體成長。 It has promoted my overall development	1	2	3	4	5	**H16**
3.17	課程涵蓋的理論、研究及概念使我明白成功的服務型領袖的基本特質。 The theories, research, and concepts covered in the course have enabled me to understand the characteristics of successful service leaders	1	2	3	4	5	**H17**

(continued)

(continued)

APSS1A21/M (Service Leadership) 對您的幫助: The extent to which the course has helped you:		沒有幫助 **Unhelpful**	幫助不大 **Not very helpful**	不確定 **Not sure**	頗有幫助 **Helpful**	有很大幫助 **Very helpful**	**CODE**
3.18	課程涵蓋的理論、研究及概念幫助我整合成功的服務型領袖的基本特質。 The theories, research, and concepts covered in the course have helped me synthesize the characteristics of successful service leaders	1	2	3	4	5	**H18**
3.19	幫助我理解和尊重其他人的不同觀點 It has helped me understand and respect the different views of others	1	2	3	4	5	**H19**
3.20	加強我與不同背景同學之間的協作 It has enhanced my collaboration with others from different backgrounds	1	2	3	4	5	**H20**
3.21	幫助我與其他人建立良好的關係 It has helped me build positive relationships with others	1	2	3	4	5	**H21**

第四部分 **Part 4**

您會否建議您的朋友報讀這個科目? 請圈出一個您認為最能夠代表您意見的數字。 Will you suggest that your friends take **this course**? Please ***circle the number*** that best describes your views					**CODE**
1	2	3	4	5	
一定不會 Definitely will not suggest	不會 Will not suggest	不確定 Not sure	會 Will suggest	一定會 Definitely will suggest	**Recommend**

第五部分 **Part 5**

您會否再次報讀這類科目? 請圈出一個您認為最能夠代表您意見的數字。 Will you take **similar courses** in future? Please ***circle the number*** that best describes your views					**CODE**
1	2	3	4	5	
一定不會 Definitely will not take	不會 Will not take	不確定 Not sure	會 Will take	一定會 Definitely will take	**Repart**

第六部分 **Part 6**

整體而言, 您對這個科目有怎樣的滿意程度? 請圈出一個您認為最能夠代表您意見的數字。 On the whole, are you satisfied with this course? Please ***circle the number*** that best describes your views					**CODE**
1	2	3	4	5	
十分不滿意 Very dissatisfied	頗不滿意 Moderately dissatisfied	中立 Neutral	滿意 Satisfied	十分滿意 Very satisfied	**Satisfaction**

第七部分 **Part 7**

請完成下列各題:

Please complete the following items:

7.1 請寫出一項或以上您從該科目中學到最重要的東西: (如沒有, 請填「沒有」。) Please write down one or more important thing(s) you have learned in this course. If there is no comment, please write "NIL."	**CODE**
______________________________	**Important**
______________________________	
______________________________	
7.2 請寫出一項或以上您認為在該科目中最值得欣賞的地方: (如沒有, 請填「沒有」。) Please write down one or more thing(s) that you appreciate most in this course. If there is no comment, please write "NIL."	**CODE**

(continued)

(continued)

____	**Appreciative**
____	
____	
7.3 您對該科目的講師有何意見? (如沒有, 請填「沒有」。) Do you have any comments about the lecturer(s)? If there is no comment, please write "NIL."	**CODE**
____	**Comments**
____	
____	
7.4 您認為該科目有哪些地方需要改善? (如沒有, 請填「沒有」。) What aspects of this course should be improved? If there is no comment, please write "NIL."	**CODE**
____	**Improve**
____	
____	

完。謝謝!
End. Thank you!

Appendix 3: Publications

Service Leadership Publication List

A. **Curriculum Development and Theories**

A1. **Journal Articles**

1. Shek, D. T. L., Yu, L., & Fu, X. (2013). Confucian virtues and Chinese adolescent development: A conceptual review. *International Journal of Adolescent Medicine and Health*, *25*(4), 335–344. https://doi.org/10.1515/ijamh-2013-0031
2. Shek, D. T. L., Yu, L., Ma, C. M. S., Sun, R. C. F., & Liu, T. T. (2013). Development of a credit-bearing Service Leadership subject for university students in Hong Kong. *International Journal of Adolescent Medicine and Health*, *25*(4), 353–361. https://doi.org/10.1515/ijamh-2013-0033
3. Shek, D. T. L., Chung, P. P. Y., Yu, L., & Merrick, J. (2015). Editorial: Service Leadership education for university students: The Hong Kong experience. *International Journal on Disability and Human Development, 14*(3), 203–204.

4. Shek, D. T. L., Chung, P. P. Y., & Leung, H. (2015). Manufacturing economy vs. service economy: Implications for Service Leadership. *International Journal on Disability and Human Development, 14*(3), 205–215.
5. Shek, D. T. L., Chung, P. P. Y., & Leung, H. (2015). How unique is the Service Leadership model? A comparison with contemporary leadership approaches. *International Journal on Disability and Human Development, 14*(3), 217–231.
6. Shek, D. T. L., & Lin, L. (2015). Core beliefs in the Service Leadership model proposed by the Hong Kong Institute of Service Leadership and Management. *International Journal on Disability and Human Development, 14*(3), 233–242.
7. Shek, D. T. L., Sun, R. C. F., & Liu, T. T. (2015). Evolution and realms of Service Leadership and leadership models. *International Journal on Disability and Human Development, 14*(3), 243–254.
8. Shek, D. T. L., & Lin, L. (2015). Intrapersonal competencies and Service Leadership. *International Journal on Disability and Human Development, 14*(3), 255–263.
9. Shek, D. T. L., Yu, L., & Siu, A. M. H. (2015). Interpersonal competence and Service Leadership. *International Journal on Disability and Human Development, 14*(3), 265–274.
10. Shek, D. T. L., Ma, C. M. S., & Liu, T. T. (2015). Adolescent developmental assets and Service Leadership. *International Journal on Disability and Human Development, 14*(3), 275–283.
11. Shek, D. T. L., & Lin, L. (2015). Nurturing university students to be social entrepreneurs: Relevance of Service Leadership education. *International Journal on Disability and Human Development, 14*(3), 285–293.
12. Shek, D. T. L., Chung, P. P. Y., Yu, L., & Merrick, J. (2015). Editorial: Service Leadership curriculum and higher education reform in Hong Kong. *International Journal on Disability and Human Development, 14*(4), 297–298.
13. Shek, D. T. L., & Yu, L. (2015). Character strengths and Service Leadership. *International Journal on Disability and Human Development, 14*(4), 299–307.
14. Shek, D. T. L., Sun, R. C. F., & Liu, T. T. (2015). Character strengths in Chinese philosophies: Relevance to Service Leadership. *International Journal on Disability and Human Development, 14*(4), 309–318.
15. Shek, D. T. L., & Li, X. (2015). The role of a caring disposition in Service Leadership. *International Journal on Disability and Human Development, 14*(4), 319–332.
16. Shek, D. T. L., & Lin, L. (2015). Factors leading to the creation, development and maintenance of positive social relationship. *International Journal on Disability and Human Development, 14*(4), 333–342.

17. Shek, D. T. L., Ma, C. M. S., Liu, T. T., & Siu, A. M. H. (2015). The role of self-leadership in Service Leadership. *International Journal on Disability and Human Development, 14*(4), 343–350.
18. Shek, D. T. L., & Lin, L. (2015). Leadership and mentorship: Service leaders as mentors of the followers. *International Journal on Disability and Human Development, 14*(4), 351–359.
19. Shek, D. T. L., & Li, X. (2015). Nurturing students to be caring service leaders. *International Journal on Disability and Human Development, 14*(4), 361–369.
20. Leung, H., Ma, C. M. S., Shek, D. T. L., & Law, M. Y. M. (2016). Nurturing service leaders through service learning for university students. *International Journal of Child and Adolescent Health, 9*(2), 211–221.
21. Shek, D. T. L., Chung, P. P. Y., Lin, L., & Merrick J. (2018). Editorial: Service Leadership education for university students. *International Journal on Disability and Human Development, 17*(1), 03–06.
22. Shek, D. T. L., Siu, A. M. H. & Merrick J. (2014). Editorial: A tale of two innovative leadership subjects in Hong Kong, People's Republic of China. *International Journal on Disability and Human Development, 13*(4), 409–411.
23. Shek, D. T. L., & Ng, E. C. W. (2017). Leadership training for university students in Hong Kong: A critical review. *International Journal of Child and Adolescent Health, 10*(1), 25–40.
24. Shek, D. T. L., Sun, R. C. F., Lin, L., Leung, H., Siu, A. M. H., Ma, C. M. S., …, & Law, Y. M. (2018). Service Leadership education at The Hong Kong Polytechnic University. *International Journal on Disability and Human Development, 17*(1), 79–84.
25. Shek, D. T. L., & Chung, P. P. Y. (2018). The quest for an alternative paradigm of STEM education for young people. *International Journal of Child and Adolescent Health, 11*(3), 259–270.
26. Shek, D. T. L., Zhu, X., Dou, D., & Merrick, J. (2021). The origin and nature of the Service Leadership theory. *International Journal of Child Health and Human Development, 14*(4), 363–365.
27. Shek, D. T. L. & Yang, Z. (2021). Origin, development, and assertions of Service Leadership theory. *International Journal of Child Health and Human Development, 14*(4), 369–380.
28. Zhu, X., Shek, D. T. L., & Ng, D. C. (2021). Humanistic leadership in service economy. *International Journal of Child Health and Human Development, 14*(4), 381–391.
29. Dou, D., Shek, D. T. L., & Zhu, Z. (2021). Moral character in the Service Leadership theory. *International Journal of Child Health and Human Development, 14*(4), 393–404.
30. Dou, D., & Shek, D. T. L. (2021). The dark side of leadership in the Service Leadership theory. *International Journal of Child Health and Human Development, 14*(4), 405–413.

31. Zhu, X., Shek, D. T. L., & Zhu, Z. (2021). Caring leadership in service economy. *International Journal of Child Health and Human Development, 14*(4), 415–424.
32. Shek, D. T. L., & Yang, Z. (2021). The Fung Service Leadership initiative in Hong Kong. *International Journal of Child Health and Human Development, 14*(4), 449–461.
33. Chai, W., & Dou, D., & Shek, D. T. L. (2021) The role of trust in the service economy. *International Journal of Child Health and Human Development, 14*(4), 425–435.
34. Chai, W., Shek, D. T. L., & Dou, D. (2021). Self-leadership in the Service Leadership theory. *International Journal of Child Health and Human Development, 14*(4), 437–447
35. Shek, D. T. L., & Wilkinson, A. D. (2022). Leadership and resilience: where should we go next? *Journal of Leader*ship Studies, 16(2), 50–55. https://doi.org/10.1002/jls.21817

A2. **Book Chapters**

1. Shek, D. T. L., & Chung, P. P. Y. (2015). Service Leadership education for university students: Seven unfinished tasks. In D. T. L. Shek & P. P. Y. Chung (Eds.), *Promoting Service Leadership qualities in university students: The case of Hong Kong. Quality of life in Asia, vol. 6* (pp. 225–232). Singapore: Springer.
2. Shek, D. T. L., & Leung, H. (2015). Service Leadership qualities in university students through the lens of student well-being. In D. T. L. Shek & P. P. Y. Chung (Eds.), *Promoting Service Leadership qualities in university students: The case of Hong Kong. Quality of life in Asia, vol. 6* (pp. 1–16). Singapore: Springer.
3. Leung, H., Ma, C. M. S., Shek, D. T. L., & Law, M. Y. M. (2015). Nurturing service leaders [Reprint]. In D. T. L. Shek, F. K. Y. Wu, & J. Merrick (Eds.), *Leadership and service learning education: Holistic development for Chinese university students* (pp. 55–74). New York: Nova Sciences Publisher.
4. Leung, H., Shek, D. T. L., & Xie, Q. (2015). Service Leadership education evaluation by university students in Hong Kong [Reprint]. In D. T. L. Shek, F. K. Y. Wu, & J. Merrick (Eds.), *Leadership and service learning education: Holistic development for Chinese university students* (pp. 95–110). New York: Nova Sciences Publisher.
5. Leung, J. T. Y., & Shek, D. T. L. (2015). To serve and to learn [Reprint]. In D. T. L. Shek, F. K. Y. Wu, & J. Merrick (Eds.), *Leadership and service learning education: Holistic development for Chinese university students* (pp. 23–40). New York: Nova Sciences Publisher.
6. Shek, D. T. L., & Liang, J. (2015). How can we know a program is effective? [Reprint]. In D. T. L. Shek, F. K. Y. Wu, & J. Merrick (Eds.), *Leadership and service learning education: Holistic development for*

Chinese university students (pp. 125–140). New York: Nova Sciences Publisher.

7. Shek, D. T. L., Chung, P. P. Y., & Leung, H. (2016). Implications of the shift from manufacturing economy to service economy [Reprint]. In D. T. L. Shek, C. M. S. Ma, L. Lin & J. Merrick (Eds.), *Education in Hong Kong: Service Leadership for university students* (pp. 9–25). New York: Nova Science Publishers.
8. Shek, D. T. L., Chung, P. P. Y., & Leung, H. (2016). The Service Leadership model [Reprint]. In D. T. L. Shek, C. M. S. Ma, L. Lin & J. Merrick (Eds.), *Education in Hong Kong: Service Leadership for university students* (pp. 27–48). New York: Nova Science Publishers.
9. Shek, D. T. L., Chung, P. P. Y., Yu, L., & Merrick, J. (2016). Leadership and management education for university students [Reprint]. In D. T. L. Shek, C. M. S. Ma, L. Lin & J. Merrick (Eds.), *Education in Hong Kong: Service Leadership for university students* (pp. 3–6). New York: Nova Science Publishers.
10. Shek, D. T. L., & Lin, L. (2016). Core beliefs and the Service Leadership model [Reprint]. In D. T. L. Shek, C. M. S. Ma, L. Lin & J. Merrick (Eds.), *Education in Hong Kong: Service Leadership for university students* (pp. 49–62). New York: Nova Science Publishers.
11. Shek, D. T. L., & Lin, L. (2016). Different forms of intrapersonal competence [Reprint]. In D. T. L. Shek, C. M. S. Ma, L. Lin & J. Merrick (Eds.), *Education in Hong Kong: Service Leadership for university students* (pp. 81–93). New York: Nova Science Publishers.
12. Shek, D. T. L., & Lin, L. (2016). University students as social entrepreneurs [Reprint]. In D. T. L. Shek, C. M. S. Ma, L. Lin & J. Merrick (Eds.), *Education in Hong Kong: Service Leadership for university students* (pp. 121–133). New York: Nova Science Publishers.
13. Shek, D. T. L., Ma, C. M. S., & Liu, T. T. (2016). Human development assets and leadership [Reprint]. In D. T. L. Shek, C. M. S. Ma, L. Lin & J. Merrick (Eds.), *Education in Hong Kong: Service Leadership for university students* (pp. 109–120). New York: Nova Science Publishers.
14. Shek, D. T. L., Sun, R. C. F., & Liu, T. T. (2016). History and evolutionary origin of leadership [Reprint]. In D. T. L. Shek, C. M. S. Ma, L. Lin & J. Merrick (Eds.), *Education in Hong Kong: Service Leadership for university students* (pp. 63–79). New York: Nova Science Publishers.
15. Shek, D. T. L., Yu, L., & Siu, A. M. H. (2016). Promotion of interpersonal competence [Reprint]. In D. T. L. Shek, C. M. S. Ma, L. Lin & J. Merrick (Eds.), *Education in Hong Kong: Service Leadership for university students* (pp. 95–108). New York: Nova Science Publishers.

16. Shek, D. T. L., Yuen-Tsang, A. W. K., & Ng, E. C. W. (2016). Global Youth Leadership Institute [Reprint]. In D. T. L. Shek, C. M. S. Ma, L. Lin & J. Merrick (Eds.), *Education in Hong Kong: Service Leadership for university students* (pp. 147–155). New York: Nova Science Publishers.
17. Shek, D. T. L., Chung, P. P. Y., Yu, L. & Merrick, J. (2016). Higher education reform and development of leaders in Hong Kong [Reprint]. In D. T. L. Shek, A. M. H. Siu, H. Leung, & J. Merrick (Eds.), *Higher education in Hong Kong: Nurturing students to be caring service leaders* (pp. 3–6). New York: Nova Sciences Publisher.
18. Shek, D. T. L., Ma, C. M. S., Liu, T. T., & Siu A. M. H. (2016). The nature of self-leadership [Reprint]. In D. T. L. Shek, A. M. H. Siu, H. Leung, & J. Merrick (Eds.), *Higher education in Hong Kong: Nurturing students to be caring service leaders* (pp. 71–82). New York: Nova Sciences Publisher.
19. Shek, D. T. L., & Li, X. (2016). Caring disposition: Awareness, love and nurturing [Reprint]. In D. T. L. Shek, A. M. H. Siu, H. Leung, & J. Merrick (Eds.), *Higher education in Hong Kong: Nurturing students to be caring service leaders* (pp. 37–54). New York: Nova Sciences Publisher.
20. Shek, D. T. L., & Li, X. (2016). Nurturing Students [Reprint]. In D. T. L. Shek, A. M. H. Siu, H. Leung, & J. Merrick (Eds.), *Higher education in Hong Kong: Nurturing students to be caring service leaders* (pp. 97–110). New York: Nova Sciences Publisher.
21. Shek, D. T. L., & Lin, L. (2016). Creation, development and maintenance of social relationship [Reprint]. In D. T. L. Shek, A. M. H. Siu, H. Leung, & J. Merrick (Eds.), *Higher education in Hong Kong: Nurturing students to be caring service leaders* (pp. 55–70). New York: Nova Sciences Publisher.
22. Shek, D. T. L., & Lin, L. (2016). Mentorship [Reprint]. In D. T. L. Shek, A. M. H. Siu, H. Leung, & J. Merrick (Eds.), *Higher education in Hong Kong: Nurturing students to be caring service leaders* (pp. 83–96). New York: Nova Sciences Publisher.
23. Shek, D. T. L., Sun, R. C. F., & Liu, T. T. (2016). Chinese philosophy and character strength [Reprint]. In D. T. L. Shek, A. M. H. Siu, H. Leung, & J. Merrick (Eds.), *Higher education in Hong Kong: Nurturing students to be caring service leaders* (pp. 23–36). New York: Nova Sciences Publisher.
24. Shek, D. T. L., & Yu, L. (2016). How to foster character strengths? [Reprint]. In D. T. L. Shek, A. M. H. Siu, H. Leung, & J. Merrick (Eds.), *Higher education in Hong Kong: Nurturing students to be caring service leaders* (pp. 9–22). New York: Nova Sciences Publisher.

25. Shek, D. T. L., Chung, P. P. Y., Lin, L., & Merrick J. (2017). Service Leadership education for university students [Reprint]. In D. T. L. Shek, P. P. Y. Chung, L. Lin, & J. Merrick (Eds.), *Service Leadership Education for University Students* (pp. 3–8). New York: Nova Sciences Publisher.
26. Shek, D. T. L., Sun, R. C. F., Lin, L., Leung, H., Siu, A. M. H., Ma, C. M. S., …, & Law, M. Y. M. (2017). Service Leadership education at The Hong Kong Polytechnic University [Reprint]. In D. T. L. Shek, P. P. Y. Chung, L. Lin, & J. Merrick (Eds.), *Service Leadership Education for University Students* (pp. 83–92). New York: Nova Sciences Publisher.
27. Shek, D. T. L., Chung, P. P. Y., Lin, L. Leung, H., & Ng, E. (2018). Service Leadership under the service economy. In J. L. Chin, J. E. Trimble, & J. E. Garcia (Eds.)., *Global and culturally diverse leaders and leadership: New dimensions and challenges for business, education and society* (pp. 143–161). Wagon Lane, Bingley: Emerald Publication.
28. Shek, D. T. L., Chung, P. P. Y., & Dou, D. (2019). The dark side of service leaders. In M. F. Brandebo, & A. Alvinius (Eds.), *Dark sides of organizational behavior and leadership* (pp. 125–146). London, UK: IntechOpen. https://doi.org/10.5772/intechopen.75086
29. Shek, D. T. L., & Chung, P. P. Y. (2018). The quest for an alternative paradigm of STEM education for young people [Reprint]. In J. Merrick (Ed.), *Childhood and adolescence.* (pp. 11–32). New York, NY: Nova Science Publishers.
30. Shek, D. T. L., Chung, P. P. Y. & Zhu, X. (2018). Service Leadership in the service era. In D. C. Poff, & A. C. Michalos (Eds.), *Encyclopedia of Business and Professional Ethics* (pp. 01–07). Cham: Springer.
31. Shek, D. T. L., Wu, J., Lin, L., & Pu, E. X. P. (2018). Qualitative evaluation of a Service Leadership subject in a Chinese context [Reprint]. In D. T. L. Shek, J. T. Y. Leung, & J. Merrick (Eds.), *Soft skills and aspirations in Chinese children and youth* (pp. 223–242). New York, NY: Nova Science Publishers.
32. Shek, D. T. L., Cheng, M. N. S., & Ma, C. M. S. (2019). Nurturing Service Leadership qualities in university students through corporate-community university partnership. In D. T. L. Shek, G. Ngai, & S. C. F. Chan (Eds.), *Service-learning for youth leadership: The case of Hong Kong* (pp. 113–132). Singapore: Springer
33. Shek, D. T. L., & Ho, W. W. L. (2019). Serving clients in a drug rehabilitation agency as a vehicle to promote Service Leadership in university students. In D. T. L. Shek, G. Ngai, & S. C. F. Chan (Eds.), *Service-learning for youth leadership: The case of Hong Kong* (pp. 65–82). Singapore: Springer.

34. Ma, C. M. S., Shek, D. T. L., & Li, P. P. K. (2019). Service Leadership through serving socially deprived student: Experience gained from corporate-community partnership (Project WeCan). In D. T. L. Shek, G. Ngai, & S. C. F. Chan (Eds.), *Service-learning for youth leadership: The case of Hong Kong* (pp. 83–112). Singapore: Springer.
35. Shek, D. T. L., Zhu, X., Dou, D., Law, M. Y. M., Yu, L., Ma, C. M. S., & Lin, L. (2019). Nurturing holistic development in university students through leadership courses: The Hong Kong experience. In G. H. Tonon (Ed.), *Teaching quality of life in different fields* (pp. 61–80). Singapore: Springer.
36. Shek, D. T. L., Zhu, X., & Merrick, J. (2021). The origin and nature of the Service Leadership theory [Reprint]. In D. T. L. Shek, X. Zhu, D. Dou, & J. Merrick (Eds.), *Service Leadership theory: Origin and nature* (pp. 3–8). New York, NY: Nova Science Publishers.
37. Shek, D. T. L., & Yang, Z. (2021). Origin, development and assertions of Service Leadership theory [Reprint]. In D. T. L. Shek, X. Zhu, D. Dou, & J. Merrick (Eds.), *Service Leadership theory: Origin and nature.* (pp. 11–34). New York, NY: Nova Science Publishers.
38. Zhu, X., Shek, D. T. L., & Yang, Z. (2021). Humanistic leadership in service economy [Reprint]. In D. T. L. Shek, X. Zhu, D. Dou, & J. Merrick (Eds.), *Service Leadership theory: Origin and nature.* (pp. 35–56). New York, NY: Nova Science Publishers.
39. Dou, D., Shek, D. T. L., & Zhu, Z. (2021). Moral character in the Service Leadership theory [Reprint]. In D. T. L. Shek, X. Zhu, D. Dou, & J. Merrick (Eds.), *Service Leadership theory: Origin and nature* (pp. 57–80). New York, NY: Nova Science Publishers.
40. Dou, D., & Shek, D. T. L. (2021). The dark side of leadership in the Service Leadership theory [Reprint]. In D. T. L. Shek, X. Zhu, D. Dou, & J. Merrick (Eds.), *Service Leadership theory: Origin and nature* (pp. 81–98). New York, NY: Nova Science Publishers.
41. Zhu, X., Shek, D. T. L., & Zhu, Z. (2021). Caring leadership in service economy [Reprint]. In D. T. L. Shek, X. Zhu, D. Dou, & J. Merrick (Eds.), *Service Leadership theory: Origin and nature* (pp. 99–118). New York, NY: Nova Science Publishers.
42. Chai, W., & Shek, D. T. L. (2021). The role of trust in the service economy [Reprint]. In D. T. L. Shek, X. Zhu, D. Dou, & J. Merrick (Eds.), *Service Leadership theory: Origin and nature* (pp. 119–140). New York, NY: Nova Science Publishers.
43. Chai, W., Shek, D. T. L., & Dou, D. (2021). Self-leadership in the Service Leadership theory [Reprint]. In D. T. L. Shek, X. Zhu, D. Dou, & J. Merrick (Eds.), *Service Leadership theory: Origin and nature* (pp. 141–162). New York, NY: Nova Science Publishers.

44. Shek, D. T. L., & Yang, Z. (2021). The Fung Service Leadership Initiative in Hong Kong [Reprint]. In D. T. L. Shek, X. Zhu, D. Dou, & J. Merrick (Eds.), *Service Leadership theory: Origin and nature* (pp. 163–187). New York, NY: Nova Science Publishers.
45. Shek, D.T.L., Chung, P., Zhu, X. (2022). Service Leadership as the Backbone of University Social Responsibility. In: Poff, D.C. (Ed.) University Corporate Social Responsibility and University Governance (pp. 105–188). Advances in Business Ethics Research, vol 8. Springer, Cham.

A3. **Conference Presentations**

1. Ma, C. M. S., Shek, D. T. L., & Liu, T. T. (2012, December 2–5). *Caring dispositions and positive youth development: Relevance to Service Leadership in university students.* Paper presented at the Third International Congress on Paediatric Chronic Diseases, Disability and Human Development, Jerusalem, Israel organized by Cincinnati Children's Hospital Medical Centre, Hadassah-Hebrew University Medical Centre, and National Institute of Child Health and Human Development, Israel.
2. Shek, D. T. L., Sun, R. C. F., Yu, L., Ma, C. M. S., & Siu, A. M. H. (2012, December 2–5). *Promotion of holistic development of university students in Hong Kong: Development of a Service Leadership course.* Paper presented at the Third International Congress on Paediatric Chronic Diseases, Disability and Human Development, Jerusalem, Israel organized by Cincinnati Children's Hospital Medical Centre, Hadassah-Hebrew University Medical Centre, and National Institute of Child Health and Human Development, Israel.
3. Yu, L., & Shek, D. T. L. (2012, December 2–5). *Confucian virtues and positive youth development: Insights for Service Leadership.* Paper presented at the Third International Congress on Paediatric Chronic Diseases, Disability and Human Development, Jerusalem, Israel organized by Cincinnati Children's Hospital Medical Centre, Hadassah-Hebrew University Medical Centre, and National Institute of Child Health and Human Development, Israel.
4. Law, M. Y. M., & Shek, D. T. L. (2013, March 22). *Development of a non-credit-bearing Service Leadership program for university students in Hong Kong: Some initial experience.* Paper presented at the Service Leadership Roundtable, The Hong Kong Polytechnic University, Hong Kong.
5. Leung, H., & Shek, D. T. L. (2013, March 22). *The development of Service Leadership models and its implications for university education in Hong Kong.* Paper presented at the Service Leadership Roundtable, The Hong Kong Polytechnic University, Hong Kong.
6. Lin, L., & Shek, D. T. L. (2013, March 22). *A good service leader, a good mentor.* Paper presented at the Service Leadership Roundtable, The Hong Kong Polytechnic University, Hong Kong.

7. Liu, T. T., & Shek, D. T. L. (2013, March 22). *Developmental assets of service leaders.* Paper presented at the Service Leadership Roundtable, The Hong Kong Polytechnic University, Hong Kong.
8. Ma, C. M. S., & Shek, D. T. L. (2013, March 22). *Caring disposition and Service Leadership among Hong Kong university students.* Paper presented at the Service Leadership Roundtable, The Hong Kong Polytechnic University, Hong Kong.
9. Shek, D. T. L., Sun, R. C. F., & Siu, A. M. H. (2013, March 22). *Helping university students to thrive: The Service Leadership initiative at The Hong Kong Polytechnic University.* Keynote speech presented at the Service Leadership Roundtable, The Hong Kong Polytechnic University, Hong Kong.
10. Yu, L., & Shek, D. T. L. (2013, March 22). *Character strengths in Chinese culture: Confucian virtues and Service Leadership.* Paper presented at the Service Leadership Roundtable, The Hong Kong Polytechnic University, Hong Kong.
11. Shek, D. T. L., Sun, R. C. F., Yu, L., Ma, C. M. S., Siu, A. M. H., Lin, L., Leung, H., & Law, M. Y. M. (2014, May 14–15). *Service Leadership education and research at The Hong Kong Polytechnic University: An overview.* Paper presented at the International Conference on Service Leadership Education for University Students: Experience in Hong Kong, Hong Kong.
12. Shek, D. T. L., Sun, R. C. F., Lin, L., Leung, H., Yu, L., Ma, C. M. S., Siu, A. M. H., & Law, M. Y. M. (2016, January 6–7). *Service Leadership Education at The Hong Kong Polytechnic University.* Paper presented at the International Conference on Service Leadership Education in Service Economies, Hong Kong.
13. Shek, D. T. L., Lin, L., Leung, H., Yu, L., Ma, C. S. M., Ma, L., & Zhu, X. (2018, June). *Development of measures of Service Leadership knowledge, attitude and behavior.* Paper presented at the 16th International Society for Quality-of-Life Studies Annual Conference—"Promotion of Quality of Life in the Changing World", The Hong Kong Polytechnic University, Hong Kong.
14. Leung, H., & Shek, D. T. L. (2018, June). *Promotion of well-being through the nurturance of Service Leadership qualities.* Paper presented at the 16th International Society for Quality-of-Life Studies Annual Conference—"Promotion of Quality of Life in the Changing World", The Hong Kong Polytechnic University, Hong Kong.
15. Zhu, X. & Shek, D. T. L. (2019, September). *Blended learning pedagogy for a Service Leadership subject in Hong Kong: Experience and challenges.* Paper presented at the 17th International Society for Quality-of-Life Studies Annual Conference, Granada, Spain.

16. Dou, D. & Shek, D. T. L. (2019, September). *Relationship between Service Leadership qualities and positive youth development in university students in Hong Kong.* Paper presented at the 17th International Society for Quality-of-Life Studies Annual Conference, Granada, Spain.
17. Chai, W. Y., Leung, H., & Shek, D. T. L. (2019, September). *Leadership qualities and life satisfaction among university students in Hong Kong.* Paper presented at the 17th International Society for Quality-of-Life Studies Annual Conference, Granada, Spain.

A4. **Other Articles**

1. 石丹理、鍾普洋、林立、黎翔. (2014). 如何培育香港大學生的領袖素質? 紫荊論壇, 5–6月號第15期, 86–94.
2. 石丹理. (2014). 香港如何培育人才? 紫荊論壇, 11–12月號第18期, 27–35.

B. **Evaluation (credit-bearing subjects)**

B1. **Journal Articles**

1. Shek, D. T. L., Yu, L., & Ma, C. M. S. (2014). The students were happy, but did they change positively? *International Journal on Disability and Human Development, 13*(4), 505–511.
2. Shek, D. T. L., Lin, L., & Liu, T. T. (2014). Service Leadership education for university students in Hong Kong: Subjective outcome evaluation. *International Journal on Disability and Human Development, 13*(4), 513–521.
3. Shek, D. T. L., Lin, L., Liu, T. T., & Law, M. Y. M. (2014). Service Leadership education for university students in Hong Kong: Qualitative evaluation. *International Journal on Disability and Human Development. 13*(4), 523–529.
4. Shek, D. T. L., Lin, L., Liu, T. T., & Law, M. Y. M. (2014). Process evaluation of a pilot subject on Service Leadership for university students in Hong Kong. *International Journal on Disability and Human Development. 13*(4), 531–540.
5. Shek, D. T. L., Law, M. Y. M., & Liu, T. T. (2015). Focus group evaluation of a Service Leadership subject in Hong Kong. *International Journal on Disability and Human Development, 14*(4), 371–376.
6. Shek, D. T. L., & Liang, J. (2015). Subjective outcome evaluation of a university subject on Service Leadership. *International Journal on Disability and Human Development, 14*(4), 385–392.
7. Shek, D.T.L., Liang, J., & Law, M.Y.M. (2016). Process evaluation of a university subject on Service Leadership in Hong Kong. *International Journal of Child and Adolescent Health, 9*(2), 253–261.
8. Shek, D.T.L., Liang, J., & Zhu, X. (2016). Subjective outcome evaluation of a Service Leadership subject for university students in Hong Kong. *International Journal of Child Health and Human Development, 9*(2), 225–232.

9. Shek, D. T. L., Lin. L., & Xie, Q. (2016). Service Leadership education for university students in Hong Kong: A qualitative evaluation study. *International Journal of Child and Adolescent Health, 9*(2), 235–243.
10. Shek, D. T. L., Chi, X., & Lin, L. (2017). Subjective outcome evaluation of a Service Leadership subject for university students in Hong Kong. *International Journal of Child and Adolescent Health, 10*(2), 213–221.
11. Shek, D. T. L., Lin, L, & Leung, H. (2018). Objective outcome evaluation of Service Leadership education for university students in Hong Kong. *International Journal on Disability and Human Development, 17*(1), 119–124.
12. Shek, D. T. L., Wu, J., Lin, L, & Pu, E. X. P. (2017). Qualitative evaluation of a Service Leadership subject in a Chinese context. *International Journal on Disability and Human Development, 16*(4), 433–441. https://doi.org/10.1515/ijdhd-2017-7012
13. Ma, C. M. S., Shek, D. T. L., Li, P., & Shek, V. (2018). Promotion of Service Leadership: An evaluation of a service learning subject in Hong Kong. *Journal of Service-Learning in Higher Education, 8*, 1–12.
14. Lin, L., & Shek, D.T.L. (2019). Does Service Leadership education contribute to student well-being? A quasi-experimental study based on Hong Kong university students. *Applied Research in Quality of Life, 14*(5), 1147–1163. https://doi.org/10.1007/s11482-018-9644-x
15. Zhu, X. & Shek, D. T. L. (2021). Promoting Service Leadership qualities and well-being among university students: Evaluation findings in Hong Kong. *Applied Research in Quality of Life,16*(6), 2475–2495. https://doi.org/10.1007/s11482-021-09922-w
16. Leung, H., Shek, D. T. L., & Dou, D. (2021). Evaluation of service-learning in Project WeCan under COVID-19 in a Chinese context. *International Journal of Environmental Research and Public Health, 18(7),* 3596. https://doi.org/10.3390/ijerph18073596
17. Zhu, X., Shek, D. T., & Chan, C. H. (2021). Promoting Service Leadership qualities and well-being among university students through an online course during COVID-19 pandemic. *International Journal of Environmental Research and Public Health, 18*(15), 8162. https://doi.org/10.3390/ijerph18158162
18. Shek D. T. L., Zhu, X., Dou, D., & Tan, L. (2023). Self-leadership as an attribute of Service Leadership: Its relationship to well-being among university students in Hong Kong. *Frontiers in Psychology, 14*, Article 1088154. https://doi.org/10.3389/fpsyg.2023.1088154

B2. **Book Chapters**

1. Shek, D. T. L., Yu, L., & Ma, C. M. S. (2015). The students were happy, but did they change positively? [Reprint]. In D. T. L. Shek, A. M. H. Siu, & J. Merrick. (Eds.), *Tomorrow's leaders: Service Leadership*

and holistic development in Chinese university students (pp. 157–168). New York: Nova Sciences Publisher.

2. Shek, D. T. L., Lin L., & Liu, T. T. (2015). Service Leadership education for university students in Hong Kong: Subjective outcome evaluation [Reprint]. In D. T. L. Shek, A. M. H. Siu, & J. Merrick. (Eds.), *Tomorrow's leaders: Service Leadership and holistic development in Chinese university students* (pp. 169–180). New York: Nova Sciences Publisher.
3. Shek, D. T. L., Lin L., Liu, T. T., & Law, M. Y. M. (2015). Service Leadership education for university students in Hong Kong: Qualitative evaluation [Reprint]. In D. T. L. Shek, A. M. H. Siu, & J. Merrick. (Eds.), *Tomorrow's leaders: Service Leadership and holistic development in Chinese university students* (pp. 181–192). New York: Nova Sciences Publisher.
4. Shek, D. T. L., Lin L., Liu, T. T., & Law, M. Y. M. (2015). Process evaluation of a pilot subject on Service Leadership for university students in Hong Kong [Reprint]. In D. T. L. Shek, A. M. H. Siu, & J. Merrick. (Eds.), *Tomorrow's leaders: Service Leadership and holistic development in Chinese university students*, (pp. 193–204). New York: Nova Sciences Publisher.
5. Shek, D. T. L., & Lin, L. (2015). Evaluating Service Leadership programs with multiple strategies. In D. T. L. Shek & P. P. Y. Chung (Eds.), *Promoting Service Leadership qualities in university students: The case of Hong Kong. Quality of life in Asia, vol. 6* (pp. 197–211). Singapore: Springer.
6. Shek, D. T. L., Chi, X., & Lin, L. (2016). Student Service Leadership program: Subjective outcome evaluation [Reprint]. In D. T. L. Shek, F. K. Y. Wu, J. T. Y. Leung, & J. Merrick (Eds.), *Adolescence: Positive youth development programs in Chinese communities* (pp. 125–136). New York: Nova Sciences Publisher.
7. Shek, D. T. L., Law, M. Y. M., & Liu, T. T. (2016). Focus group evaluation of Service Leadership [Reprint]. In D. T. L. Shek, A. M. H. Siu, H. Leung, & J. Merrick (Eds.), *Higher education in Hong Kong: Nurturing students to be caring service leaders* (pp. 111–122). New York: Nova Sciences Publisher.
8. Shek, D. T. L., & Liang, L. (2016). Student evaluation of a university subject on Service Leadership [Reprint]. In D. T. L. Shek, A. M. H. Siu, H. Leung, & J. Merrick (Eds.), *Higher education in Hong Kong: Nurturing students to be caring service leaders* (pp. 137–150). New York: Nova Sciences Publisher.
9. Shek, D. T. L., Lin, L., & Leung, H. (2017). The evaluation of Service Leadership education for university students in Hong Kong [Reprint]. In D. T. L. Shek, P. P. Y. Chung, L. Lin, & J. Merrick (Eds.), *Service Leadership Education for University Students* (pp. 151–162). New York: Nova Sciences Publisher.

10. Shek, D. T. L., Lin, L., & Xie, Q. (2017). Service Leadership education for university students in Hong Kong: A qualitative evaluation study [Reprint]. In J. Merrick (Ed.), *Child and adolescent health yearbook 2016* (pp. 119–129). New York, NY: Nova Science Publishers.
11. Shek, D. T. L., Liang, J., & Law, M. Y. M. (2017). Process evaluation of a university subject on Service Leadership in Hong Kong [Reprint]. In J. Merrick (Ed.), *Child and adolescent health yearbook 2016* (pp. 141–151). New York, NY: Nova Science Publishers.
12. Shek, D. T. L., Liang, J., & Zhu, X. (2017). Subjective outcome evaluation of a Service Leadership subject for university students in Hong Kong [Reprint]. In J. Merrick (Ed.), *Child health and human development yearbook 2016* (pp. 273–282). New York, NY: Nova Science Publishers.
13. Shek, D. T. L., Chi, X., & Lin, L. (2018). Subjective outcome evaluation of a Service Leadership subject for university students in Hong Kong [Reprint]. In J. Merrick (Ed.), *Child and adolescent health yearbook 2017* (pp. 247–257). New York, NY: Nova Science Publishers.

B3. **B3. Conference Presentations**

1. Shek, D. T. L., Lin, L., Leung, H., Law, M. Y. M., & Li, X. (2014, May 14–15). *Evaluation of Service Leadership programs using multiple evaluation methods.* Paper presented at the International Conference on Service Leadership Education for University Students: Experience in Hong Kong, Hong Kong.
2. Shek, D. T. L., Lin, L., & Leung, H. (2016, January 6–7). *Objective outcome evaluation of Service Leadership education at The Hong Kong Polytechnic University.* Paper presented at the International Conference on Service Leadership Education in Service Economies, Hong Kong.
3. Lin, L., & Shek, D. T. L. (2017, September 28–30). *Effects of a leadership course on the psychological well-being of university students.* Paper presented at the 15th International Society for Quality-of-Life Studies Annual Conference—"Quality of Life: Towards a Better Society", Innsbruck, Austria.
4. Wu, J., & Shek, D. T. L. (2018, June). *Qualitative evaluation of a university subject on Service Leadership education: Views of the students.* Paper presented at the 16th International Society for Quality-of-Life Studies Annual Conference—"Promotion of Quality of Life in the Changing World", The Hong Kong Polytechnic University, Hong Kong.
5. Ma, L., & Shek, D. T. L. (2018, June). *Promoting well-being in future leaders? Objective outcome evaluation of Service Leadership education for university students.* Paper presented at the 16th International Society for Quality-of-Life Studies Annual Conference—"Promotion of Quality of Life in the Changing World", The Hong Kong Polytechnic University, Hong Kong.

6. Leung, J. T. Y., Shek, D. T. L., & Zhao, P. X. (2019, September). *Subjective outcome evaluation of a Service Leadership subject: Findings based on university students in Hong Kong.* Paper presented at the 17th International Society for Quality-of-Life Studies Annual Conference, Granada, Spain.
7. Dou, D., & Shek, D. T. L. (2023, August). *Subjective outcome evaluation of a leadership education program for university students under the pandemic.* Paper presented at the 21st International Society for Quality-of-Life Studies Annual Conference, Rotterdam, Netherlands

C. **Evaluation (non-credit-bearing programs)**

C1. **Journal Articles**

1. Shek, D. T. L., & Li, X. (2015). Evaluation of an innovative leadership training program for Chinese students: Subjective outcome evaluation. *International Journal on Disability and Human Development, 14*(4), 393–400.
2. Shek, D. T. L., & Lin, L. (2016). Service Leadership education in the global youth leadership programme: A qualitative evaluation. *International Journal of Child and Adolescent Health, 9*(2), 245–252.
3. Shek, D. T. L., & Lin, L. (2016). Changes in university students after joining a Service Leadership program in China. *Journal of Leadership Education, 15*(1), 96–109.
4. Shek, D. T. L., Lin, L., Leung, H. & Zhu, X. (2017). The impact of an intensive Service Leadership course in Mainland China: Objective outcome evaluation. *International Journal of Child and Adolescent Health, 10*(1), 63–71.
5. Shek, D. T. L., Zhu, X., & Lin, L. (2017). Evaluation of an intensive Service Leadership course in mainland China. *International Journal of Child and Adolescent Health, 10*(2), 223–231.
6. Leung, H., Shek, D. T. L., Lin, L. (2018). Promotion of Service Leadership qualities in Chinese university students: Objective outcome evaluation based on six waves of data. *The International Journal of Child and Adolescent Health, 11*(1), 37–46.
7. Leung, J. T. Y., & Shek, D. T. L. (2019). Subjective outcome evaluation of a Service Leadership subject: Findings based on university students in Hong Kong. *International Journal of Child Health and Human Development, 12*(3), 247–257.
8. Shek, D. T. L., Zhu, X., & Merrick, J. (2020). Service Leadership education in an era of service economy. *International Journal of Child and Adolescent Health, 13*(2), 107–109
9. Chai, W. Y., Shek, D. T. L., Lee, B., & Xie, M. (2020). Impact of Service Leadership education on University students in Hong Kong. *International Journal of Child and Adolescent Health, 13* (2), 113–123.

10. Zhu, X., Shek, D. T. L., Zhu, Z. L., & Zhao, P. X. (2020). Promotion of well-being and leadership qualities among university students after taking a credit-bearing Service Leadership subject. *International Journal of Child and Adolescent Health, 13* (2), 125–135.
11. Law, M. Y. W., Shek, D. T. L., & Zhang, J. X. (2020). Evaluation of an intensive Service Leadership program using the subjective outcome evaluation approach. *International Journal of Child and Adolescent Health, 13* (2), 137–152.
12. Shek, D. T. L., Kwok, R. K. H., & Low, S. S. (2020). Promotion of Service Leadership in university students: Views of university students. *International Journal of Child and Adolescent Health, 13* (2), 153–166.
13. Law, M. Y. M., Shek, D. T. L., & Kwok, R. K. H. (2020). Impact of a leadership program on the holistic development of university students in Hong Kong. *International Journal of Child and Adolescent Health, 13* (2), 167–180.
14. Zi, Y., Shek, D. T. L., & Zhang, J. X. (2020). The effectiveness of a Service Leadership subject in Hong Kong: A qualitative evaluation study. *International Journal of Child and Adolescent Health, 13* (2), 181–194.
15. Zi, Y., Shek, D. T. L., & Zhang, J. X. (2020). A qualitative evaluation of a Service Leadership subject in a higher educational institution in Hong Kong. *International Journal of Child and Adolescent Health, 13* (2), 195–208.
16. Zhu, X., Shek, D. T. L., Dou, D., & Chai, W. Y. (2020). Development and evaluation of a Service Leadership subject in a blended learning mode. *International Journal of Child and Adolescent Health, 13* (2), 209–221

C2. **Book Chapters**

1. Shek, D. T. L., & Lin, L. (2015). "Global Youth Leadership Programme" and its evaluation [Reprint]. In D. T. L. Shek, F. K. Y. Wu, & J. Merrick (Eds.), *Leadership and service learning education: Holistic development for Chinese university students* (pp. 111–124). New York: Nova Sciences Publisher.
2. Shek, D. T. L., & Li, X. (2016). Evaluation of a leadership training program for Chinese students [Reprint]. In D. T. L. Shek, A. M. H. Siu, H. Leung, & J. Merrick (Eds.), *Higher education in Hong Kong: Nurturing students to be caring service leaders* (pp. 151–164). New York: Nova Sciences Publisher.
3. Shek, D. T. L., Lin, L., Leung, H., & Zhu, X. (2016). Impact of an intensive Service Leadership course in mainland China [Reprint]. In D. T. L. Shek, C. M. S. Ma, L. Lin & J. Merrick (Eds.), *Education in Hong Kong: Service Leadership for university students* (pp. 135–145). New York: Nova Science Publishers.

4. Shek, D. T. L., Zhu, X., & Lin, L. (2016). Service Leadership course in mainland China: An evaluation [Reprint]. In D. T. L. Shek, F. K. Y. Wu, J. T. Y. Leung, & J. Merrick (Eds.), *Adolescence: Positive youth development programs in Chinese communities* (pp. 137–148). New York: Nova Sciences Publisher.
5. Shek, D. T. L., & Lin, L. (2017). Service Leadership education in the global youth leadership programme: A qualitative evaluation [Reprint]. In J. Merrick. (Ed.), *Child and adolescent health yearbook 2016* (pp. 131–140). New York, NY: Nova Science Publishers.
6. Shek, D. T. L., Liang, J., & Law, M. Y. M. (2017). Process evaluation of a university subject on Service Leadership in Hong Kong [Reprint]. In J. Merrick. (Ed.), *Child and adolescent health yearbook 2016* (pp. 141–151). New York, NY: Nova Science Publishers.
7. Shek, D. T. L., Lin, L., Leung, H., & Zhu, X. (2018). The impact of an intensive Service Leadership course in mainland China: Objective outcome evaluation. In J. Merrick (Ed.), *Child and adolescent health yearbook 2017* (pp. 75–85). New York, NY: Nova Science Publishers.
8. Shek, D. T. L., Zhu, X., & Lin, L. (2018). Evaluation of an intensive Service Leadership course in mainland China [Reprint]. In J. Merrick (Ed.), *Child and adolescent health yearbook 2017* (pp. 259–269). New York, NY: Nova Science Publishers.
9. Shek, D. T. L., Zhu, X., & Merrick, J. (2020). Service Leadership education in an era of service economy [Reprint]. In D. T. L. Shek, X. Zhu, & J. Merrick (Eds.), *Service Leadership Education in an Era of Service Economy* (pp. 3–7). New York, NY: Nova Science Publishers.
10. Chai, W., Shek, D. T. L., Lee, B., & Xie, M. (2020). Impact of Service Leadership education on university students in Hong Kong [Reprint]. In D. T. L. Shek, X. Zhu, & J. Merrick (Eds.), *Service Leadership Education in an Era of Service Economy* (pp. 11–31). New York, NY: Nova Science Publishers.
11. Zhu, X., Shek, D. T. L., Zhu, Z. L., & Zhao, P. X. (2020). Promotion of well-being and leadership qualities among university students after taking a credit-bearing Service Leadership subject [Reprint]. In D. T. L. Shek, X. Zhu, & J. Merrick (Eds.), *Service Leadership Education in an Era of Service Economy* (pp. 33–55). New York, NY: Nova Science Publishers.
12. Law, M. Y. M., Shek, D. T. L., & Zhang, J. X. (2020). Evaluation of an intensive Service Leadership Program using the subjective outcome evaluation approach [Reprint]. In D. T. L. Shek, X. Zhu, & J. Merrick (Eds.), *Service Leadership Education in an Era of Service Economy* (pp. 57–83). New York, NY: Nova Science Publishers.
13. Shek, D. T. L., Kwok, R. K. H., & Low, S. S. (2020). Promotion of Service Leadership in university students: Views of university students [Reprint]. In D. T. L. Shek, X. Zhu, & J. Merrick

(Eds.), *Service Leadership Education in an Era of Service Economy* (pp. 85–107). New York, NY: Nova Science Publishers.

14. Law, M. Y. M., Shek, D. T. L., & Kwok, R. K. H. (2020). Impact of a Leadership Program on the holistic development of university students in Hong Kong [Reprint]. In D. T. L. Shek, X. Zhu, & J. Merrick (Eds.), *Service Leadership Education in an Era of Service Economy* (pp. 109–133). New York, NY: Nova Science Publishers.
15. Yang, Z., Shek, D. T. L., & Zhang, J. X. (2020). The effectiveness of a Service Leadership subject in Hong Kong: A qualitative evaluation study [Reprint]. In D. T. L. Shek, X. Zhu, & J. Merrick (Eds.), *Service Leadership Education in an Era of Service Economy* (pp. 135–161). New York, NY: Nova Science Publishers.
16. Yang, Z., Shek, D. T. L., & Zhang, J. X. (2020). A qualitative evaluation of a Service Leadership subject in a higher educational institution in Hong Kong [Reprint]. In D. T. L. Shek, X. Zhu, & J. Merrick (Eds.), *Service Leadership Education in an Era of Service Economy* (pp. 163–185). New York, NY: Nova Science Publishers.
17. Zhu, X., Shek, D. T. L., Dou, D., & Chai, W. (2020). Development and evaluation of a Service Leadership subject in a blended learning mode [Reprint]. In D. T. L. Shek, X. Zhu, & J. Merrick (Eds.), *Service Leadership Education in an Era of Service Economy* (pp. 187–210). New York, NY: Nova Science Publishers.
18. Leung, J. T. Y., & Shek, D. T. L. (2020). Subjective outcome evaluation of a Service Leadership subject: Findings based on university students in Hong Kong [Reprint]. In A. Tenenbaum, D. T. L. Shek, M. Y. M. Law, & J. Merrick (Eds.), *Advances in Chinese children, adolescent and family research.* (pp. 267–288). New York, NY: Nova Science Publishers.
19. Leung, H., Shek, D. T. L., & Lin, L. (2020). Promotion of Service Leadership qualities in Chinese university students: Objective outcome evaluation based on six waves of data [Reprint]. In A. Tenenbaum, D. T. L. Shek, M. Y. M. Law, & J. Merrick (Eds.), *Advances in Chinese children, adolescent and family research.* (pp. 313–329). New York, NY: Nova Science Publishers.

C3. **Conference Presentations**

1. Leung, H., Shek, D. T. L., Lin, L. (2016, August 25–27). *Promotion of Service Leadership qualities in Chinese university students: An evaluation based on six waves of data.* Paper presented at The 2016 International Society for Quality of Life Studies Annual Conference—"Bridging Quality-of-Life Experiences From East to West", Seoul, South Korea.
2. Dou, D., & Shek, D. T. L. (2018, June). *Subjective outcome evaluation of a leadership training program for university students.* Paper presented at the 16th International Society for Quality-of-Life Studies

Annual Conference—"Promotion of Quality of Life in the Changing World", The Hong Kong Polytechnic University, Hong Kong.
3. Chung, Y. Y. H., Shek, D. T. L., & Au, H. S. S. (2018, June). *Positive youth development, leadership and well-being in students participating in the Silk Road Leadership Program.* Paper presented at the 16th International Society for Quality-of-Life Studies Annual Conference—"Promotion of Quality of Life in the Changing World", The Hong Kong Polytechnic University, Hong Kong.

D. **Assessment tools**

D1. **Journal Articles**

1. Shek, D. T. L., & Lin, L. (2018). Criterion-related validation of the Service Leadership knowledge scale. *International Journal on Disability and Human Development, 17*(1), 137–145.
2. Shek, D. T. L., Lin, L., Leung, H., Yu, L. Ma, C., & Li, X. (2018). Development and validation of the Service Leadership knowledge scale in a Chinese context. *International Journal on Disability and Human Development, 17(*1), 125–136.
3. Shek, D. T. L., Lin, L., Leung, H., Yu, L. Ma, C., & Li, X. (2018). Content validation of the Service Leadership attitudes scale. *International Journal on Disability and Human Development, 17(*1), 147–158.
4. Lin, L., & Shek, D. T. L. (2018). Leadership assessment tools in different Chinese contexts. *International Journal of Child and Adolescent Health, 11*(4), 385–394.
5. Shek, D. T. L., Zhu, X., & Zhu, A. Y. F. (2018). Conceptual background and the development of Service Leadership knowledge scale. *International Journal of Child and Adolescent Health, 11*(4), 395–404.
6. Ma, C. M. S., Shek, D. T. L., & Chandra, Y. (2018). Development of the attitude to Service Leadership Scale in Hong Kong. *International Journal of Child and Adolescent Health, 11*(4), 405–414.
7. Shek, D. T. L., Zhu, X., & Chan, K. M. (2018). Development of Service Leadership Behavior Scale: Background and conceptual model. *International Journal of Child and Adolescent Health, 11*(4), 415–425.
8. Shek, D. T. L., Ma, L. K., Lin, L., & Leung, H. (2018). Psychometric properties of the Service Leadership Behavior Scale: Preliminary findings. *International Journal of Child and Adolescent Health, 11*(4), 427–444.
9. Shek, D. T. L., Wu, J., Lin, L., & Li, X. (2018). Content validation of a Service Leadership Behavior Scale in Hong Kong. *International Journal of Child and Adolescent Health, 11*(4), 445–454.

10. Shek, D. T. L., Ma, L. K., Yu, L., & Leung, L. M. K. (2018). Validation of the Service Leadership Knowledge Scale: Factorial and convergent validity. *International Journal of Child and Adolescent Health, 11*(4), 455–466.
11. Shek, D. T. L., Zhu, A. Y. F., Ma, L. K., & Lin, L. (2018). Validation of the Service Leadership Attitude Scale in Hong Kong. *International Journal of Child and Adolescent Health, 11*(4), 467–478.
12. Shek, D. T. L., Ma, L. K., Ma, C. M. S., & Hoshmand, A. R. (2018). Convergent and factorial validation of the Service Leadership Behavior Scale. *International Journal of Child and Adolescent Health, 11*(4), 479–492.
13. Shek, D. T. L., Zhu, X., & Tse, S. (2018). The Service Leadership Knowledge Scale: Norms and psychological correlates. *International Journal of Child and Adolescent Health, 11*(4), 493–504.
14. Shek, D. T. L., Wu, J., & Chan, B. Y. B. (2018). The Service Leadership Attitude Scale: Normative data and personal correlates in Chinese university students. *International Journal of Child and Adolescent Health, 11*(4), 505–516.
15. Shek, D. T. L., Dou, D., & Snell, R. S. (2018). The Service Leadership Behavior Scale: Norms and personal correlates. *International Journal of Child and Adolescent Health, 11*(4), 517–527.
16. Shek, D. T. L., Zhu, X. & Merrick, J. Editorial: Development and validation of assessment tools on Service Leadership knowledge, attitude and behavior. *International Journal of Child and Adolescent Health, 11*(4), 379–383.
17. Shek, D. T. L., & Lin, L. (2018). Validation of the Service Leadership knowledge scale: Criterion-related validity. *International Journal on Disability and Human Development, 17(*1), 137–146.
18. Shek, D. T. L., & Chai, W. Y. (2019). Psychometric properties of the Service Leadership Attitude Scale in Hong Kong. *Frontiers in Psychology, 10,* Article 1070. https://doi.org/10.3389/fpsyg.2019.01070
19. Shek, D. T. L., Dou, D., & Ma, L. K. (2019). Development and validation of a pioneer scale on Service Leadership behavior in the service economies. *Frontiers in Psychology, 10*, Article 1770. https://doi.org/10.3389/fpsyg.2019.01770

D2. **Book Chapters**

1. Shek, D. T. L., Lin, L., Leung, H., Yu, L., Ma, C. M. S., & Li, X. (2017). Development and validation of the Service Leadership knowledge scale in a Chinese context [Reprint]. In D. T. L. Shek, P. P. Y. Chung, L. Lin, & J. Merrick (Eds.), *Service Leadership Education for University Students* (pp. 163–188). New York: Nova Sciences Publisher.
2. Shek, D. T. L., & Lin, L. (2017). Validation of the Service Leadership knowledge scale: Criterion-related validity [Reprint]. In D. T. L. Shek, P. P. Y. Chung, L. Lin, & J. Merrick (Eds.), *Service Leadership*

Education for University Students (pp. 189–204). New York: Nova Sciences Publisher.

3. Shek, D. T. L., & Lin, L. Leung, H., Yu, L., Ma. C. M. S., & Li, X. (2017). Content validation of the Service Leadership attitudes scale [Reprint]. In D. T. L. Shek, P. P. Y. Chung, L. Lin, & J. Merrick (Eds.), *Service Leadership Education for University Students* (pp. 205–226). New York: Nova Sciences Publisher.
4. Shek, D. T. L., Zhu, X., & Merrick, J. (2019). Development and validation of assessment tools on Service Leadership knowledge, attitude and behavior [Reprint]. In D. T. L. Shek, X. Zhu, L. Lin, & J. Merrick (Eds.), *Service Leadership: Tools to assess knowledge, attitude and behavior* (pp. 3–7). New York, NY: Nova Science Publishers.
5. Lin, L. & Shek, D. T. L. (2019). Leadership assessment tools in different Chinese contexts [Reprint]. In D. T. L. Shek, X. Zhu, L. Lin, & J. Merrick (Eds.), *Service Leadership: Tools to assess knowledge, attitude and behavior* (pp. 11–22). New York, NY: Nova Science Publishers.
6. Shek, D. T. L., Zhu, X., & Zhu, A. Y. F. (2019). Conceptual background and the development of Service Leadership knowledge scale [Reprint]. In D. T. L. Shek, X. Zhu, L. Lin, & J. Merrick (Eds.), *Service Leadership: Tools to assess knowledge, attitude and behavior* (pp. 23–36). New York, NY: Nova Science Publishers.
7. Ma, C. M. S., Shek, D. T. L., & Chandra, Y. (2019). Development of the attitude to Service Leadership Scale in Hong Kong [Reprint]. In D. T. L. Shek, X. Zhu, L. Lin, & J. Merrick (Eds.), *Service Leadership: Tools to assess knowledge, attitude and behavior* (pp. 37–50). New York, NY: Nova Science Publishers.
8. Shek, D. T. L., Zhu, X., & Chan, K. M. (2019). Development of Service Leadership Behavior Scale: Background and conceptual model [Reprint]. In D. T. L. Shek, X. Zhu, L. Lin, & J. Merrick (Eds.), *Service Leadership: Tools to assess knowledge, attitude and behavior* (pp. 51–64). New York, NY: Nova Science Publishers.
9. Shek, D. T. L., Ma, L. K., Lin, L. & Leung, H. (2019). Psychometric properties of the Service Leadership Behavior Scale: Preliminary findings [Reprint]. In D. T. L. Shek, X. Zhu, L. Lin, & J. Merrick (Eds.), *Service Leadership: Tools to assess knowledge, attitude and behavior* (pp. 65–84). New York, NY: Nova Science Publishers.
10. Shek, D. T. L., Wu, J., Lin, L., & Li, X. (2019). Content validation of a Service Leadership Behavior Scale in Hong Kong [Reprint]. In D. T. L. Shek, X. Zhu, L. Lin, & J. Merrick (Eds.), *Service Leadership: Tools to assess knowledge, attitude and behavior* (pp. 87–100). New York, NY: Nova Science Publishers.
11. Shek, D. T. L., Ma, L. K., Yu, L., & Leung, L. M. K. (2019). Validation of the Service Leadership Knowledge Scale: Factorial and convergent validity [Reprint]. In D. T. L. Shek, X. Zhu, L. Lin, & J. Merrick

(Eds.), *Service Leadership: Tools to assess knowledge, attitude and behavior* (pp. 101–116). New York, NY: Nova Science Publishers.

12. Shek, D. T. L., Zhu, A. Y. F., Ma, L, K., & Lin, L. (2019). Validation of the Service Leadership Attitude Scale in Hong Kong. [Reprint]. In D. T. L. Shek, X. Zhu, L. Lin, & J. Merrick (Eds.), *Service Leadership: Tools to assess knowledge, attitude and behavior* (pp. 117–132). New York, NY: Nova Science Publishers.
13. Shek, D. T. L., Ma, L. K., Ma, C. M. S., & Hoshmand, A. R. (2019). Convergent and factorial validation of the Service Leadership Behavior Scale [Reprint]. In D. T. L. Shek, X. Zhu, L. Lin, & J. Merrick (Eds.), *Service Leadership: Tools to assess knowledge, attitude and behavior* (pp. 133–152). New York, NY: Nova Science Publishers.
14. Shek, D. T. L., Zhu, X. & Tse, S. (2019). The Service Leadership Knowledge Scale: Norms and psychological correlates [Reprint]. In D. T. L. Shek, X. Zhu, L. Lin, & J. Merrick (Eds.), *Service Leadership: Tools to assess knowledge, attitude and behavior* (pp. 153–170). New York, NY: Nova Science Publishers.
15. Shek, D. T. L., Wu, J., & Chan, B. Y. B. (2019). The Service Leadership Attitude Scale: Normative data and personal correlates in Chinese university students. [Reprint]. In D. T. L. Shek, X. Zhu, L. Lin, & J. Merrick (Eds.), *Service Leadership: Tools to assess knowledge, attitude and behavior* (pp. 171–188). New York, NY: Nova Science Publishers.
16. Shek, D. T. L., Dou, D., & Snell, R. S. (2019). The Service Leadership Behavior Scale: Norms and personal correlates [Reprint]. In D. T. L. Shek, X. Zhu, L. Lin, & J. Merrick (Eds.), *Service Leadership: Tools to assess knowledge, attitude and behavior* (pp. 189–206). New York, NY: Nova Science Publishers.
17. Shek, D. T. L., Ma, L. K., Low, S. S., Zhu, X., & Dou, D. (2019). A user manual for the Service Leadership Knowledge Scale. In D. T. L. Shek, X. Zhu, L. Lin, & J. Merrick (Eds.), *Service Leadership: Tools to assess knowledge, attitude and behavior* (pp. 209–226). New York, NY: Nova Science Publishers.
18. Shek, D. T. L., & Zhu, X. (2019). A user manual for Service Leadership Attitude Scale. In D. T. L. Shek, X. Zhu, L. Lin, & J. Merrick (Eds.), *Service Leadership: Tools to assess knowledge, attitude and behavior* (pp. 227–252). New York, NY: Nova Science Publishers.
19. Shek, D. T. L., Zhu, X. & Dou, D. (2019). A user manual for the Service Leadership Behavior Scale. In D. T. L. Shek, X. Zhu, L. Lin, & J. Merrick (Eds.), *Service Leadership: Tools to assess knowledge, attitude and behavior* (pp. 253–276). New York, NY: Nova Science Publishers.

20. Shek, D. T. L., Dou, D., & Ma, L. K. Y. (2020). Development and validation of a pioneer scale on Service Leadership behavior in the service economies [Reprint]. In N. C. Silver, L. Badenes-Ribera, & E. Pedroli (Eds.), *Scale Development and Score Validation.* (pp. 147–164). Lausanne: Frontiers Media SA.

E. **Books and Special Issues**

E1. **E1. Special Issues**

1. Shek, D. T. L., Siu, A. M. H., & Merrick, J. (Eds.). (2014). A tale of two innovative leadership programs in Hong Kong, China [Special issue]. *International Journal on Disability and Human Development, 13*(4), 409–543.
2. Shek, D. T. L., Chung, P. P. Y., Yu, L., & Merrick, J. (Eds.). (2015). Service Leadership education for university students: The Hong Kong experience [Special issue]. *International Journal on Disability and Human Development, 14*(3), 203–293.
3. Shek, D. T. L., Chung, P. P. Y., Yu, L., & Merrick, J. (Eds.). (2015). Service Leadership curriculum and higher education reform in Hong Kong [Special issue]. *International Journal on Disability and Human Development, 14*(4), 297–406.
4. Shek, D. T. L., Chung, P. P., Lin, L., & Merrick, J. (Eds.). (2018). Service Leadership education for university students [Special issue]. *International Journal on Disability and Human Development, 17*(1), 3–158.
5. Shek, D. T. L., Zhu, X. & Merrick, J. (Eds.). (2018). Development and validation of assessment tools on Service Leadership knowledge, attitude and behavior [Special issue]. *International Journal of Child and Adolescent Health, 11*(4), 379–527.
6. Shek, D.T. L., Zhu, X., & Merrick, J. (Eds.). (2020). Service Leadership education in an era of service economy. [Special issue]. *International Journal of Child and Adolescent Health, 13*(2), 107–221.
7. Shek, D. T. L., Zhu, X., Dou, D., & Merrick, J. (Eds.). (2021). The origin and nature of the Service Leadership theory [Special issue]. *International Journal of Child Health and Human Development, 14*(4), 363–461.

E2. **Books**

1. Shek, D. T. L., & Chung, P. P. Y. (Eds.). (2015). *Promoting Service Leadership qualities in university students: The Case of Hong Kong. Quality of life in Asia, vol. 6.* Singapore: Springer.
2. Shek, D. T. L., Siu, A. M. H., & Merrick, J. (Eds.). (2015). *Tomorrow's leaders: Service Leadership and holistic development in Chinese university students.* New York: Nova Sciences Publisher.
3. Shek, D. T. L., Wu, F. K. Y., & Merrick, J. (Eds.). (2015). *Leadership and service learning education: Holistic development for Chinese university students.* New York: Nova Sciences Publisher.

4. Shek, D. T. L., Ma, C. M. S., Lin, L., & Merrick, J. (Eds.). (2016). *Education in Hong Kong: Service Leadership for university students.* New York: Nova Sciences Publisher.
5. Shek, D. T. L., Siu, A. M. H., Leung, H., & Merrick, J. (Eds.). (2016). *Higher education in Hong Kong: Nurturing students to be caring service leaders.* New York: Nova Sciences Publisher.
6. Shek, D. T. L., Chung, P. P. Y., Lin, L., & Merrick, J. (Eds.). (2017). *Service Leadership Education for University Students.* New York: Nova Sciences Publisher.
7. Shek, D. T. L., Zhu, X., Lin, L., & Merrick, J. (Eds.) (2019). *Service Leadership: Tools to assess knowledge, attitude and behavior.* New York, NY: Nova Science Publishers.
8. Shek, D. T. L., Zhu, X., & Merrick, J. (Eds.). (2020). *Service Leadership Education in an Era of Service Economy [Reprint].* New York, NY: Nova Science Publishers.
9. Shek, D. T. L., Zhu, X., Dou, D., & Merrick, J. (Eds.). (2021). *Service Leadership theory: Origin and nature [Reprint].* New York, NY: Nova Science Publishers

F. **Conferences (organized by PolyU)**

1. Service Leadership Roundtable held on March 22, 2013 at The Hong Kong Polytechnic University, Hong Kong
2. International Conference on Service Leadership Education for University Students: Experience in Hong Kong, held on May 14–15, 2014 at The Hong Kong Polytechnic University, Hong Kong
3. International Conference on Service Leadership Education in Service Economies was held on January 6–7, 2016, at The Hong Kong Polytechnic University, Hong Kong.

Summary of publications	No.
A. Curriculum development and theory	99
B. Evaluation (credit-bearing subjects)	38
C. Evaluation (non-credit-bearing programs)	38
D. Assessment tool	39
E. Books and special issues	16
F. Conferences (organized by PolyU)	3
Total	233

Output type	Number
Books and special issues	16
Book chapters	97

(continued)

(continued)

Output type	Number
Journal articles	88
Conference presentations	27
Conferences (organized by PolyU)	3
Other articles	2
Total	233

References

Census and Statistics Department. (2023). *Gross domestic product by economic activity*. Hong Kong. https://www.censtatd.gov.hk/en/wbr.html?ecode=B10300042023QQ01&scode=250

Chai, W. Y., & Shek, D. T. L. (2021). The role of trust in the service economy. *International Journal of Child Health and Human Development, 14*(4), 425–436.

Chai, W. Y., Shek, D. T. L., Lee, B., & Xie, M. (2020). Impact of Service Leadership education on university students in Hong Kong. *International Journal of Child and Adolescent Health, 13*(2), 113–124.

Chung, P. P. Y. (2012). *Service reborn*. Lexingford Publishing.

Chung, P. P. Y., & Bell, A. H. (2015). *25 principles of service leadership*. Lexingford Publishing.

Dou, D. Y., & Shek, D. T. L. (2021). The dark side of leadership in the service leadership theory. *International Journal of Child Health and Human Development, 14*(4), 405–414.

Dou, D. Y., Shek, D. T. L., & Zhu, Z. (2021). Moral character in the service leadership theory. *International Journal of Child Health and Human Development, 14*(4), 393–404.

Grönfeldt, S., & Strother, J. B. (2006). *Service leadership: The quest for competitive advantage*. SAGE. https://doi.org/10.4135/9781452231068

Kezar, A., Carducci, R., & Contreras-McGavin, M. (2006). *Rethinking the "L" word in higher education: The revolution of research on leadership: ASHE higher education report*. John Wiley & Sons.

Law, M. Y. M., Shek, D. T. L., & Zhang, J. (2020). Evaluation of an intensive Service Leadership program using the subjective outcome evaluation approach. *International Journal of Child and Adolescent Health, 13*(2), 137–152.

Nations Encyclopedia. (2023, November 8). *Hong Kong—Services*. https://www.nationsencyclopedia.com/economies/Asia-and-the-Pacific/Hong-Kong-SERVICES.html

Peterson, C., & Seligman, M. E. (2004). *Character strengths and virtues: A handbook and classification* (Vol. 1). Oxford University Press.

Rost, J. C. (1993). *Leadership for the 21st century*. Praeger Publishers.

Shek, D. T. L., & Chung, P. P. Y. (Eds.). (2015a). *Promoting service leadership qualities in university students: The case of Hong Kong*. Springer.

Shek, D. T. L., & Chung, P. P. Y. (2015b). Service Leadership education for university students: Seven unfinished tasks. In D. T. L. Shek & P. P. Y. Chung (Eds.), *Promoting service leadership qualities in university students* (pp. 225–232). Springer.

Shek, D. T. L., Chung, P. P. Y., & Leung, H. (2015a). How unique is the service leadership model? A comparison with contemporary leadership approaches. *International Journal on Disability and Human Development, 14*(3), 217–231. https://doi.org/10.1515/ijdhd-2015-0403

Shek, D. T. L., Chung, P. P. Y., & Leung, H. (2015b). Manufacturing economy vs. service economy: Implications for Service Leadership. *International Journal on Disability and Human Development, 14*(3), 205–215. https://doi.org/10.1515/ijdhd-2015-0402

Shek, D. T. L., Chung, P. P. Y., Lin, L., & Merrick, J. (2018). Service leadership education for university students [Special issue]. *International Journal on Disability and Human Development, 17*(1), 1–168.

Shek, D. T. L., Chung, P. P. Y., Yu, L., & Merrick, J. (2015c). Service Leadership curriculum and higher education reform in Hong Kong [Special issue]. *International Journal on Disability and Human Development, 14*(4), 297–406.

Shek, D. T. L., Chung, P. P. Y., Yu, L., & Merrick, J. (2015d). Service Leadership education for university students: The Hong Kong experience. *International Journal on Disability and Human Development, 14*(3), 203–204. https://doi.org/10.1515/ijdhd-2015-0401

Shek, D. T. L., Chung, P. P. Y., Yu, L., & Merrick, J. (2015e). Service Leadership education for university students: The Hong Kong experience [Special issue]. *International Journal on Disability and Human Development, 14*(3), 203–293.

Shek, D. T. L., Chung, P. P. Y., & Zhu, X. (2022). Service leadership as the backbone of university social responsibility. In *University corporate social responsibility and university governance* (pp. 105–118). Springer.

Shek, D. T. L., Kwok, R. K. H., & Low, S. S. (2020a). Promotion of Service Leadership in university students: Views of university students. *International Journal of Child and Adolescent Health, 13*(2), 153–165.

Shek, D. T. L., & Lin, L. (2015). Evaluating service leadership programs with multiple strategies. In D. T. L. Shek & P. P. Y. Chung (Eds.), *Promoting service leadership qualities in university students* (pp. 197–212). Springer.

Shek, D. T. L., Ma, C. M. S., & Liu, T. T. (2015f). Adolescent developmental assets and service leadership. *International Journal on Disability and Human Development, 14*(3), 275–283. https://doi.org/10.1515/ijdhd-2015-0408

Shek, D. T. L., & Yang, Z. (2021). Origin, development, and assertions of service leadership theory. *International Journal of Child Health and Human Development, 14*(4), 369–380.

Shek, D. T. L., & Yuen, A. (2019). The quest for holistic youth leadership development: What should be the desired attributes of youth leaders? *International Journal of Child and Adolescent Health, 12*(1), 43–60.

Shek, D. T. L., Yu, L., & Siu, A. M. H. (2015g). Interpersonal competence and service leadership. *International Journal on Disability and Human Development, 14*(3), 265–274. https://doi.org/10.1515/ijdhd-2015-0407

Shek, D. T. L., Yu, L., Ma, C. M. S., Sun, R. C. F., & Liu, T. T. (2013). Development of a credit-bearing service leadership subject for university students in Hong Kong. *International Journal of Adolescent Medicine and Health, 25*(4), 353–361. https://doi.org/10.1515/ijamh-2013-0033

Shek, D. T. L., Zhu, X., Dou, D. Y., & Merrick, J. (2021). The origin and nature of the service leadership theory. *International Journal of Child Health and Human Development, 14*(4), 363–365.

Shek, D. T. L., Zhu, X., & Merrick, J. (2020b). Editorial: Service leadership education in an era of service economy. *International Journal of Child and Adolescent Health, 13*(2), 107–109.

Shek, D. T. L., Zhu, X., & Merrick, J. (2020c). Service Leadership education in an era of service economy. [Special issue]. *International Journal of Child and Adolescent Health, 13*(2), 107–221.

Yang, Z., Shek, D. T. L., & Zhang, J. (2020a). The effectiveness of a service leadership subject in Hong Kong: A qualitative evaluation study. *International Journal of Child and Adolescent Health, 13*(2), 181–194.

Yang, Z., Shek, D. T. L., & Zhang, J. (2020b). A qualitative evaluation of a service leadership subject in a higher educational institution in Hong Kong. *International Journal of Child and Adolescent Health, 13*(2), 195–208.

Zhu, X., Shek, D. T. L., Dou, D., & Chai, W. (2020). Development and evaluation of a service leadership subject in a blended learning mode. *International Journal of Child and Adolescent Health, 13*(2), 209–221.

Zhu, X., Shek, D. T. L., & Ng, D. C. H. (2021). Humanistic leadership in service economy. *International Journal of Child Health and Human Development, 14*(4), 381–391.

Chapter 11
A Tale of Two Cities: A Service-Learning Subject for Migrant Children in East China and Needy Youth in Hong Kong

Daniel T. L. Shek and Lu Yu

Abstract Despite the mission of providing holistic education to nurture students' sustainability competence, university education has faced criticism for failing to achieve this goal. Therefore, a curriculum-based Service-Learning (SL) Subject was developed and implemented for migrant children in East China and needy youth in Hong Kong to build their diverse developmental assets. Based on the positive youth development and strength-based approaches, multiple teaching and learning strategies and techniques are adopted in the SL subject. Moreover, after a review of the development and achievements of this SL subject over a decade, this chapter introduces the effectiveness evaluation of the SL subject from multiple perspectives (e.g., service providers, service recipients, and partnering organizations). It provides a comprehensive summary of the students' learning experiences across seven aspects (e.g., contributions to intrapersonal and interpersonal development). To date, the SL subject has benefited more than 3,000 migrant children in China and 6,400 needy youth in Hong Kong, making a tremendous social impact in promoting educational and cultural exchanges and strengthening social capital and sustainability in the served schools and communities. In future, the SL subject will be continuously refined from various aspects to bring more significant benefits to youth and serve as a "model" for counterparts in mainland China and countries along the Belt and Road, aiming to sustain support for disadvantaged youth.

Keywords Curriculum-based Service-Learning (SL) subject · Developmental assets · Migrant children · Positive youth development (PYD) · Student learning experience · Evaluation

11.1 Introduction

Unquestionably, providing holistic education for students to acquire sustainability competencies effectively is the mission of university education. Specifically, Wiek et al. (2011) defined five key competencies for sustainable development: interpersonal, systems-thinking, anticipatory, normative, and strategic competence, which

D. T. L. Shek, *Promoting Holistic Development in University Students*, Quality of Life in Asia 17, https://doi.org/10.1007/978-981-96-0251-3_11

are essential for effective leadership and citizenship. Firstly, interpersonal competence includes positive and negative development in teams, leadership, collaboration, and empathy. Normative competence covers fairness, justice, responsibility, and happiness. Of course, we should ask how university education can nurture such sustainability competencies. In particular, one should reflect on how social sustainability, which refers to "equality, well-being, and balance across the quality of life indicators between sociocultural groups over time and from one generation to the next" (Ross, 2013), can be promoted in students in the higher education sector.

Unfortunately, there are criticisms that universities have failed to promote holistic and sustainable development in students. While university students receive professional or disciplinary training, they have shown signs of dependency, a rise in egocentrism, a drop in empathy, and a lack of social responsibility (Shek, 2010; Shek & Wong, 2011). Therefore, educators must shoulder the responsibility to nurture sustainable competencies and soft skills of employability in students. Hence, we implemented curriculum-based Service-Learning (SL) subject to build up university students' personal assets, thereby enhancing their self-improvement, interpersonal communication, and future development (Shek et al., 2019).

The Hong Kong Polytechnic University (PolyU) is committed to providing education and research that can promote sustainability competencies in students. One important initiative is implementing SL subject, through which students can learn knowledge and theories from formal academic study and practice their skills and understanding through community service. Moreover, they can enhance their social responsibility after the service (Shek et al., 2020, 2021). Since 2013, a 3-credit SL subject entitled "Promotion of Children and Adolescent Development" has been offered to 2095 PolyU students from different majors. Up to now, over 3,000 migrant children in mainland China and 6400 secondary school students have benefited from this subject. This subject aims to "(1) introduce different perspectives of youth development, (2) enable students to apply the theories to design and implement appropriate service to youth in need, (3) enhance students' competencies of problem-solving, decision-making, and teamwork, (4) cultivate positive values and a strengths orientation, (5) nurture students' sense of care and compassion toward other people in the community, and (6) reflect on their own roles and social responsibilities in terms of sustainable development of oneself and the society."

11.2 Teaching and Learning Approach

Besides cognitive learning, SL also focuses on the subjective learning experience of the students. In his four-stage learning cycle theory, Kolb (1984) emphasized that learning from practice and reflective observation is vital in the cycle. As a form of experiential learning, SL subject and programs facilitate students to meaningfully reflect on their past and current education and service experiences. More importantly, they are equipped with critical thinking skills to view their experiences from various angles. Through adopting experiential learning pedagogy and guided self-reflection strategies, students learn how to explore meaning in their lives, make responsible decisions in their daily lives, drill their employability skills, develop more sustainable outcomes such as social support as well as civic responsibility, and experience positive personal changes (Leung et al., 2021).

Regarding reflection, Eyler and Giles (1999) emphasized that reflection is essential in SL practices as it builds the linkage between service and learning. Through purposeful and continuous verbal and/or written reflection, students can consolidate their service experiences, view their learning critically, and explore new insights (Eyler & Giles, 1999; Kolb, 1984). In this regard, this SL subject provided by PolyU stresses the importance of "learning through reflection" and carries out various strategies to facilitate continuous reflection in the classroom and service.

Based on the positive youth development and strength-based approaches, multiple teaching and learning strategies and techniques are adopted in the SL subject to facilitate students' engagement in two consecutive semesters, including (1) e-learning, (2) lectures, (3) preparation of service projects, (4) mock teaching, (5) program implementation and evaluation, (6) reflective journals, and (7) group presentation. The details of some of these strategies are as follows:

(a) E-learning modules: The basic concepts of SL are introduced.
(b) Experiential learning: Multiple group discussions, case studies, mock teaching, and actual direct service are arranged. "Competencies," "Aspirations," and "Resilience," which are cornerstones of individuals' strengths-building, are stressed and conveyed to the PolyU students and service participants. It also helps them develop a sense of responsibility, a caring disposition, and moral character.
(c) Collaborative learning: Strategies like group service projects, peer assessment, and recruiting student helpers from different universities as assessors and collaborators are adopted. It inspires students to learn and build up their confidence and aspirations.
(d) Guided reflection: Continuous reflective exercises are arranged, such as various in-class reflective exercises, written reflective journals, and the daily reflective meetings that help review and reflect on the whole-day service, the reflection workshops after service implementation, and the group presentation as a summary. These allow students to undergo self-exploration and enhance their self-understanding.

On top of classroom teaching and small group discussions on the university campus, real-life learning opportunities can align well with key competencies in sustainable development. Students can gain hands-on experience in linking knowledge to action for sustainability at personal and societal levels. Also, equal emphasis is placed on both mastering theoretical knowledge and its practical application in real life. Experiential learning and collaborative learning are two effective approaches to enhance student learning and participation. Students can learn to develop and consolidate sustainability strategies through experience. Moreover, learning through guided reflection is also emphasized in the subject for effective learning and to enhance students' self-understanding.

11.3 Development and Achievements

The subject was first implemented in 2013, with 40 participants providing service in Shanghai. To cater to the increased needs of students, two other service sites, Hong Kong and Hangzhou, were established in 2014 and 2015, respectively. So far, 2,095 PolyU students have taken this subject. Meanwhile, an increasing number of students living in underprivileged conditions have joined our service. Up to now, 3,050 migrant children in Shanghai and Hangzhou and 6,409 adolescents in Hong Kong have received the service provided by PolyU students through this subject. In addition, 130 universities in China participated in the service as peer collaborators.

PolyU initiated the project with collaborative efforts from multiple institutions. In the Chinese mainland two universities (East China Normal University and Zhejiang University), two NGOs serving migrant families, and a local Education Bureau participated in the project and helped arrange the service. PolyU students have provided services to migrant children from eight primary schools. In Hong Kong, we have closely collaborated with the Society of Boys' Centres and two secondary schools under Project WeCan (by Wharf Group). The service recipients are youths with social and emotional problems, learning difficulties, and socio-economically underprivileged family backgrounds.

The PolyU block grants financially supported the development, implementation, and evaluation of this subject. Since 2014, the summer service projects conducted in both Shanghai and Hangzhou have received financial support from the "Ten Thousand Student Interflow Program of the Ministry of Education" approved by the Ministry of Education, People's Republic of China (PRC). In Hong Kong, some service projects collaborating with ten schools under the Project WeCan have been financially supported by Wharf. Project WeCan is a Business-in-Community initiative launched by the Wharf (Holdings) Limited in 2011.

11.4 Evaluation of the Impact of the Subject

To evaluate the effectiveness of the subject, we routinely assess this subject from several perspectives. First, we collect data from university students who provide the service. Besides evaluating the changes of the students by collecting pretest and posttest data (see Appendix 1), we also use a subjective outcome evaluation strategy to examine students' subjective perceptions of the course and the service project (see Appendix 2). Second, we collect data from the service recipients, including objective outcome evaluation (see Appendix 3) and subjective outcome evaluation (see Appendix 4). Third, we collect feedback from partnering organizations, such as the schools involved (see Appendix 5). Moreover, we collect perceptions of subject teachers through the focus group (see Appendix 6). Finally, we engage observers to assess students using an evaluation form (see Appendix 7).

In the early years of implementing this subject, two evaluation studies were published in the International Journal of Child and Adolescent Health (Volume 9, Issue 2). Two paper presentations were also conducted at the Second International Conference on SL, which was held in December 2016. Two book chapters were published in the book "Service-Learning for Youth Leadership: The Case of Hong Kong" by Springer in 2019 (Shek et al., 2019). Different newspapers have reported on service implementation in Minhang District, Shanghai. Additionally, the service project (Journey of Hope) was awarded in the Fellowship Scheme, which is one of the brand projects run by the Communist Youth League of China Central Committee. The experience and achievement of the current SL subject have been distributed through different channels, such as newspapers in Hong Kong and mainland China, international conferences of SL, periodicals, websites, and newsletters of different collaborating schools.

Regarding the impacts of the SL subject on university students, they have full autonomy to design services that best fit the needs of the service targets. Moreover, they enjoyed what they had achieved—they taught knowledge and skills, induced hope and aspirations, and shared love and care with the migrant children in the service (Leung & Shek, 2016; Leung et al., 2021). Many students shared that their passion for life and learning has been re-ignited, and they would like to continue serving the community in future. In one of our studies, students generally agreed that the subject had enabled them to develop a strong sense of civic responsibility and enriched their overall development (Wu & Shek, 2016). Another mixed-method study reported the evaluative findings on students' performance and program effectiveness (Yu et al., 2016). The results showed that students had meaningful gains in multiple aspects, including "(a) increased empathy toward others and passion for helping needy people, (b) deeper self-understanding, (c) improved problem-solving and decision-making skills, (d) enhanced interpersonal skills, and (e) a stronger sense of responsibility and citizenship." Shek and Chak (2019) examined the perceived changes and benefits of 87 students taking the subject in the 2013–14 academic year. Results revealed that students displayed positive changes in terms of interpersonal relationship skills, team building, cognitive competence, and social responsibilities. Furthermore, most students appreciated the opportunity to engage in service and agreed that SL promoted their sense of citizenship and concern for society. As shared by a student, "One of them (the kid) even wants to study at PolyU and find us in future. These messages moved me deeply. Some of them we served lived in poor environments and were allocated limited resources. This leads me to think about underprivileged groups in Hong Kong. Many people may hesitate to help them, including me. However, now my passion is growing. If I have a chance, I may try to serve the needy in Hong Kong." In another study conducted by Yu et al. (2019), service providers (e.g., university students) responded to subjective outcome evaluation questionnaires. Almost all students regarded the subject as meaningful and contributing to their development, such as self-confidence, respect for other people, compassion, and care. Moreover, based on the responses of service recipients (355 primary school students), results showed that the service recipients were satisfied with the program and service providers, and they felt that the program was beneficial to their development. Positive comments and ratings were also observed from the primary school teachers and observers (local university).

11.5 Learning Experience of the Students

To comprehensively understand student's learning experiences, we have collected reflections from students who got scholarships for this subject (Shek & Chak, 2019; Shek & Ho, 2019). Based on the students' sharing, we can identify several observations regarding the benefits to the students and their reflections.

11.5.1 Shift in Perception: From Initial Negative or Neutral Feelings to Positive Experience

Some students shared that they did not plan to choose this subject initially. However, they eventually had very positive experiences and felt that joining this subject was rewarding:

- "'*Promotion of Children and Adolescent Development'* was not my first choice among all SL subjects, considering I do not have much experience with children and adolescents and am not confident in interacting with them. Hence, I was both afraid and excited when I took this course, especially since I had no friends studying with me in the same class. However, I gained a new perspective after studying this course. Through this course, not only did I learn new academic knowledge and theories in lectures, but I also enhanced my personal skills in holding online workshops."
- "If I were asked to describe the *Promotion of Children and Adolescent Development* with one adjective, I would say it is an 'impactful' subject. When I first registered for this course last year, I simply regarded it as a way to fulfill my graduation requirement at PolyU. However, I knew I was wrong after learning essential theoretical knowledge in lectures and tutorials and serving adolescents in need. This subject does have a tremendous impact on me."
- "Throughout the past year, I have served children with special educational needs. Children there are different from typical children. They have difficulties managing their emotions and behaviors. In the past, handling and serving children was quite a nightmare for me as I was not able to understand them, and therefore, I encountered several failures. After this course and services, I have found a passion for serving children and developed a related competence. It also inspires me to do something as a citizen."
- "Time flies. Here comes the end of the two-semester SL course. It was a long but meaningful journey for me. 'Learn to serve, serve to learn.' It was the very first statement that inspired me in this SL course. Honestly, I thought it was nothing

special but voluntary work. In fact, it was not just about delivering the service; it helped me learn and grow at the same time."

11.5.2 Contributions to Intrapersonal and Interpersonal Development

Many students shared that this subject contributed to their intrapersonal development (such as empowerment and organizational skills) and interpersonal development (such as teamwork and leadership):

- *Empowerment*: "It seems that not everyone is comfortable in praising others; some would even consider it a difficult act and need the courage to do so … Moreover, I know that sometimes, praising others can be embarrassing as well if I cannot find the appropriate moment to do so. This is also what I am worried about. I am afraid that students are not that active and unwilling to answer our questions; even though I have the heart to praise them, I cannot find the perfect timing. However, to my surprise, children attend our lessons actively and compete fiercely in order to get a chance to answer. Their passion changed my original attitude from praising them intentionally to praising them from the bottom of my heart. I do not even need to find a time to appreciate them purposely but value their answers and attitudes sincerely."
- *Empowering Other People*: "I am the final editor of our performance video. Sometimes, I needed help from others, especially when the time was limited; I had to come up with a decision immediately and seek help from the correct person; this, somehow, boosted my problem-solving skills as well. Also, since other performance planners and teachers have supported me genuinely, I know the significance of empowerment in motivating students to do better. Therefore, apart from leading the whole group, giving empathy to teammates and caring about their feelings are vital no matter which post I take, whether as the coordinator or a team player. I hope that with my willingness to empower people, those who work with me will feel less pressured and panicked, creating fewer conflicts but bringing sympathy and harmony to my future workplace after I graduate."
- *Interpersonal Competence*: "I know that I do not seem to be a passive girl who feels unconfident when chatting with boys, but then I really am! Also, I felt so insecure with the number of boys more than girls in my group. With these worries in mind, I did not take the lead at first for safety. After a few meetings with groupmates, I found out that boys are not that scary and can do more than I think. Therefore, I know that I have to put down all my biases in order to build a good team connection for the success of our service. So, I applied my practice in doing university group projects that motivated them gradually and pushed them to attend our meetings whenever we had things to discuss. What makes a good leader is not just getting all things completed but also being able to energize and influence others. I turned myself into an extrovert successfully and dominated the whole

team while encouraging them to voice out opinions simultaneously. Luckily, my groupmates are good team players who are willing to coordinate and listen. We, thus, had a satisfactory performance at last."

- *Leadership Development*: "I feel thankful to have a chance to be a leader since it proved that leading the team is not that awful, whereas I believe I have a high probability of being the coordinator in future group projects. Yet, since this was my first time, I seemed to be too harsh and demanding to my groupmates. I should have cared more about their emotions as well if I would like to be an effective group leader since the team's emotional stability is one of the factors contributing to the team's performance. Fortunately, my teammates are willing to follow my high-intensive working style for five days, but it might be inappropriate if our service period lasts longer as people's working intention and productivity will drop if they feel bored with one thing."
- *Organization Skills*: "The subject offers the opportunity to learn about organizing activities for others. We had to form a small service group, and each member had their own role. We worked together to carry out numerous tasks, including proposals, meeting minutes, session plans, service practices, and review meetings. These settings have taught me how to coordinate with other parties, such as groupmates, tutors, helpers, and teachers and students in collaborative institutions. This can help me practice interpersonal skills for society and the workplace because most job responsibilities include coordination with different internal departments and external partners. Specifically, I am an administrator in my service group, responsible for paperwork, liaison, and promotion. These tasks are closely connected to my business study as well as future administrative and office jobs."
- *Teamwork*: "Holding online workshops was a new experience for me, so it brings many challenges to me. Yet, I am grateful for this chance to do it, especially with my groupmates. While this course relies a lot on teamwork as it requires us to finish different activities and projects, I was excited but nervous about the grouping and working with groupmates."

11.5.3 Personal Reflection and Self-evaluation

Many students pointed out that SL enabled them to have personal reflection and self-evaluation, which led to changes in their behavior:

- "I am glad that I have reflected and grown a lot throughout the entire service, from pre-service preparations to post-service evaluations. This is really rewarding, and I never regret choosing this subject in 2021 Semester 2!"
- "As a primary school teacher who was not that familiar with their learning curriculum, my role of being a teacher gave me lots of pressure since I could not perform my responsibility of teaching students well … the sense of insecurity gave me thousands of stress. Yet, I know that it is no use for me to struggle with it daily, so the only thing I could do was to review the lesson recording every day in

order to identify which part of my performance could be improved and to observe how children behaved (e.g., which part of the lesson they are most interested in). I do not always reflect on myself. However, doing self-evaluation is really useful to me since one of my queries has been solved via this after-class review. It turned out that they did better than our expectations and had far more potential than we thought."

- "During the group evaluation, I found that students in every class cried during their farewells to teachers, except for those in our class who did not. My group felt questioned until we chatted with our beloved teacher that our class did not cry, which might be due to the lack of in-depth emotional connection with them. Admittedly, when compared to other groups, we shared fewer personal experiences since we played happily and crazily with them most of the time. There is no doubt that it is somehow difficult to handle children's emotions remotely if they really cry at last … Therefore, I would prefer to let them smile and have fun until the very last moment since people can normally recall positive past incidents and emotions easier than negative ones."
- "What I loved the most was that we were given so much freedom in designing the entire service. From the planning to the execution, from the content materials to the teaching methods, together with the communication with the school and the allocation of human resources, we were given plenty of space and chances to manage on our own. As a management student, it was an amazing chance for me to learn how to organize an event and develop leadership skills. There is nothing more valuable than hands-on practical experience for learning."

11.5.4 Social Responsibility and Responsible Citizenship

Many students pointed out that SL helped them rethink their social responsibility and the ways to serve as responsible citizens:

- "Other than academic knowledge and personal growth, this course allowed me to think deeper about the social responsibility I have as a young adult. As the service recipients were F.5 students this time, before the workshop, I did not know how much I could be helpful to them as we did not have a large age difference. However, the reaction of the students told otherwise. In the workshops, we shared some of our stories in studying, like our path in entering university after DSE and the difficulties we encountered during that time, which the students appreciated and felt relatable … I understand the responsibility and role I have as a university student is to help other students (mostly secondary school students) by sharing my stories and providing them with encouragement and help. With the success and the fun I had, I look forward to other opportunities to hold or participate in similar events or workshops that target children and adolescents."
- "Last but not least, this subject has enabled me to understand more about the situation of the underprivileged in Hong Kong and develop a sense of empathy towards them. Being a citizen who has more resources than them, I believe that

I have the responsibility to assist them. As the old saying goes, give more than you take. Although it is not possible for me to single-handedly help all the underprivileged, I sincerely hope that more people will offer a helping hand in the near future. Personally, I will offer more care to those in need through applying the theories and practical experiences I learned from this course both as a healthcare worker and as a caring citizen."

- "The subject taught me that I should contribute to society because we need to be responsible citizens. The subject provides the chance to practice social responsibility. Other than academic achievement, I should focus on shaping my own character in a good manner. Furthermore, I should apply my professional knowledge to contribute to and promote the corresponding industry. Even if I were located in the middle class of society in the near future, I would need to care for and respect underprivileged people such as impoverished families, elderly, lower-class workers, and adolescents who have learning difficulties. I will try my best to treat the society fairly and harmoniously."

11.5.5 Changes in Views on Social Deprivation and Social Problems

Through the study and related service, students remarked that they had changed their views on social deprivation and social problems, such as dispelling stereotypes about underprivileged students:

- "I have broken my stereotypes towards underprivileged students. Initially, I believed in the stereotypes put on them by society because they needed special education. The interest classes worsened these beliefs as I witnessed their emotional and behavioral problems. However, I changed my perceptions of them. I was able to have more personal contact with the students during the educational camp, and I evidenced that they are as normal as any other students in Hong Kong. During barbecue time, several students offered me food despite the fact that there was not much of it. They even gave me soft drinks bought from outside. Furthermore, I saw that some of them excel at sports and handcrafting and even have the knowledge to build their own mini race car. Some students even taught me how to change the motor for acceleration and speed adjustments. Although they may not be diligent inside the classroom, they have shown that they are full of hidden talents and generosity, which makes them totally normal children."
- "The most significant change in me would be my perception of underprivileged students, especially those who cannot excel academically. In the past, society labeled teenagers who could not study well as 'Band 3 students.' News, documentaries, and movies commonly associate them with negative issues, including gangster activity and behavioral problems. These long-standing biases progressively indoctrinate the public, including me, to believe that they do not possess any strength. This impression made me worried that these students may be rude

to me or even ignore me during service activities because of my identity as a university student, which is 'traditionally' believed to be substantially superior to Band 3 students."

- "Before this subject, I attended several courses about teenage development, from which the three circles of family, schools, and friends are always regarded as the main factors contributing to a healthy teenager's personal growth. However, this service experience breaks new ground and inspires me to rethink the situation in Hong Kong. Listening to the sharing from some seasoned social workers and educators, I have realized that some underprivileged adolescents are raised in problematic families, like single-parent families and grassroots families with limited resources. Through a face-to-face discussion with the teachers in the two serving secondary schools, I have better understood that teachers nowadays suffer from heavy workloads, especially administrative duties, which makes them allocate less time and effort to their students' academic performance and personal growth. From the lectures, furthermore, I have learned that the social networking of underprivileged students is comparatively weak. These learnings are like an alarm ringing to me that the importance of the three circles towards underprivileged teenagers has been reduced. Therefore, I, as a future educator, should start to seek other solutions in order to prevent the potential adversities from minimizing their resilience, aspiration, and competence."

11.5.6 Strength-Based Conceptions

Through SL, students identified strengths in themselves as well as in the service recipients, which did not exist before they took the SL subject.

- "After the lessons and the service experience, I was inspired that people, especially teenagers, possess certain hidden strengths that are unrecognizable by them but potentially beneficial to their personal growth. Along with this learning, I started to reflect on my own personality throughout the preparation process for the English camp, and the hidden strength I identified was my efficient problem-solving skills. Originally, I did not find it to be my strength because I used to be a slow decision-maker who took a long time for research to avoid uncertainty, especially when time was not limited. Recalling the memory of the service, however, I found some unexpected incidents I handled well, and one of them was about the late lunch delivery. On the first day, the 100 boxed meals arrived at 1:15 p.m., 30 minutes later than expected, but the activities were supposed to end at 1 p.m. Once I had noticed the problem, I immediately rescheduled the sessions and reallocated the manpower. After the camp, I realized that it was an effective solution based on the feedback and appreciation from others, which not only shows my ability but also demonstrates my efficiency in tackling problems."

11.5.7 Aspirations for the Future

Some students felt that the subject changed their views about the service recipients, the society, and their positive aspirations for the future in terms of volunteering:

- "The course was over. However, I did not think that it was the end of the journey. Caring for the society does not end here. I might not have time now to join a lot of services, but I will start to pay more attention to people in need in society. I will also seek opportunities to take part in event organization instead of simply volunteering in voluntary services."
- "After this course and these services, I have found a passion for serving children and developed a related competence of mine. It also inspires me to do something as a citizen."
- "I have been able to learn how my role as a student and responsible citizen can make a difference for them and to understand the difficulties faced by underprivileged children; hence, I have gained more social awareness towards them."
- "Last but not least, this subject has enabled me to understand more about the situation of the underprivileged in Hong Kong and develop a sense of empathy towards them. Being a citizen who has more resources than them, I believe that I have the responsibility to assist them. Personally, I will offer more care to those in need by applying the theories and practical experiences I learned from this course both as a healthcare worker and as a caring citizen … 'Promotion of Children and Adolescent Development' has completely changed my views towards the underprivileged and had a strong impact on my future."

11.6 Achievement and the Way Forward

To date, we have served more than 3000 migrant children in the Chinese mainland and 6,400 needy youth in Hong Kong. The programs are generally well-received. All the service participants appreciated the companionship and experienced the formulation of their own goals, whereas some service targets would usually sacrifice their own dreams for their family's own good. The teachers from the participating schools were also amazed by the university students' innovative teaching methods and designs, which positively stimulated and influenced their own teaching. Over the past five years, it has been observed that the SL project has had a tremendous social impact in promoting educational and cultural exchanges and strengthening the social capital and sustainability in the schools and communities served. The implementation had caught the attention of different areas, newspapers, and government education officials in both Hong Kong and the Chinese mainland. In 2016, the project launched in Shanghai, "Journey of Hope" Summer Camp, was one of the awarded projects in the Fellowship Scheme, which is one of the brand projects run by the Communist Youth League Central Committee, PRC.

To further understand how the subject has impacted the students and the service targets, we plan to conduct more comprehensive evaluation work. In particular, evaluation data will be collected from the service recipients and organizations involved in the initiative. For the subject, the continuation is not a repetition of what has been done in the past years but continuing to polish the teaching materials that best fit the needs of the university students, migrant children, and needy youth, improve the collaboration with the partners in both Hong Kong and China that could maximize the benefits to the service participants.

Besides conducting post-course subjective outcome evaluation and qualitative evaluation of students' reflective journals, longitudinal and exploratory studies should be administered to understand the impacts of the subject upon the university students, the service participants, and the community served at a deeper level. In addition, our SL practices could serve as a "model" for China's counterparts to sustain the assistance to the migrant children. We may consider setting additional sites in other countries along the Belt (Kyrgyzstan) and Road (Cambodia) to strengthen the connectivity and continuity of the subject. In particular, our focus will be placed on serving students with social deprivation. Systematic and professional training for teachers, particularly teachers outside Hong Kong, contributes to the sustainability of the subject as well. We have already established an SL and Leadership Training Centre at the Royal University of Phnom Penh. An e-learning package will be developed to help teachers better understand the rationale and resources used in the subject.

Acknowledgements The preparation of this chapter is financially supported by The Hong Kong Polytechnic University (ZZ4U and ZZUE), Li and Fung Endowed Professorship in Service Leadership Education, Wofoo Foundation, and the Matching Fund of Research Grants Council (ZECL and ZH4Q).

Appendix 1: Objective Outcome Evaluation Form

學生問卷調查

Student Questionnaire

親愛的同學:

較早時我們成功獲得您的同意填寫這份問卷。問卷的內容主要是幫助我們了解Promotion of Children and Adolescent Development科目的成效及你的發展特質。問卷內的問題沒有對或錯的答案，請您憑著對自己的認識或感覺誠實作答。為了了解您作答的情況，請保留已完成的問卷副本以作日後課堂討論之用。我們將為完成填寫的問卷進行計分，並把您所填寫的問卷和其他人的問卷合併作整體統計分析之用。我們向您保證，您所提供的一切意見及資料，均絕對保密且只用作教學和研究之用。謝謝您的幫忙!

Dear Students,

We have previously obtained your consent to complete this questionnaire, which will help us understand the impacts of the Promotion of Children and Adolescent Development and your developmental characteristics. There are **no correct or incorrect answers** to these questions. **Please answer them honestly based on your knowledge and impression of yourself.** For a better understanding of yourself, please keep a copy of the completed questionnaire for further use in class discussion. Marks will be given for successful completion. Please be assured that your data will be analyzed in an aggregated manner, and the information you provide will be **kept strictly confidential and solely used for education and research purposes**. Thank you for your help!

第一部分 **Part 1**

請小心閱讀下列各句子， 然後在下表圈出一個您認為最能夠代表您的想法的數字。

Please read each sentence carefully and ***circle the number*** that best describes your thoughts.

		非常不同意 **Strongly disagree**	不同意 **Disagree**	有點不同意 **Slightly disagree**	有點同意 **Slightly agree**	同意 **Agree**	非常同意 **Strongly agree**
1.	我懂得怎樣與人溝通。 I know how to communicate with others	1	2	3	4	5	6
2.	我了解人與人相處的規則和要求。 I understand the rules and expectations in interacting with others	1	2	3	4	5	6
3.	我能夠與其他人融洽相處。 I can get along well with others	1	2	3	4	5	6
4.	當我不開心時, 我能夠適當地表達我的情緒。 When I am unhappy, I can appropriately express my emotions	1	2	3	4	5	6

(continued)

(continued)

		非常 不同意 **Strongly disagree**	不同意 **Disagree**	有點 不同意 **Slightly disagree**	有點 同意 **Slightly agree**	同意 **Agree**	非常 同意 **Strongly agree**
5.	在與人發生衝突時, 我通常能夠處理我的情緒。 When I have conflict with others, I can usually manage my emotions	1	2	3	4	5	6
6.	我能夠站在別人的角度看問題和了解他們的感受。 I can stand in the shoes of others	1	2	3	4	5	6
7.	我懂得從不同角度去看事物。 I know how to see things from different angles	1	2	3	4	5	6
8.	我會嘗試用創新的方法去解決我面對的問題。 I try new ways to solve my problems	1	2	3	4	5	6
9.	我懂得分析問題的成因和尋找解決的方法。 I know how to find the causes of and solutions to a problem	1	2	3	4	5	6
10.	我能夠分辨事情的好與壞。 I can differentiate between the good and the bad aspects of things	1	2	3	4	5	6
11.	我能夠以開放的態度面對批評。 I can face criticisms with an open mind	1	2	3	4	5	6

(continued)

(continued)

		非常不同意 **Strongly disagree**	不同意 **Disagree**	有點不同意 **Slightly disagree**	有點同意 **Slightly agree**	同意 **Agree**	非常同意 **Strongly agree**
12.	我能夠表達與其他人不同的意見。 I can express views that are different from others	1	2	3	4	5	6
13.	對於自己的行為,我有較高的道德要求。 I have high moral standards for my behavior	1	2	3	4	5	6
14.	我向他人承諾了會做的事,我會把它完成。 I fulfill my promises	1	2	3	4	5	6
15.	為了賺錢而放棄一些道德原則,並沒有太大問題。(Reverse keyed) It is no big deal to give up some of our moral principles in exchange for money	1	2	3	4	5	6
16.	我有自我檢討的習慣。 I have a habit of self-reflection	1	2	3	4	5	6
17.	我有能力作出明智的抉擇。 I am capable of making wise choices	1	2	3	4	5	6
18.	我對自己所作的決定有信心。 I am confident about my decisions	1	2	3	4	5	6

(continued)

(continued)

		非常 不同意 **Strongly disagree**	不同意 **Disagree**	有點 不同意 **Slightly disagree**	有點 同意 **Slightly agree**	同意 **Agree**	非常 同意 **Strongly agree**
19.	我相信將來發生在我身上的事情,大部分取決於我自己。 I believe that the things that will happen in my life are mostly determined by myself	1	2	3	4	5	6
20.	我是一個有自信的人。 I am a person with self-confidence	1	2	3	4	5	6
21.	我相信自己有領袖的特質及能力。 I believe I have the qualities and abilities of a leader	1	2	3	4	5	6
22.	我有信心解決我將來會面對的問題。 I have the confidence to solve my future problems	1	2	3	4	5	6
23.	我有信心能夠大學畢業。 I have the confidence to graduate from university	1	2	3	4	5	6
24.	我有信心畢業後能夠成為一個有用的人。 I have confidence that I will be a useful person after I graduate	1	2	3	4	5	6

(continued)

(continued)

		非常不同意 **Strongly disagree**	不同意 **Disagree**	有點不同意 **Slightly disagree**	有點同意 **Slightly agree**	同意 **Agree**	非常同意 **Strongly agree**
25.	在很多方面, 我的生活接近我理想中的狀態。 In most ways, my life is close to my ideal	1	2	3	4	5	6
26.	我的生活狀況是極好的。 The conditions of my life are excellent	1	2	3	4	5	6
27.	我對自己的人生感到滿意。 I am satisfied with my life	1	2	3	4	5	6
28.	到目前為止, 我已經取得生命中我想得到的重要東西。 So far, I have gotten the important things I want in life	1	2	3	4	5	6
29.	如果我能夠再活一次, 我依然會選擇現有的生活。 If I could live my life over, I would still choose the life I have now	1	2	3	4	5	6
30.	我的生命很有意義。 My life is meaningful	1	2	3	4	5	6
31.	我已經找到人生的目標。 I have found my purpose in life	1	2	3	4	5	6
32.	我考慮過自殺。 I have considered committing suicide before	1	2	3	4	5	6

(continued)

(continued)

		非常 不同意 **Strongly disagree**	不同意 **Disagree**	有點 不同意 **Slightly disagree**	有點 同意 **Slightly agree**	同意 **Agree**	非常 同意 **Strongly agree**
33.	我相信心靈上的富有比物質上的富有更為重要。 I believe spiritual riches are more important than material prosperity	1	2	3	4	5	6
34.	面對困難時, 我不會輕易放棄。 When I face difficulties, I do not give up easily	1	2	3	4	5	6
35.	我的信念是:「就算明天變得更差, 我仍會好好地生活下去。」 My belief is that even though tomorrow becomes worse, I will still live in a good manner	1	2	3	4	5	6
36.	我相信人生中的困難是可以解決的。 I believe problems in life can be solved	1	2	3	4	5	6
37.	我明白自我發展的重要性。 I understand the importance of self-development	1	2	3	4	5	6
38.	我清楚知道自己的優點和缺點。 I know my strengths and weaknesses	1	2	3	4	5	6
39.	我有能力管理自己的生活。 I am capable of managing my own life	1	2	3	4	5	6

(continued)

(continued)

		非常 不同意 **Strongly disagree**	不同意 **Disagree**	有點 不同意 **Slightly disagree**	有點 同意 **Slightly agree**	同意 **Agree**	非常 同意 **Strongly agree**
40.	我對自己的生活有好的規劃。 I have good planning for my life	1	2	3	4	5	6
41.	我控制自己的言行以免言行失當。 I control my own behavior to avoid stepping out of line	1	2	3	4	5	6
42.	我容易察覺到別人的需求。 I am sensitive to others' needs	1	2	3	4	5	6
43.	別人和我說話時,我會專心聽。 I pay attention to others when they are talking to me	1	2	3	4	5	6
44.	當他人有需要時,我會為他人提供建議。 I offer advice to others when there is a need	1	2	3	4	5	6
45.	我時刻願意幫助有需要的人。 I am always ready to lend a hand to those in need	1	2	3	4	5	6
46.	我懂得如何欣賞他人,即使是那些與我很不相同的人。 I know how to appreciate others, even those who are completely different from me	1	2	3	4	5	6

(continued)

(continued)

		非常 不同意 **Strongly disagree**	不同意 **Disagree**	有點 不同意 **Slightly disagree**	有點 同意 **Slightly agree**	同意 **Agree**	非常 同意 **Strongly agree**
47.	我以尊重的態度對待他人。 I treat others with dignity and respect	1	2	3	4	5	6
48.	我關心他人。 I care about others	1	2	3	4	5	6
49.	我對他人很友善。 I am kind and friendly to others	1	2	3	4	5	6
50.	我樂於學習新知識。 I open my mind to embrace new knowledge	1	2	3	4	5	6
51.	我對生活中的許多事情心懷感恩。 I am grateful for many things in my life	1	2	3	4	5	6
52.	我不喜歡說謊和欺騙。 Lying or cheating is not my way	1	2	3	4	5	6
53.	即使我遇到挫折,我也會堅持不懈地追求我的目標。 I persist in pursuing my goals even though I encounter setbacks	1	2	3	4	5	6
54.	我不喜歡炫耀發生在我身上的好事。 I do not like to show off good things happening to me	1	2	3	4	5	6

(continued)

(continued)

		非常不同意 **Strongly disagree**	不同意 **Disagree**	有點不同意 **Slightly disagree**	有點同意 **Slightly agree**	同意 **Agree**	非常同意 **Strongly agree**
55.	即使遭受反對, 我也會毫不猶豫地抗議我認為錯誤的事情。 I do not hesitate to fight against what I think is wrong despite opposition	1	2	3	4	5	6
56.	我把他人的利益放於自己的利益之前。 I place my interests after the interests of others	1	2	3	4	5	6
57.	我視誠信為人生最重要的部份。 I regard integrity as the most important aspect of life	1	2	3	4	5	6
58.	我樂於尊重規則。 It is my pleasure to obey rules and regulations	1	2	3	4	5	6
59.	如果我做錯了事, 我會感到羞恥。 I would feel ashamed if I had done something wrong	1	2	3	4	5	6
60.	我儘量維持人際交往中的和諧。 I try to maintain harmony in interpersonal relationships	1	2	3	4	5	6
61.	看到不公義的事, 我會挺身而出。 I will fight against injustice	1	2	3	4	5	6

(continued)

(continued)

		非常 不同意 **Strongly disagree**	不同意 **Disagree**	有點 不同意 **Slightly disagree**	有點 同意 **Slightly agree**	同意 **Agree**	非常 同意 **Strongly agree**
62.	我不去嘗試佔有不應得的東西。 I do not attempt to possess anything undeserved	1	2	3	4	5	6
63.	我的所言與所行是一致的。 I live my life in the way I have claimed	1	2	3	4	5	6
64.	在面對得失時, 我通常能保持內心的平靜。 Most of the time, I can keep my mind peaceful in face of gains or losses	1	2	3	4	5	6
65.	領導是一種對自我、他人、團體以及社會的服務。 Leadership is a service for self, others, groups, and society	1	2	3	4	5	6
66.	每一個人每天都有機會實踐領導能力。 Everyone has opportunities to practice leadership every day	1	2	3	4	5	6
67.	領導的效能取決於專業能力、個人品德和關愛他人的能力。 Leadership effectiveness is determined by situational task competencies, character strength, and caring ability	1	2	3	4	5	6

(continued)

(continued)

		非常不同意 **Strongly disagree**	不同意 **Disagree**	有點不同意 **Slightly disagree**	有點同意 **Slightly agree**	同意 **Agree**	非常同意 **Strongly agree**
68.	成功的領袖必須竭盡所能,提升自己的能力及滿足他人的需求。 A successful leader should try his/her best to improve his/her competencies and satisfy others' needs	1	2	3	4	5	6
69.	作為服務型領袖,要向每天接觸到的人提供高品質的服務,不論對方的地位和能力。 A service leader needs to provide high-quality service to the people he/ she contacts, regardless of their position and capacity	1	2	3	4	5	6
70.	服務型領袖需要不斷地提升自己的品德和關愛他人的能力。 A service leader needs to improve his/her character strength and caring ability continuously	1	2	3	4	5	6

第二部分 **Part 2**

這部分將問及一些個人資料, 您提供的資料會絕對保密。請在合適位置選出或填上答案。

This part will ask about your personal information; the information you provide will be kept strictly confidential. Please **choose or fill in your answer** in the space provided.

OFFICIAL USE ONLY

1. 性別 Sex:= 男 male; = 女 female

2. 年齡 Age: ______________

3. 出生日期 Date of birth: ______/_____ / ______ (yyyy/ mm/ dd)
(例子: 如你於 1992 年 1 月 9 日出生, 請填 1992/01/09)
(Example: If you were born on the 9th of January 1992, please fill in 1992/01/09)

4. 學生証編號(中間三個號碼): XXX ___ ___ ___ XXX
Middle three digits of student ID card number
(例子: 如你學生証編號是 09123456d, 請填 XXX 234 XXX)
(Example: If your student ID card number is 09123456d, please fill in XXX 234 XXX)

5. 您父母現時的婚姻狀況是怎樣?
What is the current marital status of your parents?

父親與母親已離婚 Divorced	父親與母親已分居 Separated	父親與母親是夫婦 (第一段婚姻) Married (first marriage)	父親與母親是夫婦 (第二段婚姻) Married (second marriage)	其他 (請註明) Others (please specify)

parent Sex

6. 您覺得您的家庭生活愉快嗎?
Do you think you have a happy family life?

很不愉快 Very unhappy	不愉快 Unhappy	普通 Average	愉快 Happy	很愉快 Very Happy

happiness

完。謝謝!

End. Thank you!

Scoring

Subscales	Variables	Items	Item number
1. Social competence	SC	1–3	3
2. Emotional competence	EC	4–6	3
3. Cognitive competence	CC	7–10	4
4. Behavioral competence	BC	11–12	2
5. Moral competence	MC	13, 14, 15r, 16	4

(continued)

(continued)

Subscales	Variables	Items	Item number
6. Self-determination	SD	17–19	3
7. Clear and positive identity	CPI	20–21	2
8. Belief in future	BF	22–24	3
9. Spirituality	SP	30, 31, 32r, 33	4
10. Resilience	RE	34–36	3
• Composite scores			
• Cognitive-behavioral competencies (CBC)	CC + BC + SD	7–12, 17–19	9
• Positive identity (PI)	CPI + BF	20–24	5
• Positive youth development qualities (PYDQ)	SC + EC + MC + SP + RE	1–6, 13–16, 30–36	17
11. Life satisfaction	LS	25–29	5
12. Service Leadership Scale			
• Self-leadership	SL	37–41	5
• Caring disposition	CD	42–49	8
• Character strengths	CS	50–64	15
• Beliefs and values of Service Leadership	SLV	65–70	6
Total			**70**

Note r = reversed item

Appendix 2: Subjective Outcome Evaluation Form

課程檢討問卷調查

Course Evaluation Form

親愛的同學:

為了幫助我們了解 Promotion of Children and Adolescent Development 課程的成效, 現懇請您完成此問卷。問卷內的問題沒有對或錯的答案, 所以請您憑著您的觀感誠實作答。當您完成這份問卷後, 請將問卷直接交給在場的工作人員。您無需在問卷寫下您的名字, 您所提供的一切意見及資料, 均絕對保密。有關講師在日後絕對不會知道個別同學的答案, 所有的資料只會供研究人員作整體分析之用。如有任何疑問, 請詢問在場的工作人員。謝謝您的幫忙!

Dear Students,

In order to better understand the impacts of the course of Promotion of Children and Adolescent Development, we sincerely invite you to complete this questionnaire.

The questions in the questionnaire **do not have correct or incorrect answers.** Please **honestly answer them based on your views**. After completing the questionnaire, please give it back to our staff directly. You do not need to provide your name on the questionnaire, and the information you provide will be **kept strictly confidential**. The lecturer(s) concerned will not know the responses of individual students, and the data will be used for overall analyses only. Should you have any questions, please contact the staff conducting this survey. Thank you for your help!

第一部分 **Part 1**

請回想一下您對Promotion of Children and Adolescent Development課程內容的觀感, 然後在下表圈出一個您認為最能夠代表您觀感的數字。

Please think about your impression concerning the curriculum contents of the Promotion of Children and Adolescent Development, and then ***circle the number*** that best describes your views.

		非常不同意 Strongly Disagree	不同意 Disagree	中立 Neutral	同意 Agree	非常同意 Strongly Agree	OFFICIAL USE ONLY
1.1	課程的目標很清楚。 The objectives of the curriculum are very clear.	1	2	3	4	5	Cou_01
1.2	課程內容設計得很好。 The content design of the curriculum is very good.	1	2	3	4	5	Cou_02
1.3	教學活動安排得很有條理。 The activities were carefully arranged.	1	2	3	4	5	Cou_03
1.4	課程進行時的氣氛很好。 The classroom atmosphere was very pleasant.	1	2	3	4	5	Cou_04
1.5	在課堂中，同學間有很多交流。 There was much peer interaction amongst the students.	1	2	3	4	5	Cou_05
1.6	我積極參與課程內的活動（包括：討論、分享、遊戲等）。 I participated in class activities actively (including discussions, sharing, games, etc.).	1	2	3	4	5	Cou_06
1.7	在課堂中，我獲得鼓勵去做到最好。 I was encouraged to do my best.	1	2	3	4	5	Cou_07
1.8	課堂中的學習經驗，增加我對這個課程的興趣。 The learning experience enhanced my interest in the course.	1	2	3	4	5	Cou_08
1.9	整體而言，我對這個課程有非常正面的評價。 Overall speaking, I have a very positive evaluation of the course.	1	2	3	4	5	Cou_09
1.10	整體而言，我很喜歡這個課程。 On the whole, I like this course very much.	1	2	3	4	5	Cou_10

第二部分 **Part 2**

請回想一下您對Promotion of Children and Adolescent Development課程講師的觀感, 然後在下表圈出一個您認為最能夠代表您觀感的數字。

Please think about your impression concerning the lecturer(s) of the Promotion of Children and Adolescent Development, and then ***circle the number*** that best describes your views.

		非常不同意 Strongly Disagree	不同意 Disagree	中立 Neutral	同意 Agree	非常同意 Strongly Agree	OFFICIAL USE ONLY
2.1	講師對這個課程有充分的掌握。 The lecturer(s) had a good mastery of the course.	1	2	3	4	5	Lec_01
2.2	講師的準備功夫充足。 The lecturer(s) was (were) well prepared for the lessons.	1	2	3	4	5	Lec_02
2.3	講師的教學技巧良好。 The teaching skills of the lecturer(s) were good.	1	2	3	4	5	Lec_03
2.4	講師的專業態度很好。 The lecturer(s) showed good professional attitudes.	1	2	3	4	5	Lec_04
2.5	講師表現很投入。 The lecturer(s) was (were) very involved.	1	2	3	4	5	Lec_05
		非常不同意 Strongly Disagree	不同意 Disagree	中立 Neutral	同意 Agree	非常同意 Strongly Agree	OFFICIAL USE ONLY
2.6	講師鼓勵同學參與課堂活動。 The lecturer(s) encouraged students to participate in the activities.	1	2	3	4	5	Lec_06
2.7	講師關心同學。 The lecturer(s) cared for the students.	1	2	3	4	5	Lec_07
2.8	同學有需要時，講師樂意提供協助。 The lecturer(s) was (were) ready to offer help to students when needed.	1	2	3	4	5	Lec_08
2.9	導師與同學有很多交流。 The lecturer(s) had much interaction with the students.	1	2	3	4	5	Lec_09
2.10	我對講師的整體表現有非常正面的評價。 Overall speaking, I have a very positive evaluation of the lecturer(s).	1	2	3	4	5	Lec_10

第三部分 **Part 3**

請評估Promotion of Children and Adolescent Development課程對您的幫助有多大, 然後在下表圈出一個您認為最能夠代表您觀感的數字。

Please evaluate to what extent you have benefited from the Promotion of Children and Adolescent Development, and then ***circle the number*** that best describes your views.

		沒有幫助 Unhelpful	幫助不大 Not Very Helpful	不確定 Not sure	頗有幫助 Helpful	有很大幫助 Very Helpful	OFFICIAL USE ONLY
3.1	促進我與人相處的能力。 It has enhanced my social competence.	1	2	3	4	5	eff_01
3.2	增強我表達及處理情緒的能力。 It has improved my ability to express and handle my emotions.	1	2	3	4	5	eff_02
3.3	加強我批判思考的能力。 It has enhanced my critical thinking.	1	2	3	4	5	eff_03
3.4	加強我作出明智抉擇的能力。 It has increased my competence in making sensible and wise choices.	1	2	3	4	5	eff_04
3.5	幫助我作出合符道德標準的決定。 It has helped me make ethical decisions.	1	2	3	4	5	eff_05
3.6	加強我面對逆境的能力。 It has strengthened my resilience in adverse conditions.	1	2	3	4	5	eff_06
3.7	加強我的自信。 It has strengthened my self-confidence.	1	2	3	4	5	eff_07
3.8	幫助我更積極面對將來。 It has helped me face the future with a positive attitude.	1	2	3	4	5	eff_08
3.9	提升我對生活的熱愛。 It has enhanced my love for life.	1	2	3	4	5	eff_09
3.10	幫助我探索人生的意義。 It has helped me explore the meaning of life.	1	2	3	4	5	eff_10
3.11	增強我領導自我的能力。 It has enhanced my ability of self-leadership.	1	2	3	4	5	eff_11
3.12	培養我對他人的憐憫和愛護。 It has helped me cultivate compassion and care for others.	1	2	3	4	5	eff_12
3.13	有助於全面地提升我的品質。 It has helped me enhance my character strengths comprehensively.	1	2	3	4	5	eff_13
3.14	使我明白專業能力、個人品質和關愛他人對於成功領袖的重要性。 It has enabled me to understand the importance of situational task competencies, character strength, and caring disposition in successful leadership.	1	2	3	4	5	eff_14
3.15	培養我貢獻社會的責任感。 It has promoted my sense of responsibility in serving the society.	1	2	3	4	5	eff_15
3.16	促進我的整體成長。 It has promoted my overall development.	1	2	3	4	5	eff_16
3.17	課程涵蓋的理論、研究及概念使我明白成功的服務型領袖的基本特質。 The theories, research, and concepts covered in the course have enabled me to understand the characteristics of successful service leaders.	1	2	3	4	5	eff_17
3.18	課程涵蓋的理論、研究及概念幫助我整合成功的服務型領袖的基本特質。 The theories, research, and concepts covered in the course have helped me synthesize the characteristics of successful service leaders.	1	2	3	4	5	eff_18

第四部分 **Part 4**

您會否建議您的朋友報讀這個課程？請***圈出***一個您認為最能夠代表您意見的***數字***。
Will you suggest your friends to take this course? Please ***circle the number*** that best describes your views.

1	2	3	4	5
一定不會 Definitely Will Not Suggest	不會 Will Not Suggest	不確定 Not Sure	會 Will Suggest	一定會 Definitely Will Suggest

OFFICIAL USE ONLY
Q_04

第五部分 Part 5

如果將來有機會，您會否再報讀這類課程？請***圈出***一個您認為最能夠代表您意見的***數字***。
Will you participate in similar courses again in the future? Please ***circle the number*** that best describes your views.

1	2	3	4	5
一定不會 Definitely Will Not Suggest	不會 Will Not Suggest	不確定 Not Sure	會 Will Suggest	一定會 Definitely Will Suggest

OFFICIAL USE ONLY
Q_05

第六部分 Part 6

整體而言，您對這個課程有怎樣的滿意程度？請***圈出***一個您認為最能夠代表您意見的***數字***。
On the whole, are you satisfied with this course? Please ***circle the number*** that best describes your views.

1	2	3	4	5
十分不滿意 Very Dissatisfied	頗不滿意 Moderately Dissatisfied	中立 Neutral	滿意 Satisfied	十分滿意 Very Satisfied

OFFICIAL USE ONLY
Q_06

第七部分 Part 7

請完成下列各題:

Please complete the following items:

7.1 請寫出**一項或以上**您從該課程中學到最重要的東西：（如沒有，請填「沒有」。）
Please write down one or more important thing(s) you have learned in this course. If there is no comment, please write "NIL".

OFFICIAL USE ONLY

Q_7.1

7.2 請寫出**一項或以上**您認為在該課程中最值得欣賞的地方：（如沒有，請填「沒有」。）
Please write down one or more thing(s) that you appreciate most in this course. If there is no comment, please write "NIL".

OFFICIAL USE ONLY

Q_7.2

7.3 您對該課程的講師有何意見？（如沒有，請填「沒有」。）
Do you have any comments about the lecturer(s)? If there is no comment, please write "NIL".

OFFICIAL USE ONLY

Q_7.3

7.4 您認為該課程有哪些地方需要改善？（如沒有，請填「沒有」。）
What aspects of this course should be improved? If there is no comment, please write "NIL".

OFFICIAL USE ONLY

Q_7.4

第八部分 **Part 8**

請提供您的個人資料:

Please provide your demographic information:

1	出生日期 Date of birth: / / (yyyy/mm/dd) (例子：如您於 1992 年 1 月 9 日出生， 請填 1992/01/09) (Example: If you were born on the 9th of January 1992, please fill in1992/01/09)
3	學號最后四个数字 (Last 4 digits of Student ID) (北大的學生，請填你在北大的學號；香港理工大學的學生，請填你在香港理工大學的學號) (For the students of Peking University, please fill in your SID of PekingU; For the students of The Hong Kong Polytechnic University, please fill in your SID of PolyU)
5	日期 Date: ______ / ______ / ______ (yyyy/mm/dd)

完。謝謝！
End. Thank you!

Appendix 3: Objective Outcome Evaluation-Service Recipient

服务学习夏令营 (问卷 **I**)

Service-Learning Summer Camp (Questionnaire I)

小朋友们好:

为了解儿童成长及评估希望旅程服务学习夏令营的成效， 我们现邀请你完成这份问卷。你所提供的答案会绝对保密, 并仅作为这次评估使用, 请放心填写。你的家长和老师都不会看到你所填写的内容。

每页问卷都有答题指引, 回答问题前, 请确定你已经清楚问卷的答题要求。

本问卷没有对错之分，只需如实作答即可。回答问题时，请不要花太多时间思考每道题目, 只要根据你的第一反应来回答, 并且不要和别人讨论问卷内容, 谢谢你的合作!

Dear all,

To understand how the children grow after the Service-Learning activities and assess the effectiveness of the Journey for Hope Service-Learning Camp, we now invite you to complete this questionnaire. The answers you provide will be kept confidential and used only for this assessment; please feel free to fill them out. Neither your parents nor your teachers will see your answers.

There are instructions on each page of the questionnaire. Before answering questions, make sure you have understood the requirements of the questionnaire.

There are no right or wrong answers in this questionnaire; please answer truthfully. When answering questions, please do not spend too much time thinking about each question and answer them according to your first reaction. Do not discuss the questionnaire with others. Thank you for your cooperation.

第一部分（A）

请如实填写你的个人资料，你提供的答案会绝对保密。你可以在横线上填上适当的答案，或在□_内打√。

1. 你现在所就读的年级：___ 班级：______ 座号：_______
2. 你在2021年7月希望旅程服务学习夏令营中所在的班级：_______
3. 你的性别： 1）□男 2）□女
4. 你的年龄：____ 周岁 出生年月：_______
5. 你的出生地点： 杭州 杭州以外地区 - 请注明省、市、县、乡：_______
6. 你的户籍： 1）□农村户口 2）□城市户口
7. 你已在杭州居住多长时间： ____年
8. 与你同住的家庭成员有：（可选择多于一个的答案）
   1）父亲 2）继父 3）母亲
   4）继母 5）爷爷 6）奶奶
   7）外公 8）外婆 9）哥哥
   10）姐姐 11）弟弟 12）妹妹
   13）其他人：_____
9. 平时谁是你的主要照顾者：（可选择多于一个的答案）
   1）父亲 2）继父 3）母亲
   4）继母 5）爷爷 6）奶奶
   7）外公 8）外婆 9）哥哥
   10）姐姐 11）其他人：______
10. 父亲目前的工作状况：（单选）
   1）全职工作 2）兼职工作 3）无业
   4）退休 5）不知道
11. 母亲目前的工作状况：（单选）
   1）全职工作 2）兼职工作 3）无业
   4）退休 5）不知道
12. 父亲的教育程度：（单选）
   1）没有接受任何正式教育 2）小学一年级至五年级 3）小学毕业
   4）初中毕业 5）高中毕业 6）大专
   7）大学或以上 8）不知道
13. 母亲的教育程度：（单选）
   1）没有接受任何正式教育 2）小学一年级至五年级 3）小学毕业
   4）初中毕业 5）高中毕业 6）大专
   7）大学或以上 8）不知道
14. 你的家庭每月收入大约：
   1）3000 元或以下 2）3001 元-5000 元 3）5001 元-10000 元
   4）10000 元或以上 5）不知道

Part One (A)

Please fill in your personal information truthfully. The answers you provide will be kept confidential. You can fill in the appropriate answer on the horizontal line or type √ inside. □

1.	Your current grade:	Class: _______	Seat number: _______
2.	Which class were you in during the Journey for Hope Service-Learning Summer Camp:		
3.	Your gender:	1) Male	2) Female
4.	Your age: _______	Date of birth: Year:_______ Month:_______ Date: _______	
5.	Your place of birth:	Hangzhou	Areas outside Hangzhou—Please specify province, city, county, and township:
6.	Your household registration:	1) Rural	2) Urban
7.	How long have you lived in Hangzhou:		_______ Years
8.	The family members you live with: (you can choose more than one answer)		
	1) Father	2) Stepfather	3) Mother
	4) Stepmother	5) Grandfather	6) Grandmother
	7) Grandfather	8) Grandmother	9) Older brother
	10) Older sister	11) Younger brother	12) Younger sister
	13) Others: _______		
9.	Who is your primary caregiver: (you can choose more than one answer)		
	1) Father	2) Stepfather	3) Mother
	4) Stepmother	5) Grandfather	6) Grandmother
	7) Grandfather	8) Grandmother	9) Older brother
	10) Older sister	11) Others: _______	
10.	Father's current work status: (choose one answer)		
	1) Full-time employment	2) Part-time employment	3) Unemployed
	4) Retired	5) I don't know	
11.	Mother's current work status: (choose one answer)		
	1) Full-time employment	2) Part-time employment	3) Unemployed
	4) Retired	5) I don't know	
12.	Father's educational background: (choose one answer)		
	1) No formal education	2) Primary 1 to 5	3) Primary school graduation
	4) Junior high school graduation	5) High school graduation	6) College
	7) University or above	8) I don't know	
13.	Mother's educational background: (choose one answer)		
	1) No formal education	2) Primary 1 to 5	3) Primary school graduation

(continued)

(continued)

	4) Junior high school graduation	5) High school graduation	6) College
	7) University or above	8) I don't know	
14.	Your family monthly income is approximately:		
	1) 3000 RMB or less	2) 3001 RMB-5000 RMB	3) 5001 RMB-10000 RMB
	4) 10,000 RMB or more	5) I don't know	

第二部分 (B) Part Two (B)

请仔细阅读下列句子， 然后圈出一个你认为最能够代表你的想法或真实情况的答案。

Please read the following sentences carefully, and then circle one answer that you think best represents what you think or what is true.

		非常不同意 **Strongly disagree**	不同意 **Disagree**	有点不同意 **Slightly disagree**	有点同意 **Slightly agree**	同意 **Agree**	非常同意 **Strongly agree**
1	我对学习知识很感兴趣。 I am very interested in learning knowledge	1	2	3	4	5	6
2	我对英语方面的课程很感兴趣。 I am very interested in the English courses	1	2	3	4	5	6
3	我对科学方面的课程很感兴趣。 I am very interested in the Science courses	1	2	3	4	5	6
4	我对健康教育方面的课程很感兴趣。 I am very interested in the Health Education courses	1	2	3	4	5	6
5	我对个人成长方面的课程很感兴趣。 I am very interested in the courses on personal growth	1	2	3	4	5	6
6	我掌握了很多知识。 I have mastered a lot of knowledge	1	2	3	4	5	6

(continued)

(continued)

		非常 不同意 **Strongly disagree**	不同意 **Disagree**	有点 不同意 **Slightly disagree**	有点 同意 **Slightly agree**	同意 **Agree**	非常 同意 **Strongly agree**
7	我掌握了很多英语知识。 I have mastered a lot of English knowledge	1	2	3	4	5	6
8	我掌握了很多科学知识。 I have mastered a lot of scientific knowledge	1	2	3	4	5	6
9	我掌握了很多关于健康教育方面的知识。 I have learned a lot about health education	1	2	3	4	5	6
10	我掌握了很多关于个人成长方面的知识。 I have acquired a lot of knowledge about my personal growth	1	2	3	4	5	6

Subscales	**Items**
Study interest	B1–B5
Knowledge	B6–B10

第三部分 **(C) Part Three (C)**

请仔细阅读下列句子， 然后圈出一个你认为最能够代表你的想法或真实情况的答案。

Please read the following sentences carefully, and then circle one answer that you think best represents what you think or what is true.

		非常 不同意 **Strongly disagree**	不同意 **Disagree**	有点 不同意 **Slightly disagree**	有点 同意 **Slightly agree**	同意 **Agree**	非常 同意 **Strongly agree**
1.	我懂得怎样与人沟通。 I know how to communicate with people	1	2	3	4	5	6

(continued)

(continued)

		非常 不同意 **Strongly disagree**	不同意 **Disagree**	有点 不同意 **Slightly disagree**	有点 同意 **Slightly agree**	同意 **Agree**	非常 同意 **Strongly agree**
2.	我了解人与人相处的规则和要求。 I understand the rules and requirements of getting people together	1	2	3	4	5	6
3.	我能够与其他人融洽相处。 I can get along well with other people	1	2	3	4	5	6
4.	当我不开心时，我能够适当地表达我的情绪。 When I am unhappy, I can express my emotions appropriately	1	2	3	4	5	6
5.	在与人发生冲突时，我通常能够处理我的情绪。 I am usually able to deal with my emotions in conflicts with people	1	2	3	4	5	6
6.	我能够站在别人的角度看问题和了解他们的感受。 I can look at other people's point of view and understand their feelings	1	2	3	4	5	6

(continued)

(continued)

		非常不同意 **Strongly disagree**	不同意 **Disagree**	有点不同意 **Slightly disagree**	有点同意 **Slightly agree**	同意 **Agree**	非常同意 **Strongly agree**
7.	我懂得从不同角度去看事物。 I know how to see things from different angles	1	2	3	4	5	6
8.	我会尝试用创新的方法去解决我面对的问题。 I try new ways to solve my problems	1	2	3	4	5	6
9.	我懂得分析问题的成因和寻找解决的方法。 I know how to find the causes of and solutions to a problem	1	2	3	4	5	6
10.	我能够分辨事情的好与坏。 I can differentiate between the good and the bad aspects of things	1	2	3	4	5	6
11.	我能够以开放的态度面对批评。 I can face criticisms with an open mind	1	2	3	4	5	6
12.	我能够表达与其他人不同的意见。 I can express views that are different from others	1	2	3	4	5	6

(continued)

(continued)

		非常 不同意 **Strongly disagree**	不同意 **Disagree**	有点 不同意 **Slightly disagree**	有点 同意 **Slightly agree**	同意 **Agree**	非常 同意 **Strongly agree**
13.	对于自己的行为, 我有较高的道德要求。 I have high moral standards for my behaviors	1	2	3	4	5	6
14.	我向他人承诺了会做的事, 我会把它完成。 I fulfill my promises	1	2	3	4	5	6
15.	为了赚钱而放弃一些道德原则, 并没有太大问题。 It is no big deal to give up some of our moral principles in exchange for money	1	2	3	4	5	6
16.	我有自我检讨的习惯。 I have a habit of self-reflection	1	2	3	4	5	6
17.	面对困难时, 我不会轻易放弃。 In the face of difficulties, I will not give up easily	1	2	3	4	5	6

(continued)

(continued)

		非常 不同意 **Strongly disagree**	不同意 **Disagree**	有点 不同意 **Slightly disagree**	有点 同意 **Slightly agree**	同意 **Agree**	非常 同意 **Strongly agree**
18.	我的信念是: "就算明天变得更差, 我仍会好好地生活下去。" My belief is: "Even if tomorrow becomes worse, I will still live a better life."	1	2	3	4	5	6
19.	我相信生活中的困难是可以解决的。 I believe that the difficulties in life can be solved	1	2	3	4	5	6
20.	当我需要帮助时, 我相信我的父母 (或监护人)一定会帮助我。 When I need help, I believe that my parents (or guardian) will help me	1	2	3	4	5	6
21.	当我需要帮助时, 我相信我的朋友一定会帮助我。 When I need help, I am sure that my friends will help me	1	2	3	4	5	6

(continued)

(continued)

		非常不同意 **Strongly disagree**	不同意 **Disagree**	有点不同意 **Slightly disagree**	有点同意 **Slightly agree**	同意 **Agree**	非常同意 **Strongly agree**
22.	当我需要帮助时, 我相信我的老师一定会帮助我。 When I need help, I am sure that my teachers will help me	1	2	3	4	5	6
23.	我喜欢我的老师和同学。 I like my teachers and classmates	1	2	3	4	5	6
24.	在我的生活里, 有很多关心我的好朋友。 In my life, there are many good friends who care about me	1	2	3	4	5	6
25.	我的父母 (或监护人) 十分关心我。 My parents (or guardians) care very much about me	1	2	3	4	5	6
26.	我关心社会上遭遇不幸的人。 I care about those who encounter misfortune in society	1	2	3	4	5	6
27.	如有机会, 我会参加志愿者服务。 If I have the opportunity, I will participate in the volunteer service	1	2	3	4	5	6

(continued)

(continued)

		非常不同意 **Strongly disagree**	不同意 **Disagree**	有点不同意 **Slightly disagree**	有点同意 **Slightly agree**	同意 **Agree**	非常同意 **Strongly agree**
28.	我同意每个人都应该受到法律的约束。 I agree that everyone should be bound by the law	1	2	3	4	5	6
29.	我乐于遵守校规。 I am happy to follow the school rules	1	2	3	4	5	6
30.	如果我做错事,我会感到羞耻。 I will feel ashamed if I do something wrong	1	2	3	4	5	6
31.	我与他人相处得很好。 I get along very well with other people	1	2	3	4	5	6
32.	我会做对集体 (例如: 班级、小组) 有益的事情。 I will do something beneficial for the group (for example, class, group)	1	2	3	4	5	6
33.	我会用自己喜欢被对待的方式去对待朋友。 I will treat my friends in the way that I like to be treated	1	2	3	4	5	6

(continued)

(continued)

		非常 不同意 **Strongly disagree**	不同意 **Disagree**	有点 不同意 **Slightly disagree**	有点 同意 **Slightly agree**	同意 **Agree**	非常 同意 **Strongly agree**
34.	我会友善对待与自己不同的孩子。 I will be friendly to the children who are different from myself	1	2	3	4	5	6
35.	当别的孩子不开心时，我会尝试让他们高兴起来。 When the other kids are not happy, I will try to make them happy	1	2	3	4	5	6
36.	我是别人的好朋友。 I am someone else's good friend	1	2	3	4	5	6

Subscales	**Items**
Social competence	C1–C3
Emotional competence	C4–C6
Cognitive competence	C7–C10
Behavioral competence	C11–C12
Moral competence	C13–C16
Resilience	C17–C19
Bonding	C20–C25
Prosocial norms	C26–C30
Prosocial behavior	C31–C36

第四部分 **(D) Part Four (D)**

请仔细阅读下列句子， 然后圈出一个你认为最能够代表你的想法或真实情况的答案。

Please read the following sentences carefully, and then circle one answer that you think best represents what you think or what is true.

		非常 不同意 **Strongly disagree**	不同意 **Disagree**	有点 不同意 **Slightly disagree**	有点 同意 **Slightly agree**	同意 **Agree**	非常 同意 **Strongly agree**
1.	我有能力作出明智的抉择。 I am capable of making wise choices	1	2	3	4	5	6
2.	我对自己所作的决定有信心。 I am confident about my decisions	1	2	3	4	5	6
3.	我相信将来发生在我身上的事情, 大部分取决于我自己。 I believe things that will happen in my life are mostly determined by my efforts	1	2	3	4	5	6
4.	我是一个有自信的人。 I am a person with self-confidence	1	2	3	4	5	6
5.	我相信自己有领袖的特质及能力。 I believe I have the qualities and abilities of a leader	1	2	3	4	5	6
6.	我有信心解决我将来会面对的问题。 I have the confidence to solve my future problems	1	2	3	4	5	6
7.	我有信心能够大学毕业。 I have the confidence to graduate from university	1	2	3	4	5	6

(continued)

(continued)

		非常 不同意 **Strongly disagree**	不同意 **Disagree**	有点 不同意 **Slightly disagree**	有点 同意 **Slightly agree**	同意 **Agree**	非常 同意 **Strongly agree**
8.	我有信心毕业后能够成为一个有用的人。 I have confidence that I will be a useful person after I graduate	1	2	3	4	5	6
9.	在很多方面, 我的生活接近我理想中的状态。 In most ways, my life is close to my ideal	1	2	3	4	5	6
10.	我的生活状况是极好的。 The conditions of my life are excellent	1	2	3	4	5	6
11.	我对自己的人生感到满意。 I am satisfied with my life	1	2	3	4	5	6
12.	到目前为止, 我已经取得生命中我想得到的重要东西。 So far, I have gotten the important things I want in life	1	2	3	4	5	6
13.	如果我能够再活一次, 我依然会选择现有的生活。 If I could live my life over, I would still choose the life I have now	1	2	3	4	5	6

Subscales	**Items**
Self-determination	D1–D3
Clear and positive identity	D4–D5

(continued)

(continued)

Subscales	Items
Belief in future	D6–D8
Life satisfaction	D9–D13

第五部分 (E) Part Five (E)

请仔细阅读下列句子， 然后圈出一个你认为最能够代表你的想法或真实情况的答案。

Please read the following sentences carefully, and then circle one answer that you think best represents what you think or what is true.

		非常 不同意 **Strongly disagree**	不同意 **Disagree**	有点 不同意 **Slightly disagree**	有点 同意 **Slightly agree**	同意 **Agree**	非常 同意 **Strongly agree**
1.	我明白自我发展的重要性。 I understand the importance of self-development	1	2	3	4	5	6
2.	我清楚知道自己的优点和缺点。 I know my strengths and weaknesses	1	2	3	4	5	6
3.	我有能力管理自己的生活。 I am capable of managing my own life	1	2	3	4	5	6
4.	我对自己的生活有好的规划。 I have good planning for my life	1	2	3	4	5	6
5.	我控制自己的言行以免言行失当。 I control my own behavior to avoid stepping out of line	1	2	3	4	5	6
6.	我容易察觉到别人的需求。 I am sensitive to others' needs	1	2	3	4	5	6

(continued)

(continued)

		非常 不同意 **Strongly disagree**	不同意 **Disagree**	有点 不同意 **Slightly disagree**	有点 同意 **Slightly agree**	同意 **Agree**	非常 同意 **Strongly agree**
7.	别人和我说话时,我会专心听。 I pay attention to others when they are talking to me	1	2	3	4	5	6
8.	当他人有需要时,我会为他人提供建议。 I offer advice to others when there is a need	1	2	3	4	5	6
9.	我时刻愿意帮助有需要的人。 I am always ready to lend a hand to those in need	1	2	3	4	5	6
10.	我懂得如何欣赏他人, 即使是那些与我很不相同的人。 I know how to appreciate others, even those who are completely different from me	1	2	3	4	5	6
11.	我以尊重的态度对待他人。 I treat others with dignity and respect	1	2	3	4	5	6
12.	我关心他人。 I care about others	1	2	3	4	5	6
13.	我对他人很友善。 I am kind and friendly to others	1	2	3	4	5	6
14.	我乐于学习新知识。 I open my mind to embrace new knowledge	1	2	3	4	5	6

(continued)

(continued)

		非常不同意 **Strongly disagree**	不同意 **Disagree**	有点不同意 **Slightly disagree**	有点同意 **Slightly agree**	同意 **Agree**	非常同意 **Strongly agree**
15.	我对生活中的许多事情心怀感恩。 I am grateful for many things in my life	1	2	3	4	5	6
16.	我不喜欢说谎和欺骗。 Lying or cheating is not my way	1	2	3	4	5	6
17.	即使我遇到挫折，我也会坚持不懈地追求我的目标。 I persist in pursuing my goals even though I encounter setbacks	1	2	3	4	5	6
18.	我不喜欢炫耀发生在我身上的好事。 I do not like to show off good things happening to me	1	2	3	4	5	6
19.	即使遭受反对，我也会毫不犹豫地抗议我认为错误的事情。 I do not hesitate to fight against what I think is wrong despite opposition	1	2	3	4	5	6
20.	我把他人的利益放于自己的利益之前。 I place my interests after the interests of others	1	2	3	4	5	6
21.	我视诚信为人生最重要的部份。 I regard integrity as the most important aspect of life	1	2	3	4	5	6

(continued)

(continued)

		非常 不同意 **Strongly disagree**	不同意 **Disagree**	有点 不同意 **Slightly disagree**	有点 同意 **Slightly agree**	同意 **Agree**	非常 同意 **Strongly agree**
22.	我乐于尊重规则。 It is my pleasure to obey rules and regulations	1	2	3	4	5	6
23.	如果我做错了事，我会感到羞耻。 I would feel ashamed if I have done something wrong	1	2	3	4	5	6
24.	我尽量维持人际交往中的和谐。 I try to maintain harmony in interpersonal relationships	1	2	3	4	5	6
25.	看到不公义的事，我会挺身而出。 I will fight against injustice	1	2	3	4	5	6
26.	我不去尝试占有不应得的东西。 I do not attempt to possess anything undeserved	1	2	3	4	5	6
27.	我的所言与所行是一致的。 I live my life in the way I have claimed	1	2	3	4	5	6
28.	在面对得失时，我通常能保持内心的平静。 Most of the time, I can keep my mind peaceful in face of gains or losses	1	2	3	4	5	6

Subscales	**Items**
Self-leadership	E1–E5
Caring disposition	E6–E13
Character strength	E14–E28

完, 谢谢
End. Thank you!

Appendix 4: Recipients' View of the Camp

"希望旅程" 夏令营评估问卷

"Journey for Hope" Summer Camp

Assessment Questionnaire

請仔細閱讀下列句子， 然後圈出一個你認為最能夠代表你的想法或真實情況的答案。

Please read the following sentences carefully, and then circle one answer that you think best represents what you think or what is true.

1. 对服务项目的观感: **Views about the service program:**	非常不同意 **Strongly disagree**	不同意 **Disagree**	有点不同意 **Slightly disagree**	有点同意 **Slightly agree**	同意 **Agree**	非常同意 **Strongly agree**
1.1. 服务项目设计的很好。 This service program was well-designed	1	2	3	4	5	6
1.2. 提供的服务形式适宜。 The form of service provided was appropriate	1	2	3	4	5	6
1.3. 服务中活动的气氛很好。 The atmosphere of the activities in the service was good	1	2	3	4	5	6
1.4. 服务中我们同学之间有很多交流。 There was a lot of communication between our classmates during the service	1	2	3	4	5	6

(continued)

(continued)

1. 对服务项目的观感: **Views about the service program:**	非常不同意 **Strongly disagree**	不同意 **Disagree**	有点不同意 **Slightly disagree**	有点同意 **Slightly agree**	同意 **Agree**	非常同意 **Strongly agree**
1.5. 我积极参与服务中的活动。 I actively participated in activities during the services	1	2	3	4	5	6
1.6. 我获得鼓励去做到最好。 I was encouraged to do my best	1	2	3	4	5	6
1.7. 这次的学习经验增进了我对这个项目的兴趣。 This learning experience increased my interest in this project	1	2	3	4	5	6
1.8. 整体而言，我对这次的服务项目有正面评价。 Overall, I have a positive evaluation of this service	1	2	3	4	5	6

2. 对老师的观感 (理大大学学生): **Views about the service provider (PolyU students):**	非常不同意 **Strongly disagree**	不同意 **Disagree**	有点不同意 **Slightly disagree**	有点同意 **Slightly agree**	同意 **Agree**	非常同意 **Strongly agree**
2.1. 老师对服务的准备功夫充足。 The teachers were well prepared for the service	1	2	3	4	5	6

(continued)

(continued)

2. 对老师的观感 (理大大学学生): **Views about the service provider (PolyU students):**	非常不同意 **Strongly disagree**	不同意 **Disagree**	有点不同意 **Slightly disagree**	有点同意 **Slightly agree**	同意 **Agree**	非常同意 **Strongly agree**
2.2. 老师的专业态度很好。 The teacher's professional attitude was very good	1	2	3	4	5	6
2.3. 老师理解我的需求和潜力。 The teachers understood my needs and potential	1	2	3	4	5	6
2.4. 老师表现的很投入。 The teachers were very engaged	1	2	3	4	5	6
2.5. 老师关心我。 The teachers cared about me	1	2	3	4	5	6
2.6. 在我有需要的时候, 老师随时乐意提供帮助。 The teachers were always willing to help me when I needed it	1	2	3	4	5	6
2.7. 老师与我们有很多交流。 The teachers communicated a lot with us	1	2	3	4	5	6

(continued)

(continued)

2. 对老师的观感 (理大大学学生): **Views about the service provider (PolyU students):**	非常不同意 **Strongly disagree**	不同意 **Disagree**	有点不同意 **Slightly disagree**	有点同意 **Slightly agree**	同意 **Agree**	非常同意 **Strongly agree**
2.8. 我对老师的整体表现有正面评价。 I had a positive opinion of the teachers' overall performance	1	2	3	4	5	6

3. 服务项目对我的帮助: **The extent to which the service program has helped me:**	毫无帮助 **Not helpful at all**	没有帮助 **Unhelpful**	帮助不大 **Not very helpful**	有些帮助 **Slightly helpful**	颇有帮助 **Helpful**	有很大帮助 **Very helpful**
3.1. 加强我面对逆境的能力。 It has strengthened my resilience	1	2	3	4	5	6
3.2. 帮助我积极面对未来。 It has helped me face the future with a positive attitude	1	2	3	4	5	6
3.3. 提高我的自信。 It has improved my self-confidence	1	2	3	4	5	6
3.4. 开阔了我的视野。 It has broadened my horizons	1	2	3	4	5	6
3.5. 增强了我对学习的兴趣。 It has reinforced my interest in learning	1	2	3	4	5	6

(continued)

(continued)

3. 服务项目对我的帮助: **The extent to which the service program has helped me:**	毫无帮助 **Not helpful at all**	没有帮助 **Unhelpful**	帮助不大 **Not very helpful**	有些帮助 **Slightly helpful**	颇有帮助 **Helpful**	有很大帮助 **Very helpful**
3.6. 提高了我关心他人的能力。 It has strengthened my ability to care for other people	1	2	3	4	5	6
3.7. 帮助我与健康的成人建立良好关系 (例如, 老师, 父母, 等等)。 It has helped me build good relationships with healthy adults. (e.g., teachers, parents, etc.)	1	2	3	4	5	6
3.8. 提升了我对未来生活的抱负。 It has promoted my aspirations in life	1	2	3	4	5	6
3.9. 促进我的整体发展。 It has enriched my overall development	1	2	3	4	5	6
3.10. 总体而言, 我对这次的服务项目感到满意。 Overall speaking, I have a positive evaluation of the service program	1	2	3	4	5	6

4.	请回答以下问题: **Please complete the following questions:**	
4.1	我会用以下三个词或短语(例如,有趣,有活力,温暖,等等)来形容我对这次服务项目的感受,看法,和体验: I would use the following THREE words or phrases (e.g., fun, energetic, warm, etc.) to describe my feeling, perception, or experience of this program: 1) ____________________ 2) ____________________ 3) ____________________	
4.2	请用一个比喻(例如某个物品,事件,或状态)来代表这次服务项目(例如,生活中的指南针,一次愉快的旅行,等),并简要说明这个比喻的含义是甚么。 Consider a metaphor (e.g., an object, event, or state) that can represent the service program (e.g., a compass in life, a pleasant trip, etc.). Give a brief explanation of the meaning of the metaphor.	
	我会用 ________________ I would use ____________________	来代表这次的服务项目,因为: ____________ to represent this service project because: ______ ________

Appendix 5: Service Partner Evaluation Questionnaire

服务合作单位评估问卷

Service Partner Evaluation Questionnaire

請仔細閱讀下列句子, 然後圈出一個你認為最能夠代表你的想法或真實情況的答案。

Please read the following sentences carefully, and then circle one answer that you think best represents what you think or what is true.

1. 对服务项目的观感: **Views about the service program:**	非常不同意 **Strongly disagree**	不同意 **Disagree**	有点不同意 **Slightly disagree**	有点同意 **Slightly agree**	同意 **Agree**	非常同意 **Strongly agree**
1.1. 服务项目设计的很好。 This service program was well-designed	1	2	3	4	5	6
1.2. 提供的服务形式适宜。 The form of the service provided was appropriate	1	2	3	4	5	6

(continued)

(continued)

1. 对服务项目的观感: **Views about the service program:**	非常不同意 **Strongly disagree**	不同意 **Disagree**	有点不同意 **Slightly disagree**	有点同意 **Slightly agree**	同意 **Agree**	非常同意 **Strongly agree**
1.3. 服务中活动的气氛很好。The process of delivering the service activities was pleasant	1	2	3	4	5	6
1.4. 提供的服务能迎合服务对象的需要。The services provided could meet the needs of the clients	1	2	3	4	5	6
1.5. 服务项目提升了社区 (例如, 学校) 积极的氛围。Service projects promoted a positive atmosphere in the community (e.g., school)	1	2	3	4	5	6
1.6. 对本次服务项目的观察和了解提高了我对参与这类项目的兴趣。The observation and understanding of this service project had increased my interest in participating in such projects	1	2	3	4	5	6

(continued)

(continued)

1. 对服务项目的观感: **Views about the service program:**	非常不同意 **Strongly disagree**	不同意 **Disagree**	有点不同意 **Slightly disagree**	有点同意 **Slightly agree**	同意 **Agree**	非常同意 **Strongly agree**
1.7. 整体而言，这次的项目对服务对象有所裨益。 Overall speaking, the project has benefited the clients	1	2	3	4	5	6
1.8. 整体而言，我对这次的服务项目有正面评价。 Overall speaking, I have a positive evaluation of the service program	1	2	3	4	5	6

2. 对服务者的观感 (理大大学学生): **Views about the service provider (PolyU students):**	非常不同意 **Strongly disagree**	不同意 **Disagree**	有点不同意 **Slightly disagree**	有点同意 **Slightly agree**	同意 **Agree**	非常同意 **Strongly agree**
2.1. 理工学生对服务的准备功夫充足。 The teachers were well prepared for the service	1	2	3	4	5	6
2.2. 理工学生的专业态度很好。 The teachers' professional attitude was very good	1	2	3	4	5	6

(continued)

(continued)

2. 对服务者的观感 (理大大学生): **Views about the service provider (PolyU students):**	非常不同意 **Strongly disagree**	不同意 **Disagree**	有点不同意 **Slightly disagree**	有点同意 **Slightly agree**	同意 **Agree**	非常同意 **Strongly agree**
2.3. 理工学生理解服务对象的需求和潜力。 The teachers understood the clients' needs and potential	1	2	3	4	5	6
2.4. 理工学生表现的很投入。 The teachers were very engaged	1	2	3	4	5	6
2.5. 理工学生关心服务对象。 The teachers cared about the clients	1	2	3	4	5	6
2.6. 在服务对象有需要的时候,理工学生随时乐意提供帮助。 The teachers were always willing to help the clients when they needed it	1	2	3	4	5	6
2.7. 理工学生与服务对象有很多交流。 The teachers communicated a lot with the clients	1	2	3	4	5	6
2.8. 我对理工学生在服务中的整体表现有正面评价。 I had a positive opinion of the teachers' overall performance	1	2	3	4	5	6

3. 服务项目对服务对象的帮助: **The extent to which the service program has helped the clients:**	毫无帮助 **Not helpful at all**	没有帮助 **Unhelpful**	帮助不大 **Not very helpful**	有些帮助 **Slightly helpful**	颇有帮助 **Helpful**	有很大帮助 **Very helpful**
3.1. 加强服务对象面对逆境的能力。 It has strengthened the clients' resilience	1	2	3	4	5	6
3.2. 帮助服务对象积极面对未来。 It has helped the clients face the future with a positive attitude	1	2	3	4	5	6
3.3. 提高服务对象的自信。 It has improved the clients' self-confidence	1	2	3	4	5	6
3.4. 开阔了服务对象的视野。 It has broadened the clients' horizons	1	2	3	4	5	6
3.5. 增强了服务对象对学习的兴趣。 It has reinforced the clients' interest in learning	1	2	3	4	5	6
3.6. 提高了服务对象关心他人的能力。 It has strengthened the clients' ability to care for other people	1	2	3	4	5	6

(continued)

(continued)

3. 服务项目对服务对象的帮助: **The extent to which the service program has helped the clients:**	毫无帮助 **Not helpful at all**	没有帮助 **Unhelpful**	帮助不大 **Not very helpful**	有些帮助 **Slightly helpful**	颇有帮助 **Helpful**	有很大帮助 **Very helpful**
3.7. 帮助服务对象与健康的成人建立良好关系 (例如, 老师, 父母, 等等)。 It has helped the clients build good relationships with healthy adults (e.g., teachers, parents)	1	2	3	4	5	6
3.8. 提升了服务对象对未来生活的抱负。 It has promoted the clients' aspirations in life	1	2	3	4	5	6
3.9. 促进服务对象的整体发展。 It has enriched the overall development of the clients	1	2	3	4	5	6
3.10. 总体而言, 我对这次的服务项目感到满意。 Overall speaking, I am satisfied with this service program	1	2	3	4	5	6

4.	请回答以下问题: **Please answer the following questions:**
4.1	本次服务项目中有哪些方面您认为对服务对象最有益处? In what aspects of this service project do you think will be most beneficial to the clients? ________________________________ ________________________________
4.2	本次服务项目可以怎样改进,从而更好的帮助服务对象? How can this service be improved to help the clients better? ________________________________ ________________________________

Appendix 6: Focus Group

訪談大綱

Interview outline

謝謝你們來參加焦點小組訪談。訪談旨在更多地了解你們在本學期 “服務學習” 這門課程的教學體驗。為了更詳盡分析訪談的內容, 我們會進行錄音。如果老師們不介意, 請大家先在研究同意書上簽名。這項研究僅僅為了學術和研究目的。大家的隱私將會得到嚴格保密。

Thank you for joining this focus group. The interview aims to learn more about your experience teaching the Service-Learning course this semester. In order to analyze the contents of the interview thoroughly, we will make a recording. Please sign the research consent form first if you don't mind. This research is for academic and research purposes only. Your privacy will be kept strictly confidential.

<u>基本個人資料收集</u>

<u>Basic Personal Data Collection</u>

(以下四項將于訪談開始前與研究同意書一併收集)

• 姓名:	• 學系及職位:
• 性別:	• 教授專案: 杭州

(The following four items will be collected with the study consent form prior to the interview)

• Name:	• Department and position:
• Gender:	• Service-Learning course taught: Hangzhou

在教授本學期 "服務學習"這門學科之前，有沒有其他教學經驗？如果有的話，

Do you have any other teaching experience before teaching the subject of "Service-Learning" this semester?

1. 你有多少年的教學經驗 (不論面授或網上)?
   How many years of teaching experience do you have (whether face-to-face or online)?
2. 你于香港理工大學任教多少年?
   How many years have you been teaching at The Hong Kong Polytechnic University?
3. 你之前有沒有教授"服務學習"這門學科的經驗嗎?
   Have you ever taught the subject of "Service-Learning" before?
   a. 如果有的話, 可以分享一下你之前的經驗嗎?
      If yes, can you share your previous experience?
   b. 如果沒有的話，在教授這門學科之前，你對服務學習的看法和感受是怎樣的?
      If not, what were your views and feelings about Service-Learning before teaching the subject?

個人教學

Individual Teaching

1. 對於本學期以網上形式進行七節的工作坊教學， 你對這個安排有什麼看法?
   What are your thoughts on the seven-session workshop to be conducted online this semester?
2. 你可否簡單介紹一下你所教授的課節內容?
   Can you share more about the contents of each workshop?
3. 對於七節工作坊每節約三小時的安排方面, 你對於這個安排有什麼看法? 是否足夠教授所有課程目標的內容?
   What are your thoughts on the seven sessions of three-hour workshop? Were they sufficient to achieve all the objectives of the course?
4. 你用了什麼教學手法來維持教學質素及提升理大學生的學習體驗嗎? 請舉例說明。
   What teaching methods have you used to maintain the quality of teaching and enhance the learning experience of PolyU students?
5. 你個人比較喜歡面對面教學還是網上教學?
   Do you personally prefer face-to-face or online teaching?

6. 你覺得學生是否喜歡網上教學?
   Do you think students enjoy online teaching?
7. 進行教授期間, 當中有沒有遇到什麼困難? 如果有的話, 可否分享1-2個例子? 你怎樣應對相關困難?
   Were there any difficulties during the teaching process? If yes, could you share 1-2 examples, and how did you deal with them?
8. 你認為工作坊教學內容對理大學生設計服務夏令營的內容有沒有説明? 請舉例說明。
   Do you think the content of the workshop has helped PolyU students to design the contents of the Summer Camp?
9. 你認為工作坊教學內容對理大學生應對小朋友課堂的表現有沒有幫助? 請舉例說明。
   Do you think the contents of the workshop has helped PolyU students cope with the performance of children in class?
10. 對於本學期邀請內地大學的評估員參與工作坊， 你對這個安排有什麼看法?
   What do you think about inviting evaluators from mainland China University to participate in the workshop this semester?

提供的支援及鼓勵

Support and Encouragement Provided

1. 在七節工作坊的教學期間, 你有沒有向理大學生提供支持及鼓勵?
   During the seven workshops, did you provide support and encouragement to PolyU students?
   a. 如果有提供的話, 可以分享一下你提供哪些方面的支持及鼓勵呢? 那麼, 所提供的支持及鼓勵是否足夠呢?
      If yes, can you share what kind of support and encouragement you have offered? Was the support and encouragement provided sufficient?
   b. 如果沒有提供的話, 你覺得為什麼沒有呢?
      If not, why don't you think it's provided?
2. 在五天網上服務夏令營進行期間, 你有沒有向理大學生提供支持及鼓勵?
   Did you provide support and encouragement to PolyU students during the five-day online service summer camp?
   a. 如果有提供的話, 可以分享一下你提供哪些方面的支持及鼓勵呢? 那麼, 所提供的支持及鼓勵是否足夠呢?
      If yes, can you share what kind of support and encouragement you have offered? Was the support and encouragement provided sufficient?
   b. 如果沒有提供的話, 你覺得為什麼沒有呢?
      If not, why don't you think it's provided?

個人得到的支持和鼓勵

The Support and Encouragement that Individuals Received

1. 在本學期的教學中, 你是否有得到任何的支持或鼓勵? 比如: 你是否從大學、學系得到支持? 如有, 你所得到的支持是否足夠?
   Did you receive any support from universities or departments in this semester? If yes, was the support and encouragement provided sufficient?
2. 如有, 你是如何運用所得的支持在你的教學當中?
   If yes, how did you use the support you received in your teaching?
3. 如果你所得到的支援不充分, 你希望可以得到哪些方面的支持? 在沒有這些支援的情況下, 你是如何自行解決所面臨的困難的? 可以舉例說明。
   If you didn't receive enough support, what kind of support or encouragement do you hope to receive? Without the support, how did you solve the difficulties you face on your own?
4. 你個人與合作的內地大學、小學的合作經驗是否愉快?
   Did you enjoy your personal experience working with universities and primary schools in mainland China?

對服務提供者的觀感

Perception of Service Providers

1. 你認為理大同學怎樣看待自己所設計的課程呢?
   What do you think PolyU students think of the courses they have designed?
2. 你認為理大同學修讀服務學習及參與五天網上服務夏令營後, 對他們的全人發展方面有沒有幫助呢? 如果有的話, 可不可以分享幾個例子?
   Do you think PolyU students have helped their whole-person development by taking service-learning and participating in the five-day online service summer camp? If yes, would you please share few examples?
3. 你認為理大學生在修讀這個服務學習學科後會有一些改變?
   Do you think PolyU students will change after studying this service-learning course?

   a. 如果有的話, 有哪些方面的改變? 你覺得哪些什麼因素導致他們有以上的改變?
      If yes, what have changed? What factors contributed to the above changes?
   b. 如果沒有的話, 你認為有什麼因素導致他們沒有改變?
      If not, what do you think is the reason why they haven't changed?

對服務使用者的觀感

Perception of Service Users

1. 你認為小朋友們怎樣看待理大同學所設計的課程呢?
   What do you think the service users think of the curriculum designed by PolyU students?

2. 你認為小朋友們參與這些課程後有沒有進步呢? 如果有的話, 在哪些方面有進步?

   Do you think the service users have made any progress after participating in these lessons? If so, in what areas?
3. 你認為小朋友們對作為服務提供者的大哥哥大姐姐有什麼看法和感受?

   What do you think the service users think and feel about the brothers and the sisters (PolyU students) as service providers?
4. 你認為小朋友們經歷整個網上服務學習夏令營, 對他們的全人發展方面有沒有幫助呢? 如果有的話, 可不可以分享幾個例子?

   Do you think the children's experience of the online service-learning summer camp has helped them in their whole-person development?

對內地大學評估員及小學老師的觀感

Perception of mainland China University Assessors and the Primary School Teachers

1. 在準備網上服務夏令營的期間, 你覺得內地大學的評估員提供的支持及鼓勵是否足夠? 如果足夠的話, 哪些方面的支持足夠呢? 如果不足夠的話, 哪些方面的支援不足夠或需要改進呢?

   During the preparation of the online service summer camp, do you think the support and encouragement provided by the evaluators at mainland China University is sufficient? If yes, which areas of support were sufficient? If not, which areas were insufficient or needed improvement?
2. 在五天網上服務夏令營進行期間, 你覺得內地大學的評估員提供的支持及鼓勵是否足夠? 如果足夠的話, 哪些方面的支持足夠呢? 如果不足夠的話, 哪些方面的支援不足夠或需要改進呢?

   During the five-day online service summer camp, do you think the support and encouragement provided by the evaluators at mainland China University was sufficient?
3. 在準備網上服務夏令營的期間, 你覺得內地小學的老師提供的支持及鼓勵是否足夠? 如果足夠的話, 哪些方面的支持足夠呢? 如果不足夠的話, 哪些方面的支持不足夠呢?

   During the preparation of the online service summer camp, do you think the support and encouragement provided by the teachers of mainland China Primary School were sufficient?
4. 在五天網上服務夏令營進行期間, 你對內地小學的老師的看法和感受是怎樣的?

   During the five-day online service summer camp, what were your feeling and thoughts about the teachers of mainland China Primary School?

對整個網上夏令營服務的觀感

Perception of the Entire Online Summer Camp Service

1. 對於本學期以網上形式進行五天的服務學習夏令營，你對這個安排有什麼看法?

   What are your thoughts on the five-day service-learning summer online camp this semester?
2. 對今後改進完善服務學習這個學科，不論是教學內容或服務內容，你有什麼建議嗎?

   Do you have any suggestions for improving the subject of service learning in future, whether it is about teaching content or service content?
3. 你對整個服務學習計畫的印象是什麼? 請分享給你留下印象最深刻的一件事情。

   What are your impressions of the overall service-learning program? Please share one thing that most impressed you.
4. 你可不可以分享這個計畫的獨特之處?

   Can you share the uniqueness of this program?
5. 如果可以情況許可,你會選擇網上服務學習還是面對面提供教學及服務呢? 為什麼?

   If available, whether you would choose online service-learning or face-to-face teaching and services, and why?
6. 你有沒有其他想補充的內容?

   Do you have anything else that you'd like to add?

Appendix 7: Field Observation Form

服务学习计划（2021）学生表现评估表格

Service-Learning Program (2021)
Student Performance Assessment Form

机密 Confidential

谢谢您与香港理工大学合作提供服务学习计划。我们恳请您就理大学生的服务表现作出评估。
评估后，请把表格于每天下课后直接交予理工大学老师________________________。

Thank you for partnering with The Hong Kong Polytechnic University to provide a Service-Learning program. We kindly invite you to evaluate the service performance of PolyU students. After the assessment, please submit the form directly to the Polytechnic University teacher ______________

服务学习计划名称:
Service-Learning Program Name: ____
服务学习日期:
Service-Learning Dates: ____
理大学生姓名:
PolyU Student Name: ____
评估项目内容
Lesson Content: ____

请就学生的服务表现作出评估 (在适当的空格中加上√号):

Please evaluate the student's performance (Put a √ sign in the appropriate spaces):

		Very good 很好	Good 好	Fair 一般	Poor 差	Very Poor 很差	N/A 不适用
		(5)	(4)	(3)	(2)	(1)	(0)
1.	服务态度 Service Attitude	□	□	□	□	□	□
2.	责任感 Sense of Responsibility	□	□	□	□	□	□
3.	服务对象需要掌握 Awareness of Needs	□	□	□	□	□	□
4.	对服务对象之关心 Sense of Care	□	□	□	□	□	□
5.	文化触觉 Cultural Sensitivity	□	□	□	□	□	□
6.	合作性 Teamwork	□	□	□	□	□	□
7.	解决问题技巧 Problem Solving Skills	□	□	□	□	□	□
8.	与服务对象沟通技巧 Communication Skills with Service Targets	□	□	□	□	□	□
9.	教授内容技巧 Teaching Skills	□	□	□	□	□	□
10.	有关知识之应用 Application of discipline-related Knowledge	□	□	□	□	□	□
11.	反思态度 Reflective Attitude	□	□	□	□	□	□
12.	准时 Punctuality	□	□	□	□	□	□
13.	整体表现 Overall Performance	□	□	□	□	□	□

Comments:

评估员签名 Signature of the evaluator: ______________ 日期 Date： ______________

评估员姓名 Name of the evaluator： ________________ 职位 Position： ____________

联络方式 Contact Method： __________________

References

Eyler, J., & Giles, D. (1999). *Where's the learning in service-learning?* Jossey-Bass.

Kolb, D. A. (1984). *Experiential learning: Experience as the source of learning and development.* Prentice-Hall.

Leung, J. T., & Shek, D. T. L. (2016). To serve and to learn: Students' reflections of the service learning experience in serving the migrant children in Shanghai. *International Journal of Child and Adolescent Health, 9*(2), 165–175.

Leung, H., Shek, D. T. L., & Dou, D. (2021). Evaluation of service-learning in project WeCan under COVID-19 in a Chinese Context. *International Journal of Environmental Research and Public Health, 18*(7), 3596. https://doi.org/10.3390/ijerph18073596

Ross, D. (2013). Social sustainability. In S. Idowu, N. Capaldi, & A. D. Gupta, & L. Zu (Eds.), *Encyclopedia of corporate social responsibility* (pp. 2245–2249). Springer. https://doi.org/10.1007/978-3-642-28036-8_58

Shek, D. T. L. (2010). Nurturing holistic development of university students in Hong Kong: Where are we and where should we go? *The Scientific World Journal, 10*, 563–575. https://doi.org/10.1100/tsw.2010.62

Shek, D. T. L., & Chak, Y. L. Y. (2019). Perceived changes and benefits of a service-learning subject for underprivileged children in Shanghai: Views of university students. In D. T. L. Shek, G. Ngai, & S. C. F. Chan (Eds.), *Service-learning for youth leadership: The case of Hong Kong* (pp. 33–47). Springer.

Shek, D. T. L., Chak, Y., Li, X., Leung, E., Li, P., Mok, B., & Shek, V. (2021). Service-learning under COVID-19: Experience gained from project WeCan in Hong Kong. *International Journal of Child & Adolescent Health, 14*(2), 155–164.

Shek, D. T. L., & Ho, W. W. L. (2019). Serving clients in a drug rehabilitation agency as a vehicle to promote service leadership in university students. In D. T. L. Shek, G. Ngai, & S. C. F. Chan (Eds.), *Service-learning for youth leadership: The case of Hong Kong* (pp. 65–82). Springer.

Shek, D. T. L., Ma, C. M. S., & Yang, Z. (2020). Transformation and development of university students through service-learning: A corporate-community-university partnership initiative in Hong Kong (Project WeCan). *Applied Research in Quality of Life, 15*(5), 1375–1393. https://doi.org/10.1007/s11482-019-09738-9

Shek, D. T. L., Ngai, G., & Chan, C. F. (2019). *Service-learning for youth leadership: The case of Hong Kong*. Springer.

Shek, D. T. L., & Wong, K. K. (2011). Do adolescent developmental issues disappear overnight? Reflections about holistic development in university students. *The Scientific World Journal, 11*(1), 353–361. https://doi.org/10.1100/tsw.2011.5

Wiek, A., Withycombe, L., & Redman, C. L. (2011). Key competencies in sustainability: A reference framework for academic program development. *Sustainability Science, 6*, 203–218. https://doi.org/10.1007/s11625-011-0132-6

Wu, K. Y. F., & Shek, D. T. L. (2016). Subjective outcome evaluation of a service learning subject in a Chinese context. *International Journal of Child and Adolescent Health, 9*(2), 177–185.

Yu, L., Shek, D. T. L., Liu, Q. Y., Chen, H. J., & Zhi, H. (2016, December). *Promoting positive development of migrant children in Hangzhou: Pioneering experience and preliminary evaluation findings.* [Paper presentation]. The 2nd International Conference on Service-Learning [ICSL], Hong Kong, China.

Yu, L., Shek, D. T. L., & Xing, K. Y. (2019). Impact of a service-learning programme in Mainland China: Views of different stakeholders. In D. T. L. Shek, G. Ngai, & S. C. F. Chan (Eds.), *Service-learning for youth leadership: The case of Hong Kong* (pp. 49–63). Springer.

Chapter 12
Service Leadership Through Service-Learning

Daniel T. L. Shek and Diya Dou

Abstract The demand for service industry leaders is growing, requiring adaptability and customer-focused skills. Traditional academic settings often overlook soft skills and social responsibility. In response to this emerging demand, Service-Learning (SL) courses are offered to enable students' holistic development. This chapter uses mixed methods to explore the impact of the SL course entitled "Service Leadership through Serving Children and Families with Special Needs" implemented at The Hong Kong Polytechnic University (PolyU) on student development and community well-being. Multiple stakeholders were involved in the evaluation process, including university students, schools and communities, school students (e.g., service recipients), teachers, and the business sector. Based on evaluation data and stakeholder feedback, it was found that the SL course facilitated positive changes in students' personal development, leadership, and other competencies. Equally important, the shift to online SL activities not only extended service opportunities but also enhanced student-community engagement. Results indicate that both service providers and service recipients positively evaluated the course. Parents and teachers have found positive changes in children's growth through participating in SL activities. Children became more vibrant and learned essential life skills like managing stress and caring for the environment. Parents understood the significance of providing opportunities for personal growth. Teachers believe that SL promotes holistic development, civic responsibility, community awareness, teamwork, and problem-solving skills. In line with previous studies, the SL course successfully cultivated service leadership qualities among university students, fostered personal growth and community impact, and affirmed the significance of experiential learning for nurturing service leaders.

Keywords Service-learning (SL) · Service leadership · Evaluation · Higher education · Hong Kong

12.1 Introduction

There is a call for nurturing leaders in service industries in the contemporary world. There are two factors leading to such a change. First, service production has become a dominant component of the economy in many countries and regions. For example,

D. T. L. Shek, *Promoting Holistic Development in University Students*, Quality of Life in Asia 17, https://doi.org/10.1007/978-981-96-0251-3_12

in Hong Kong, the service sector contributes to 93% of its gross domestic product (GDP) (Shek et al., 2014b). With the rise of the service economy, leaders need to adapt to an ever-changing environment and acquire expertise and competencies that emphasize the sensitivity and flexibility to deploy the resources to meet customers' needs and demands (Hirschhorn, 1988). Chung (2014) noted the need to nurture high-performance service leaders in higher education.

The question is how to nurture service leaders in the universities. Besides developing intellectual competence, it was argued that university students should master "soft skills" such as resilience, emotional competence, interpersonal communication, and moral competence to achieve holistic development (Ngai & Shek, 2022). Nevertheless, the cultivation of soft skills has been neglected in many universities nowadays, as their main focus is to increase the academic performance of students and their international ranking. In addition, universities should strive to help youngsters develop social responsibility and enhance their civic engagement to address social problems, global issues, and the needs of vulnerable groups. However, the teaching and learning activities in traditional classrooms were not experiential and reflective enough to promote the holistic development and social responsibility of university students. The demand for experiential learning is increasing (Kuh, 2008).

As an experiential learning pedagogy, Service-Learning (SL) can consolidate the knowledge of the students by providing appropriate service to people and communities in need (Eyler & Giles, 1999; Jacoby, 1996). The SL course highlights interactive, reflective, and active learning and emphasizes the active role of participants. By exposing students to conflict-filled situations and scenarios, they are inspired to develop skills and insights to tackle challenges effectively (Kerins, 2010). SL has been proven to promote positive values and individual development and facilitate reflective learning (Astin et al., 2000). Therefore, promoting SL courses in universities can improve students' abilities to address real-life problems and enhance their well-being (Batchelder & Root, 1994; Cress et al., 2013; Prentice & Robinson, 2010).

To promote service leadership among university students, an SL course entitled "Service Leadership through Serving Children and Families with Special Needs" was implemented at The Hong Kong Polytechnic University (PolyU) in the 2013/14 academic year. This subject carries three credits and lasts for two semesters. It intends to develop students' Service Leadership by encouraging them to deepen their learning and provide high-quality services in the community, which benefits both service providers and service targets.

Traditionally, the subject was provided in a face-to-face format. With COVID-19, this subject has transformed into online and hybrid modes. Online SL played a vital role during the pandemic as the service recipients had limited access to extracurricular activities and services (Li et al., 2023; Lin et al., 2022). More importantly, offsite SL activities enabled university students to provide innovative and effective services to the community and enhance the well-being of themselves and service recipients.

12.2 Overview of the Subject

Like other university academic subjects, SL is embedded with well-designed objectives and learning outcomes. The teaching methods and assessment tools align with the university's teaching requirements. Moreover, the "Service Leadership and Management Model (SLAM)" and its seven core beliefs lay the theoretical foundation of this course. In this model, service leadership is described as "Satisfying needs by consistently providing quality personal service to everyone that one comes into contact with, including oneself, others, groups, communities, systems, and environments" (Chung, 2011, 2012). More importantly, this framework highlights the qualities of being a service leader, including leadership competencies (e.g., intrapersonal and interpersonal competencies), caring disposition, and moral character (Shek et al., 2013). Based on its course outline, this course is designed to enable students to:

(a) Understand the core attributes of service leaders;
(b) Apply the core components of service leadership through the engagement in community-based service activities;
(c) Develop self-awareness of sharing and empathy with others and the community;
(d) Reflect on their service leadership qualities, particularly intrapersonal and interpersonal competencies.

Psychosocial competence is closely related to students' well-being. Notably, the objectives of this course are essential indicators of students' lifelong learning and well-being. Firstly, this course gives the students deep exposure to a broader vision, helps them form their value system, and facilitates them to understand the importance of positive values and essential skills, which aligns with the goal of higher education proposed by the Hong Kong Education Commission (2000). Specifically, in this course, apart from integrating their professional learning and skills into community service, students' abilities to link the theories to address real-life problems and establish a strong sense of civic responsibility are also highlighted.

12.2.1 Approach

In terms of pedagogy, as a form of experiential learning, students who take this course experience the Four Stage Learning Cycle proposed by Kolb (1984), namely Do/Act (developing concrete experience), Reflect (conducting reflective observation), Think (forming abstract conceptualization), and Apply (implementing active experimentation). Specifically, reflective observation is essential in this cycle, which distinguishes this course from subjects that emphasize factual knowledge. Purposeful reflection after service activities can facilitate students' development of multiple perspectives based on their past experiences and help them gain meaning for future behaviors. Equally important, students have the opportunity to experience personal growth (Felten & Clayton, 2011).

Specifically, the design of SL activities was based on the Self-Determination Theory (Deci & Ryan, 2013; Deci et al., 1991), which emphasizes the autonomy, competence, and relatedness of the participants. For autonomy and relatedness, although the students must take SL courses, they can choose a wide range of subjects and programs that interest them. Regarding autonomy and competence, the students can learn and practice their psychosocial skills based on the general outlines of their chosen SL course, which can link the students' learning needs to the community's service needs. Therefore, this course is considerably different from volunteering and other service programs (Tam, 2014).

12.2.2 Engagement

According to Tyler (1949, p. 63), "Learning takes place through the active behavior of the student: it is what he does that he learns, not what the teacher does." Throughout decades in higher education, attempts have been made to relocate emphasis from teacher-centered approaches to student-centered approaches in teaching and learning activities. Active learning gains a positive view in higher education as it promotes student learning in relation to deep learning and long-term engagement with learning tasks (Biggs, 1999; Eitington, 2002; Kember, 2002; Ramsden, 2003). Kember and Leung (2005) further argued that a good teacher-student relationship would exert a mutually reinforcing effect to foster student learning, in addition to requiring active student involvement in teaching and learning.

This subject utilizes various teaching and learning strategies to engage the student, including "(1) a 10-hour e-learning module to acquire knowledge about the concepts of SL, (2) lectures on the teaching of service leadership, (3) small group discussions to prepare for the service project, (4) service provided to service targets, (5) reflective journal writings to allow students to deepen their learning experience" (Shek & Yuen, 2019, p. 49). Additionally, students will form small groups and do group presentations to consolidate their learning experiences. Teachers will assess their performance based on presentations and assignments and provide timely feedback for students to enhance their learning.

There are multiple elements in this subject, including lectures, workshops, and community-based services. Firstly, by attending three lectures, students can acquire a general understanding of Service Leadership, such as its definitions, theories, and concepts, to guide their future services. Specifically, Lecture One introduces the subject, service arrangements, and background information. The model, theory, and core beliefs of Service Leadership will also be covered. Additionally, Lecture Two and Lecture Three introduce the three components of effective service leadership, "leadership competencies, caring disposition, and moral character" (Shek & Yuen, 2019, p. 47). Then, seven workshops will be arranged to assist students in designing their service proposals and planning their engagement strategies. Moreover, engagement skills and the needs of the service recipients will be discussed attentively, and students can learn specific knowledge and skills for providing effective and appropriate services to the service recipients and practice their learning and skills through community-based service activities. The lectures and workshops are effective in engaging the students and inspiring them to plan and provide practical service activities for their service recipients in future.

More importantly, collaborative learning is embedded in the course, which provides more room for student–student interaction in planning, implementing, and evaluating the services conducted. First, students work in groups to come up with their service proposals. Second, students work closely with each other during the direct services based on the service proposals. Additionally, groups of students gather their learning experiences and share the difficulties they encounter and the gains they achieve during the services. Through the service delivery from preparation to evaluation, teachers act as facilitators who provide timely feedback at different stages. Semi-structured guidance is provided as an overarching framework for the services that are to be done. Collaborative learning gives the students the autonomy to design the activities by exercising their creativity. It also ensures a high level of feasibility in service implementation.

12.2.3 Impact

Remarkably, PolyU took the initiative among universities in Hong Kong to make SL courses mandatory for all full-time undergraduate students. Initially, 145 students enrolled in "Service Leadership through Serving Children and Families with Special Needs" when it was first launched in the 2013/14 academic year. From the 2013/14 school year onwards, an increasing number of students have taken this subject yearly. Since 2014, this subject has been working with one of the SL partners of "Project WeCan." Up to now, over 4900 students have taken this subject. Remarkably, this subject formed partnerships with two non-government organizations, the Society of Boys' Centre and Heep Hong Society, which aim to provide quality services and promote the well-being of underprivileged secondary school students through multi-dimensional collaboration. Based on the report of Shek and Yuen (2019, p. 49), this subject provided services to ten schools or centers in Hong Kong, including "(1) special schools admitting boys with behavioral and emotional problems (Society of Boys' Centres), (2) a non-governmental organization providing service for preschool children with developmental disorders and mental retardation (Heep Hong Society), (3) a drug rehabilitation agency (Christian Zheng Sheng College), and (4) schools admitting students with social and economic deprivation (schools in Project WeCan)." With a growing number of service sites, more schools and students will benefit from the services, and the partnerships also highlight that the need for SL courses and programs in the community is high. Moreover, the services have a beneficial impact on both service providers and service targets.

Notably, this subject is innovative in involving multiple stakeholders, including university students (e.g., service providers), schools and communities, school students (e.g., service recipients), teachers, and the business sector (e.g., Wharf).

Therefore, it is necessary to employ diversified evaluation methods to evaluate its impact. Specifically, objective outcome evaluation, subjective outcome evaluation, and qualitative evaluation are applied for assessment. Multi-faceted evaluation methods are more effective at capturing an integrative and holistic picture of the impact and effectiveness of this subject. Specifically, the assessment tools include:

(1) Objective outcome evaluation is employed to evaluate the effectiveness of the subject. At the beginning and the end of this subject, PolyU students are invited to respond to a questionnaire with 70 items to assess their positive development constructs, service leadership, and other psychosocial variables (see Appendix 1). Moreover, service recipients are also invited to complete an objective outcome evaluation (see Appendix 2).
(2) Subjective outcome evaluation is implemented (see Appendix 3). At the end of this course, students are invited to report their views of the subject, their perceptions toward the instructor teaching the subject, and their perceived benefits after taking this subject.
(3) Partnership evaluation is employed. When the service activities end, service recipients are invited to evaluate their views of the SL activities (see Appendix 4). Moreover, the community partners are also invited to share their perceptions of the activities and the overall university-community collaboration (see Appendix 5).
(4) Subject teachers are invited to share their experience of teaching this subject by attending focus group interviews. They are guided to share their thoughts on individual teaching, the support and encouragement they received, and the difficulties they encountered (see Appendix 6).
(5) Field observation is conducted when PolyU students are providing services. This method is used to assess the quality of services and the performance of university students (see Appendix 7).
(6) Students' feedback questionnaires are delivered at the end of the course to understand the university students' perceptions of the subject and their gains after taking this subject (see Appendix 8).
(7) Qualitative evaluation. After completing this SL subject, PolyU students are invited to attend focus group interviews and write reflections to consolidate their overall learning experience (see Appendix 9).

12.2.3.1 Objective Outcome Evaluation

Firstly, the Chinese Positive Youth Development Scale, which covers different domains of Positive Youth Development (PYD), is utilized to assess the qualities of students before and after taking this subject (Leung et al., 2021; Lin & Shek, 2021). Different studies have been conducted, and the findings were encouraging. Shek and Yuen (2019, p. 29) presented their findings in their research, including "(1) the agencies were highly satisfied with the students regarding their positive service attitudes, caring disposition, service leadership towards service targets, problem-solving skills, and reflective attitude in delivering services; (2) the PolyU students provided highly positive responses about the course. In a quantitative evaluation, over 90% of the respondents rated positively the professional quality of teaching staff, effectiveness in promoting service leadership, and holistic personal development; and (3) students were praised by stakeholders for the generic competencies such as emotional competence, critical thinking, social competence, and sense of responsibility." In another study conducted by Shek et al., (2014a), 316 students completed the Objective Outcome Evaluation Questionnaire. The findings showed that the students improved in all attributes of PYD, service leadership, and life satisfaction after taking the course. This study reinforced the evidence that the subject is compelling.

12.2.3.2 Subjective Outcome Evaluation

Subjective outcome evaluation helps understand how different stakeholders view the qualities of the SL subjects, including their perceptions of the quality of the subject, the qualities of teachers, and the perceived benefits of this subject. Moreover, PolyU students are invited to take subjective outcome evaluations after taking the subjects. In one study, Shek et al. (2020) collected quantitative and qualitative data from 138 university students. The findings indicated that the students experienced positive changes in social-emotional competence, self-leadership, and civic engagement.

In addition, service partners and service recipients are also invited to take subjective outcome evaluations after receiving the services in terms of their perceptions of the program, the service providers, and the benefits gained from the SL activities. Several evaluation studies for service partners were also carried out after the implementation of SL. For example, Ma et al., (2019) evaluated two SL subjects in the 2016/17 academic year. They showed that the service partners were satisfied with the implementation of SL activities, and the service recipients exhibited positive changes in some of the outcome indicators. Moreover, the field observations were encouraging as well. In another study, Shek et al. (2021) examined the data collected over three years ($N = 1854$) and revealed that most service recipients benefited from the SL services. For example, over 90% of service recipients rated the activities positively. Moreover, 92.5% of the participants agreed that the experience broadened their horizons, and 97.7% showed overall satisfaction with the services. The satisfaction ratings of the service recipients also supported the fact that they had significant changes and growth across different attributes, such as in the areas of resilience, self-confidence, and care. The study reinforced the evidence that SL activities benefited both the service providers and service recipients (Shek et al., 2019).

12.2.3.3 Qualitative Evaluation

Since diverse assessment components are involved in this subject, it is necessary to apply qualitative evaluation for SL assessment to understand the experiences of different stakeholders. Firstly, for the qualitative study, all service providers (e.g., PolyU students) are required to submit a 1000–1200-word reflective paper upon completing the course. Reflection should be based on what they have learned in this subject, their changes before and after taking this subject, and their insights gained from providing services to groups in need.

Qualitatively speaking, by writing reflective journals, students can share their insights regarding the values of leadership competence and moral competence. Moreover, they learn to demonstrate care and empathy, to listen actively, and to shoulder responsibilities while providing services. Additionally, Shek and Yuen (2019) revealed that taking this subject helped students be more well-prepared for future challenges. Apart from consolidating their reflection in their journals, students who provided services at the Christian Zheng Sheng College were also asked to use three descriptions and one metaphor to reflect on their SL experiences of the day camp. The students reported that the journey was enjoyable and meaningful, and their worldviews were changed after the service. Overall, the research showed that the integration of service leadership and SL is beneficial in enhancing the holistic development of university students and serving the needs of the community (Shek & Yuen, 2019).

From the students' narratives, most students had positive learning experiences and found the subject helpful. Moreover, they learned to be grateful for their own lives, and they treasured the chance to help underprivileged groups (Ma et al., 2016). Some examples are shown below (Shek, 2019, p. 14):

- "My SL experience was very unforgettable. The service process was very unforgettable … [Therefore,] I think the general education subjects should include more experiential learning like this. Why do I have very deep impressions of the subject? Because I really did something! … If the subject only lectured some 'empty talk' knowledge to us, we would forget the knowledge quickly."
- "Since I had never been a leader before when I studied in mainland China, I wanted to change myself this summer. So, I took the initiative to be a group leader in my SL subject. However, because I avoided responsibility, our group eventually failed [in our group project] … So, although I have learned this concept (of leadership) since my freshman year, it was my sophomore year this summer, and from this lesson (in SL) that I realized the importance of responsibility and team spirit. Otherwise, not only one person but the whole team will fail."

Equally important, take metaphor writing as an example. From 2015 to 2017, at the end of the service activities in a Drug Rehabilitation Agency, Shek and Ho (2018) collected 207 descriptors from the students, and over 95% of them were talking about positive learning experiences. Descriptors including "unexpected/amazing" ($N = 22$), "surprising" ($N = 12$), "satisfying" ($N = 12$), and "meaningful/thought-provoking/valuable" ($N = 11$) were the top four with high frequencies. Moreover, the PolyU students utilized interesting metaphors like "sponge," "durian," "ship/ferry," and "magic stone" to consolidate their learning experience. To illustrate, one shared, "Before the PolyU visit and Christian Zheng Sheng College camp, I didn't know much about Zheng Sheng students. I was afraid about what was going to happen and how I should communicate with them, just like the outlook of the durian makes people scared. However, after I knew more about them, I loved to talk to them and made good friends with them like a tasty durian" (Shek & Ho, 2018, p. 72). The descriptors and metaphors reflected the challenges and gains of PolyU students.

SL is a high-impact educational practice that can benefit both service providers and teachers. Qualitative evaluations were carried out to investigate its effectiveness and understand how different stakeholders viewed SL projects. In one study, Shek et al. (2019) collected data to understand teachers' perceptions. The results showed that their experiences with SL implementation and their evaluation of SL were positive, as both teachers and students benefited from the subjects.

As SL subjects involve multifaceted learning outcomes, the assessment of performance can be challenging for the teaching staff. Therefore, qualitative study also involves interviewing the teachers of the subject, and there is a need to assess the challenges, benefits, and needs of teachers during the process. For instance, Camus et al. (2022) interviewed teachers from four universities in Hong Kong who taught academic SL courses or programs. They were asked to share their teaching experience in a short questionnaire before the interviews. The qualitative study encouraged the teachers to apply traditional and experiential assessment tools and indicated that the reflections of students were used well. The combination of assessment tools facilitates the integration of students' learning into community practice and also enhances the quality of community service. More importantly, the research revealed that the teaching staff faced multiple challenges, including on-site observation, working with various parties, and a heavy workload. Understanding the difficulties the teachers face can develop a better understanding of the implementation of SL and show the importance of implementing effective tools to guide grading practices (Camus et al., 2022).

In another study, 124 university teachers of SL subjects were involved in investigating their ways of assessment in this course. In line with the previous findings, these participants agreed that grading the performance was more challenging than other courses or programs. Remarkably, the study revealed that university teachers became more aware of the beneficial impact of SL on the holistic development of university students. Moreover, adequate support, training, and resources were needed to help teachers conquer challenges while teaching this subject. Multifaceted research involving different stakeholders in this subject showed how SL impacts students' outcomes and the community as a whole (Ngai et al., 2022).

Although multiple assessment tools are employed to assess the effectiveness of SL projects, the studies have some limitations, such as small sample sizes and a lack of randomized control groups. The conclusions would be more convincing if randomized control trials were added in future and the impacts of the projects were investigated over a more extended period.

12.3 Electronic Service-Learning Under COVID-19

The COVID-19 pandemic has brought about considerable changes in education, particularly the forced adoption of online teaching and learning. For SL, the pandemic has created difficulties in service projects because SL typically requires face-to-face service delivery. Besides, travel restrictions also created additional problems for offshore SL activities. As such, there are only two possible solutions—suspension of the service or delivery of the service online. Waldner et al. (2012) classified four types of SLs based on onsite versus online teaching and onsite versus online service, which include the traditional form of SL (onsite teaching and onsite service), e-SL Type 1 (online instruction and onsite SL), e-SL Type 2 (onsite instruction and online SL), and extreme e-SL (both instruction and service are online).

In the summer of 2020–2022, students conducted summer camps for primary school students in Hangzhou, Chengdu, and Xi'an in the context of two SL subjects. While the "Promotion of Children and Adolescent Development" subject was implemented in Hangzhou, students taking "Service Leadership through serving children and families with special needs" served primary school students in Xi'an and Chengdu. Because of social distancing measures during the pandemic, students implemented online SL projects in these three sites in the summer of 2020, 2021, and 2022. As few studies have been conducted to evaluate the effectiveness of online SL projects, we collected evaluation data on online SL from different stakeholders, including PolyU students, PolyU teachers, service partners, and service recipients, particularly in the summer of 2021 (Li et al., 2023; Lin et al., 2022; Shek et al., 2022). In addition, we collected pretest–posttest data, subjective outcome evaluation data on the SL subject, satisfaction data on the SL projects, and focus group data from PolyU students. To illustrate, we successfully collected data from the three sites in the summer of 2021, which is shown in Table 12.1.

The evaluation data showed that PolyU students changed positively after taking the subjects and had positive views of the subject and the SL projects. Other stakeholders also had positive evaluations of the performance of PolyU students and the value of online SL projects to the service recipients (Lin & Shek, 2021; Lin et al., 2022). Moreover, in the study conducted by Leung et al. (2021), they examined the changes in university students and their perceptions of the SL experience. They also found that service recipients' satisfaction with the SL activities was generally positive. For instance, 93.2% of the university students agreed that the SL subject nurtured care and compassion among them, and 90.6% agreed that this course enhanced their social competence. From the perspectives of the service recipients, they were satisfied with the performance of their service providers. Specifically, 85.7% reported active participation, and 83.9% agreed that the activities were appropriate and the atmosphere was pleasant. The research showed that both the university students and recipients benefited from the activities, which also demonstrated the positive impact of online SL activities under COVID-19.

Different stakeholders were also invited to qualitatively share their views and reflections after they participated in the SL activities. For example, in Chengdu

Table 12.1 Evaluation data from three service sites in the summer of 2021

Evaluation design	Evaluation method Content of assessment	Status	Chengdu ($N = 85$)	Hangzhou ($N = 87$)	Xi'an (N = 88)
PolyU Students					
Quantitative	Objective outcome evaluation (Pretest–posttest evaluation): To assess the impacts of SL on students' personal development using validated measures	Completed	Pretest: 85 Posttest: 84 Matched: 84	Pretest: 63 Posttest: 74 Matched: 52	Pretest: 88 Posttest: 87 Matched: 87
Quantitative	Subjective outcome evaluation: To assess students' views toward the quality of the course, instructors, and benefits	Completed	84	69	87
Quantitative	Post-service evaluation: For students to evaluate their service program	Completed	84	73	87
Qualitative	Focus group interview: To collect students' feedback on their evaluation of the learning and service as well as their gains and problems	Completed	13	15	15
Subject Teachers					
Qualitative	Focus group interview: To collect teachers' feedback on the teaching and service as well as their challenges and gains	Completed	3	3	4

(continued)

Table 12.1 (continued)

Evaluation design	Evaluation method Content of assessment	Status	Chengdu ($N = 85$)	Hangzhou ($N = 87$)	Xi'an (N = 88)
Service Partners (Student assessors and primary school teachers)					
Quantitative	Post-service evaluation: To understand student assessors' evaluation of PolyU students' performance after each lecture	Completed	240	46	194
Quantitative	Post-service evaluation: To understand the evaluation of teachers in the collaborating schools on PolyU students' performance	Completed	17	15	17
Service Recipients					
Quantitative	Objective outcome evaluation (Pretest–posttest evaluation): To assess the impacts of SL on students' personal development	Completed	Pretest: 467 Posttest: 485	Pretest: 258 Posttest: 264	Pretest: 383 Posttest: 341
Quantitative	Subjective outcome evaluation: To assess service recipients' views toward the quality of the service program, service providers' performance, and service effectiveness	Completed	485	257	339

(continued)

Table 12.1 (continued)

Evaluation design	Evaluation method Content of assessment	Status	Chengdu ($N = 85$)	Hangzhou ($N = 87$)	Xi'an (N = 88)
Qualitative	Self-reflection (What have I learned from the summer camp?): To understand service recipients' gains from the service program	Completed	185	257	342
Qualitative	Letter to big brothers and sisters: To understand service recipients' feelings and perceptions about PolyU students	Completed	178	244	337

Summer Online Service (2019–2020), we collected reflections from the service recipients, the parents, the school teachers, and the service providers. Some reflections are shown in the next section.

12.3.1 Sharing by Migrant Children

- "The camp taught me a lot outside of class and also allowed me to get to know my older brothers and sisters: Jack, David, Cloth, Jojo, and Jasmine. The summer camp has benefited me a lot. For example, today, we took a health class with Cloth and learned how to prevent the virus better. In Jasmine's English class, we learned how to describe our hometown; Jack's lesson taught us empathy. What I most enjoyed was David's science class. We first learned about gravity and knew that people cannot live without gravity. After learning about inertia, I understand that in sudden stops, killing cars will suddenly all fall forward. Also learned buoyancy, which makes things float at sea. I learned about friction and knew that it is divided into rolling friction, sliding friction, and static friction. Action force = reaction force, force = mass × acceleration are all taught to us by David. I hope that I can apply what I have learned in this summer camp and become a more useful person!"
- "Thank you, brothers and sisters, for your careful care and for bringing me much new knowledge. It gave me a new understanding of the outside world and my health. It also brought us to discover something that surprised us, something we

had never seen before. I also know how important my health is, and finally, thank you again, brothers and sisters, you have worked hard."

- "Thank you for spending five unforgettable days with me. I remember the shyness and excitement of the first day we met. Although every day we are separated by a cold screen, this does not make us lose our enthusiasm. Time flies by, five days together are about to pass, and humorous language and familiar faces will leave me. Thank you for passing on your knowledge to me. This time is woven by me, and you will be an unforgettable and fond memory."
- "Thank you, sister, for teaching me a lot in these short five days; I benefited a lot. I enjoyed the science class because it was really fun. Thank you for your hard work and companionship. We went from strange to familiar, and every greeting is so warm. Finally, I would like to express my heartfelt thanks to the hard-working teachers! I wish my brothers and sisters success in their studies (or work)! Remember to be happy every day!"
- "Thank you for giving us a week of lessons; I learned some new English words, seven handwashing techniques, and some health knowledge for everyday life. I rarely spoke in class, but I also listened carefully to the new and interesting classes you brought to me. The small games between classes are also fun. Thank you for preparing the classes! Thank you for the props and classes, and you gave us your own book at The Hong Kong Polytechnic University. I think this should be your proof of The Hong Kong Polytechnic University. There is also a pen case, which is cute and easy to use, and ten pencils and an atom pen with a logo on it. I love those. And your carefully prepared classes, thank you for this week to take care of us, brothers and sisters!"
- "I'm sorry I didn't write with the paper sent by the summer camp, but I'm sure you'll forgive me. Because you guys have a big belly, although we met in Tencent Video online classes, it's really nice to meet you. You are interesting and inclusive big brothers and sisters, and I'm really happy. Why is it fun and inclusive? Tolerance is because I didn't hear a single bad word and bad word from your mouth from start to finish, so it's good. Then, every time I go to class, I have a lot of fun and want to laugh, so it's fun. Finally, we kept giving our opinions during the class, and you guys not only didn't get angry but also commented and said it was great and so accommodating. In the end, I just want to say one thing: we will definitely meet again for two reasons: first, we have a good relationship; Second, the earth is round."

12.3.2 Sharing by Parents

- "This year's summer camp is very special because, due to the pandemic, we can only meet the big brothers and sisters of The Hong Kong Polytechnic University through online classes. In this summer camp activity, not only have the children gained growth, but we, as parents, have also received more enlightenment, harvest, and reflection. I used to say: Why do children do everything at school but do

nothing in their own homes? That's because I can't see the brilliance of my own children, but only other children. Because I often say, 'You go to do your homework, I'll do these things,' depriving children of the opportunity to do their own things. Let's treat our own children with the same appreciative eyes as other people's children and also return the responsibility to the child, believing that he will do it. Through these few days of classroom learning, I have seen the growth of the child, and he has learned how to face pressure, control his temper, and manage his finances. Moreover, he also took the sorted garbage downstairs and threw it into different garbage cans, learning how to care for the environment and protect the earth. This is more important than what is learned in textbooks, and perhaps this activity delayed the trip, but these are not as good as children who know life because children who can live will definitely learn. This online summer camp activity is very meaningful, and it brings me not only superficial educational guidance but also a spirit deeply rooted in people's hearts. This spirit is the spirit of struggle, hard work, and being enterprising, and the child gains a lot. Here, I would like to thank the leaders and teachers of The Hong Kong Polytechnic University, Sichuan University, and Xishu Experimental School for their hard work! Thank you also to the big brothers and sisters for their hard work! Thank you!"
- "My child said that the activities were wonderful. I observed that the children became more vibrant after two days. The sisters and brothers from PolyU really did a great job of teaching the lessons effectively and efficiently. As parents, we always share the knowledge with our children, but they do not have the patience to listen to us."

12.3.3 Sharing by Teachers

- "The students said that it was great; after listening to the class for these two days, everyone was much more active than usual! Big brothers and big sisters worked hard! Parents can also tell these truths, but the children do not listen to them much, and the effect is not as effective and comprehensive as the brothers and sisters!"
- "Thank you for your hard work on behalf of the children! Children will remember your teachings, and they will always miss you. Thank you for taking them on an extraordinary journey."
- "After a few days of getting along, we learned more about Hong Kong and the young people in Hong Kong. You guys are serious in class. Well-prepared and well-designed lessons before class. You are very knowledgeable, and the class is wonderful. Health classes let children understand the meaning of life and guide them to form independent personalities. English classes enrich children's knowledge of grammar; science classes fully stimulate children's curiosity and teach children to focus on science and practice. The personal development course is new for us, which has inspired me to integrate it into our teaching in future and treat every child equally so that children feel loved. Thank you, PolyU, Sichuan

University youth; from you, I see the sunshine, cooperation, responsibility, and love. The Motherland has you. How can it not be strong?! I love you. Because of you, children's holidays are even more exciting! Our kids are in love with you, too! Thank you!"

12.3.4 Sharing by PolyU Students

- "I would use virtual reality to stand for the service program because I never thought that I would ever have a chance to give lessons to students in mainland China as a teacher. I was blessed that I learned a lot throughout the service. The whole process is unrealistic, just like an experience of a virtual reality game."
- "I would use sculptor to stand for the service program because both service leaders and service recipients may develop skills, acquire new knowledge, reshape characters, and make self-reflection to become better individuals due to the service experience. This process is like the work of a sculptor. A sculptor may start with clay and overwork away at it to show something more refined and sculpted within."
- "I would use a profound debate to stand for the service program because several opposing ideas clashed in my mind, and finally, I chose to deliver the most appropriate content to the service target. At the same time, I listened to the opinions of many others and learned more knowledge."
- "I would use tree planting to stand for the service program because we cultivate students/potential and strength to reach their maximum carefully and patiently. That is rewarding and meaningful. The students are our future, just like planting trees for the future community."

Specifically, the above findings and sharing highlighted several observations. First, objective outcome evaluation findings showed that PolyU students revealed positive changes after joining the online SL projects (Lin et al., 2022; Shek et al., 2022; Zhu et al. 2022). Second, PolyU students evaluated the subject positively. Third, PolyU teachers had positive perceptions of the SL projects (Shek et al., 2022). Fourth, service recipients perceived that they had benefited from the SL programs. Fifth, service collaborators (e.g., teachers in primary schools) evaluated SL programs positively. Finally, observers (university students from the local university) had positive perceptions of the quality of the service provided.

The research findings have the following implications. First, the findings collected underscore the meaningfulness and viability of conducting online SL projects. It demystified the common myth that it is impossible to conduct meaningful and impactful online SL programs. Second, academically, as the studies on the effectiveness of online SL are limited, the research contributes to the scientific literature on SL, particularly in the Chinese context. Third, theoretically, the findings would help us construct models on the usefulness of online SL, predictors of student satisfaction in SL, student development, and teacher development under online SL. Fourth, practically, we have gained much experience from online SL in these two years. We have also trained teachers for online SL. Such experience can help us understand the facilitating factors and hurdles for implementing online SL in future.

Based on the experiences we gained from the e-SL projects in three summers, we suggest several follow-up actions. Firstly, there is a need to consolidate online SL experiences. We may invite the teachers to document their experiences and work out some guidelines for e-SL programs. Second, it would be helpful to disseminate the e-SL experiences by organizing seminars to share successful SL experiences and form a Community of Practice on e-SL activities. Third, more data is needed to strengthen the evaluation database.

12.4 Student Learning Experiences

In the past years, we have used different methods to encourage students to share their learning experiences and perceptions of the subject. Besides asking students to write reflections on the subject, we also invited the scholarship holders to write reflections about the subject. In the following section, we present some of the students' salient views on SL.

12.4.1 Promotion of Personal Development

Some students shared that they found it was a valuable experience to take this subject. Some examples are presented below.

- "This SL subject was a very meaningful and fruitful experience for me. Although we could not go to XXX and provide the service to the children in person, I am still happy that we had the opportunity to help the people in need. This subject has enabled me to serve, lead, and learn at the same time. It also inspired my personal development in many ways."
- "I really treasure the taste of serving others in the subject of Service-Learning, the acknowledgment of my work, and the opportunity to discover myself on personal and professional enhancement."
- "Through this subject, my personal development improved, and I gained a deeper understanding of service leadership, which is providing a high-quality service to meet the needs of the target and the needs of our group, like self-development and a sense of achievement. During the services, I could integrate my professional knowledge into practice."
- "This service experience inspired me greatly and increased my personal capabilities in several ways. Moreover, it also changed my values regarding underprivileged children and adolescents and forced me to think more about my personal development."

- "Some may view this as a waste of time or the fulfillment for graduation, but I think how you feel this is actually showing your dedication to the subject. I am happy I was involved, so I gained."

12.4.2 Leadership

Students generally believed their leadership skills were enhanced and developed after taking this subject. Some comments are presented below.

- "Through the study of theoretical knowledge first, I have learned the capabilities required by service leaders, that is, effective service leadership includes competencies, caring disposition, and moral character. I have gained a profound understanding of these three aspects through practice after theoretical learning. The next is the service preparation process."
- "In the service process, my flexibility, innovation, communication skills, coordination skills, and problem-solving abilities have been fully utilized and significantly enhanced. I acted as a coordinator in the team, responsible for the promotion of collective tasks, giving feedback and suggestions to members, as well as communicating and coordinating with all parties."
- "I enhanced my interpersonal skills in collaboration with others through this service journey, as I experienced the role of the leader in this service."
- "I used to think that becoming a leader is difficult; only talented people can do it. However, learning about service leadership changed my beliefs. Service Leadership emphasizes that everybody is a leader for at least 15 minutes every day. This belief gave me strong support and strengthened my confidence in the leadership team."

12.4.3 Competence

Students generally felt that the subject could promote their knowledge, attitudes, and skills about leadership. In particular, the subject was able to nurture their leadership competence. Some student narratives are presented below.

- *Use of One's Strengths*: "I could learn to use my own strengths and abilities to help team members complete tasks together, as well as find and make use of my own ability and potential."
- *Communication*: "Instead of keeping everything to myself, I voiced my opinions and tried to initiate discussions within my team. We knew each other better, and so communication became smoother. I learned that it is vital to build a friendly relationship with my teammates to ensure good teamwork. I also realized the importance of communication and cooperation in service provision."
- *Putonghua*: "Language was another challenge. I was not proficient in Putonghua and simplified Chinese characters, so I had to put in extra effort to practice my

Putonghua. Before each lesson I was responsible for, I always rehearsed my teaching to make sure that I could speak fluently without pronunciation problems. Through this service, my Putonghua has improved a lot, and I am also very grateful for working with such a helpful and nice groupmate."

- *Care About Others*: "During the services, it also inspired me to develop my caring disposition so that I can think more from others' perspectives, especially from the service recipients' perspectives. In order to target others' genuine needs, not only should we pay attention to the expressed needs, but we should also observe their unexpressed needs."
- *Empathy*: "Apart from personal development, I have also developed a sense of empathy by investigating and observing the problems or difficulties that teenagers nowadays face. By learning more about the difficulties they were facing, I started to understand what I could do for them. I started to be more passionate about helping children as I know that what I have done to them can help them a lot."
- "I have also further developed a sense of empathy. Before organizing the workshops, I didn't have too many opportunities to get along with students with Special Educational Needs, which led me to misunderstand them, believing they could not follow instructions and communicate with me smoothly."
- *Cultural Competence*: "My cultural competence was improved, too. The most important point of cultural competence is respecting other cultures and accepting their differences. Another important point is the ability to communicate and interact with people having different backgrounds."
- "This SL experience not only helped me strengthen my passion for helping people with special needs in society but also helped me recognize my strengths and potential in emotional competence and event management. During the service preparation, although I was nervous due to the unexpected arrangements, such as the shortened time of leadership training, I managed my emotions by taking a deep breath in order to ensure that our activities could continue smoothly."
- "In addition to intrapersonal and interpersonal leadership competencies, this SL experience has also improved my problem-solving and decision-making capacities."
- *Altruism*: "I have further developed a sense of altruism. Due to my experience in video making, I undertook the relatively heavy work of editing videos. At first, compared with others, I was a little dissatisfied with the workload. However, after editing the video, I got compliments from my teammates and tutor, which made me feel that my contribution was meaningful. I started to change my mind, thinking that they gave me the heavy task because they believed in my capacity, and I realized mutual appreciation and altruism are needed for team efficiency."
- "SL is a course that builds my thinking skills, and it is a way to change my personality. As I mentioned in the beginning, we rise by lifting others. Through helping others, I was able to discover both my positive and negative self-regulation abilities and find out how my group collaboration was great by having problems and solving issues. Finally, by serving the client, my group and I were able to get countless benefits."

- *Communication*: "By continuously communicating with my groupmates, professors, and the service targets, my communication skills improved gradually. When talking to different people, our word choice and tone have to be different. This inspired me to learn how to adjust my communication strategies when facing people from different walks of life in the future."
- *Resilience*: "While facing so many difficulties in this SL subject, I developed resilience. My adaptability to challenges improved a lot as I had to face a number of unexpected situations in the service. In the years to come, I will have to cope with more and more challenges and difficulties. I am confident that with the higher level of resilience and adaptability gained in this subject, I am fully equipped to jump over all the obstacles I am going to face in life."
- *Problem-solving and Decision-making Skills*: "I also improved my problem-solving skills, hosting skills, and decision-making capacities through the service ... Through this service experience and solving other problems, my problem-solving skills, hosting skills, and decision-making capacities have been enhanced a lot."
- *Ethical Consideration*: "Before the services, I thought that decision-making was an easy step and that we did not need many considerations. For instance, I had forced participants to respond to my questions before. If no one answered my question, I would name one. This decision did not respect their rights and created a stressful atmosphere. Participants became even more pessimistic than before. After the services, I learned that before making a decision, we should always consider whether it is ethical or not. We shall also speculate who will be affected and how they will be affected before carrying out the decision."
- *Gratitude*: "Through the SL course, I got a precious chance to give back to my beloved place and deeply realized the saying that 'it is more blessed to give than to receive.'"
- *Value One's Life*: "I found that I have become more mature and cherish life more after this service. Compared with Zheng Sheng students and other underprivileged children, my life is much luckier and more comfortable than theirs."

12.4.4 Learning from Failures

Many students shared that the subject was able to facilitate them to learn and reflect on failures, which contributed to their overall personal development. Some reflections are shown below.

- "Before the commencement of the service, all groups were required to submit lesson plans to the professor to make sure that all the teaching materials and activities were suitable and feasible for the service. My lesson plans were not perfect at first, and one of them was banned for its infeasibility. I was quite frustrated at that time as I put a lot of time and effort into completing the lesson plans. I also found it hard to modify my lesson plans because all the teaching materials that I had prepared beforehand could no longer be used. However, I still tried my best to amend the lesson plans to make my teaching more feasible and intriguing. The process was tough as I had to tidy up my thoughts from various perspectives and give up on some of my original teaching ideas, but I see this as a valuable learning experience to learn how to accept my own mistakes and courageously rectify them."

12.4.5 Success Experience

- "Besides teaching, I was a member of the performance team. Our team was in charge of the farewell performance at the closing ceremony. As I know how to play the piano, I volunteered to play the piano and sing as part of my performance. The performance preparation process was fun and rewarding. I was happy that I could contribute to my team using my piano and singing skills. I also had the chance to help in the closing ceremony as one of the IT supporters. I was responsible for playing videos during the closing ceremony. It was my first time taking up such a role, so I was quite nervous that I would make mistakes and ruin the ceremony. Nevertheless, during the rehearsal sessions, the professors and student helpers all showed their understanding of my mistakes and encouraged me to do better. I am very thankful to all the people who helped and supported me. Helping out in the closing ceremony was one of the most memorable moments I had in the subject. I was glad to be on the closing ceremony team."

12.4.6 Learning from the Service Recipients

As the subject focuses on providing services to needy groups, students generally shared that they also got the opportunity to learn from their service recipients. Some comments are presented below.

- "In addition, I gained a deeper understanding of this SL, that is, learning and growing is a two-way street. The process of helping and teaching children is a two-way process of learning and growing for both the service provider and the service recipient. I have learned and gained a lot from the preparation, execution, and reflection process in the service. I also learned a lot from the children. Although their families are underprivileged, they always maintain a positive attitude. They study hard and hope to change their lives through their own efforts. I am acutely aware that I should be grateful for what I have now, learn from their optimistic attitude toward life and their diligent attitude toward learning, and continue to improve myself and help more people in need through my abilities."

12.4.7 Changing Perceptions of the Needs of the Clients

Some students shared that their original views of the needs and attributes of service recipients needed to be corrected. However, their subsequent experiences have changed their views during the process. Some examples are presented below.

- "One of the most important values that I learned from this service is that I should not label anyone easily before I get along with them. Before the service, I searched for some background information and heard from my relatives about XXX students, which affected my view of them. Thinking they may be shy, naughty, or pessimistic. However, after spending three days with XXX students, I found they are talkative, positive, friendly, and motivated in their future studies."
- "Another gain in this course is that this service delivery inspired me to know that there are many underprivileged children and adolescents who require my help. Society needs to face this situation and offer more help to them. In fact, there are many 'bad children' who are not bad. I think they are just unlucky and cannot get enough care or help from their parents or society only, like Zheng Sheng's students."
- "As a matter of fact, SEN students are mistakenly labeled as 'naughty' or children with behavioral problems. In my opinion, these prejudices can be solved by showing care, concern, and appreciation for oneself and others. From now on, I hope I can be more sensitive to people in need around me."

12.4.8 Perceptions of Service-Learning

Some students shared that they initially held the view that the subject was not meaningful, and they were merely taking this compulsory subject to fulfill the university requirement. Nevertheless, their perceptions were proved wrong after the whole process. Some examples are presented below.

- "Originally, to me, the SL subject was just credit-bearing volunteer work and was registered for this subject because it is compulsory. At the very beginning, frankly speaking, I had no incentive to be dedicated to this subject. However, after studying this subject, I realized that what I learned was actually more than what I had paid for. I see the value in it, and this is a precious experience to me."
- "When I was informed that the service center is located in XXX, I thought the arrangement was inappropriate since the voluntary work should be convenient to both the service recipients and the providers, as the traveling time to go to the center will be wasted. However, I was inspired by the tutor that the suburban district often lacks volunteers due to inconvenient transportation. I believe that with great power comes great responsibility. Also, educating autistics always requires some specialized knowledge, so university students may be more suitable to take the post. While in contact with those needy, I can know more about their situation and action."

- "Working as a volunteer in this subject, I enjoyed helping people learn about community services available to them. I was very surprised that the service only lasted four days, but my insight is that my whole life is long. To be honest, some students serve SL as a mandatory requirement before they graduate or take a course, and I did not expect that it would profoundly affect my values."
- "Before attending this course, my classmates and I talked about this Service Leadership program and assumed that it was a kind of volunteering work, that it was just fulfilling some work hours we needed to be able to graduate. By now, as I had finished my service, I came to understand that it is more than just putting in hours. The foundation of service is the deeds performed by a person with the purpose of helping or bringing benefits to one's community and self at the same time. Leadership elements and qualities can also be practiced and reflected in service provision."

12.4.9 Social Responsibility

As the subject focuses on promoting civic responsibility of university students, students generally shared that the subject was able to promote their understanding of the needs of society, and they were motivated to shoulder more social responsibility in future. Some comments are presented below.

- "As university students, we receive many resources from society; this means we have the responsibility to contribute to society when we have professional knowledge and related experiences. Although SL is a credit-bearing subject, it is much more meaningful than a grade on those three credits in our lives."
- "This SL experience is my beacon; it guides me to practice effective service leadership, to develop a sense of responsibility as a professional and passion toward people in need, to recognize my strengths and weaknesses, and to enhance my intrapersonal and interpersonal competences as well as my problem-solving skills."
- "Apart from learning and applying the knowledge on effective service leadership, I recognized my role and responsibility as a professional and citizen in helping the children and their families in need from this SL."
- "On the whole, SL is seen as an invaluable opportunity for me to practice the know-how in the frontline services before my graduation. Also, as Hong Kong citizens, we do have a civic responsibility to treasure and serve our community."
- "Before joining the SL course, Service Leadership through Serving Children and Families with Special Needs, I thought Service Leadership was all about consecration. But now, I would say Service Leadership is not only utilizing our competence in providing services but also aiming at ethically satisfying the needs of oneself and other stakeholders in the community. It is a chance for us to learn the knowledge, which cannot be learned from books, to unleash our potential and get to know ourselves better."

- "In the beginning, I had not set up any goals for this course; I just wanted to pass this subject in order to let me graduate. However, as time flies, the more time I have spent trying to understand my service target, the higher expectations I had set for myself for this course. This also led to my reflection on my civil responsibility and future career."

12.4.10 Application to Real Life

Some students shared that they were surprised that the subject motivated them to be a better person in future, and they believed that this subject was helpful for their future career. Some examples are presented below.

- "Overall, I am thankful that I have learned different theories on lessons, and I can apply them during services. I am surprised that I can explore myself and learn from my mistakes to become a better me. It is amazing that I can always learn to serve while serving to learn. I believe that what I have learned is not limited to volunteering but can always be applied anytime and anywhere."
- *Future Career*: "The knowledge I gained in the aspect of service leadership, such as moral character, leadership competences, etc., is also helpful to my future career development as a physiotherapist. As a future healthcare professional, I am a service leader. By providing healthcare services, I am leading my patients at the same time."

12.4.11 Serving Others in Future

In SL, we strongly emphasize the importance of serving others as service leaders. Students also underscored the value of providing services to others in future. Some narratives are shown below.

- "This SL experience inspired me a lot in values, personal capabilities, and personal development and increased my passion for providing voluntary work in the future."
- "It seems that SL is not only a subject learning but a distinctive experience that further brings me with a deeper self-reflection on personal and professional enhancement, which are significant in my lifelong commitment to learning from and serving others and myself."
- "This trip made me earn a lot, not only academically but also in terms of my moral character, interpersonal skills, and the competencies of service leadership. I also understand more about the importance of communication and teamwork. At the same time, this trip gave me a memorable and joyful experience. I gained some valuable relationships last summer. If I am capable and available, I would like to join these kinds of trips again; I may get different rewards and experiences at that time."

- "In the future, hopefully, I can utilize my professional skills to help different parties regarding housing issues or living quality."
- "These proved the effort from all of us during the whole SL experience was worth it. The SL course ended, but serving and learning would be continued."
- "By joining every activity, I became more and more passionate. Therefore, although I achieved 100 hours, I continued to be a student helper without accompanying by my group members. In future, I would like to maintain my passion and improve myself to be a good citizen."

12.5 Teacher Experiences

Besides the students, the teachers also showed positive views of the subject. They used descriptors and metaphors to describe their experiences, such as "a strong sense of achievement," "a strong sense of satisfaction," "happy to witness the (personal) growth of students," and "co-walker." Moreover, the teachers agreed that the subject can develop the holistic development and civic responsibility of students (Ma et al., 2016). One teacher shared in the narrative.

- "My students mentioned that the home visit or getting along with the elder people ... this kind of ... real touch, real feeling was crucial. Books could not provide this experience. The sense of community in Hong Kong, diversity, empowerment, and all these things are different from textbook knowledge. Students could feel this when they really get in touch with the old people, and this contact provided them with genuine feelings [towards the needy]."
- "Students have developed a great sense of civic responsibility and realized the importance of a concerted effort by different stakeholders in the society to work toward environmental sustainability. For many students, the experience of working with students with different academic backgrounds not only created synergy in problem-solving but also enabled them to polish their teamwork skills and to appreciate the strengths of other professionals."
- "In order to develop the well-being of adolescents, SL is therefore a valuable vehicle for adolescents to know about their lives by doing. The cultivation and transformation of life cannot be done by paperwork nor by passing any examination to demonstrate the competence acquired, but through exercising the will. Throughout facilitating the service trips, I know that SL has been beneficial not only to the service targets and the PolyU students as the service providers but also to myself. The teaching of this subject enabled me to reflect on my life and my calling every time. The teaching has also driven me to continue my vigorous search from my mind and heart to answer the question of why I still enjoy serving people around me. The service with Zheng Sheng helped to identify my weaknesses, mostly in terms of my character and my leadership skills."

12.5.1 Views on Service-Learning

Some teachers agreed that SL can link university students and the community together, and university students can experience personal growth during this process (Shek et al., 2019). Some narratives are shown below.

- "When we put too much focus on developing our professions, we forget our obligation to serve our community. SL guided them to think more about how to use their professional knowledge to contribute to the community."
- "It is not only about fulfilling the service hours required or teaching students about adolescent development. I think our course aims to enhance students' self-understanding and help them understand what it means to serve and to contribute. Of course, we need to ensure the quality of the service provided, but the most important thing is not for them (university students) to create activities; the most important thing is they learn how to connect with others."

12.5.2 Obstacles in Undertaking Service-Learning

When discussing the challenges encountered, the teachers shared that time conflict and communication problems among different stakeholders are the most significant obstacles. Nevertheless, the teachers also reflected that the subject has positive influences on both university students and secondary school students (Shek et al., 2019). Some teachers shared below.

- "There was a student whose major was not fashion design, but he was responsible for sewing clothes. He stayed in the secondary school and worked until 11 p.m. a few days in a row. He eventually received the scholarship. Many secondary school teachers remembered him and asked about him in the next two academic years."
- "A PolyU student who graduated from an underprivileged secondary school was emotional while providing service. In the debriefing, the student expressed feeling disappointed when he saw some of the secondary school teachers have given up on teaching the secondary school students. This student shared with his classmates, 'They (secondary school students) will actually listen to what you teach; you just have to find the right method.'"

12.6 Next Steps

First, the nurturance of service leadership is transformational and, as the foremost important goal, aims to change the students' worldview. Although the SL pedagogy and the use of reflection are, to some extent, effective ways to foster students' learning in application and synthesis, the effect on the changed worldview would be even more substantial, especially if the level of complexity of knowledge formation in the current subject materials by using the Structure of Observed Learning Outcomes taxonomy (Biggs & Collis, 1982) would be reviewed. Second, as there are more than ten service sites in four agencies, the teaching materials should be more contextualized to address the different needs of various communities and maintain the unity of the teaching of Service Leadership attributes.

Subjective outcome evaluation using surveys is involved in evaluating the impact of the course. Feedback from the service agencies regarding students' performance and reflective writings of students are also collected to understand the perceptions of the overall SL and Service Leadership experiences from different perspectives. However, although it is efficient to evaluate the outcomes by using quantitative methods with some qualitative evidence to support the findings, the quantitative data cannot show comprehensive subjective experiences of learning (Thomas & Beauchamp, 2011). In addition, Parlett and Hamilton (1972) argued that many formal evaluations cannot provide an accurate picture of educational life. As such, the teaching team invited students to use metaphors to describe their service experience in one of the service sites, Christian Zheng Sheng College, during the summer of 2015. This method has been used and validated in Project P.A.T.H.S. (Positive Adolescent Training through Holistic Social Programs) in Hong Kong (Shek & Sun, 2012). The next step will be to extend this method to evaluate all the students who participated in this course. Moreover, a longitudinal case study should also be adopted to learn about the development of Service Leadership and the impact of the SL experiences on students.

Acknowledgements The preparation of this chapter is financially supported by The Hong Kong Polytechnic University (ZZ4U and ZZUE), Li and Fung Endowed Professorship in Service Leadership Education, Wofoo Foundation, and the Matching Fund of Research Grants Council (ZECL and ZH4Q).

Appendix 1 Objective Outcome Evaluation Form

學生問卷調查

Student Questionnaire

親愛的同學:

較早時我們成功獲得您的同意填寫這份問卷。問卷的內容主要是幫助我們瞭解Service Leadership through Serving Children and Families with Special Needs科目的成效及你的發展特質。問卷內的問題沒有對或錯的答案，請您憑著對自己的認識或感覺誠實作答。為了瞭解您作答的情況，請保留已完成的問卷副本以作日後課堂討論之用。我們將為完成填寫的問卷進行計分，並把您所填寫的問卷和其他人的問卷合併作整體統計分析之用。我們向您保證，您所提供的一切意見及資料，均絕對保密且只用作教學和研究之用。謝謝您的幫忙!

Dear Students,

We have previously obtained your consent to complete this questionnaire, which helps us understand the impact of service leadership through serving children and families with special needs and your developmental characteristics. There are **no correct or incorrect answers** to these questions. **Please answer them honestly based on your knowledge and impression of yourself.** For a better understanding of yourself, please keep a copy of the completed questionnaire for further use in class discussion. Marks will be given for successful completion. Please be assured that your data will be analyzed in an aggregated manner, and the information you provide will be **kept strictly confidential and solely used for education and research purposes**. Thank you for your help!

第一部分 **Part 1**

請小心閱讀下列各句子， 然後在下表圈出一個您認為最能夠代表您的想法的數字。

Please read each sentence carefully and ***circle the number*** that best describes your thoughts.

		非常 不同意 **Strongly disagree**	不同意 **Disagree**	有點 不同意 **Slightly disagree**	有點 同意 **Slightly agree**	同意 **Agree**	非常 同意 **Strongly agree**
1.	我懂得怎樣與人溝通。 I know how to communicate with others	1	2	3	4	5	6
2.	我了解人與人相處的規則和要求。 I understand the rules and expectations in interacting with others	1	2	3	4	5	6
3.	我能夠與其他人融洽相處。 I can get along well with others	1	2	3	4	5	6
4.	當我不開心時, 我能夠適當地表達我的情緒。 When I am unhappy, I can appropriately express my emotions	1	2	3	4	5	6

(continued)

(continued)

		非常 不同意 **Strongly disagree**	不同意 **Disagree**	有點 不同意 **Slightly disagree**	有點 同意 **Slightly agree**	同意 **Agree**	非常 同意 **Strongly agree**
5.	在與人發生衝突時, 我通常能夠處理我的情緒。 When I have conflict with others, I can usually manage my emotions	1	2	3	4	5	6
6.	我能夠站在別人的角度看問題和瞭解他們的感受。 I can stand in the shoes of others	1	2	3	4	5	6
7.	我懂得從不同角度去看事物。 I know how to see things from different angles	1	2	3	4	5	6
8.	我會嘗試用創新的方法去解決我面對的問題。 I try new ways to solve my problems	1	2	3	4	5	6
9.	我懂得分析問題的成因和尋找解決的方法。 I know how to find the causes of and solutions to a problem	1	2	3	4	5	6
10.	我能夠分辨事情的好與壞。 I can differentiate between the good and the bad aspects of things	1	2	3	4	5	6
11.	我能夠以開放的態度面對批評。 I can face criticisms with an open mind	1	2	3	4	5	6

(continued)

(continued)

		非常不同意 **Strongly disagree**	不同意 **Disagree**	有點不同意 **Slightly disagree**	有點同意 **Slightly agree**	同意 **Agree**	非常同意 **Strongly agree**
12.	我能夠表達與其他人不同的意見。 I can express views that are different from others	1	2	3	4	5	6
13.	對於自己的行為, 我有較高的道德要求。 I have high moral standards for my behaviors	1	2	3	4	5	6
14.	我向他人承諾了會做的事, 我會把它完成。 I fulfill my promises	1	2	3	4	5	6
15.	為了賺錢而放棄一些道德原則, 並沒有太大問題。(Reverse keyed) It is no big deal to give up some of our moral principles in exchange for money	1	2	3	4	5	6
16.	我有自我檢討的習慣。 I have a habit of self-reflection	1	2	3	4	5	6
17.	我有能力作出明智的抉擇。 I am capable of making wise choices	1	2	3	4	5	6
18.	我對自己所作的決定有信心。 I am confident about my decisions	1	2	3	4	5	6

(continued)

(continued)

		非常 不同意 **Strongly disagree**	不同意 **Disagree**	有點 不同意 **Slightly disagree**	有點 同意 **Slightly agree**	同意 **Agree**	非常 同意 **Strongly agree**
19.	我相信將來發生在我身上的事情,大部分取決於我自己。 I believe things that will happen in my life are mostly determined by myself	1	2	3	4	5	6
20.	我是一個有自信的人。 I am a person with self-confidence	1	2	3	4	5	6
21.	我相信自己有領袖的特質及能力。 I believe I have the qualities and abilities of a leader	1	2	3	4	5	6
22.	我有信心解決我將來會面對的問題。 I have confidence to solve my future problems	1	2	3	4	5	6
23.	我有信心能夠大學畢業。 I have confidence to graduate from university	1	2	3	4	5	6
24.	我有信心畢業後能夠成為一個有用的人。 I have confidence that I will be a useful person after I graduate	1	2	3	4	5	6
25.	在很多方面, 我的生活接近我理想中的狀態。 In most ways, my life is close to my ideal	1	2	3	4	5	6

(continued)

(continued)

		非常不同意 **Strongly disagree**	不同意 **Disagree**	有點不同意 **Slightly disagree**	有點同意 **Slightly agree**	同意 **Agree**	非常同意 **Strongly agree**
26.	我的生活狀況是極好的。 The conditions of my life are excellent	1	2	3	4	5	6
27.	我對自己的人生感到滿意。 I am satisfied with my life	1	2	3	4	5	6
28.	到目前為止, 我已經取得生命中我想得到的重要東西。 So far I have gotten the important things I want in life	1	2	3	4	5	6
29.	如果我能夠再活一次, 我依然會選擇現有的生活。 If I could live my life over, I would still choose the life I have now	1	2	3	4	5	6
30.	我的生命很有意義。 My life is meaningful	1	2	3	4	5	6
31.	我已經找到人生的目標。 I have found my purpose in life	1	2	3	4	5	6
32.	我考慮過自殺。 I have considered committing suicide before	1	2	3	4	5	6
33.	我相信心靈上的富有比物質上的富有更為重要。 I believe spiritual riches are more important than material prosperity	1	2	3	4	5	6

(continued)

(continued)

		非常不同意 **Strongly disagree**	不同意 **Disagree**	有點不同意 **Slightly disagree**	有點同意 **Slightly agree**	同意 **Agree**	非常同意 **Strongly agree**
34.	面對困難時, 我不會輕易放棄。 When I face difficulties, I do not give up easily	1	2	3	4	5	6
35.	我的信念是:「就算明天變得更差, 我仍會好好地生活下去。」 My belief is that even though tomorrow becomes worse, I will still live in a good manner	1	2	3	4	5	6
36.	我相信人生中的困難是可以解決的。 I believe problems in life can be solved	1	2	3	4	5	6
37.	我明白自我發展的重要性。 I understand the importance of self-development	1	2	3	4	5	6
38.	我清楚知道自己的優點和缺點。 I know my strengths and weaknesses	1	2	3	4	5	6
39.	我有能力管理自己的生活。 I am capable of managing my own life	1	2	3	4	5	6
40.	我對自己的生活有好的規劃。 I have good planning for my life	1	2	3	4	5	6

(continued)

(continued)

		非常 不同意 **Strongly disagree**	不同意 **Disagree**	有點 不同意 **Slightly disagree**	有點 同意 **Slightly agree**	同意 **Agree**	非常 同意 **Strongly agree**
41.	我控制自己的言行以免言行失當。 I control my own behavior to avoid stepping out of line	1	2	3	4	5	6
42.	我容易察覺到別人的需求。 I am sensitive to others' needs	1	2	3	4	5	6
43.	別人和我說話時，我會專心聽。 I pay attention to others when they are talking to me	1	2	3	4	5	6
44.	當他人有需要時，我會為他人提供建議。 I offer advice to others when there is a need	1	2	3	4	5	6
45.	我時刻願意幫助有需要的人。 I am always ready to lend a hand to those in need	1	2	3	4	5	6
46.	我懂得如何欣賞他人，即使是那些與我很不相同的人。 I know how to appreciate others, even those who are completely different from me	1	2	3	4	5	6
47.	我以尊重的態度對待他人。 I treat others with dignity and respect	1	2	3	4	5	6
48.	我關心他人。 I care about others	1	2	3	4	5	6

(continued)

(continued)

		非常 不同意 **Strongly disagree**	不同意 **Disagree**	有點 不同意 **Slightly disagree**	有點 同意 **Slightly agree**	同意 **Agree**	非常 同意 **Strongly agree**
49.	我對他人很友善。 I am kind and friendly to others	1	2	3	4	5	6
50.	我樂於學習新知識。 I open my mind to embrace new knowledge	1	2	3	4	5	6
51.	我對生活中的許多事情心懷感恩。 I am grateful for many things in my life	1	2	3	4	5	6
52.	我不喜歡說謊和欺騙。 Lying or cheating is not my way	1	2	3	4	5	6
53.	即使我遇到挫折，我也會堅持不懈地追求我的目標。 I persist in pursuing my goals even though I encounter setbacks	1	2	3	4	5	6
54.	我不喜歡炫耀發生在我身上的好事。 I do not like to show off good things happening to me	1	2	3	4	5	6
55.	即使遭受反對，我也會毫不猶豫地抗議我認為錯誤的事情。 I do not hesitate to fight against what I think wrong despite opposition	1	2	3	4	5	6

(continued)

(continued)

		非常 不同意 **Strongly disagree**	不同意 **Disagree**	有點 不同意 **Slightly disagree**	有點 同意 **Slightly agree**	同意 **Agree**	非常 同意 **Strongly agree**
56.	我把他人的利益放於自己的利益之前。 I place my interests after the interests of others	1	2	3	4	5	6
57.	我視誠信為人生最重要的部份。 I regard integrity as the most important aspect of life	1	2	3	4	5	6
58.	我樂於尊重規則。 It is my pleasure to obey rules and regulations	1	2	3	4	5	6
59.	如果我做錯了事，我會感到羞恥。 I would feel ashamed if I had done something wrong	1	2	3	4	5	6
60.	我儘量維持人際交往中的和諧。 I try to maintain harmony in interpersonal relationships	1	2	3	4	5	6
61.	看到不公義的事，我會挺身而出。 I will fight against injustice	1	2	3	4	5	6
62.	我不去嘗試佔有不應得的東西。 I do not attempt to possess anything undeserved	1	2	3	4	5	6
63.	我的所言與所行是一致的。 I live my life in the way I have claimed	1	2	3	4	5	6

(continued)

(continued)

		非常 不同意 **Strongly disagree**	不同意 **Disagree**	有點 不同意 **Slightly disagree**	有點 同意 **Slightly agree**	同意 **Agree**	非常 同意 **Strongly agree**
64.	在面對得失時, 我通常能保持內心的平靜。 Most of the time, I can keep my mind peaceful in face of gains or losses	1	2	3	4	5	6
65.	領導是一種對自我, 他人, 團體以及社會的服務。 Leadership is a service for self, others, groups, and society	1	2	3	4	5	6
66.	每一個人每天都有機會實踐領導能力。 Everyone has opportunities to practice leadership every day	1	2	3	4	5	6
67.	領導的效能取決於專業能力、個人品德和關愛他人的能力。 Leadership effectiveness is determined by situational task competencies, character strength, and caring ability	1	2	3	4	5	6
68.	成功的領袖必須竭盡所能, 提升自己的能力及滿足他人的需求。 A successful leader should try his/her best to improve his/her competencies and satisfy others' needs	1	2	3	4	5	6

(continued)

(continued)

		非常 不同意 **Strongly disagree**	不同意 **Disagree**	有點 不同意 **Slightly disagree**	有點 同意 **Slightly agree**	同意 **Agree**	非常 同意 **Strongly agree**
69.	作為服務型領袖，要向每天接觸到的人提供高品質的服務，不論對方的地位和能力。 A service leader needs to provide high-quality service to the people he/ she contacts, regardless of their position and capacity	1	2	3	4	5	6
70.	服務型領袖需要不斷地提升自己的品德和關愛他人的能力。 A service leader needs to improve his/her character strength and caring ability continuously	1	2	3	4	5	6

第二部分 **Part 2**

這部分將問及一些個人資料，您提供的資料會絕對保密。請在合適位置選出或填上答案。

This part will ask about your personal information; the information you provide will be kept strictly confidential. Please **choose or fill in your answer** in the space provided.

OFFICIAL USE ONLY

1. 性別 Sex:= 男 male; = 女 female

2. 年齡 Age：______________

3. 出生日期 Date of birth：_____ / ____ / ______ (yyyy/ mm/ dd)
(例子： 如你於 1992 年 1 月 9 日出生， 請填 1992/01/09)
(Example: If you were born on the 9th of January 1992, please fill in 1992/01/09)

4. 學生証編號(中間三個號碼)： XXX ___ ____ ___ XXX
Middle three digits of student ID card number
(例子： 如你學生証編號是 09123456d, 請填 XXX 234 XXX)
(Example: If your student ID card number is 09123456d, please fill in XXX 234 XXX)

parent Sex

5. 您父母現時的婚姻狀況是怎樣？
What is the current marital status of your parents?

父親與母親已離婚 Divorced	父親與母親已分居 Separated	父親與母親是夫婦(第一段婚姻) Married (first marriage)	父親與母親是夫婦 (第二段婚姻) Married (second marriage)	其他（請註明） Others (please specify)

6. 您覺得您的家庭生活愉快嗎？
Do you think you have a happy family life?

happiness

很不愉快 Very unhappy	不愉快 Unhappy	普通 Average	愉快 Happy	很愉快 Very Happy

完。謝謝！
End. Thank you!

Scoring

Subscales	Variables	Items	Item number
1. Social competence	SC	1–3	3
2. Emotional competence	EC	4–6	3
3. Cognitive competence	CC	7–10	4
4. Behavioral competence	BC	11–12	2
5. Moral competence	MC	13, 14, 15r, 16	4
6. Self-determination	SD	17–19	3
7. Clear and positive identity	CPI	20–21	2
8. Belief in future	BF	22–24	3

(continued)

(continued)

Subscales	Variables	Items	Item number
9. Spirituality	SP	30, 31, 32r, 33	4
10. Resilience	RE	34–36	3
• Composite scores			
• Cognitive-behavioral competencies (CBC)	CC + BC + SD		9
• Positive identity (PI)	CPI + BF		5
• Positive youth development qualities (PYDQ)	SC + EC + MC + SP + RE		17
11. Life satisfaction	LS	25–29	5
12. Service leadership scale			
• Self-leadership	SL	37–41	5
• Caring disposition	CD	42–49	8
• Character strengths	CS	50–64	15
• Beliefs and values of service leadership	SLV	65–70	6
Total			**70**

Note r = reversed item

Appendix 2 Objective Outcome Evaluation-Service Recipient

服务学习夏令营

Service-Learning Summer Camp

小朋友们好:

为了解儿童成长及评估希望旅程服务学习夏令营的成效， 我们现邀请你完成这份问卷。你所提供的答案会绝对保密, 并仅作为这次评估使用, 请放心填写。你的家长和老师都不会看到你所填写的内容。

每页问卷都有答题指引, 回答问题前, 请确定你已经清楚问卷的答题要求。

本问卷没有对错之分, 只需如实作答即可。回答问题时, 请不要花太多时间思考每道题目, 只要根据你的第一反应来回答, 并且不要和别人讨论问卷内容, 谢谢你的合作!

Dear all,

To understand how the children grow after the Service-Learning activities and assess the effectiveness of the Journey for Hope Service-Learning Camp, we now invite you to complete this questionnaire. The answers you provide will be kept confidential and used only for this assessment; please feel free to fill them out. Neither your parents nor your teachers will see your answers.

There are instructions on each page of the questionnaire. Before answering questions, make sure you have understood the requirements of the questionnaire.

There are no right or wrong answers in this questionnaire; please answer truthfully. When answering questions, please do not spend too much time thinking about each question and answer them according to your first reaction. Do not discuss the questionnaire with others. Thank you for your cooperation.

第一部分**(A)**

请如实填写你的个人资料, 你提供的答案会绝对保密。你可以在横线上填上适当的答案, 或在□ 内打√。

1.	你现在所就读的年级: ____	班级: ____	座号: ____
2.	你在 2021年 7月希望旅程服务学习夏令营中所在的班级:		____
3.	你的性别:	1) □男	2) □女
4.	你的年龄: ____周岁	出生年月: ____	
5.	你的出生地点:	成都	成都以外地区 - 请注明省、市、县、乡: ____
6.	你的户籍:	1) □农村户口	2) □城市户口
7.	你已在成都居住多长时间:	____年	
8.	与你同住的家庭成员有: (可选择多于一个的答案)		
	1) 父亲	2) 继父	3) 母亲
	4) 继母	5) 爷爷	6) 奶奶
	7) 外公	8) 外婆	9) 哥哥
	10) 姐姐	11) 弟弟	12) 妹妹
	13) 其他人: ____		
9.	平时谁是你的主要照顾者: (可选择多于一个的答案)		
	1) 父亲	2) 继父	3) 母亲
	4) 继母	5) 爷爷	6) 奶奶
	7) 外公	8) 外婆	9) 哥哥
	10) 姐姐	11) 其他人: ____	
10.	父亲目前的工作状况: (单选)		
	1) 全职工作	2) 兼职工作	3) 无业
	4) 退休	5) 不知道	
11.	母亲目前的工作状况: (单选)		
	1) 全职工作	2) 兼职工作	3) 无业

(continued)

(continued)

	4) 退休	5) 不知道	
12.	父亲的教育程度: (单选)		
	1) 没有接受任何正式教育	2) 小学一年级至五年级	3) 小学毕业
	4) 初中毕业	5) 高中毕业	6) 大专
	7) 大学或以上	8) 不知道	
13.	母亲的教育程度: (单选)		
	1) 没有接受任何正式教育	2) 小学一年级至五年级	3) 小学毕业
	4) 初中毕业	5) 高中毕业	6) 大专
	7) 大学或以上	8) 不知道	
14.	你的家庭每月收入大约:		
	1) 3000 元或以下	2) 3001 元–5000 元	3) 5001 元–10,000 元
	4) 10,000 元或以上	5) 不知道	

Part One (A)

Please fill in your personal information truthfully. The answers you provide will be kept confidential. You can fill in the appropriate answer on the horizontal line or type √ inside.

1.	Your current grade: ____	Class: ____	Seat number: ____
2.	Which class were you in during the Journey for Hope Service-Learning Summer Camp: ____		
3.	Your gender:	1) Male	2) Female
4.	Your age: ____	Date of birth: Year: ____Month: ____Date: ____	
5.	Your place of birth:	Chengdu	Areas outside Chengdu—Please specify province, city, county, and township: ____
6.	Your household registration:	1) Rural	2) Urban
7.	How long have you lived in Chengdu:		____ Years
8.	The family members you live with: (you can choose more than one answer)		
	1) Father	2) Stepfather	3) Mother
	4) Stepmother	5) Grandfather	6) Grandmother
	7) Grandfather	8) Grandmother	9) Older brother
	10) Older sister	11) Younger brother	12) Younger sister
	13) Others: ____		

(continued)

(continued)

9.	Who is your primary caregiver: (you can choose more than one answer)		
	1) Father	2) Stepfather	3) Mother
	4) Stepmother	5) Grandfather	6) Grandmother
	7) Grandfather	8) Grandmother	9) Older brother
	10) Older sister	11) Others: ____	
10.	Father's current work status: (choose one answer)		
	1) Full-time employment	2) Part-time employment	3) Unemployed
	4) Retired	5) I don't know	
11.	Mother's current work status: (choose one answer)		
	1) Full-time employment	2) Part-time employment	3) Unemployed
	4) Retired	5) I don't know	
12.	Father's educational background: (choose one answer)		
	1) No formal education	2) Primary 1–5	3) Primary school graduation
	4) Junior high school graduation	5) High school graduation	6) College
	7) University or above	8) I don't know	
13.	Mother's educational background: (choose one answer)		
	1) No formal education	2) Primary 1–5	3) Primary school graduation
	4) Junior high school graduation	5) High school graduation	6) College
	7) University or above	8) I don't know	
14.	Your family monthly income is approximately:		
	1) 3000 RMB or less	2) 3001 RMB–5000 RMB	3) 5001 RMB–10,000 RMB
	4) 10,000 RMB or more	5) I don't know	

第二部分 **(B) Part Two (B)**

请仔细阅读下列句子， 然后圈出一个你认为最能够代表你的想法或真实情况的答案。

Please read the following sentences carefully, and then circle one answer that you think best represents what you think or what is true.

		非常 不同意 **Strongly disagree**	不同意 **Disagree**	有点 不同意 **Slightly disagree**	有点 同意 **Slightly agree**	同意 **Agree**	非常 同意 **Strongly agree**
1.	我对学习知识很感兴趣。 I am very interested in learning knowledge	1	2	3	4	5	6
2.	我对英语方面的课程很感兴趣。 I am very interested in the English courses	1	2	3	4	5	6
3.	我对科学方面的课程很感兴趣。 I am very interested in the Science courses	1	2	3	4	5	6
4.	我对健康教育方面的课程很感兴趣。 I am very interested in the Health Education courses	1	2	3	4	5	6
5.	我对个人成长方面的课程很感兴趣。 I am very interested in the courses on personal growth	1	2	3	4	5	6
6.	我掌握了很多知识。 I have mastered a lot of knowledge	1	2	3	4	5	6
7.	我掌握了很多英语知识。 I have mastered a lot of English knowledge	1	2	3	4	5	6
8.	我掌握了很多科学知识。 I have mastered a lot of scientific knowledge	1	2	3	4	5	6
9.	我掌握了很多关于健康教育方面的知识。 I have learned a lot about health education	1	2	3	4	5	6
10.	我掌握了很多关于个人成长方面的知识。 I have acquired a lot of knowledge about my personal growth	1	2	3	4	5	6

第三部分 **(C) Part Three (C)**

请仔细阅读下列句子， 然后圈出一个你认为最能够代表你的想法或真实情况的答案。

Please read the following sentences carefully, and then circle one answer that you think best represents what you think or what is true.

		非常不同意 **Strongly disagree**	不同意 **Disagree**	有点不同意 **Slightly disagree**	有点同意 **Slightly agree**	同意 **Agree**	非常同意 **Strongly agree**
1.	我懂得怎样与人沟通。 I know how to communicate with people	1	2	3	4	5	6
2.	我了解人与人相处的规则和要求。 I understand the rules and expectations in interacting with others	1	2	3	4	5	6
3.	我能够与其他人融洽相处。 I can get along well with others	1	2	3	4	5	6
4.	当我不开心时，我能够适当地表达我的情绪。 When I am unhappy, I can appropriately express my emotions	1	2	3	4	5	6
5.	在与人发生冲突时，我通常能够处理我的情绪。 When I have conflict with others, I can usually manage my emotions	1	2	3	4	5	6

(continued)

(continued)

		非常 不同意 **Strongly disagree**	不同意 **Disagree**	有点 不同意 **Slightly disagree**	有点 同意 **Slightly agree**	同意 **Agree**	非常 同意 **Strongly agree**
6.	我能够站在别人的角度看问题和了解他们的感受。 When I have conflict with others, I can usually manage my emotions	1	2	3	4	5	6
7.	我懂得从不同角度去看事物。 I know how to see things from different angles	1	2	3	4	5	6
8.	我会尝试用创新的方法去解决我面对的问题。 I try new ways to solve my problems	1	2	3	4	5	6
9.	我懂得分析问题的成因和寻找解决的方法。 I know how to find the causes of and solutions to a problem	1	2	3	4	5	6
10.	我能够分辨事情的好与坏。 I can differentiate between the good and the bad aspects of things	1	2	3	4	5	6
11.	我能够以开放的态度面对批评。 I can face criticisms with an open mind	1	2	3	4	5	6

(continued)

(continued)

		非常不同意 **Strongly disagree**	不同意 **Disagree**	有点不同意 **Slightly disagree**	有点同意 **Slightly agree**	同意 **Agree**	非常同意 **Strongly agree**
12.	我能够表达与其他人不同的意见。 I can express views that are different from others	1	2	3	4	5	6
13.	对于自己的行为, 我有较高的道德要求。 I have high moral standards for my behaviors	1	2	3	4	5	6
14.	我向他人承诺了会做的事, 我会把它完成。 I fulfill my promises	1	2	3	4	5	6
15.	为了赚钱而放弃一些道德原则, 并没有太大问题。 It is no big deal to give up some of our moral principles in exchange for money	1	2	3	4	5	6
16.	我有自我检讨的习惯。 I have a habit of self-reflection	1	2	3	4	5	6
17.	面对困难时, 我不会轻易放弃。 In the face of difficulties, I will not give up easily	1	2	3	4	5	6

(continued)

(continued)

		非常 不同意 **Strongly disagree**	不同意 **Disagree**	有点 不同意 **Slightly disagree**	有点 同意 **Slightly agree**	同意 **Agree**	非常 同意 **Strongly agree**
18.	我的信念是: "就算明天变得更差, 我仍会好好地生活下去。" My belief is: "Even if tomorrow becomes worse, I will still live in a good manner."	1	2	3	4	5	6
19.	我相信生活中的困难是可以解决的。 I believe that the difficulties in life can be solved	1	2	3	4	5	6
20.	当我需要帮助时, 我相信我的父母 (或监护人) 一定会帮助我。 When I need help, I believe that my parents (or guardian) will help me	1	2	3	4	5	6
21.	当我需要帮助时, 我相信我的朋友一定会帮助我。 When I need help, I am sure that my friends will help me	1	2	3	4	5	6

(continued)

(continued)

		非常 不同意 **Strongly disagree**	不同意 **Disagree**	有点 不同意 **Slightly disagree**	有点 同意 **Slightly agree**	同意 **Agree**	非常 同意 **Strongly agree**
22.	当我需要帮助时, 我相信我的老师一定会帮助我。 When I need help, I am sure that my teachers will help me	1	2	3	4	5	6
23.	我喜欢我的老师和同学。 I like my teachers and classmates	1	2	3	4	5	6
24.	在我的生活里, 有很多关心我的好朋友。 In my life, there are many good friends who care about me	1	2	3	4	5	6
25.	我的父母 (或监护人) 十分关心我。 My parents (or guardians) care very much about me	1	2	3	4	5	6
26.	我关心社会上遭遇不幸的人。 I care about those who encounter misfortune in society	1	2	3	4	5	6
27.	如有机会, 我会参加志愿者服务。 If I have the opportunity, I will participate in the volunteer service	1	2	3	4	5	6

(continued)

(continued)

		非常 不同意 **Strongly disagree**	不同意 **Disagree**	有点 不同意 **Slightly disagree**	有点 同意 **Slightly agree**	同意 **Agree**	非常 同意 **Strongly agree**
28.	我同意每个人都应该受到法律的约束。 I agree that everyone should be bound by the law	1	2	3	4	5	6
29.	我乐于遵守校规。 I am happy to follow the school rules	1	2	3	4	5	6
30.	如果我做错事,我会感到羞耻。 I will feel ashamed if I do something wrong	1	2	3	4	5	6
31.	我与他人相处得很好。 I get along very well with other people	1	2	3	4	5	6
32.	我会做对集体(例如: 班级, 小组) 有益的事情。 I will do something beneficial for the group (for example, a class, group)	1	2	3	4	5	6
33.	我会用自己喜欢被对待的方式去对待朋友。 I will treat my friends in the way that I like to be treated	1	2	3	4	5	6

(continued)

(continued)

		非常 不同意 **Strongly disagree**	不同意 **Disagree**	有点 不同意 **Slightly disagree**	有点 同意 **Slightly agree**	同意 **Agree**	非常 同意 **Strongly agree**
34.	我会友善对待与自己不同的孩子。 I will be friendly to the children who are different from myself	1	2	3	4	5	6
35.	当别的孩子不开心时, 我会尝试让他们高兴起来。 When the other kids are not happy, I will try to make them happy	1	2	3	4	5	6
36.	我是别人的好朋友。 I am someone else's good friend	1	2	3	4	5	6

第四部分 **(D) Part Four (D)**

请仔细阅读下列句子， 然后圈出一个你认为最能够代表你的想法或真实情况的答案。

Please read the following sentences carefully, and then circle one answer that you think best represents what you think or what is true.

		非常 不同意 **Strongly disagree**	不同意 **Disagree**	有点 不同意 **Slightly disagree**	有点 同意 **Slightly agree**	同意 **Agree**	非常 同意 **Strongly agree**
1.	我有能力作出明智的抉择。 I am capable of making wise choices	1	2	3	4	5	6

(continued)

(continued)

		非常 不同意 **Strongly disagree**	不同意 **Disagree**	有点 不同意 **Slightly disagree**	有点 同意 **Slightly agree**	同意 **Agree**	非常 同意 **Strongly agree**
2.	我对自己所作的决定有信心。 I am confident about my decisions	1	2	3	4	5	6
3.	我相信将来发生在我身上的事情，大部分取决于我自己。 I believe things that will happen in my life are mostly determined by myself	1	2	3	4	5	6
4.	我是一个有自信的人。 I am a person with self-confidence	1	2	3	4	5	6
5.	我相信自己有领袖的特质及能力。 I believe I have the qualities and abilities of a leader	1	2	3	4	5	6
6.	我有信心解决我将来会面对的问题。 I have confidence to solve my future problems	1	2	3	4	5	6
7.	我有信心能够大学毕业。 I have confidence to graduate from university	1	2	3	4	5	6

(continued)

(continued)

		非常不同意 **Strongly disagree**	不同意 **Disagree**	有点不同意 **Slightly disagree**	有点同意 **Slightly agree**	同意 **Agree**	非常同意 **Strongly agree**
8.	我有信心毕业后能够成为一个有用的人。 I have confidence that I will be a useful person after I graduate	1	2	3	4	5	6
9.	在很多方面，我的生活接近我理想中的状态。 In most ways, my life is close to my ideal	1	2	3	4	5	6
10.	我的生活状况是极好的。 The conditions of my life are excellent	1	2	3	4	5	6
11.	我对自己的人生感到满意。 I am satisfied with my life	1	2	3	4	5	6
12.	到目前为止，我已经取得生命中我想得到的重要东西。 So far, I have gotten the important things I want in life	1	2	3	4	5	6
13.	如果我能够再活一次，我依然会选择现有的生活。 If I could live my life over, I would still choose the life I have now	1	2	3	4	5	6

第五部分 **(E) Part Five (E)**

请仔细阅读下列句子， 然后圈出一个你认为最能够代表你的想法或真实情况的答案。

Please read the following sentences carefully, and then circle one answer that you think best represents what you think or what is true.

		非常 不同意 **Strongly disagree**	不同意 **Disagree**	有点 不同意 **Slightly disagree**	有点 同意 **Slightly agree**	同意 **Agree**	非常 同意 **Strongly agree**
1.	我明白自我发展的重要性。 I understand the importance of self-development	1	2	3	4	5	6
2.	我清楚知道自己的优点和缺点。 I know my strengths and weaknesses	1	2	3	4	5	6
3.	我有能力管理自己的生活。 I am capable of managing my own life	1	2	3	4	5	6
4.	我对自己的生活有好的规划。 I have a good planning on my life	1	2	3	4	5	6
5.	我控制自己的言行以免言行失当。 I control my own behavior to avoid stepping out of line	1	2	3	4	5	6
6.	我容易察觉到别人的需求。 I am sensitive to others' needs	1	2	3	4	5	6
7.	别人和我说话时，我会专心听。 I pay attention to others when they are talking to me	1	2	3	4	5	6
8.	当他人有需要时，我会为他人提供建议。 I offer advice to others when there is a need	1	2	3	4	5	6

(continued)

(continued)

		非常 不同意 **Strongly disagree**	不同意 **Disagree**	有点 不同意 **Slightly disagree**	有点 同意 **Slightly agree**	同意 **Agree**	非常 同意 **Strongly agree**
9.	我时刻愿意帮助有需要的人。 I am always ready to lend a hand to those in need	1	2	3	4	5	6
10.	我懂得如何欣赏他人, 即使是那些与我很不相同的人。 I know how to appreciate others, even those who are completely different from me	1	2	3	4	5	6
11.	我以尊重的态度对待他人。 I treat others with dignity and respect	1	2	3	4	5	6
12.	我关心他人。 I care about others	1	2	3	4	5	6
13.	我对他人很友善。 I am kind and friendly to others	1	2	3	4	5	6
14.	我乐于学习新知识。 I open my mind to embrace new knowledge	1	2	3	4	5	6
15.	我对生活中的许多事情心怀感恩。 I am grateful for many things in my life	1	2	3	4	5	6
16.	我不喜欢说谎和欺骗。 Lying or cheating is not my way	1	2	3	4	5	6

(continued)

(continued)

		非常 不同意 **Strongly disagree**	不同意 **Disagree**	有点 不同意 **Slightly disagree**	有点 同意 **Slightly agree**	同意 **Agree**	非常 同意 **Strongly agree**
17.	即使我遇到挫折，我也会坚持不懈地追求我的目标。 I persist in pursuing my goals even though I encounter setbacks	1	2	3	4	5	6
18.	我不喜欢炫耀发生在我身上的好事。 I do not like to show off good things happening to me	1	2	3	4	5	6
19.	即使遭受反对，我也会毫不犹豫地抗议我认为错误的事情。 I do not hesitate to fight against what I think wrong despite opposition	1	2	3	4	5	6
20.	我把他人的利益放于自己的利益之前。 I place my interests after the interests of others	1	2	3	4	5	6
21.	我视诚信为人生最重要的部份。 I regard integrity as the most important aspect of life	1	2	3	4	5	6
22.	我乐于尊重规则。 It is my pleasure to obey rules and regulations	1	2	3	4	5	6
23.	如果我做错了事，我会感到羞耻。 I would feel ashamed if I have done something wrong	1	2	3	4	5	6

(continued)

(continued)

		非常 不同意 **Strongly disagree**	不同意 **Disagree**	有点 不同意 **Slightly disagree**	有点 同意 **Slightly agree**	同意 **Agree**	非常 同意 **Strongly agree**
24.	我尽量维持人际交往中的和谐。 I try to maintain harmony in interpersonal relationships	1	2	3	4	5	6
25.	看到不公义的事,我会挺身而出。 I will fight against injustice	1	2	3	4	5	6
26.	我不去尝试占有不应得的东西。 I do not attempt to possess anything undeserved	1	2	3	4	5	6
27.	我的所言与所行是一致的。 I live my life in the way I have claimed	1	2	3	4	5	6
28.	在面对得失时,我通常能保持内心的平静。 Most of the time, I can keep my mind peaceful in face of gains or losses	1	2	3	4	5	6

完, 谢谢
End. Thank you!

Appendix 3 Subjective Outcome Evaluation Form

課程檢討問卷調查

Course Evaluation Form

親愛的同學:

為了幫助我們瞭解 Service Leadership through Serving Children and Families with Special Needs課程的成效, 現懇請您完成此問卷。問卷內的問題沒有對或錯的答案, 所以請您憑著您的觀感誠實作答。當您完成這份問卷後, 請將問卷直接交給在場的工作人員。您無需在問卷寫下您的名字，您所提供的一切意見及資料，均絕對保密。有關講師在日後絕對不會知道個別同學的答案，所有的資料只會供研究人員作整體分析之用。如有任何疑問，請詢問在場的工作人員。謝謝您的幫忙！

Dear Students,

In order to better understand the impacts of the course of Service Leadership through Serving Children and Families with Special Needs, we sincerely invite you to complete this questionnaire. The questions in the questionnaire **do not have correct or incorrect answers.** Please **honestly answer them based on your views**. After completing the questionnaire, please give it back to our staff directly. You do not need to provide your name on the questionnaire, and the information you provide will be **kept strictly confidential**. The lecturer(s) concerned will not know the responses of individual students, and the data will be used for overall analyses only. Should you have any questions, please contact the staff conducting this survey. Thank you for your help!

第一部分 **Part 1**

請回想一下您對Service Leadership through Serving Children and Families with Special Needs課程內容的觀感，然後在下表圈出一個您認為最能夠代表您觀感的數字。

Please think about your impression concerning the curriculum contents of this course, and then ***circle the number*** that best describes your views.

		非常不同意 Strongly Disagree	不同意 Disagree	中立 Neutral	同意 Agree	非常同意 Strongly Agree	OFFICIAL USE ONLY
1.1	課程的目標很清楚。 The objectives of the curriculum are very clear.	1	2	3	4	5	Cou_01
1.2	課程內容設計得很好。 The curriculum's content design is very good.	1	2	3	4	5	Cou_02
1.3	教學活動安排得很有條理。 The activities were carefully arranged.	1	2	3	4	5	Cou_03
1.4	課程進行時的氣氛很好。 The classroom atmosphere was very pleasant.	1	2	3	4	5	Cou_04
1.5	在課堂中，同學間有很多交流。 There was much peer interaction amongst the students.	1	2	3	4	5	Cou_05
1.6	我積極參與課程內的活動（包括：討論、分享、遊戲等）。 I participated in class activities actively (including discussions, sharing, games, etc.).	1	2	3	4	5	Cou_06
1.7	在課堂中，我獲得鼓勵去做到最好。 I was encouraged to do my best in the course	1	2	3	4	5	Cou_07
1.8	課堂中的學習經驗，增加我對這個課程的興趣。 The learning experience enhanced my interest in the course.	1	2	3	4	5	Cou_08
1.9	整體而言，我對這個課程有非常正面的評價。 Overall speaking, I have a very positive evaluation of the course.	1	2	3	4	5	Cou_09
1.10	整體而言，我很喜歡這個課程。 On the whole, I like this course very much.	1	2	3	4	5	Cou_10

第二部分 **Part 2**

請回想一下您對Service Leadership through Serving Children and Families with Special Needs課程講師的觀感，然後在下表圈出一個您認為最能夠代表您觀感的數字。

Please think about your impression concerning the lecturer(s) of this course, and then ***circle the number*** that best describes your views.

		非常不同意 Strongly Disagree	不同意 Disagree	中立 Neutral	同意 Agree	非常同意 Strongly Agree	OFFICIAL USE ONLY
2.1	講師對這個課程有充分的掌握。 The lecturer(s) had a good mastery of the course.	1	2	3	4	5	Lec_01
2.2	講師的準備功夫充足。 The lecturer(s) was (were) well prepared for the lessons.	1	2	3	4	5	Lec_02
2.3	講師的教學技巧良好。 The teaching skills of the lecturer(s) were good.	1	2	3	4	5	Lec_03
2.4	講師的專業態度很好。 The lecturer(s) showed good professional attitude.	1	2	3	4	5	Lec_04
2.5	講師表現很投入。 The lecturer(s) was (were) very involved.	1	2	3	4	5	Lec_05
2.6	講師鼓勵同學參與課堂活動。 The lecturer(s) encouraged students to participate in the activities.	1	2	3	4	5	Lec_06
2.7	講師關心同學。 The lecturer(s) cared for the students.	1	2	3	4	5	Lec_07
2.8	同學有需要時，講師樂意提供協助。 The lecturer(s) was (were) ready to offer help to students when needed.	1	2	3	4	5	Lec_08
2.9	導師與同學有很多交流。 The lecturer(s) had much interaction with the students.	1	2	3	4	5	Lec_09
2.10	我對講師的整體表現有非常正面的評價。 Overall speaking, I have a very positive evaluation of the lecturer(s).	1	2	3	4	5	Lec_10

第三部分 **Part 3**

請評估Service Leadership through Serving Children and Families with Special Needs課程對您的幫助有多大，然後在下表圈出一個您認為最能夠代表您觀感的數字。

Please evaluate to what extent you have benefited from the course, and then ***circle the number*** that best describes your views.

		沒有幫助 Unhelpful	幫助不大 Not Very Helpful	不確定 Not sure	頗有幫助 Helpful	有很大幫助 Very Helpful	OFFICIAL USE ONLY
3.1	促進我與人相處的能力。 It has enhanced my social competence.	1	2	3	4	5	eff_01
3.2	增強我表達及處理情緒的能力。 It has improved my ability to express and handle my emotions.	1	2	3	4	5	eff_02
3.3	加強我批判思考的能力。 It has enhanced my critical thinking.	1	2	3	4	5	eff_03
3.4	加強我作出明智抉擇的能力。 It has increased my competence in making sensible and wise choices.	1	2	3	4	5	eff_04
3.5	幫助我作出合符道德標準的決定。 It has helped me make ethical decisions.	1	2	3	4	5	eff_05
3.6	加強我面對逆境的能力。 It has strengthened my resilience in adverse conditions.	1	2	3	4	5	eff_06
3.7	加強我的自信。 It has strengthened my self-confidence.	1	2	3	4	5	eff_07
3.8	幫助我更積極面對將來。 It has helped me face the future with a positive attitude.	1	2	3	4	5	eff_08
3.9	提升我對生活的熱愛。 It has enhanced my love for life.	1	2	3	4	5	eff_09
3.10	幫助我探索人生的意義。 It has helped me explore the meaning of life.	1	2	3	4	5	eff_10
3.11	增強我領導自我的能力。 It has enhanced my ability of self-leadership.	1	2	3	4	5	eff_11
3.12	培養我對他人的憐憫和愛護。 It has helped me cultivate compassion and care for others.	1	2	3	4	5	eff_12
3.13	有助於全面地提升我的品質。 It has helped me enhance my character strengths comprehensively.	1	2	3	4	5	eff_13
3.14	使我明白專業能力、個人品質和關愛他人對於成功領袖的重要性。 It has enabled me to understand the importance of situational task competencies, character strength, and caring disposition in successful leadership.	1	2	3	4	5	eff_14
3.15	培養我貢獻社會的責任感。 It has promoted my sense of responsibility to serve society.	1	2	3	4	5	eff_15
3.16	促進我的整體成長。 It has promoted my overall development.	1	2	3	4	5	eff_16
3.17	課程涵蓋的理論、研究及概念使我明白成功的服務型領袖的基本特質。 The theories, research, and concepts covered in the course have enabled me to understand the characteristics of successful service leaders.	1	2	3	4	5	eff_17
3.18	課程涵蓋的理論、研究及概念幫助我整合成功的服務型領袖的基本特質。 The theories, research, and concepts covered in the course have helped me synthesize the characteristics of successful service leaders.	1	2	3	4	5	eff_18

第四部分 **Part 4**

您會否建議您的朋友報讀這個課程？請***圈出***一個您認為最能夠代表您意見的***數字***。
Will you suggest that your friends take this course? Please ***circle the number*** that best describes your views.

1	2	3	4	5
一定不會 Definitely Will Not Suggest	不會 Will Not Suggest	不確定 Not Sure	會 Will Suggest	一定會 Definitely Will Suggest

OFFICIAL USE ONLY
Q_04

第五部分 Part 5

如果將來有機會，您會否再報讀這類課程？請***圈出***一個您認為最能夠代表您意見的***數字***。
Will you participate in similar courses again in the future? Please ***circle the number*** that best describes your views.

1	2	3	4	5
一定不會 Definitely Will Not Suggest	不會 Will Not Suggest	不確定 Not Sure	會 Will Suggest	一定會 Definitely Will Suggest

OFFICIAL USE ONLY
Q_05

第六部分 Part 6

整體而言，您對這個課程有怎樣的滿意程度？請***圈出***一個您認為最能夠代表您意見的***數字***。
On the whole, are you satisfied with this course? Please ***circle the number*** that best describes your views.

1	2	3	4	5
十分不滿意 Very Dissatisfied	頗不滿意 Moderately Dissatisfied	中立 Neutral	滿意 Satisfied	十分滿意 Very Satisfied

OFFICIAL USE ONLY
Q_06

第七部分 Part 7

請完成下列各題:

Please complete the following items:

7.1	請寫出**一項或以上**您從該課程中學到最重要的東西：（如沒有，請填「沒有」。） Please write down one or more important thing(s) you have learned in this course. If there is no comment, please write "NIL". ____ ____ ____	OFFICIAL USE ONLY Q_7.1
7.2	請寫出**一項或以上**您認為在該課程中最值得欣賞的地方：（如沒有，請填「沒有」。） Please write down one or more thing(s) that you appreciate most in this course. If there is no comment, please write "NIL". ____ ____ ____	OFFICIAL USE ONLY Q_7.2
7.3	您對該課程的講師有何意見？（如沒有，請填「沒有」。） Do you have any comments about the lecturer(s)? If there is no comment, please write "NIL". ____ ____ ____	OFFICIAL USE ONLY Q_7.3
7.4	您認為該課程有哪些地方需要改善？（如沒有，請填「沒有」。） What aspects of this course should be improved? If there is no comment, please write "NIL". ____ ____ ____	OFFICIAL USE ONLY Q_7.4

第八部分 **Part 8**

請提供您的個人資料:

Please provide your demographic information:

1	出生日期 Date of birth: / / (yyyy/mm/dd) (例子:如您於1992年1月9日出生, 請填1992/01/09) (Example: If you were born on the 9th of January 1992, please fill in1992/01/09)

(continued)

(continued)

3	學號最后四个数字 (Last 4 digits of Student ID) (北大的學生, 請填你在北大的學號; 香港理工大學的學生, 請填你在香港理工大學的學號) (For the students of Peking University, please fill in your SID of PekingU; For the students of The Hong Kong Polytechnic University, please fill in your SID of PolyU)
5	日期 Date: ____/_____/_____(yyyy/mm/dd)

完。謝謝!
End. Thank you!

Appendix 4 Service Recipients' Views of the Camp

"希望旅程"夏令营评估问卷

"Journey of Hope" Summer Camp

Assessment Questionnaire

1. 对服务项目的观感: **Views about the service program:**	非常不同意 **Strongly disagree**	不同意 **Disagree**	有点不同意 **Slightly disagree**	有点同意 **Slightly agree**	同意 **Agree**	非常同意 **Strongly agree**
1.1 服务项目设计的很好。 This service program was well-designed						
1.2 提供的服务形式适宜。 The form of service provided was appropriate						
1.3 服务中活动的气氛很好。 The atmosphere of the activities in the service was good						

(continued)

(continued)

1. 对服务项目的观感: **Views about the service program:**	非常不同意 **Strongly disagree**	不同意 **Disagree**	有点不同意 **Slightly disagree**	有点同意 **Slightly agree**	同意 **Agree**	非常同意 **Strongly agree**
1.4 服务中我们同学之间有很多交流。 There was a lot of communication between our classmates during the service						
1.5 我积极参与服务中的活动。 I actively participated in activities during the services						
1.6 我获得鼓励去做到最好。 I was encouraged to do my best						
1.7 这次的学习经验增进了我对这个项目的兴趣。 This learning experience increased my interest in this project						
1.8 整体而言, 我对这次的服务项目有正面评价。 Overall, I have a positive evaluation of this service						

2. 对老师的观感(理大大学学生): **Views about the service provider (PolyU students):**	非常不同意 **Strongly disagree**	不同意 **Disagree**	有点不同意 **Slightly disagree**	有点同意 **Slightly agree**	同意 **Agree**	非常同意 **Strongly agree**
2.1 老师对服务的准备功夫充足。 The teachers were well prepared for the service						
2.2 老师的专业态度很好。 The teacher's professional attitude was very good						
2.3 老师理解我的需求和潜力。 The teachers understood my needs and potential						
2.4 老师表现的很投入。 The teachers were very engaged						
2.5 老师关心我。 The teachers cared about me						
2.6 在我有需要的时候, 老师随时乐意提供帮助。 The teachers were always willing to help me when I needed it						
2.7 老师与我们有很多交流。 The teachers communicated a lot with us						

(continued)

(continued)

2. 对老师的观感(理大大学学生): **Views about the service provider (PolyU students):**	非常不同意 **Strongly disagree**	不同意 **Disagree**	有点不同意 **Slightly disagree**	有点同意 **Slightly agree**	同意 **Agree**	非常同意 **Strongly agree**
2.8 我对老师的整体表现有正面评价。 I had a positive opinion of the teachers' overall performance						

3. 服务项目对我的帮助: **The extent to which the service program has helped me:**	毫无帮助 **Not helpful at all**	没有帮助 **Unhelpful**	帮助不大 **Not very helpful**	有些帮助 **Slightly helpful**	颇有帮助 **Helpful**	有很大帮助 **Very helpful**
3.1 加强我面对逆境的能力。 It has strengthened my resilience						
3.2 帮助我积极面对未来。 It has helped me face the future with a positive attitude						
3.3 提高我的自信。 It has improved my self-confidence						
3.4 开阔了我的视野。 It has broadened my horizons						
3.5 增强了我对学习的兴趣。 It has reinforced my interest in learning						

(continued)

(continued)

3. 服务项目对我的帮助: **The extent to which the service program has helped me:**	毫无帮助 **Not helpful at all**	没有帮助 **Unhelpful**	帮助不大 **Not very helpful**	有些帮助 **Slightly helpful**	颇有帮助 **Helpful**	有很大帮助 **Very helpful**
3.6 提高了我关心他人的能力。 It has strengthened my ability to care for other people						
3.7 帮助我与健康的成人建立良好关系(例如, 老师, 父母, 等等)。 It has helped me build good relationships with healthy adults. (e.g., teachers, parents, etc.)						
3.8 提升了我对未来生活的抱负。 It has promoted my aspirations in life						
3.9 促进我的整体发展。 It has enriched my overall development						
3.10 总体而言, 我对这次的服务项目感到满意。 Overall speaking, I have a positive evaluation of the service program						

4. 请回答以下问题:
Please complete the following questions:

(continued)

(continued)

4.1 我会用以下三个词或短语 (例如, 有趣, 有活力, 温暖, 等等) 来形容我对这次服务项目的感受, 看法, 和体验: I would use the following THREE words or phrases (e.g., fun, energetic, warm, etc.) to describe my feeling, perception, or experience of this program:
1) ________________ 2) ________________ 3) ________________
4.2 请用一个比喻 (即某个物品, 事件, 或状态) 来代表这次服务项目 (例如, 生活中的指南针, 一次愉快的旅行, 等) , 并简要说明这个比喻的含义是什么。 Consider a metaphor (i.e., an object, event, or state) that can represent the service program (e.g., a compass in life, a pleasant trip, etc.). Give a brief explanation of the meaning of the metaphor

我会用 ________________ I would use ________________	来代表这次的服务项目, 因为: ________________ to represent this service project because: ________________ ___

Appendix 5 Service Partner Evaluation Questionnaire

服务合作单位评估问卷

Service Partner Evaluation Questionnaire

1. 对服务项目的观感: **Views about the service program:**	非常不同意 **Strongly disagree**	不同意 **Disagree**	有点不同意 **Slightly disagree**	有点同意 **Slightly agree**	同意 **Agree**	非常同意 **Strongly agree**
1.1 服务项目设计的很好。 This service program was well-designed						
1.2 提供的服务形式适宜。 The form of the service provided was appropriate						
1.3 服务中活动的气氛很好。 The process of delivering the service activities was pleasant						

(continued)

(continued)

1. 对服务项目的观感: **Views about the service program:**	非常不同意 **Strongly disagree**	不同意 **Disagree**	有点不同意 **Slightly disagree**	有点同意 **Slightly agree**	同意 **Agree**	非常同意 **Strongly agree**
1.4提供的服务能迎合服务对象的需要。 The services provided could meet the needs of the clients						
1.5 服务项目提升了社区 (例如, 学校) 积极的氛围。 Service projects promoted a positive atmosphere in the community (e.g., school)						
1.6 对本次服务项目的观察和了解提高了我对参与这类项目的兴趣。 The observation and understanding of this service project increased my interest in participating in such projects						
1.7 整体而言, 这次的项目对服务对象有所裨益。 Overall speaking, the project has benefited the clients						

(continued)

(continued)

1. 对服务项目的观感: **Views about the service program:**	非常不同意 **Strongly disagree**	不同意 **Disagree**	有点不同意 **Slightly disagree**	有点同意 **Slightly agree**	同意 **Agree**	非常同意 **Strongly agree**
1.8 整体而言，我对这次的服务项目有正面评价。 Overall speaking, I have a positive evaluation of the service program						

2. 对服务者的观感 (理大大学学生): **Views about the service provider (PolyU students):**	非常不同意 **Strongly disagree**	不同意 **Disagree**	有点不同意 **Slightly disagree**	有点同意 **Slightly agree**	同意 **Agree**	非常同意 **Strongly agree**
2.1 理工学生对服务的准备功夫充足。 The teachers were well prepared for the service						
2.2 理工学生的专业态度很好。 The teachers' professional attitude was very good						
2.3 理工学生理解服务对象的需求和潜力。 The teachers understood the client's needs and potential						
2.4 理工学生表现的很投入。 The teachers were very engaged						

(continued)

(continued)

2. 对服务者的观感 (理大大学学生): **Views about the service provider (PolyU students):**	非常不同意 **Strongly disagree**	不同意 **Disagree**	有点不同意 **Slightly disagree**	有点同意 **Slightly agree**	同意 **Agree**	非常同意 **Strongly agree**
2.5 理工学生关心服务对象。 The teachers cared about the clients						
2.6 在服务对象有需要的时候，理工学生随时乐意提供帮助。 The teachers were always willing to help the clients when they needed it						
2.7 理工学生与服务对象有很多交流。 The teachers communicated a lot with the clients						
2.8 我对理工学生在服务中的整体表现有正面评价。 I had a positive opinion of the teachers' overall performance						

3. 服务项目对服务对象的帮助: **The extent to which the service program has helped the clients:**	毫无帮助 **Not helpful at all**	没有帮助 **Unhelpful**	帮助不大 **Not very helpful**	有些帮助 **Slightly helpful**	颇有帮助 **Helpful**	有很大帮助 **Very helpful**
3.1 加强服务对象面对逆境的能力。 It has strengthened the clients' resilience						
3.2 帮助服务对象积极面对未来。 It has helped the clients face the future with a positive attitude						
3.3 提高服务对象的自信。 It has improved the clients' self-confidence						
3.4 开阔了服务对象的视野。 It has broadened the clients' horizons						
3.5 增强了服务对象对学习的兴趣。 It has reinforced the client's interest in learning						
3.6 提高了服务对象关心他人的能力。 It has strengthened the clients' ability to care for other people						

(continued)

(continued)

3. 服务项目对服务对象的帮助: **The extent to which the service program has helped the clients:**	毫无帮助 **Not helpful at all**	没有帮助 **Unhelpful**	帮助不大 **Not very helpful**	有些帮助 **Slightly helpful**	颇有帮助 **Helpful**	有很大帮助 **Very helpful**
3.7 帮助服务对象与健康的成人建立良好关系 (例如, 老师, 父母, 等等)。 It has helped the clients build good relationships with healthy adults (e.g., teachers and parents)						
3.8 提升了服务对象对未来生活的抱负。 It has promoted the clients' aspirations in life						
3.9 促进服务对象的整体发展。 It has enriched the overall development of the clients						
3.10 总体而言, 我对这次的服务项目感到满意。 Overall speaking, I am satisfied with this service program						

4. 请回答以下问题: **Please answer the following questions:**
4.1 本次服务项目中有哪些方面您认为对服务对象最有益处? In what aspects of this service project do you think will be most beneficial to the clients?
____
____
4.2 本次服务项目可以怎样改进, 从而更好的帮助服务对象? How can this service be improved to help the clients better?
____
____

Appendix 6 Focus Group (Teacher)

訪談大綱

Interview outline

謝謝你們來參加焦點小組訪談。訪談旨在更多地瞭解你們在本學期 "服務學習" 這門課程的教學體驗。為了更詳盡分析訪談的內容, 我們會進行錄音。如果老師們不介意, 請大家先在研究同意書上簽名。這項研究僅僅為了學術和研究目的。大家的隱私將會得到嚴格保密。

Thank you for joining this focus group. The interview aims to learn more about your experience teaching the Service-Learning course this semester. In order to analyze the contents of the interview thoroughly, we will make a recording. Please sign the research consent form first if you don't mind. This research is for academic and research purposes only. Your privacy will be kept strictly confidential.

基本個人資料收集

Basic Personal Data Collection

(以下四項將于訪談開始前與研究同意書一併收集)

• 姓名:	• 學系及職位:
• 性別:	• 教授專案:成都/西安/杭州

(The following four items will be collected with the study consent form prior to the interview)

• Name:	• Department and Position:
• Gender:	• Service-Learning course taught: Chengdu/Xi'an/Hangzhou

在教授本學期 "服務學習"這門學科之前, 有沒有其他教學經驗?如果有的話,

Do you have any other teaching experience before teaching the subject of "Service-Learning" this semester?

1. 你有多少年的教學經驗 (不論面授或網上)?

How many years of teaching experience do you have (whether face-to-face or online)?

2. 你于香港理工大學任教多少年?

How many years have you been teaching at The Hong Kong Polytechnic University?

3. 你之前有沒有教授"服務學習"這門學科的經驗嗎?

Have you ever taught the subject of "Service-Learning" before?

a. 如果有的話, 可以分享一下你之前的經驗嗎?
   If yes, can you share your previous experience?
b. 如果沒有的話, 在教授這門學科之前, 你對服務學習的看法和感受是怎樣的? If not, what were your views and feelings about Service-Learning before teaching the subject?

<u>個人教學</u>

<u>Individual Teaching</u>

1. 對於本學期以網上形式進行七節的工作坊教學, 你對這個安排有什麼看法?

What are your thoughts on the seven-session workshop to be conducted online this semester?

2. 你可否簡單介紹一下你所教授的課節內容?

Can you share more about the contents of each workshop?

3. 對於七節工作坊每節約三小時的安排方面, 你對於這個安排有什麼看法? 是否足夠教授所有課程目標的內容?

What are your thoughts on the seven sessions of the three-hour workshop? Were they sufficient to achieve all the objectives of the course?

4. 你用了什麼教學手法來維持教學質素及提升理大學生的學習體驗嗎? 請舉例說明

What teaching methods have you used to maintain the quality of teaching and enhance the learning experience of PolyU students?

5. 你個人比較喜歡面對面教學還是網上教學?

Do you personally prefer face-to-face or online teaching?

6. 你覺得學生是否喜歡網上教學?

Do you think students enjoy online teaching?

7. 進行教授期間，當中有沒有遇到什麼困難? 如果有的話，可否分享1-2個例子? 你怎樣應對相關困難?

Were there any difficulties during the teaching process? If yes, could you share 1–2 examples, and how did you deal with them?

8. 你認為工作坊教學內容對理大學生設計服務夏令營的內容有沒有幫助? 請舉例說明。

Do you think the content of the workshop has helped PolyU students to design the contents of the Summer Camp?

9. 你認為工作坊教學內容對理大學生應對小朋友課堂的表現有沒有幫助? 請舉例說明。

Do you think the contents of the workshop have helped PolyU students cope with the performance of children in class?

10. 對於本學期邀請四川大學的評估員參與工作坊， 你對這個安排有什麼看法?

What do you think about inviting evaluators from Sichuan University to participate in the workshop this semester?

提供的支援及鼓勵

Support and Encouragement Provided

1. 在七節工作坊的教學期間, 你有沒有向理大學生提供支持及鼓勵?

During the seven workshops, did you provide support and encouragement to PolyU students?

a. 如果有提供的話, 可以分享一下你提供哪些方面的支持及鼓勵呢? 那麼, 所提供的支持及鼓勵是否足夠呢?
If yes, can you share what kind of support and encouragement you have offered? Was the support and encouragement provided sufficient?
b. 如果沒有提供的話, 你覺得為什麼沒有呢?
If not, why don't you think it's provided?

2. 在五天網上服務夏令營進行期間, 你有沒有向理大學生提供支持及鼓勵?

Did you provide support and encouragement to PolyU students during the five-day online service summer camp?

a. 如果有提供的話, 可以分享一下你提供哪些方面的支持及鼓勵呢? 那麼, 所提供的支持及鼓勵是否足夠呢?
   If yes, can you share what kind of support and encouragement you have offered? Was the support and encouragement provided sufficient?
b. 如果沒有提供的話, 你覺得為什麼沒有呢?
   If not, why don't you think it's provided?

個人得到的支持和鼓勵

The Support and Encouragement that Individuals Received

1. 在本學期的教學中, 你是否有得到任何的支持或鼓勵? 比如: 你是否從大學、學系得到支持? 如有, 你所得到的支持是否足夠?

Did you receive any support from universities or departments in this semester? If yes, was the support and encouragement provided sufficient?

2. 如有, 你是如何運用所得的支持在你的教學當中?

If yes, how did you use the support you received in your teaching?

3. 如果你所得到的支援不充分, 你希望可以得到哪些方面的支持? 在沒有這些支援的情況下, 你是如何自行解決所面臨的困難的? 可以舉例說明。

If you didn't receive enough support, what kind of support or encouragement do you hope to receive? Without the support, how did you solve the difficulties you face on your own?

4. 你個人與合作的內地大學、小學的合作經驗是否愉快?

Did you enjoy your personal experience working with universities and primary schools in mainland China?

對服務提供者的觀感

Perception of Service Providers

1. 你認為理大同學怎樣看待自己所設計的課程呢?

What do you think PolyU students think of the courses they have designed?

2. 你認為理大同學修讀服務學習及參與五天網上服務夏令營後, 對他們的全人發展方面有沒有幫助呢? 如果有的話, 可不可以分享幾個例子?

Do you think PolyU students have helped their whole-person development by taking service-learning and participating in the five-day online service summer camp? If yes, would you please share a few examples?

3. 你認為理大學生在修讀這個服務學習學科後會有一些改變?

Do you think PolyU students will change after studying this service-learning course?

a. 如果有的話, 有哪些方面的改變? 你覺得什麼因素導致他們有以上的改變?
   If yes, what has changed? What factors contributed to the above changes?
b. 如果沒有的話, 你認為有什麼因素導致他們沒有改變?
   If not, what do you think is the reason why they haven't changed?

對服務使用者的觀感

Perception of the Service Users

1. 你認為小朋友們怎樣看待理大同學所設計的課程呢?

What do you think the service users think of the curriculum designed by PolyU students?

2. 你認為小朋友們參與這些課程後有沒有進步呢? 如果有的話, 在哪些方面有進步?

Do you think the service users have made any progress after participating in these lessons? If so, in what areas?

3. 你認為小朋友們對作為服務提供者的大哥哥大姐姐有什麼看法和感受?

What do you think the service users think and feel about the brothers and the sisters (PolyU students) as service providers?

4. 你認為小朋友們經歷整個網上服務學習夏令營, 對他們的全人發展方面有沒有幫助呢? 如果有的話, 可不可以分享幾個例子?

Do you think the children's experience of the online service-learning summer camp has helped them in their whole-person development?

對川大評估員及小學老師的觀感

Perception of Sichuan University Assessors and the Primary School Teachers

1. 在準備網上服務夏令營的期間, 你覺得四川大學的評估員提供的支持及鼓勵是否足夠? 如果足夠的話, 哪些方面的支持足夠呢? 如果不足夠的話, 哪些方面的支援不足夠或需要改進呢?

During the preparation of the online service summer camp, do you think the support and encouragement provided by the evaluators at Sichuan University is sufficient? If yes, which areas of support were sufficient? If not, which areas were insufficient or needed improvement?

2. 在五天網上服務夏令營進行期間，你覺得四川大學的評估員提供的支持及鼓勵是否足夠? 如果足夠的話, 哪些方面的支持足夠呢? 如果不足夠的話, 哪些方面的支援不足夠或需要改進呢?

During the five-day online service summer camp, do you think the support and encouragement provided by the evaluators at Sichuan University was sufficient?

3. 在準備網上服務夏令營的期間，你覺得成都西蜀實驗小學的老師提供的支持及鼓勵是否足夠? 如果足夠的話, 哪些方面的支持足夠呢? 如果不足夠的話, 哪些方面的支持不足夠呢?

During the preparation of the online service summer camp, do you think the support and encouragement provided by the teachers of Chengdu Xishu Experimental Primary School were sufficient?

4. 在五天網上服務夏令營進行期間，你對成都西蜀實驗小學的老師的看法和感受是怎樣的?

During the five-day online service summer camp, what were your feeling and thoughts about the teachers of Chengdu Xishu Experimental Primary School?

對整個網上夏令營服務的觀感

Perception of the Entire Online Summer Camp Service

1. 對於本學期以網上形式進行五天的服務學習夏令營，你對這個安排有什麼看法?

What are your thoughts on the five-day service-learning summer online camp this semester?

2. 對今後改進完善服務學習這個學科，不論是教學內容或服務內容，你有什麼建議嗎?

Do you have any suggestions for improving the subject of service learning in future, whether it is about teaching content or service content?

3. 你對整個服務學習計畫的印象是什麼? 請分享給你留下印象最深刻的一件事情。

What are your impressions of the overall service-learning program? Please share one thing that most impressed you.

4. 你可不可以分享這個計畫的獨特之處?

Can you share the uniqueness of this program?

5. 如果情況許可，你會選擇網上服務學習還是面對面提供教學及服務呢? 為什麼?

If available, whether you would choose online service-learning or face-to-face teaching and services, and why?

6. 你有没有其他想補充的内容?

Do you have anything else that you'd like to add?

Appendix 7 Field Observation Form

服务学习计划 **(2021)** 学生表现评估表格

Service-Learning Program (2021)

Student Performance Assessment Form

机密 Confidential

请就学生的服务表现作出评估 (在适当的空格中加上√号):

Please evaluate the student's performance (Put an √ sign in the appropriate spaces):

	Very good 很好	**Good** 好	**Fair** 一般	**Poor** 差	**Very Poor** 很差	**N/A** 不适用
	(5)	**(4)**	**(3)**	**(2)**	**(1)**	**(0)**
1. 服务态度Service Attitude	☐	☐	☐	☐	☐	☐
2. 责任感Sense of Responsibility	☐	☐	☐	☐	☐	☐
3. 服务对象需要掌握Awareness of Needs	☐	☐	☐	☐	☐	☐
4. 对服务对象之关心 Sense of Care	☐	☐	☐	☐	☐	☐
5. 文化触觉 Cultural Sensitivity	☐	☐	☐	☐	☐	☐
6. 合作性Teamwork	☐	☐	☐	☐	☐	☐
7. 解决问题技巧Problem Solving Skills	☐	☐	☐	☐	☐	☐
8. 与服务对象沟通技巧Communication Skills with Service Targets	☐	☐	☐	☐	☐	☐
9. 教授内容技巧 Teaching Skills	☐	☐	☐	☐	☐	☐

(continued)

(continued)

	Very good 很好	**Good** 好	**Fair** 一般	**Poor** 差	**Very Poor** 很差	**N/A** 不适用
	(5)	**(4)**	**(3)**	**(2)**	**(1)**	**(0)**
10. 有关知识之应用Application of discipline-related Knowledge	☐	☐	☐	☐	☐	☐
11. 反思态度Reflective Attitude	☐	☐	☐	☐	☐	☐
12. 准时Punctuality	☐	☐	☐	☐	☐	☐
13. 整体表现Overall Performance	☐	☐	☐	☐	☐	☐
Comments:						

评估员签名Signature of the evaluator: __________ 日期 Date: __________
评估员姓名Name of the evaluator: __________ 职位Position: __________
联络方式Contact Method: __________

Appendix 8 Students' Feedback Form

Post-Service Evaluation Form for Service Providers (PolyU Students)

1.	**Views about the service program:**	**Strongly disagree**	**Disagree**	**Slightly disagree**	**Slightly agree**	**Agree**	**Strongly agree**
1.1	This service program was well-designed						
1.2	The form of the service we provided was appropriate						
1.3	The process of delivering the service activities was pleasant						
1.4	There was much peer interaction among the clients						

(continued)

(continued)

1.5	The clients participated actively during our service						
1.6	The clients were encouraged to do their best						
1.7	We had a good collaboration with different parties (school teachers, staff, etc.) during the service						
1.8	The service experience I encountered enhanced my interest in this subject						
1.9	The service experience increased my passion for helping people in need						
1.10	Overall speaking, I have a positive evaluation of the service program						
2.	**Views about the service provider (i.e., yourself):**	**Strongly disagree**	**Disagree**	**Slightly disagree**	**Slightly agree**	**Agree**	**Strongly agree**
2.1	I prepared well for the service						
2.2	I showed good professional attitudes in my service						
2.3	I understood the needs and potentials of my clients						
2.4	I was very involved in the service						

(continued)

(continued)

2.5	I cared for the clients I served						
2.6	I was ready to offer help to the clients whenever needed						
2.7	I had much interaction with the clients						
2.8	Overall speaking, I have positive evaluation of myself in serving the clients						
3	**The extent to which the service program has helped the clients:**	**Not helpful at all**	**Unhelpful**	**Not very helpful**	**Slightly helpful**	**Helpful**	**Very helpful**
3.1	It has strengthened our clients' resilience						
3.2	It has helped our clients face the future with a positive attitude						
3.3	It has improved our clients' self-confidence						
3.4	It has broadened our clients' horizons						
3.5	It has reinforced our clients' interest in learning						
3.6	It has strengthened our clients' ability to care for other people						

(continued)

(continued)

3.7	It has helped our clients build good relationships with healthy adults						
3.8	It has promoted our clients' aspirations in life						
3.9	It has enriched the overall development of our clients						

4	**The extent to which the service learning program has helped the service provider:**	**Not helpful at all**	**Unhelpful**	**Not very helpful**	**Slightly helpful**	**Helpful**	**Very helpful**
4.1	It has enabled me to understand the needs and potentials of the service recipients						
4.2	It has helped me integrate academic knowledge into real-life situations through service delivery						
4.3	It has enhanced my competences in problem-solving and decision-making						
4.4	It has helped me appreciate and respect people from diverse backgrounds						

(continued)

(continued)

4	**The extent to which the service learning program has helped the service provider:**	**Not helpful at all**	**Unhelpful**	**Not very helpful**	**Slightly helpful**	**Helpful**	**Very helpful**
4.5	It has helped me develop a sense of care and compassion toward other people						
4.6	It has improved my interpersonal skills						
4.7	It has boosted my self-confidence						
4.8	It has enabled me to apply the knowledge and skills I acquired in university to solve complex issues in the service						
4.9	It has inspired me to reflect on my roles and responsibilities as both a professional and a responsible citizen						
4.10	On the whole, I am satisfied with this service program						

5. Please complete the following questions:

5.1 I would use the following THREE words or phrases (e.g., inspiring, meaningful, rewarding … etc.) to describe my feeling, perception or experience of this program:

__________;__________;__________;

5.2 Think about a metaphor (e.g., an object, event, or state) that can stand for the service program (e.g., an enjoyable tour, tree planting, etc.). Give a brief explanation of the meaning of the metaphor.

I would use __________to stand for the service program because:

____

____

____

Appendix 9 Qualitative Evaluation Form

訪談大綱

Interview Guide

謝謝你們來參加焦點小組訪談。訪談旨在更多地瞭解你們在本學期 "服務學習" 這門課程的學習體驗。為了更詳盡分析訪談的內容, 我們會進行錄音。如果同學不介意, 請大家先在研究同意書上簽名。這項研究僅僅為了學術和研究目的。大家的隱私將會得到嚴格保密。

Thank you for joining this focus group. The interview aims to learn more about your experience teaching the Service-Learning course this semester. In order to analyze the contents of the interview thoroughly, we will make a recording. Please sign the research consent form first if you don't mind. This research is for academic and research purposes only. Your privacy will be kept strictly confidential.

個人學習體驗

Your Learning Experiences

1. 對於本學期以網上形式進行五天的服務學習夏令營, 你對這個安排有什麼看法?

How do you like this year's five-day Service-Learning summer camp, given its being held online?

2. 在經歷整個網上服務學習夏令營, 你認為對你的全人發展方面有沒有幫助呢? 如果有的話, 可不可以分享幾個例子?

Would you say the Service-Learning summer camp is helpful with your whole-person development? If yes, would you share concrete examples of how it is helpful?

3. 在本科目的網上服務夏令營中, 作為服務提供者, 你最大的收穫是什麼? 請舉例說明。

As a service provider, what would be the most beneficial things on your behalf during this online Service-Learning summer camp? Please elaborate with concrete examples.

4. 在本科目的網上服務夏令營中, 作為服務提供者, 你有沒有遇到一些困難? 你是如何解決的? 請舉例說明。

As a service provider, what challenges have you encountered during this online Service-Learning summer camp? If any, how did you deal with them? Please elaborate with concrete examples.

5. 在修讀這個服務學習學科後, 你有沒有察覺到自己有些改變? 如果有的話, 在哪些方面有改變呢? 有什麼改變呢? 你認為是哪些因素導致你出現這些改變呢?

Have you identified any changes inside yourself after taking this Service-Learning subject? If any, what would be the things that have changed and how? In your opinion, what would be the factors that have entailed these changes?

6. 你認為網上服務夏令營和面對面的夏令營有什麼不同?你覺得網上夏令營是好處多還是壞處多?為什麼? 請舉例說明。

In your opinion, what would be the differences between online and in-person Service-Learning summer camps? Would you say there are more pros than cons of online summer camps, or vice versa? Please elaborate with concrete examples.

<u>對服務使用者的觀感</u>

<u>Perceptions of Service Recipients</u>

1. 作為服務提供者, 可否簡單介紹一下你所負責的課程?

As a service provider, would you please give a brief introduction to the courses you were in charge of?

2. 你認為小朋友們怎樣看待你所設計的課堂呢? 比如: 他們是否喜歡你的課堂? 他們是否在你的課堂上有所收穫?

In your opinion, what would the students say about classes you designed? For example, do they like these classes, and have they benefited from them?

3. 你認為小朋友上完這些課程有沒有進步?如果有的話, 在哪些方面有進步?

In your opinion, have these students made satisfactory progress after taking the classes? If they have, what are those?

4. 你認為小朋友們對作為服務提供者的大哥哥大姐姐有什麼看法和感受?

In your opinion, how would the students feel about you and other service providers?

<u>對支持及協助的川大評估員和小學老師的觀感</u>

Perceptions of SCU Assessors and Primary School Teachers Who Have Provided Supports

1. 在準備網上服務夏令營的期間，你覺得四川大學的評估員提供的支持及鼓勵是否足夠? 如果足夠的話, 哪些方面的支持足夠呢? 如果不足夠的話, 哪些方面的支援不足夠或需要改進呢?

Would you say that SCU assessors provided sufficient support during preparations for the online Service-Learning summer camp? If yes, what are the supports that you find satisfactory? If no, what are the supports that you find insufficient and would like more?

2. 在五天網上服務夏令營進行期間，你覺得四川大學的評估員提供的支持及鼓勵是否足夠? 如果足夠的話, 哪些方面的支持足夠呢? 如果不足夠的話, 哪些方面的支援不足夠或需要改進呢?

Would you say that SCU assessors provided sufficient supports during the five-day online Service-Learning summer camp? If yes, what are the supports that you find satisfactory? If no, what are the supports that you find insufficient and would like more?

3. 在準備網上服務夏令營的期間，你覺得成都西蜀實驗小學的老師提供的支持及鼓勵是否足夠? 如果足夠的話, 哪些方面的支持足夠呢? 如果不足夠的話, 哪些方面的支持不足夠呢?

Would you say that Xishu Experimental Primary School teachers provided sufficient support during preparations for the online Service-Learning summer camp? If yes, what are the supports that you find satisfactory? If no, what are the supports that you find insufficient and would like more?

4. 在五天網上服務夏令營進行期間，你對成都西蜀實驗小學的老師的看法和感受是怎樣的?

Would you say that Xishu Experimental Primary School teachers provided sufficient support during the five-day online Service-Learning summer camp? If yes, what are the supports that you find satisfactory? If no, what are the supports that you find insufficient and would like more?

對理大老師

Perceptions of PolyU Instructors

1. 在準備網上服務夏令營的期間，你覺得理大老師提供的支持及鼓勵是否足夠? 如果足夠的話, 哪些方面的支持足夠呢? 如果不足夠的話, 哪些方面的支援不足夠或需要改進呢?

Would you say that PolyU instructors provided sufficient support during preparations for the online Service-Learning summer camp? If yes, what are the supports that you find satisfactory? If no, what are the supports that you find insufficient and would like more?

2. 在五天網上服務夏令營進行期間, 你覺得理大老師提供的支持及鼓勵是否足夠? 如果足夠的話, 哪些方面的支持足夠呢? 如果不足夠的話, 哪些方面的支持不足夠呢?

Would you say that PolyU instructors provided sufficient support during the five-day online Service-Learning summer camp? If yes, what are the supports that you find satisfactory? If no, what are the supports that you find insufficient and would like more?

3. 你對理大老師的看法和感受是怎樣的?

What would you say about PolyU instructors?

評估和建議

Evaluation and Suggestions

1. 整體而言, 你對這個學科的印象怎麼樣? 請分享給你留下印象最深的一件事情。

Overall, what would be your impressions of this subject? Please share an incident that impressed you the most.

2. 對今後改進完善網上服務學習, 你有什麼建議嗎?

Would you offer some suggestions for further improving online Service-Learning?

3. 如果你可以選擇,你會選擇網上服務學習還是面對面提供服務?為什麼?

If possible, would you take online or in-person Service Learning? Why?

4. 你有沒有其他想補充的內容?

Are there any other things that you want to share with us?

References

Astin, A. W., Vogelgesang, L. J., Ikeda, E. K., & Yee, J. A. (2000). *How service learning affects students*. Higher Education Research Institute. https://www.heri.ucla.edu/PDFs/HSLAS/HSLAS.PDF

Batchelder, T. H., & Root, S. (1994). Effects of an undergraduate program to integrate academic learning and service: Cognitive, prosocial cognitive, and identity outcomes. *Journal of Adolescence, 17*(4), 341–355. https://doi.org/10.1006/jado.1994.1031

Biggs, J. B. (1999). *Teaching for quality learning at university: What the student does?* Society for Research into Higher Education and Open University Press.
Biggs, J. B., & Collis, K. F. (1982). *Evaluating the quality of learning: The SOLO taxonomy.* Academic Press. https://doi.org/10.1016/C2013-0-10375-3
Camus, R. M., Ngai, G., Kwan, K. P., & Shek, D. T. L. (2022). Assessing students in academic service-learning: Faculty experiences and challenges. In G. Ngai & D. T. L. Shek (Eds.), *Service-learning capacity enhancement in Hong Kong higher education* (pp. 47–69). Springer. https://doi.org/10.1007/978-981-19-2437-8_4
Chung, P. (2011). Hong Kong Institution of Service Leadership & Management (HKI-SLAM) curriculum framework. *Unpublished document.*
Chung, P. (2012). *Service reborn:The knowledge, skills and attitudes of service companies.* Lexingford Publishing.
Chung, P. (2014, May 23). Hong Kong must work harder to maintain its service-industry edge. *South China Morning Post.* https://www.scmp.com/comment/article/1518546/hong-kong-must-work-harder-maintain-its-service-industry-edge
Commission, H. K. E. (2000). *Learning for life, learning through life: Reform proposals for the education system in Hong Kong.* Hong Kong Education Commission. https://www.e-c.edu.hk/wp-content/uploads/2000/09/Proposal_Edu_Reform_2000.pdf
Cress, C. M., Collier, P. J., & Reitenauer, V. L. (2013). *Learning through serving: A student guidebook for service-learning and civic engagement across academic disciplines and cultural communities.* Stylus Publishing.
Deci, E. L., & Ryan, R. M. (2013). *Intrinsic motivation and self-determination in human behavior.* Springer Science+Business Media. https://doi.org/10.1007/978-1-4899-2271-7
Deci, E. L., Vallerand, R. J., Pelletier, L. G., & Ryan, R. M. (1991). Motivation and education: The self-determination perspective. *Educational Psychologist, 26*(3–4), 325–346. https://doi.org/10.1080/00461520.1991.9653137
Eitington, J. E. (2002). *The winning trainer: Winning ways to involve people in learning* (4th ed.). Butterworth-Heinemann.
Eyler, J., & Giles, Jr. D. E. (1999). *Where's the learning in service-learning? Jossey-Bass higher and adult education series.* ERIC.
Felten, P., & Clayton, P. H. (2011). Service-learning. *New Directions for Teaching and Learning, 2011*(128), 75–84. https://doi.org/10.1002/tl.470
Hirschhorn, L. (1988). The post-industrial economy: Labour, skills and the new mode of production. *The Service Industries Journal, 8*(1), 19–38. https://doi.org/10.1080/02642068800000003
Jacoby, B. (1996). *Service-learning in higher education: Concepts and practices. The Jossey-Bass higher and adult education series.* ERIC.
Kember, D. (2002). Long-term outcomes of educational action research projects. *Educational Action Research, 10*(1), 83–104. https://doi.org/10.1080/09650790200200174
Kember, D., & Leung, D. Y. (2005). The influence of active learning experiences on the development of graduate capabilities. *Studies in Higher Education, 30*(2), 155–170. https://doi.org/10.1080/03075070500043127
Kerins, A. T. (2010). *An adventure in service-learning: Developing knowledge, values and responsibility.* Gower Publishing Limited.
Kolb, D. (1984). *Experiential learning: Experience as the source of learning and development.* Prentice-Hall.
Kuh, G. D. (2008). Excerpt from high-impact educational practices: What they are, who has access to them, and why they matter. *Association of American Colleges and Universities, 14*(3), 28–29.
Leung, H., Shek, D. T. L., & Dou, D. Y. (2021). Evaluation of service-learning in project WeCan under COVID-19 in a Chinese context. *International Journal of Environmental Research and Public Health, 18*(7), 3596. https://doi.org/10.3390/ijerph18073596
Li, X., Shek, D. T. L., Mok, B. P. W., Shek, E. Y. W., & Bai, Y. P. (2023). Effectiveness of electronic service-learning (e-SL) in primary school children in China during the COVID-19 Pandemic.

Applied Research in Quality of Life, 19, 3081–3108. https://doi.org/10.1007/s11482-023-10244-2

Lin, L., & Shek, D. T. L. (2021). Serving children and adolescents in need during the COVID-19 Pandemic: Evaluation of service-learning subjects with and without face-to-face interaction. *International Journal of Environmental Research and Public Health, 18*(4), 2114. https://doi.org/10.3390/ijerph18042114

Lin, L., Shek, D. T. L., & Li, X. (2022). Who benefits and appreciates more? An evaluation of online service-learning projects in Mainland China during the COVID-19 pandemic. *Applied Research in Quality of Life,18*, 625–646. https://doi.org/10.1007/s11482-022-10081-9

Ma, C. M. S., Shek, D. T. L., & Li, P. (2016). *Promoting service leadership through service leadership learning among Chinese university students* [Paper Presentation]. Second International Conference on Service-Learning Organized by The Hong Kong Polytechnic University, University Social Responsibility Network together with Office of Service-Learning, Hong Kong, China. https://ira.lib.polyu.edu.hk/bitstream/10397/64578/2/Ma_Promoting_Service_Leadership.pdf

Ma, C. M. S., Shek, D. T. L., & Li, P. P. K. (2019). Service leadership through serving socially deprived students: Experience gained from corporate-community-university partnership (project WeCan). In D. T. L. Shek, G. Ngai & C. F. Chan (Eds.), *Service-learning for youth leadership: The case of Hong Kong* (pp. 83–112). Springer. https://doi.org/10.1007/978-981-13-0448-4_6

Ngai, G., Lau, K. H., Kwan, K. P., Chan, S. C. F., & Shek, D. T. L. (2022). How Hong Kong university teachers assess students in service-learning: An exploratory study. In G. Ngai & D. T. L. Shek (Eds.), *Service-learning capacity enhancement in Hong Kong higher education* (Vol. 14, pp. 71–97). Springer. https://doi.org/10.1007/978-981-19-2437-8_5

Ngai, G., & Shek, D. T. L. (2022). *Service-learning capacity enhancement in Hong Kong higher education* (Vol. 14). Springer Nature. https://doi.org/10.1007/978-981-19-2437-8

Parlett, M., & Hamilton, D. (1972). *Evaluation as illumination: A new approach to the study of innovatory programmes*. University Centre for Research in Educational Science. https://files.eric.ed.gov/fulltext/ED167634.pdf

Prentice, M., & Robinson, G. (2010). *Improving student learning outcomes with service learning*. American Association of Community Colleges. https://files.eric.ed.gov/fulltext/ED535904.pdf

Ramsden, P. (2003). *Learning to teach in higher education*. Routledge. https://doi.org/10.4324/9780203507711

Shek, D. T. L. (2019). Development of the new 4-year Undergraduate program in Hong Kong. In D. T. L. Shek, G. Ngai & C. F. Chan (Eds.), *Service-learning for youth leadership: The case of Hong Kong* (pp. 1–17). Springer. https://doi.org/10.1007/978-981-13-0448-4_1

Shek, D. T. L., Cheng, M. N. S., & Ma, C. M. S. (2019). Nurturing service leadership qualities in university students through corporate-community-university partnership. In D. T. L. Shek, G. Ngai & C. F. Chan (Eds.), *Service-learning for youth leadership: The case of Hong Kong* (pp.113–131). Springer. https://doi.org/10.1007/978-981-13-0448-4_7

Shek, D. T. L., & Ho, W. W. L. (2018). Serving clients in a drug rehabilitation agency as a vehicle to promote Service Leadership in university students. In D. T. L. Shek, G. Ngai & C. F. Chan (Eds.), *Service-learning for youth leadership: The case of Hong Kong* (pp. 65–82). Springer. https://doi.org/10.1007/978-981-13-0448-4_5

Shek, D. T. L., Li, X., Chak, Y. L. Y., & Lin, L. (2022). Service-learning in the context of business-community-university partnership: The project Wecan in Hong Kong. In G. Ngai & D. T. L. Shek (Eds.), *Service-learning capacity enhancement in Hong Kong higher education* (Vol. 14, pp. 181–201). Springer. https://doi.org/10.1007/978-981-19-2437-8_10

Shek, D. T. L., Lin, L., & Liu, T. T. (2014a). Service leadership education for university students in Hong Kong: Subjective outcome evaluation. *International Journal on Disability and Human Development, 13*(4), 513–521. https://doi.org/10.1515/ijdhd-2014-0349

Shek, D. T. L., Ma, C. M. S., & Yang, Z. (2020). Transformation and development of university students through service-learning: A corporate-community-university partnership initiative in Hong Kong (Project WeCan). *Applied Research in Quality of Life, 15*, 1375–1393. https://doi.org/10.1007/s11482-019-09738-9

Shek, D. T. L., & Sun, R. C. F. (2012). Qualitative evaluation of a positive youth development course in a university setting in Hong Kong. *International Journal on Disability and Human Development, 11*(3), 243–248. https://doi.org/10.1515/ijdhd-2012-0040

Shek, D. T. L., Sun, R. C. F., Yu, L., Ma, C. M. S., Siu, A. M. H., Leung, H., & Law, M. Y. M., (2014b). Service leadership education and research at The Hong Kong Polytechnic University: An overview. In D. T. L. Shek & P. Chung (Eds.), *Promoting service leadership qualities in university students* (Vol. 6). Springer. https://doi.org/10.1007/978-981-287-515-0_8

Shek, D. T. L., Yang, Z., Ma, C., & Chai, C. (2021). Subjective outcome evaluation of service-learning by the service recipients: Scale development, normative profiles and predictors. *Child Indicators Research, 14*(1), 411–434. https://doi.org/10.1007/s12187-020-09765-1

Shek, D. T. L., Yu, L., Ma, C. M., Sun, R. C., & Liu, T. T. (2013). Development of a credit-bearing service leadership subject for university students in Hong Kong. *International Journal of Adolescent Medicine and Health, 25*(4), 353–361. https://doi.org/10.1515/ijamh-2013-0033

Shek, D. T. L., & Yuen, A. (2019). The quest for holistic youth leadership development: What should be the desired attributes of youth leaders? *International Journal of Child and Adolescent Health, 12*(1), 43–60. https://ira.lib.polyu.edu.hk/bitstream/10397/93756/1/APSS-0282_Shek_Quest_Holistic_Youth.pdf

Tam, M. (2014). Intergenerational service learning between the old and young: What, why and how. *Educational Gerontology, 40*(6), 401–413. https://doi.org/10.1080/03601277.2013.822201

Thomas, L., & Beauchamp, C. (2011). Understanding new teachers' professional identities through metaphor. *Teaching and Teacher Education, 27*(4), 762–769. https://doi.org/10.1016/j.tate.2010.12.007

Tyler, R. W. (1949). *Basic principles of curriculum and instruction*. University of Chicago Press.

Waldner, L. S., Widener, M. C., & McGorry, S. Y. (2012). E-service learning: The evolution of service-learning to engage a growing online student population. *Journal of Higher Education Outreach and Engagement, 16*(2), 123–150. https://openjournals.libs.uga.edu/jheoe/article/view/936/935

Zhu, X., Chai, W., Shek, D. T. L., & Lin, L. (2022). Promotion of meaning in life and well-being among university students during the COVID-19 Pandemic via a service-learning subject. *Frontiers in Public Health, 10*, 924711. https://doi.org/10.3389/fpubh.2022.924711

Chapter 13
Law Abidance Leadership for University Students—What Do the Evaluation Findings Tell Us?

Daniel T. L. Shek and Xiang Li

Abstract The Hong Kong National Security Law (HKNSL) is new to the Special Administrative Region of China. Thus, to help young people understand the importance of national security and enhance their law abidance awareness, it is explicitly stated in the HKNSL that education institutions, including universities, have the responsibility to implement HKNSL-related education programs. At The Hong Kong Polytechnic University (PolyU), we have developed three national education programs on the HKNSL. First, we have developed a face-to-face program on law-abiding leadership for 4-year undergraduate students. Second, we have designed an online program on the same content for senior-year and advanced-standing students. Third, an e-learning course on "Understanding China and the Hong Kong Special Administrative Region, P.R.C" is delivered for both taught and research postgraduate students. During the two years of project implementation, we continued to understand the impact of the project on different student groups through objective outcome evaluations, subjective outcome evaluations, and qualitative evaluations. Research confirms that both undergraduate and postgraduate students generally have positive views of the course and affirm its effectiveness. They believe that the program benefits their personal development in critical thinking, problem-solving ability, moral competence, interpersonal communication skills, law-abiding leadership, and understanding of the significance of national security. Most importantly, the majority of them expressed the desire to become law-abiding citizens and take on social responsibility. The series of studies enriches the scientific database of teaching politically sensitive topics in the higher education context.

Keywords Law abidance leadership · National education · Evaluation · University students · Hong Kong National Security Law (HKNSL)

13.1 Introduction

The social event taking place from spring 2019 to spring 2020 in Hong Kong was unprecedented. Besides peaceful demonstrations against the Hong Kong Extradition Bill by the majority of the protestors, there was massive vandalism, violence,

D. T. L. Shek, *Promoting Holistic Development in University Students*, Quality of Life in Asia 17, https://doi.org/10.1007/978-981-96-0251-3_13

doxing, harming those with different political views, and riot behavior displayed by some protestors, including high school and university students. To regain order and stability in Hong Kong, the National People's Congress enacted the "Law of the People's Republic of China on Safeguarding National Security in the Hong Kong Special Administrative Region (HKSAR)" (commonly referred to as the "Hong Kong National Security Law" or "HKNSL"). Specifically, the HKNSL stated that educational institutions (including universities) should educate students on the importance of the HKNSL.

At The Hong Kong Polytechnic University (PolyU), to implement national security education in a quality manner, we include the HKNSL education under the Leadership subjects (including "Tomorrow's Leaders"). Besides a 3-h lecture on "law abidance leadership," students are required to spend around 7hs on self-study on topics related to modern Chinese history, the founding of the People's Republic of China, the Hong Kong Basic Law, the Constitution, and the HKNSL. In terms of assessment, students must take a test with 20 multiple-choice questions with a pass mark of 16 (out of 20). To assess the impact of the HKNSL education curricula and the experiences of different stakeholders, we have conducted several studies based on the responses of different stakeholders.

13.2 Post-lecture Evaluation of "Tomorrow's Leaders" via a Hyflex Mode (Shek et al., 2022e)

Since the outbreak of COVID-19, face-to-face teaching in the university has been changed to online mode and HyFlex mode that integrates both face-to-face and online modes. HyFlex learning is flexible; students can attend lectures in the classroom or online. Nevertheless, it has many disadvantages and is challenging for teachers and students. Many studies have been conducted to evaluate the effects of online teaching, but fewer studies have been carried out regarding the effectiveness of HyFlex learning. Therefore, understanding students' academic quality of life under the HyFlex teaching mode is necessary, as learning quality will influence the well-being of students.

To understand students' views of HyFlex teaching and the HKNSL lecture, Shek et al. (2022e) utilized post-lecture evaluation to investigate the perceptions of university students on a leadership subject entitled "Tomorrow's Leaders" at PolyU. Moreover, a 3-h lecture regarding law-abiding leadership and national security education was designed and incorporated into this subject. Specifically, we intended to understand students' perceptions of the overall lecture delivery, particularly of the aspects regarding national security education. More importantly, exploring whether students perceive the lecture as beneficial for their well-being, such as improved psychosocial competence, is essential. At the same time, conducting evaluations provides an opportunity for teachers to reflect on their teaching and empower them, which finally has a positive impact on the well-being of teachers.

In the first semester of the 2021–22 academic year, 1146 students enrolled in the "Tomorrow's Leaders" subject. From lectures 1 to 11, students were invited to respond anonymously and voluntarily to a post-lecture evaluation questionnaire online. The questionnaire contains 28 items that have high internal consistency among different lectures. To investigate students' views toward the lecture on law-abiding leadership, we revised the original questionnaire and formed a 27-item measure with good reliability. This scale has several variables, including lecture design and implementation, law-abiding leadership, national security, the benefits, and overall impression of this lecture. Additionally, students can share their comments anonymously and voluntarily. Altogether, 813 questionnaires were valid in reliability analyses, resulting in a response rate of over 70%.

This study aimed to test three hypotheses, including: (1) "students would have positive perceptions of the lectures;" (2) "most of the students would give positive quantitative and qualitative responses regarding the 3-h HyFlex lecture on law-abiding leadership;" and (3) "the perceived quality of the lecture (e.g., design and class attributes), teacher attributes, law-abiding leadership content, and benefits of the lecture would be positively related to the overall perception of the lecture."

Reliability analyses revealed that the post-lecture evaluation scale was internally consistent across all lectures. In all lectures except for Lecture 8, evaluation findings are generally positive based on frequency analyses. To begin with, the students had positive evaluations of the performance of teachers. For instance, over 90% of students agreed that "the teachers encouraged and cared about the students" and that "the teachers were well-prepared for the lectures." Students also held positive views on the lectures, including "the good design of the lectures," "the good atmosphere of the classes," and "the opportunities for interaction and reflection." For example, more than 93% of them responded that peer interactions were adequate.

Moreover, the students responded that the lectures were beneficial for them, including "improvements in problem-solving," "critical thinking," "personal development," and "understanding of the qualities of successful leaders." To illustrate, over 96% of the students agreed that the lectures enhanced their critical thinking skills and moral competence. Additionally, more than 94% stated that their communication skills had improved after the lectures. Finally, compared with traditional in-class teaching and online teaching, students preferred the HyFlex learning mode. Nearly 90% agreed that HyFlex teaching was smooth, efficient, and flexible, and more than 91% preferred the HyFlex teaching mode. In short, Hypothesis 1, "students had positive perceptions of the different aspects of the subject," was supported by the findings.

Similar positive findings can be found in the lecture on law-abiding leadership. Firstly, over 92% of respondents evaluated teachers' performance positively, including "teacher's preparation," "assistance to the students to understand the subject matter," and "encouragement and care given to students." Moreover, the lecture design and attributes, such as "class atmosphere" and "students' interaction, participation, and reflection opportunities," were recognized by the students. For instance, over 85% of the participants reported that "the lecture design was good" and "the classroom atmosphere was very pleasant." Additionally, more than 88% of them shared that there was much student participation during the class, and 87% agreed that "there were many opportunities for reflection in this lecture." Evidently, involving intensive discussion, interaction, sharing, and reflection in leadership courses like "Tomorrow's Leaders" can help the students learn sensitive topics like HKNSL. The students can be more open-minded to accept the concept of national security. More importantly, they will be encouraged and inspired to be socially responsible and law-abiding citizens in future (Ridley, 2011). The responses from the students also supported this argument. 90% of students agreed that "their understanding of national security was enhanced," around 91% shared that "they knew more about the HKNSL in Hong Kong," and nearly 90% reported that "they became more aware of the importance of law abidance leadership." Moreover, 92% of respondents shared that "they would strive to serve as socially responsible leaders."

Equally important, students were satisfied with HyFlex teaching, including its efficiency and flexibility. More than 93% of students responded that "The hybrid teaching of lecture 8 was smooth," and 94% agreed that "The hybrid teaching facilitated them to learn more efficiently about this lecture." Overall speaking, nearly 94% of students shared that they like the hybrid learning experience. Finally, the students perceived that the lecture could promote their personal development, including "problem-solving," "interpersonal communication," "critical thinking," and "understanding of the attributes of successful leaders." For example, more than 83% of the respondents reported that they became more aware that self-development is essential and that their problem-solving ability has improved. Nearly 85% of students claimed that their interpersonal communication skills improved after this lecture and that this lecture was beneficial for their personal development. Around 86% reported that their critical thinking skills were enhanced as well. These soft skills are significant elements of students' well-being (Ngai & Shek, 2022).

Remarkably, the qualitative responses (e.g., general comments on lectures) were mainly positive, with very few negative ones. We have received 70 positive responses. Apart from general positive comments like "good," "great," and "nice," some in-depth descriptive sharing was also observed. Some students shared, "I agree with the content," "I think today's lesson is educational and meaningful," "The atmosphere is very good," and "The game in the lesson is fun and helps us more engage in class." Nevertheless, we also received some negative responses such as "Though it is sort of boring, it is our responsibility to know the law," "The mic is too loud," and "This lesson is too long for me." These comments also highlighted the need to enhance our teaching and arrangement in future.

The findings are interesting for three reasons. Firstly, it demystifies the common belief that students would have negative experiences regarding national security law education. Additionally, many people assumed that the lecture would impair students' well-being, which was not supported by the findings. Quite the opposite, the students agreed that the lecture promoted their psychosocial competence, law-abiding leadership knowledge, and behavioral intention to be socially responsible leaders. Thirdly, there was no evidence to support that students felt that they were being "brainwashed." On the contrary, the students appreciated the lecture and recognized that they acquired meaningful insights from this lecture.

All in all, the findings reveal that the students had positive evaluations of the lecture design, class activities and interaction, lecture content, benefits, and overall quality. The quantitative and qualitative data of Lecture 8 also suggested that students received the lecture well. The present study highlights that HyFlex teaching and integrating HyFlex mode into the leadership framework to teach law-abiding leadership and national security are effective. It also underscores the importance of conducting evaluation studies to understand students' views toward HyFlex teaching.

13.3 Post-lecture Evaluation of "Tomorrow's Leaders" via an Online Mode (Shek et al., 2022c)

In Semester 2 of the 2021/22 academic year, because of the new wave of COVID-19 (Omicron strain), the subject "Tomorrow's Leaders" was taught online completely. Hence, there is a need to understand the students' views of the HKNSL lecture in online mode. With this objective in mind, Shek et al. (2022c) focused on how students responded to the law abidance lecture via post-lecture evaluation. To promote law abidance leadership among university students in Hong Kong, we developed a law abidance leadership program with a 3-h face-to-face lecture and a 7-h self-study. On its first implementation via hybrid mode, a study showed that students generally reacted positively to the HKNSL lecture (Shek et al., 2022e). We adopted a fully online mode in the second semester. Therefore, it is necessary to understand the difference in students' reactions to in-person versus online teaching modes affecting their satisfaction with the HKNSL education.

In this study, we conducted a post-lecture evaluation study focusing on student responses to the 3-h lecture using a 26-item measure plus open-ended questions. The lecture was conducted online without face-to-face teaching. After attending the 3-h lecture on law abidance leadership, all students were invited to reflect on and evaluate their learning experiences in terms of perceptions of lecture attributes, teacher attributes, and appreciation of law abidance in the post-lecture evaluation survey. 914 students (around 70% of 1308 registered students) completed the survey. Irrelevant personal information was not collected to minimize the sensitivity involved in participation, and the students' mean age was around 18 years.

Specifically, we intended to explore four Hypotheses based on the perspective of the students: (1) concerning the conceptual model that the measure covers lecture attributes, teacher attributes, and appreciation of law abidance, we expected that there would be support for the 3-factor model of the subjective outcome evaluation tool; (2) we expected that most students would have positive perceptions of different aspects of the lecture; (3) we expected that perceived lecture attributes, teacher attributes, and appreciation of law abidance leadership would predict overall satisfaction with the lecture; and (4) we expected that the profile of qualitative responses would be with more positive responses than negative responses.

The analyses of quantitative and qualitative data supported the four Hypotheses. For Hypothesis 1, confirmatory factor analyses showed three dimensions intrinsic to the 26-item scale assessing the students' perceptions, and the factors are stable across the two random subsamples. The present findings provided support for the factorial validity of the measure. Reliability analyses also showed that the total scale and subscales were reliable. There was also support for the convergent and discriminant validity of the measure. In this way, results showed the scale's reliability and validity. Therefore, Hypothesis 1 was supported.

Secondly, consistent with our expectation, students generally showed positive evaluation of the attributes of teachers, including their mastery of lecture materials (95%), encouragement of students to learn via different methods (95%), creation of mutual respect in class (96%), and able to help students to understand the subject matter (95%). Altogether, the findings supported Hypothesis 2 that students positively evaluated the lecture and teachers and appreciated law abidance leadership.

Regarding the predictors of overall satisfaction with the lecture, multiple regression analysis with lecture attributes, teacher attributes, and appreciation of law abidance as predictors and overall satisfaction with the lecture as the criterion variable was performed. In line with our predictions, lecture attributes (beta = 0.272, $p < 0.001$), teacher attributes (beta = 0.069, $p < 0.05$), and appreciation of law abidance (beta = 0.604, $p < 0.001$) were significant predictors of overall satisfaction with the lecture. These findings supported Hypotheses 3a, 3b, and 3c. Finally, an examination of the qualitative comments of the students showed several observations. Firstly, the number of positive responses (109 comments) outnumbered the negative (6 responses), neutral and unclassified responses (5 comments). The comments were classified into different categories, such as general positive comments, appreciation of the lecture, appreciation of the teacher, law abidance leadership, and the HKNSL. Students had positive views about the lecture attributes (such as positive attributes of the lecture), teacher attributes (such as appreciation of the teachers), and appreciation of law abidance (such as acquiring knowledge about the HKNSL).

In terms of students' feedback, 47 students gave positive responses regarding the lecture. Some comments were, "The lesson let us view it comprehensively; the lesson let us think deeply and decide our position on this law," "I have learned the importance of HKNSL and what would be the consequences of violating it," "I like the last part of 'myth'; it clarifies some information," "I have learned the difference between reform and revolution and the HKNSL in Hong Kong," "It is good to let students know that many countries (including the US and UK) have the HKNSL," and "It is good to let students understand the implementation objectives of the HKNSL. Otherwise, we will selectively ignore some knowledge." Moreover, some students appreciated the lecture and the arrangement, and some responses were, "This lecture is very informative," "Originally, law-abiding leadership should be a topic that is difficult to understand, but the design of the lesson facilitates my understanding of this topic," "The lecture notes contain some well-organized content," and "The concepts are clearly delivered." Additionally, some students shared that their sense of belonging to Hong Kong and China was enhanced, and they became more aware of the importance of law-abiding leadership. Significantly, the qualitative picture based on the students was generally positive, which supported Hypothesis 4.

This study is unique in several ways. First, as education on the HKNSL is very new in Hong Kong, it is essential to collect evidence to understand the views of the students who have taken such courses and to demystify the myth that related education is "brainwashing." The present findings showed that the participants' responses are generally positive, which is generally in line with the findings reported by Shek et al. (2022e). Thus, the available evidence demystifies the myth that students resent national security education. Second, during the pandemic, there is a need to understand the effectiveness of different forms of teaching and learning. From a replication perspective, the present findings replicated the studies (Shek et al., 2022e) in a new sample of students taking the subject via another mode at another time. Hence, the present study constitutes a modest attempt to replicate the previous findings in national security education. Moreover, the present study suggests that this evaluation measure can be objectively used to assess national security education in future. As research on national security education needs to be more extensive in the scientific literature, the present study contributes to the field.

The study also has several implications for future research. Firstly, since qualitative findings are only partially positive, they provide a good pointer for pedagogical refinement. Additionally, as only around 70% of the students joined the post-lecture evaluation, interpretations of the findings should be cautious. We need to explore diversified and practical ways to promote law-abiding leadership. Besides enriching students' knowledge in this area, we need to realize the foundational skills underlying law abidance, such as cognitive competence, social competence, and moral competence. Finally, as law abidance leadership education concerning the HKNSL is politically sensitive, there is a need to help young people understand the law and respect the need for law abidance. Teaching sensitive and controversial topics is challenging, and teachers face many issues. Studies of the perception of teachers are needed as well.

In conclusion, evaluation and replication of findings are essential in shaping the pedagogies and teaching processes. The results revealed that students were generally satisfied with the lecture attributes and agreed that the lecture helped them understand the importance and value of law abidance and national security. Nevertheless, studies should be replicated in future to understand the impact of law-abiding leadership educational programs.

13.4 Qualitative Evaluation Based on Focus Groups (Shek et al., 2023b)

As stated in Article 10 of the Hong Kong National Security Law (HKNSL), institutions, including universities, are responsible for promoting the HKNSL education. Nevertheless, there are difficulties in implementation, such as negative sentiments, feelings of uncertainty, and anxiety created by its implementation. Besides the post-lecture evaluation studies mentioned above, we also conducted a qualitative study using the focus group method aiming to evaluate students' views on a law abidance leadership program covering the HKNSL. The researchers adopted a general qualitative research design to collect data via semi-structured interviews. The present findings suggest that students perceived their learning experiences in the program and the benefits of the program positively and indicate that the program promoted the students' well-being.

Specifically, this study explored the following research questions: (1) What are the views of the students on the lecture, including its content, arrangement, atmosphere, interaction, and the teacher? (2) What are the students' views on the 60 lecture notes? (3) What are the students' views on the assessment? (4) What are the experiences of the students in the lecture, including their views on the benefits and understanding of the subject matter? (5) What are the students' perceptions of the views of classmates on National Security Law education? and (6) Do students regard National Security Law education as "brainwashing"?

The participants were selected randomly from 18 classes of Year 1 students. Three students from each class, including a total of 71 students, were invited. Finally, 52 students participated in the focus group, as some students dropped out because of a time clash, resulting in a participation rate of 73.2%. As the data collection was carried out after the completion of the subject, the students were assured that their responses would not affect their grades. Altogether, six focus group interviews were conducted via ZOOM, with six to eleven participants in each group. The discussion session utilized a semi-structured interview guide to understand students' subjective experiences with the law abidance leadership program. Although there are criticisms regarding the subjective and non-scientific nature of focus group interviews, this study employed various measures to increase its rigor, such as involving professional staff in different stages and data analysis, conducting inter-rater reliability on the positivity of the derived themes, and examining negative evidence. During the focus groups, the students were invited to answer questions about perceptions of the program, instructors, benefits, and experience (Yu et al., 2022; Zhu & Shek, 2021), including (1) their views on the different aspects of the lecture (e.g., content and interaction), notes, and assessment; (2) their perceptions of the teacher; (3) their views of the benefits and necessity of the program; and (4) their experiences, perception of the related experiences of their classmates, and whether the program was "brainwashing."

After the interviews, the verbal data was analyzed using thematic analyses. To understand the reliability of the analyses, we re-coded 20 randomly selected narratives to determine the inter-rater reliability of the narratives, particularly their positivity (Shek et al., 2005). Firstly, the data analysis showed mixed views on different aspects of the lecture. For example, some students agreed that the lecture content is "straightforward" and is the "promotion of understanding," but some argued that "the linkage between each part was not clear." In contrast, others presented neutral comments, such as "surprise to have this topic in this course." Similarly, mixed positive comments can be found in lecture arrangements, notes, and assessments.

Remarkably, overwhelmingly positive views regarding teacher performance, learning experience, perceived benefits, and the need for law-abiding leadership education can be identified. For instance, many participants commented that this course "enhanced students' understanding of the HKNSL" and "promoted students' learning motivation." Moreover, students agreed that understanding the HKNSL is "the students' responsibility" and can "help them integrate into Hong Kong culture." Regarding the performance of the teachers, one student shared, "My lecturer used various examples to help illustrate the point she was making, which I found helped me understand the topics more … it made it a lot easier for me to gauge the various topics that were being discussed … helped us apply it to real-life situations, which I thought was very useful." When talking about their learning experience, one student responded, "I am positive about the lecture, which is conducive to my understanding of the law, can avoid the wrong law, and can also deepen my understanding of the law. I will not be affected by the negative remarks about the law." Another commented, "I think the content is quite OK … everything is clear, and the material is introduced step by step."

Most importantly, the findings suggest that students agreed that the related education was not brainwashing. To illustrate, one student commented, "I feel that there is no brainwashing because the lecture time is short, and the concepts are legal facts. Actually, university students have independent thinking. Besides Year 1 students, probably Years 2, 3, and 4 students should acquire such knowledge." One student added, "I think that in the classroom, including the teacher and the content of the class, there is no promotion of a subjective idea; in fact, it is only some laws and examples of harmful behavior in society. These things do not have a subjective view, but indeed destructive behavior, so I don't think it is said that the brainwashing point of view is transmitted." Another student agreed, "There are some group discussion sessions in the classroom; there are these opportunities for us to think for ourselves so that we can accept that knowledge through our thinking." This finding provides some pioneer qualitative support to the issue that there are criticisms and polarized views about implementing the HKNSL (Shek et al., 2022c). Finally, this study also treasures the suggestions made by students, although there are difficulties in implementing them. One example could be using Chinese as a medium of instruction, which is not applicable to teaching according to the university teaching requirements.

The findings suggest that students had positive learning experiences, and the program promoted their well-being. The students did not find the program anxious and stressful. Instead, according to some students, they "really enjoy this course," "are super happy," and "the lecture and notes are comfortable." For example, one student shared, "I think the whole lecture in Tomorrow's Leaders is really useful. It gives us a chance to know more about ourselves and what kind of skills we need to develop in the universities. Yeah, and also learn like the laws in Hong Kong." Moreover, the positive learning experience and perceived benefits contributed to the academic well-being of the students, such as "promoting their knowledge on law abidance leadership" and "enhancing motivation to learn and appreciation of the learning involved." Sharing from international students also supported this conclusion, "Being a foreigner, I did not hear much about the national security law. So, coming to this lecture definitely gave me a brief idea of what this national security law is about. So, I think that will be helpful." Additionally, the findings showed that the program cultivated positive attitudes (e.g., "care about others" and "enhanced love for the Nation") and skills (e.g., "critical thinking skills" and "sharpen one's mind"). For instance, one student responded, "I think it will expand my critical thinking through this course. I have a deeper understanding of what National Security Law really is. Then, there is the difference between helping individuals and helping the State. Then, I feel like I'm going to think more multi-dimensional. Good, thanks."

Regarding different dimensions of health (Van Druten et al., 2022), the present study demonstrated that law abidance leadership education promoted cognitive health (increase in the HKNSL knowledge), social health (well-being related to social phenomena), and environmental health (well-being related to political events) of the students and contributed to social integrity (e.g., safe community) and social contribution (e.g., abiding by the HKNSL) (Keyes, 1998). Essentially, the findings align with other evaluation studies conducted before, including the post-lecture evaluations in two semesters (Shek et al., 2022c, 2022e) and the examination of views of teachers in two semesters (Shek et al. 2022d). The studies showed that both the students and teachers appreciated the benefits of the HKNSL education.

Essentially, the present findings have several implications for future research. Firstly, it is necessary to further understand students' ambivalence in expressing their views during class. Moreover, other studies are needed to investigate how lecture content, arrangement, and teacher-student relationships may shape students' learning experience. Additionally, more research can explore how teaching politically sensitive topics may impact students. Finally, this study contributes to the knowledge base of teaching politically sensitive topics. Equally important, to address the limitations in future, more students can be recruited to increase the generalizability of the findings. Furthermore, individual interviews could be conducted along with the focus group interview. Additionally, combining quantitative and qualitative data across related studies would increase the rigor of the studies.

In conclusion, the present study contributes to our understanding of the students' views on the law abidance leadership program in response to the HKNSL. Notably, different measures were utilized in this focus group evaluation study to promote its methodological rigor. In conjunction with previous findings (Shek et al., 2022b, 2022c, 2022d, 2022e), the findings suggest that the program promoted the students' knowledge about law abidance leadership and nurtured their positive attitudes toward law abidance.

13.5 Evaluation Based on the Views of the Teachers (Shek et al., 2022d)

As mentioned above, we have conducted two post-lecture evaluation studies (Shek et al. 2022c, 2022e) and one focus group study (Shek et al., 2023b) to understand the students' responses to law abidance and HKNSL education. While it is desirable to understand the students' views, it is equally important to explore the views and experiences of the teachers. To offer an additional perspective on the perceived effectiveness of education on law abidance leadership, we examined the teachers' views in this study. Examination of teachers' views is essential because the HKNSL education is a highly sensitive topic in Hong Kong, and teachers are normally not trained to teach related topics. To date, we have conducted three studies to understand the views of the teachers (Shek et al., 2023a, 2022d).

In the first study, eight teachers who taught the law abidance leadership lecture in Semester 1 of the 2021–22 academic year via HyFlex mode joined the study. After teaching this lecture, we invited them to respond to several open-ended questions about the lecture and related arrangements voluntarily and anonymously. Eventually, six teachers joined the study. Specifically, the qualitative evaluation was adopted to understand the experience of teachers teaching this subject, including their initial reactions, preparation, teaching experience, responses of the students, benefits for students, challenges encountered, professional teacher development, and their well-being. Results generally showed that the teachers had positive teaching experiences and perceived that the lecture was beneficial to the students.

We analyzed the teachers' written responses to each question and categorized them into different themes. Based on their written responses, we have several conclusions. To begin with, regarding the initial feelings when knowing the teaching assignment, the teachers generally showed negative emotions, such as ambivalence, anxiety, and nervousness. For instance, one teacher expressed uncomfortable feelings because of the belief that most students do not accept the HKNSL. Another teacher commented, "I had mixed feelings about teaching this lecture … Not only did I not want to recall the political incidents that took place in that period, but I also worried the teaching materials and discussion might provoke students' emotions." Some teachers suffered from anxiety for several weeks, and some had no appetite for a few days. Additionally, some teachers lacked familiarity with related law and its contents, which was another primary concern. They were not confident enough to teach this lecture.

Regarding the preparation process, colleagues used different means to prepare for this lecture. Sure enough, most teachers expressed that conquering anxious feelings would be a must. After that, a thorough study of the materials would be essential. Some teachers studied the materials, made physical and mental rehearsals, and revised the materials to ensure they deeply mastered the knowledge and contents. One teacher wrote, "I started to prepare this lecture and my teaching early and spent much time on it. Particularly, I studied each slide of the PPTs carefully to ensure I understood and mastered the knowledge and content at a deeper level. I gradually built up my confidence in delivering this lecture." Additionally, some colleagues utilized various platforms to enrich their knowledge about the related issues and facilitate the students' in-depth understanding, such as searching for online forums, comparing with international cases, designing interactive activities, or integrating videos. Equally important, some teachers made good use of mock teaching and reflected that the feedback from other colleagues was constructive in evaluating their teaching. One colleague shared, "The mock teaching helped me understand and evaluate my own teaching based on the feedback of my colleagues … whether my way to interact with students is appropriate or not, and whether I could explain the knowledge clearly and confidently to students."

In terms of the teaching experiences, the teachers shared that the lecture was generally smooth and positive. For instance, one teacher shared, "I was fluent in elaborating the knowledge points and content of the lecture." Additionally, some teachers shared that the generally smooth teaching might be due to the efforts made in thorough preparation. To illustrate, one teacher wrote, "I utilized some polling, games, quizzes, and climbing exercises. I also prepared little gifts for the participants. The students liked these games."

However, they also highlighted some negative experiences, such as the difficulty in motivating students to participate in the discussion. One teacher shared, "The anxiety certainly has affected the teaching performance negatively. I noticed the pace of my speech was a lot faster than usual; I made less eye contact with my students, and the lecture was much less interactive than usual due to my anxiety. It was not ideal." Additionally, some teachers were not satisfied with the pace of the lecture, the interaction during the course, and the time management issue.

Concerning the students' responses, both positive and negative responses were mentioned. Most teachers expressed that the students were generally active, cooperative, and responsive. The teacher was encouraged by students' positive sharing and active involvement in class. One teacher wrote, "I noticed that some of them had a good understanding of the history, and they could give me some examples of social instability worldwide. Additionally, they were able to talk about the concepts of social order, Chinese history, morality, law-abiding, and security. I was really impressed and encouraged by them. The sharing and involvement from students also encouraged me to keep on teaching confidently." Moreover, the interaction between students and groups was also encouraging in some lectures.

Nonetheless, some teachers found that some students were hesitant to express their views during class. For instance, one teacher reported, "Some students were not ready or open-minded in accepting the teaching content … Some students were passive." One teacher found that the students in the two classes were relatively silent compared to the previous lectures, as "Most of them were not involved in group discussion in the beginning. They had hesitation to talk about their opinions." Nonetheless, the negative response of students did not demotivate the teacher but encouraged the teacher to reflect more on the teaching. One teacher shared, "This helped me to understand that students are discontented, and they are unwilling to be attentive in class." Moreover, the teachers tried to understand the students' situation, which facilitated the teacher-student interaction. As one teacher wrote, "I guessed that they were worried about other students' response, so they chose not to say anything during lectures." One teacher shared how he/she engaged the student successfully, "Then I chose to walk around the classroom, approached every single student, and invited them to answer the questions. After that, most of the students in the classroom were involved in the discussion."

The teachers also perceived that the students benefitted from the lecture, particularly their understanding of law abidance leadership and the HKNSL. Some teachers were glad that the students were eager to learn and had developed an understanding of this topic. Moreover, another teacher observed that some students expressed their feelings in the post-class evaluation questionnaire, which were generally positive. One teacher believed that "The theories and concepts included in the lecture had stimulated students' thinking and helped them understand the importance of sustaining political and economic stability in Hong Kong, especially after what happened in our society in 2019 and 2020." Another teacher perceived that "All students got the chance to know more about the HKNSL and understand the offenses covered in the HKNSL. A number of students found the lecture educational and meaningful. Some students also reflected that they had reviewed the quality of law abidance from a new perspective."

When discussing the challenges, the teachers highlighted several obstacles in teaching this lecture, particularly in engaging the students in discussing this sensitive topic. One teacher shared, "Some students are quite worried that their answers will be recorded, and they are unwilling to share their views in class." Moreover, some teachers shared difficulties in the allocation of time for the different parts of the lecture appropriately, managing two groups of students simultaneously (face-to-face and online modes under Hybrid learning), engaging the students, realizing the need to have more real-life applications, and exploring ways to promote student interest and motivation to learn. For instance, one teacher wrote, "It is quite challenging to find some relevant materials related to their discipline … in other faculties, it is difficult to find evidence to show how it is directly related to their professions." The challenges also facilitated the teachers to think about how to engage the students effectively. For instance, one teacher shared two areas to improve, namely, utilizing the first part of law-abiding leadership as the foundation for introducing this topic and focusing more on the facts and information instead of adding personal viewpoints and interpretations in the HKNSL part.

Finally, despite their initial negative experience, teachers felt that the HKNSL teaching helps to promote their professional development and well-being. For instance, some teachers reflected that "It is important to keep in mind what our standpoint is when we deliver the message to the students. Also, I need to understand and clarify my goals in that lesson." Additionally, the concepts of national security also facilitated the teachers to reflect and understand social issues from a much wider angle. One teacher wrote, "In the past, I have not given much thought to concepts such as law abidance and the importance of stability; I realized these are indeed important elements if one were to lead a big team, to manage a company, or even a country." Some teachers also reflected on their teaching style attentively, as one wrote, "I learned to execute different teaching styles when I am facing different kinds of students … I need to slow down my pace and repeat the questions before I invite some students to share their answers." Moreover, some teachers talked about ways to improve their teaching in future. To illustrate, one teacher shared that early preparation, better time management, building up confidence, and active practice and reflection are useful in teaching this topic. Additionally, one teacher claimed that "It is necessary to have a smooth transition and build the linkage between each topic in this leadership course." Another teacher reflected, "This experience helped me see my weaknesses and pushed me to reflect on my professionalism as an educator."

This study is important for Hong Kong for several reasons. Firstly, the present findings are generally consistent with the post-lecture evaluation findings based on the students' feedback (Shek et al., 2022e). From a triangulation point of view, the findings based on different stakeholders underscored the positive perceptions of both students and teachers using different methods (post-lecture evaluation versus qualitative written responses). Although the effort to understand students' responses to teaching and learning is widespread in education, related data based on teachers are sparse. Still, the teacher is a significant stakeholder responsible for teaching. As national security education is a very new and sensitive topic, teaching this topic is challenging. Moreover, as the "social event may emotionally influence the teachers," we need to understand their teaching experience. Additionally, understanding the teachers' teaching experience can help us develop appropriate training for them (Shek & Wai, 2008; Shek et al., 2017), such as reducing their negative experiences and promoting their positive experiences in teaching law abidance leadership. Equally important, understanding teachers' views can help provide an alternative perspective on program evaluation, which can help triangulate findings based on different sources. Thus, there is a need to understand the views of teachers thoroughly. This study can contribute to examining the perceived effectiveness of national security and law abidance education.

In short, we conducted a qualitative evaluation study to understand teachers' experiences of teaching National Security Law. Results generally showed that the teachers had positive teaching experiences and perceived that the lecture was beneficial to the students.

13.6 Evaluation Based on the Views of the Teachers (Shek et al., 2022b)

Obviously, asking teachers to teach the HKNSL curriculum is also an anxiety-provoking task for them. In the evaluation study (Shek et al., 2022d), eight teachers shared that they generally had negative emotions when they knew that they had to teach a 3-h lecture on law abidance leadership and the HKNSL. These negative emotions included surprise, uncomfortable feelings, mixed feelings, panic feelings, anxiety, as well as nervousness. Some teachers even suffered from insomnia and loss of appetite for several weeks before teaching this topic. Therefore, there is a need to understand the feedback of the teachers teaching this subject. A previous study demonstrated that teachers generally had positive perceptions of the curriculum, the lecture, and students' benefits. They also agreed that the teaching helped their personal and professional development (Shek et al., 2022d). As the previous study was based on a HyFlex teaching mode, there is a need to replicate the findings under the online mode. Therefore, the study conducted by Shek et al. (2022b) intended to examine the views of the teachers of the HKNSL education via a qualitative methodology in Semester 2 of the 2021/22 academic year.

Eight teachers who taught this subject were invited to complete an open-ended questionnaire, and all teachers responded anonymously. They were invited to talk about different perspectives regarding teaching, including (1) the preparation, (2) the responses of the students, (3) the teaching experience, (4) the challenges encountered, (5) the benefits for students, (6) the benefits for teachers, and (7) reflections after teaching this subject. The qualitative data demonstrated that the teachers had positive experiences with teaching the HKNSL.

To begin with, the teachers agreed that preparation before the lecture helped them be physically and psychologically prepared for the teaching, including reviewing the teaching materials, memorizing the Articles, revising the PPT slides, searching for online information, and seeking advice from colleagues and professionals. For example, one teacher reflected, "I reviewed all the PowerPoint materials a few times and tried to strengthen the linkages between different parts of the contents." Another teacher stated that they "searched for information from all kinds of discussion forums and news regarding this topic. As the HKNSL is new to Hong Kong, we need more cases to illustrate the application of the HKNSL to real life." The participants also highlighted the importance of mock teaching and remarked that the design and quality of the lecture could be continuously reviewed and improved. To illustrate, one teacher stated that "With comments from different colleagues in the mock teaching, I have understood more about my problems and shortcomings, which helped me to improve my teaching further." Moreover, some teachers did mental and physical rehearsals before teaching and utilized various online platforms to engage students.

From the students' perspectives, the teachers observed that the students showed positive responses. However, some were "passive" and "quiet," probably because of the topic's sensitive nature. For instance, some teachers recalled that "many students had active participation in the class," "the students freely expressed their views during the lecture," and "those non-local students, for instance, students from mainland China, were more active in responding to my questions, and foreign students were more likely to share their personal views." Nevertheless, some teachers remarked that the students might feel uneasy sharing their ideas. For example, one teacher commented that students preferred listening when the contents were related to ordinances and cases. Another teacher said that "Local Hong Kong students tended to accept the HKNSL passively since they thought that the general public had no say in the HKNSL." Despite all the difficulties, most teachers agreed that patience, respect, and acceptance would promote student engagement.

Additionally, teachers generally had positive teaching experiences. One teacher was glad that "My positive experience comes from students' generally active participation in the lecture. Their sharing demonstrated their serious and careful thinking about the issue and understanding of the importance of abiding by the law." Equally important, some interactive games and activities could facilitate students' participation. For example, one teacher shared that the students enjoyed different activities that helped them understand and enjoy the lecture.

Despite the positive responses, the teachers also shared some challenges. One significant area for improvement is delivering the content interactively and interestingly. Moreover, some students participated passively in the discussion as the topic was quite sensitive. Delivering rich content within a limited time also required appropriate time management skills.

Significantly, the teachers generally perceived that the students benefitted from law-abiding education. Some teachers reflected that "The content of the lecture would encourage the students to think about the importance of abiding by the law, the importance of law to society, and the importance of being law-abiding citizens as university students." One teacher shared, "The lecture would provide more comprehensive and objective information about the HKNSL, which may challenge their previous concepts or understanding. In addition, based on the post-lecture evaluation of this lecture, most of the students had positive ratings on the design, teaching, and benefits of this lecture." More importantly, since the discussion of myths and realities was an essential part of this lecture, more students shared that "This lecture helped them clarify some myths and misconceptions about the law." However, students may not be able to reveal what they really think about the HKNSL, one teacher believed that "The subject can provide a platform to create dialogues for students with different political stands. As the university is a place for students to acquire knowledge, it is good to have such an academic platform to discuss the HKNSL." Equally important, one teacher claimed that "Some misconceptions toward the HKNSL were somehow eliminated by receiving useful materials and acquiring new knowledge." Additionally, some sharing from students was received as well. For instance, one student wrote in the post-lecture evaluation, "This lecture facilitated us to shoulder up our civil responsibilities after attending the lecture."

Essentially, the teachers experienced personal and professional growth in the process. For example, one teacher shared "This lecture has broadened my horizon and enhanced my law-abiding quality." The teachers were facilitated to reflect on their role as educators. As one wrote, "Good teacher both teaches students solid knowledge and inspires students by their characters, thoughts, and behaviors." Another teacher commented, "We share responsibility for the peace and welfare of the whole country. Moreover, this teaching increased my citizenship awareness and social responsibility and benefited my well-being as a good citizen." Regarding professional development, one teacher said, "I should be open-minded and show my acceptance to my students, and be ready to respond to their questions, opinions, and emotional responses." Additionally, some teachers reported they had enhanced time management and planning skills. One teacher also shared that resilience has been promoted in teaching the HKNSL education and that teaching this lecture helped him/her overcome challenges and manage some psychological hurdles (e.g., uncertainty and instability). The sharing demonstrated that the teachers experienced personal and professional development of themselves and their students, including shouldering great responsibility in educating the students on the HKNSL and gaining more knowledge and positive changes in their attitudes.

Remarkably, the study summarized several factors in invitational education (e.g., 7Ps) that contributed to positive learning outcomes of implementing a law-abiding leadership program, which included (1) physical and psychological "preparation" before the lecture; (2) "practice makes perfect" as mock teaching or rehearsal helped them understand their limitations and areas for improvement; (3) reflecting upon constantly "preconceptions" about the HKNSL and related education; (4) supporting teachers to have "professional and personal development" can help them eliminate anxiety and stress; (5) "perceptions of students" regarding their views on the program, teacher, benefits, and law abidance leadership are equally important; (6) "positive interaction" facilitates active discussion and reflection in class, including respect, acceptance, building up trust, and open exchange of views; and (7) "post-lecture evaluation" through different strategies is needed to understand the impact of law-abiding leadership education. Adequate training and support for teachers teaching the HKNSL education are essential.

Above all, the findings suggest that teachers have positive experiences with the HKNSL education based on law-abiding leadership for university students, although some challenges should be addressed and resolved.

13.7 Evaluation Based on the Views of the Teachers (Shek et al., 2023a)

The HKNSL was enacted in 2020. According to Article 10, educational institutions, including universities, are responsible for educating students with a basic understanding of the HKNSL. We have launched a 3-h law-abiding leadership education program to promote law abidance in university students. Thus, a qualitative evaluation of the programs was conducted to understand teachers' perceptions of the program. In contrast to the previous two studies based on HyFlex and online teaching, this lecture was delivered face-to-face in the first semester of the 2022/23 academic year. As the delivery mode differs from the hybrid mode and online mode adopted before, there is a need to explore whether the teachers' views differ from the previous study.

Nine teachers were invited to respond to several open-ended questions where they were free to narrate their teaching experience, and seven teachers responded to the questionnaire voluntarily and anonymously. The questionnaire contained several aspects, including (1) the preparation and the role of previous teaching; (2) own teaching experience; (3) challenges encountered; (4) responses of the students; (5) perceived benefits to students; (6) professional development and well-being of teachers; and (7) reflections and learning from teaching.

The study summarized their response into the following perspectives. In terms of preparation, teachers generally use a wide range of strategies to prepare for the class, and they consider their previous teaching experience to be helpful. For instance, one teacher responded, "The previous teaching is beneficial and meaningful as I became more familiar with the lecture content." In addition, one teacher stated that "both the positive and negative experiences helped me possess a certain technique in teaching the HKNSL and gave me some sense of reassurance." Another teacher said, "My previous teaching experiences gave me lots of insights on how to prepare for the contents and acquire the related information more systematically."

Regarding their teaching process, teachers generally reported positive experiences. To illustrate, one teacher said, "The teaching experiences were very positive, and my students paid much attention during the case discussion." Moreover, another teacher responded, "In general, my experience is quite positive as both lectures went smoothly, and the overall atmosphere was quite positive." Nevertheless, a few teachers presented negative experiences as well. For example, "Some students shook their head slowly when I introduced the court cases" and "A few students were not ready for this lecture and showed some emotions toward the teaching content."

Nevertheless, the teachers also demonstrated challenges from different categories, including (1) the challenges from the students, such as some students falling asleep, some students stating that they were too tired to try the quiz, and some students having difficulty in attending the morning class punctually; (2) the challenges arose from the teaching process as previously stated. For example, students tended to keep silent in class and avoid discussion when they had some solid political stands on critical cases. Moreover, some students even refused to answer questions in class when the teacher invited them; and (3) challenges related to the teacher. For instance, their prejudice made the teachers need to be more open during discussions and take more initiative in inviting students to give feedback. Moreover, some teachers experienced anxiety as they could not predict students' responses and reactions.

Concerning how to cope with the challenges, the teachers reflected that better preparation is the key to conquering challenges. To illustrate, one teacher would "have detailed planning on each part of the lesson. In this way, the allocation of time was considered carefully, and my pace in face-to-face teaching was well-adjusted. More interactive and vivid pedagogical design was developed to attract students' attention and allow them to participate and share their views." Furthermore, some reflected that teachers should accept students' standpoints and be proud of the students' braveness and openness on such issues. One teacher shared the technique for engaging the student, "I struggled to balance the space for students' authentic sharing and the concerns of keeping class order. To overcome this challenge, I followed three principles when designing relevant in-class activities, namely anonymous response, unconventional format, and neutral feedback."

From the students' responses, the teachers reflected that many students agreed that the lecture was educational and meaningful. The students' responses were generally positive, and the teachers believed that law abidance leadership education was helpful to the students. Specifically, the teachers received feedback from the students after the lecture, such as "the HKNSL protects our country," "I learn more about the actual benefits of the HKNSL," and "I have learned more concepts about national security and its importance." From the responses of students, a teacher perceived that "Students showed a good understanding of the HKNSL, potential behaviors that might violate the law, and the consequences of a law violation. Some students admitted that they think the HKNSL limits individual freedom. It allowed the class to discuss and recap the logic behind the social contract theory." Moreover, one teacher was glad that "students were cooperative and responsive. I prepared some interactive games and activities, and the students were keen to participate. The students mainly considered that the activities conducted helped them understand and enjoy the lecture." More students shared their appreciation and gain in the post-lecture evaluation. For instance, one student agreed that this lecture helped them to clarify some misconceptions about the HKNSL. Some students also reflected that they had the chance to review their law-abiding qualities from a new perspective. More importantly, some international students also showed their appreciation of this lecture as they were able to gain a good understanding of the HKNSL. Remarkably, students' positive responses encouraged the teachers to prepare well and teach confidently.

Besides, the teachers also reflected positively on professional development, pedagogy development, and teaching methods. To present some examples, one teacher said, "This lecture provided a chance for me to understand what the HKNSL is and the four offenses more specifically." Moreover, one teacher agreed that "the whole process is beneficial to me as well. In particular, I did benefit a lot from our team's mock teaching training sessions. During the process, very useful feedback and constructive suggestions were collected from the supervisor and teammates. I can refresh my understanding of the HKNSL through my teaching." Additionally, one teacher learned to be more open-minded in discussing sensitive content with students, and this experience also helped the teacher explore his/her strengths and weaknesses in teaching. Equally important, the teachers had the opportunity to reflect on their emotions, values, and teaching careers. Instead of being nervous and stressed for several weeks, one teacher shared, "I followed my pace this time. Specifically, I added some personal experiences to share, and these personal elements made me feel comfortable." Moreover, one teacher responded, "I have developed a higher acceptance of uncertainty since teachers could not have developed the intention to predict and control the students' reactions." More importantly, some teachers became "more aware that facilitating students' development should be the priority in teaching and learning, although such priority may not always align with their political stance." The teachers agreed that this lecture has enhanced their law-abiding quality and understanding of the importance of national security law in safeguarding Hong Kong's interests and people's well-being.

One unique feature of this study is to examine the perceived impact of teaching on one's professional development and well-being. Three reasons are shown for the well-being of teachers. Firstly, teachers may encounter challenges in teaching without well-being. For example, a teacher overwhelmed by anxiety would have reduced teaching efficacy in teaching law abidance leadership. One teacher reflected that he/she experienced headaches and insomnia in the previous semesters and was too nervous and scared to say something wrong or trigger the students' emotions. They realized that it was not right to anticipate that the lectures would be accepted and liked by everyone. The teacher agreed that unpredictable reactions from the students made the classes exciting and inspirational, and they were inspired to think about how to respect others' views and express their opinions peacefully. Secondly, intrinsic rewarding experiences may facilitate the development of teachers' well-being. As one new teacher shared, "I was glad I could adopt student-centered learning in my classes. Although my teaching experience was limited, I could utilize the opportunities to recognize and accommodate different learning modalities in my three classes." If teaching has a negative impact on teachers, there is a need to review the pedagogies and teaching methods. Finally, poor teacher well-being suggests the need to enhance training for teachers. The teachers appreciated the arrangement of mock teaching and writing post-teaching reflection, which helped them critically evaluate and improve their teaching. Concerning these considerations, the teachers were invited to conduct this qualitative study to understand their views.

Remarkably, the present study highlights several observations. To begin with, the teachers perceived law-abiding leadership education to be beneficial to the students. However, some students showed negative responses, and most shared positive experiences. Teachers also had positive teaching experiences, although they also experienced different challenges. Moreover, teachers gained experience while preparing and teaching, which also contributed to their positive teaching experiences. Overall, the findings supported the value of law-abiding leadership education from the teachers' perspective. From the replication perspective, the current findings echoed the previous findings (Shek et al., 2022b, 2022d). Together with the evaluation findings on the hybrid and online modes (Shek et al., 2021, 2022a), the present findings also provide additional insights into the value of law abidance leadership education in face-to-face teaching and learning.

The evidence implies that the teachers had a positive learning experience, and law abidance leadership education benefits their development. The findings also demonstrate that the program was well-designed and the teaching process was positive. There are few studies on teaching law abidance leadership in the scientific literature, so the present findings constitute constructive evidence in this field.

13.8 A Recent Evaluation Study Based on Post-lecture Evaluation (Li et al., 2023)

One important attribute of science is replicability. That is, research findings can be found in different studies involving different samples and time. To further consolidate the evaluation findings based on the face-to-face law abidance leadership program, we conducted another post-lecture evaluation study with the involvement of 1285 undergraduate students who responded to a post-lecture evaluation measure with 26 items. Consistent with the previous findings, factor analyses showed that there were three dimensions underlying the 26 items (program attributes, teacher attributes, and attitudes toward law-abiding education).

To understand the perceptions of university students taking the program ($N = 1285$), we employed a 26-item post-lecture evaluation questionnaire to conduct a subjective outcome evaluation. Using two randomly generated samples, multi-group confirmatory factor analyses (CFA) showed that there are three dimensions intrinsic to the scale (e.g., lecture attributes, teachers' qualities, and appreciation of law abidance). The findings replicated the previous findings and provided support for the construct validity of the instrument. Concerning the perceptions of the 3-h module, students generally had positive views of the program and the teachers. Most importantly, most students perceived that the program had a positive impact on their psychosocial competencies, including critical thinking, problem-solving abilities, moral competence, and appreciation of the importance of national security. Besides, almost all students indicated their willingness to be law-abiding and responsible citizens. The qualitative responses are also overwhelmingly positive. In particular, students generally felt that they learned much about law abidance and national security.

13.9 Special Issue on Law Abidance Leadership

The above papers are based on the responses of undergraduate students as well as the teachers teaching the 3-h law abidance leadership. Besides the HKNSL program for undergraduate students, we have also developed several other programs for other students. First, a 3-h online program (as well as a 7-h self-study) was developed for Senior Year and Articulation Degree Program students. Second, we have developed two 3-h programs (as well as 3-h self-study) designed for Taught Postgraduate Degree programs, with one program in English and another program in Chinese. Finally, another 3-h program (as well as 3-h self-study) was developed for Research Postgraduate Students. Consistent with our belief about the importance of evaluation, we have also conducted evaluations and prepared a special issue (Shek & Merrick, 2023) with the following papers:

- Focus group evaluation of national education in Hong Kong: Postgraduate students' perceptions
- Evaluating the impact of a National Education program on taught postgraduate students in Hong Kong
- Online National Security Law (NSL) education in Hong Kong: Qualitative evaluation based on focus groups
- Evaluating the effectiveness of an online National Education program for research postgraduate students in Hong Kong: A multidimensional approach
- Qualitative evaluation of law abidance leadership education for undergraduate students in Hong Kong: Focus groups
- Subjective outcome evaluation of an online program on law-abiding leadership
- Effectiveness of a National Education program for undergraduate students in Hong Kong: Subjective outcome evaluation.

The findings based on the above studies suggested that students generally had positive views toward the course attributes, law-abiding leadership, and the self-paced online learning mode. Based on the qualitative and quantitative findings, several observations can be drawn. First, the results indicated that the course attributes were viewed positively by students, and they perceived the course as positively impacting their personal and interpersonal development. Specifically, students found the design and content of the course appealing and believed that it provided opportunities for reflection and critical thinking, which are important for shaping them into successful leaders. Second, most students held positive views toward the self-paced online learning mode, as they believed it could enable them to assimilate knowledge more efficiently according to their circumstances. Meanwhile, they are allowed to access the course video and lecture notes quickly. As pointed out by Tullis and Benjamin (2011), allowing students to allocate their learning time and contents freely can help promote positive learning performance and outcomes while enhancing their memory. Therefore, it can be inferred that students gained a positive learning experience and benefited from the self-paced learning mode, which is conducive to their learning motivation and outcomes and their understanding of national education. Moreover, as some postgraduate students choose to obtain a professional diploma part-time in addition to their regular work, self-paced online learning provides them with flexible time without moving to the site of study. Third, given that national education involves politically sensitive topics, some students in Hong Kong may have opposing or controversial views, expressing resistance toward law-abiding education regarding national security and the HKNSL (Yiu, 2022). Therefore, e-learning mode is a good choice to create a safe and comfortable environment for students to explore knowledge themselves. Asbury and Orsborn (2020) argued in their study of cultural safety e-learning that "A private and independent e-learning package can provide students with a safe environment to encounter challenging concepts and improve their understanding of sensitive topics." Flexible e-learning modules are beneficial for students who have already been familiar with these sensitive topics as well as those encountering the concepts for the first time. Students significantly improved their knowledge and understanding of national security law while being comfortable with the course content and delivery mode.

13.10 Discussion and the Way Forward

We can draw several observations based on these studies. First, different stakeholders had positive views of the design of the lecture, although there were different views on the need to cover modern Chinese history. Our view is that to help students understand the HKNSL, there is a need to give students an understanding of what happened from the Opium War until the founding of the People's Republic of China (e.g., a century of national humiliation). The students' responses showed that they did not seem to have a good understanding of modern Chinese history. Also, there were different views on whether there is a need for a 3-h lecture. We respond that face-to-face interaction is important for teaching politically sensitive topics. Taken as a whole, most of the students and teachers were optimistic about the design of the subject, which is encouraging in view of the highly sensitive nature of the topic.

The second observation is that students were generally satisfied with the class arrangement. In particular, they appreciated the interactive nature of the classes. As the topics are politically sensitive, having interaction and discussion among the students is very important. Besides, although some students mentioned that the level of interaction among the students and involvement of the students was lower than in the other lectures, the ratings for the overall class atmosphere were generally positive. Students also participated positively during class. As the HKNSL is a very sensitive topic, interaction through discussion and sharing among students is very important. Even if there are different viewpoints, constructive interaction is the key to understanding the nature of the HKNSL and the related issues better.

The third observation is that the students had positive views about the teachers. Teachers are important agents in HKNSL education. First, they teach the knowledge of national security and the HKNSL. Second, they clarify issues and questions surrounding the HKNSL. Third, they facilitate discussion and sharing among the students. Fourth, they help to integrate different views. Fifth, they strive to empower the students and help them deal with related issues in a balanced manner. Sixth, they encourage and admonish the students to be law-abiding leaders. Finally, teachers support students in gaining an understanding of national security and the HKNSL.

The fourth observation is that both quantitative and qualitative findings showed that students experienced the benefits of the HKNSL education, including personal development, problem-solving skills, critical thinking, interpersonal communication skills, and understanding of the crucial attributes of successful leaders. These gains in "soft skills" are essential skills for the holistic development of university students. In fact, these qualities are consistent with the desired graduate attributes of PolyU and are essential leadership qualities for future leaders.

The fifth observation is that the students showed positive perceptions of the importance of law abidance as leadership qualities, and they realized the importance of law-abiding behavior for the stability of a society. Besides, students and teachers felt that the HKNSL education program promoted the students' knowledge and understanding of national security. Furthermore, different stakeholders agreed that they understood the nature, related offenses, importance, and myths of the HKNSL. Most importantly, students responding to the surveys and participating in the focus groups pointed out that they would try their best to serve as a law-abiding citizen and a socially responsible leader.

The sixth observation is that students did not feel that the HKNSL education was brainwashing. The teachers also felt that the HKNSL education was helpful to students in understanding more about the HKNSL. From the teachers' narratives, they did not feel that they had the duty to brainwash the students. The position we keep on reiterating has several elements. First, it is the choice of an individual as far as law-abiding behavior is concerned. Second, as freedom is not unlimited, one should seriously consider not to "step the red line" because there would be legal consequences. Third, students should understand national security and the HKNSL. Fourth, as educators, we encourage and admonish students to follow the HKNSL.

Finally, from the three studies involving the sharing of the teachers, we noticed that teachers showed development in teaching the HKNSL. In the beginning, teachers were stressed and anxious, and they had difficulties in taking up the teaching. However, with peer support, training, and mock teaching (Shek et al., 2022b), the teachers eventually acquired the skills to teach the 3-h program. Of course, one issue faced by some teachers is that they had to orientate to the HKNSL because of the complex feelings surrounding the social event. As time went on, we witnessed the positive experiences and feelings expressed by the teachers.

Concerning the way forward, we should consider several tasks. First, we need more evaluation work, such as conducting a controlled trial involving a control group and collecting longitudinal data across time. Second, we have to keep on refining the curriculum because there is a new development in the cases violating the HKNSL. Besides, based on the comments of the students, we should re-think about trimming the curriculum and re-organizing the materials. Third, as teachers are essential in teaching knowledge and facilitating student discussion and sharing, training is necessary. It would be helpful to develop a training manual so that new teachers can benefit from systematic training. Finally, as part of the scholarship of teaching and learning, it would be helpful to disseminate the research findings regarding pedagogy development and evaluation.

Acknowledgements The preparation of this chapter is financially supported by The Hong Kong Polytechnic University (ZZ4U and ZZUE), Li and Fung Endowed Professorship in Service Leadership Education, Wofoo Foundation, and the Matching Fund of Research Grants Council (ZECL and ZH4Q).

References

Asbury, E., & Orsborn, G. (2020). Teaching sensitive topics in an online environment: An evaluation of cultural safety e-learning. *Whitireia Nursing and Health Journal,* (27), 23–31. https://doi.org/10.3316/informit.116170908231195

Keyes, C. L. M. (1998). Social well-being. *Social Psychology Quarterly, 61*(2), 121–140.https://doi.org/10.2307/2787065

Li, X., Shek, D. T. L., Dou, D. Y., Zhu, X. Q., & Wu, X. (2024). Law abidance leadership education for university students in Hong Kong: Subjective outcome evaluation. *Applied Research in Quality of Life, 19*, 683–708. https://doi.org/10.1007/s11482-023-10260-2

Ngai, G., & Shek, D. T. L. (2022). *Service-learning capacity enhancement in Hong Kong higher education* (Vol. 14). Springer Nature. https://www.polyu.edu.hk/apss/docdrive/2022award/5.5.7.pdf

Ridley, G. (2011). National security as a corporate social responsibility: Critical infrastructure resilience. *Journal of Business Ethics, 103*, 111–125. https://doi.org/10.1007/s10551-011-0845-6

Shek, D. T. L., Chan, C. H. M., & Zhu, L. Z. (2022a). Online teaching of a leadership course under COVID-19: Evidence based on two semesters. *International Journal of Child and Adolescent Health, 15*(1), 29–40.

Shek, D. T. L., Chau, C. C., Mok, B. P., Chai, W. Y., Cheng, N. S., Shek, V., Ho, W., Chiu, T. Y., & Chak, Y. (2022b). Teachers' experience in law-abiding leadership education: Replication across time. *International Journal of Child Health and Human Development, 16*(1), 27–39.

Shek, D. T. L., Chau, C. C., Mok, B. P., Chak, L. Y., Cheng, N. S., Shek, K. F., Li, P. K., & Xiao, Z. (2023a). Education on law-abidance leadership: Does face-to-face teaching matter? *International Journal of Child Health and Human Development, 16*(1), 89–102.

Shek, D. T. L., Dou, D. Y., Zhu, X. Q., & Li, X. (2022c). Law abidance leadership education for university students in Hong Kong: Post-lecture evaluation. *Frontiers in Psychology, 13*, Article 994448. https://doi.org/10.3389/fpsyg.2022.994448

Shek, D. T. L., Ho, W., Leung, E., Li, P., Mok, B., Shek, V., & Shek, E. (2021). Nurturing leadership qualities under COVID-19: Student perceptions of the qualities and effectiveness of online teaching and learning on leadership development. *International Journal of Child and Adolescent Health, 14*(1), 89–100. https://ira.lib.polyu.edu.hk/bitstream/10397/93770/1/Shek_Nurturing_Leadership_Qualities.pdf

Shek, D. T. L., Li, X., Dou, D. Y., & Zhu, X. Q. (2022d). Teachers' experiences in law abidance leadership education: A qualitative study. *International Journal of Child Health and Human Development, 15*(1), 73–84. https://www.polyu.edu.hk/apss/docdrive/2022award/5.2.5.pdf

Shek, D. T. L. & Merrick, J. (2023). Hong Kong National Security Law education programs [special issue]. *International Journal of Child and Adolescent Health, 16*(4).

Shek, D. T. L., Pu, E. X. P., & Wu, F. K. Y. (2017). Evaluation of the training program of the Tin Ka Ping PATHS Project in mainland China. *International Journal of Child and Adolescent Health, 10*(2), 189–199.

Shek, D. T. L., Tang, V. M. Y., & Han, X. Y. (2005). Evaluation of evaluation studies using qualitative research methods in the social work literature (1990–2003): Evidence that constitutes a wake-up call. *Research on Social Work Practice, 15*(3), 180–194. https://doi.org/10.1177/1049731504271603

Shek, D. T. L., & Wai, C. L. Y. (2008). Training workers implementing adolescent prevention and positive youth development programs: What have we learned from the literature. *Adolescence, 43*(172), 823–845.

Shek, D. T. L., Zhu, X. Q., Dou, D. Y., & Li, X. (2023b). National security law education in Hong Kong: Qualitative evaluation based on the perspective of the students. *International Journal of Environmental Research and Public Health, 20*(1), 553. https://doi.org/10.3390/ijerph20010553

Shek, D. T. L., Zhu, X. Q., Li, X., & Dou, D. Y. (2022e). Satisfaction with HyFlex teaching and law-abiding leadership education in Hong Kong university students under COVID-19. *Applied Research in Quality of Life, 17*(5), 2833–2858. https://doi.org/10.1007/s11482-022-10040-4

Tullis, J. G., & Benjamin, A. S. (2011). On the effectiveness of self-paced learning. *Journal of Memory and Language, 64*(2), 109–118. https://doi.org/10.1016/j.jml.2010.11.002

Van Druten, V., Bartels, E., Van de Mheen, D., De Vries, E., Kerckhoffs, A., & Nahar-van Venrooij, L. (2022). Concepts of health in different contexts: A scoping review. *BMC Health Services Research, 22*(1), 389. https://doi.org/10.1186/s12913-022-07702-2

Yiu, W. (2022, December 09). Universities in Hong Kong will require students to pass national education courses before graduating. *South China Morning Post.* https://www.scmp.com/news/hong-kong/education/article/3202750/universities-hong-kong-will-require-students-pass-national-education-courses-graduating

Yu, L., Lin, L., Shek, D. T. L., & Chai, W. Y. (2022). Students' perceived attributes and benefits of a leadership course: Subjective outcome evaluation. *Research on Social Work Practice, 32*(2), 199–214. https://doi.org/10.1177/10497315211042823

Zhu, X. Q., & Shek, D. T. L. (2021). Subjective outcome evaluation of a positive youth development program in Mainland China. *Research on Social Work Practice, 31*(3), 285–297. https://doi.org/10.1177/1049731520980802

Chapter 14
Reflections and the Way Forward

Daniel T. L. Shek

Abstract This chapter starts by introducing and then discussing the criticisms of the four credit-bearing subjects on leadership and Service-Learning (SL). Then, several responses to these criticisms are presented. In particular, we highlight the importance of non-cognitive and 21st-century skills in response to the growing service economy and growing student mental health issues in the higher education sector. Finally, we highlight several lessons learned from using credit-bearing leadership and SL subjects to promote the holistic development of university students. These include the use of good conceptual frameworks, utilizing innovative pedagogies, embracing positive teaching philosophy, value evaluation, disseminating teaching experience and impact, rethinking sustainability, and deepening the impact of the credit-bearing leadership and SL subjects.

Keywords Credit-bearing subjects · Leadership · Service-learning · Non-cognitive skills · Holistic development · University students

14.1 Introduction

In the early days, when we proposed to offer credit-bearing subjects on leadership and service-learning (SL), colleagues always asked why there was a need to develop such subjects. For the leadership subjects, colleagues argued that not every student is (and can be) a leader, and we do not have adequate time to train leaders within a subject. Some also believed that leadership is the monopoly of elite students and that those with mediocre academic achievement do not possess leadership qualities. For the SL subjects, colleagues argued that community service is a waste of time and that it would be better to allocate the related credit hours to the major subjects. These comments have been made not just at the beginning but also throughout the past decade. In particular, when the undergraduate program is so packed with many subjects, everybody wants to free up some credits for their major programs. While we genuinely respect such views, we always invite colleagues to consider the following responses.

D. T. L. Shek, *Promoting Holistic Development in University Students*, Quality of Life in Asia 17, https://doi.org/10.1007/978-981-96-0251-3_14

14.2 The Need for Leadership and Service-Learning Subjects

14.2.1 *Higher Education is Facing Tremendous Changes*

The first response is that students in the higher education sector are facing a changing global ecology. These changes include the emergence and growing service economy, increased emphasis on the importance of technology and innovation, and growing demand for entrepreneurship skills and start-up experiences for graduates. Such changes in the economic and technological landscape obviously demand new skill sets in university students. When we talk about "Industry 4.0," what matters most are innovative thoughts, creativity, problem-solving, resilience, emotional management, teamwork, and conflict-resolution skills, which are usually referred to as "non-cognitive," "soft skills," or 21st-Century skills. Besides economic transformation, graduates are expected to engage in entrepreneurial activities such as start-ups. Again, to start a business, intellectual skills alone are not enough. Graduates working in start-ups need to possess resilience, emotional competence (e.g., keep calm when facing setbacks), self-discipline, self-leadership, spirituality (e.g., clear goals and meaning in their work), and interpersonal communication skills.

With particular reference to China, its economy is shifting from manufacturing to service economy, with roughly half of the GDP arising from service industries, which highlights the growing demand for Service Leadership qualities in young people. In particular, for a considerable number of university graduates in China, nurturing Service Leadership qualities is an important task. The same situation applies to Hong Kong, where service industries contribute to 93% of the GDP. When Hong Kong's economy relies heavily on service industries, we should ask whether undergraduates possess adequate Service Leadership qualities. In one case reported by the media, a university graduate with a Master's degree could not find a job after sending over 200 application letters. He said in an interview that he might lack communication skills, but the teachers did not teach such skills. Hence, this case reminds us about the importance of cultivating soft skills in undergraduate students.

Besides, we should not neglect the changing and dynamic political landscape in the international, regional, and local contexts. As such, university students should also acquire skills such as cultural competence, respect, acceptance, and communication skills. In particular, conflict resolution skills are at the top of the agenda, namely how to have healthy competition and peace at the same time. Essentially, service leaders should be able to resolve conflicts among different parties and arrive at a "win–win" instead of a "lose-lose" situation.

14.2.2 Adolescent Developmental Issues

The second response is that we should constructively respond to adolescent developmental issues. In Hong Kong, students in high school have many developmental challenges (Shek et al., 2011), including mental health problems, materialism, and sexuality issues. In a study on adolescent materialism, we found that a high proportion of young people were materialistic, although they thought that they were not as materialistic as the general adolescent group in Hong Kong (Shek et al., 2019c). In another study on adolescent egocentrism, many young people were found to be egocentric, although they also perceived that they were less egocentric than the general adolescent population in Hong Kong. Furthermore, we found some character issues in young people, such as cheating, dishonesty, and integrity problems (Zhou et al., 2021). Developmentally speaking, we have to note the challenges faced by university students who are commonly transiting from adolescence to early adulthood. According to Shek et al. (2019a), emerging adulthood is a period with many challenges, including personal, interpersonal, vocational, family, and social adjustment.

Obviously, although university administrators commonly assume that university students are "problem-free," Shek and Wong (2011) argued that adolescents' developmental challenges do not disappear by themselves. In fact, there are tons of studies highlighting that college students are suffering from various mental health concerns, such as depression, suicide, and substance abuse (American College Health Association, 2022; Lipson et al., 2022). In fact, specific mental health programs are instituted in universities in the West (Breet et al., 2021), including suicide prevention programs (American Foundation for Suicide Prevention n.d.), substance abuse prevention programs (NCSSLE, 2017), and depression prevention programs (Rith-Najarian et al., 2019).

Specifically, Shek and Cheung (2013) outlined that university students are suffering from behavioral problems, including addiction (e.g., alcohol, Internet addiction, and cyber-pornography addiction), sleep problems, and interpersonal conflicts. Moreover, psychological well-being issues such as depression, anxiety, and suicide are not uncommon in university students. The third issue surrounds the development of personal goals, confidence about oneself, and materialism. The final issue is their relationship to society, which includes egocentrism and civic engagement. During the COVID-19 pandemic, some research suggested that the prevalence of depression, anxiety, and Internet addiction among university students is worrying (Li et al., 2021). Due to online teaching and economic constraints, the pandemic has also imposed many problems for university students (Shek et al., 2021, 2023b). We also observed that the problem continues during the post-pandemic era (Shek, 2024).

In a paper examining the developmental context of children and adolescents in Hong Kong, Shek and Siu (2019) summarized several risk factors that contribute to their "unhappiness," which include "unhealthy values," "lack of emphasis on holistic development," "hopelessness," "morbid emphasis on academic excellence," "economic disadvantage," and "problematic family development." Obviously, such developmental influences persist when young people study in universities. While it is not easy to change the external ecological environment, it would be helpful and feasible to strengthen the competencies and leadership qualities through leadership and SL subjects.

Besides, as emerging adults, university students also encounter developmental issues, such as the transition from high school to university, gradual disengagement from the family and the parents, preparation for work life, and transition to the dynamic adult world (Shek et al., 2019a). Such transitions are intense for adolescents when they begin to disengage from the family and parents. Hence, we propose that credit-bearing Leadership and SL subjects can help promote adolescent psychological well-being and holistic development.

14.2.3 The Importance of Cultivating Soft Skills

The third response is that there are theories supporting the importance of cultivating soft skills in young people. Using developmental assets as building blocks, the Search Institute highlights the importance of soft skills presented under 40 developmental assets. These include competence, positive values, and positive identity that can be cultivated by Leadership and Service Leadership subjects. In the 5C/6C model proposed by Richard Lerner, the building blocks of healthy development include "connection, competence, character, confidence, and contribution," which are intimately related to leadership and SL subjects. With respect to 21st-century skills, many theorists argue for the importance of non-cognitive skills, including emotional competence, resilience, social relationships, and cultural competence. For example, in the model on transversal skills proposed by UNESCO (2013), six sets of transversal skills are proposed, including "critical and innovative thinking skills," "interpersonal skills," "intrapersonal skills," "global citizenship skills," "media and information literacy skills," and "competencies valued by one's country or economy." According to the concept of "non-cognitive" skills, multifaceted levels of skills, such as "creativity, innovation, reflection, communication, flexibility, optimism, resilience, empathy, and self-awareness," are emphasized (Shek et al., 2023a). Finally, character and virtues are emphasized. For example, in the Value in Action model, 24 character strengths are fundamental to human development, such as "creativity, gratitude, honesty, bravery, hope, and humility" (Peterson & Seligman, 2004).

14.2.4 The Lack of Psychosocial Competence Courses in Universities

The fourth response is that leadership skills in terms of psychosocial competencies are emphasized in primary and secondary school education in many countries and regions. For example, SEL programs have been implemented worldwide (Corcoran et al., 2018), including in European countries (Berg et al., 2022) and Australia and Asia–Pacific (Collie et al., 2017). In Singapore, the SEL framework has been adopted since 2005 to enhance the positive development of children and adolescents in schools. The framework acts as the "organizing structure" for schools to implement and evaluate programs and courses to enhance students' learning experiences (Chong & Lee, 2015). It has been adopted across different levels of schools and formulated as the "Framework for Twenty-First Century Competencies and Student Outcomes" (Liem et al., 2017). In China, scholars have refined the original SEL framework and designed a "six-dimensional SEL framework." The MoE-UNICEF SEL program was officially implemented in 2012 in 11 provinces and regions with the aim to address changes and challenges in the current curriculum and enhance students' SEL competencies (Yu & Jiang, 2017). Moreover, SEL education in Korea, which began with moral and ethical education, has been closely embedded in character education since early 2010. When came to 2015, more K-12 schools were integrating "whole-person education" to cultivate the SEL skills of students, such as "Promoting Alternative Thinking Strategies and Strong Kids" for Grade 3–8 students and "Thinking-Feeling-Behaving" for K-12 students (Lee & Bong, 2017).

Nevertheless, most SEL frameworks or approaches mainly focus on children and youth at the K-12 level, and few attempts have been made to tackle the social and emotional issues faced by adolescents and emergent adults in higher education (Conley, 2015). Obviously, the need for SEL education does not decrease or diminish when students enter universities. Hence, schools and practitioners need to recognize the value of SEL in higher education to cultivate adolescents to be healthy, caring, and contributing citizens.

14.2.5 Chinese Culture Reinforces the Value of Non-cognitive Skills

Fifth, Chinese culture highlights the importance of character and virtues, which are essentially non-cognitive skills. For example, "*Di Zi Gui*" ("*Standards for Being a Good Student and Child*") outlines the desired qualities of a child, such as modeling people with virtues and compassion and loving other people. Based on an analysis of the different chapters in the book, Shek and Law (2019) pointed out the importance of self-cultivation, self-reflection, and learning from people with virtues. In another family instruction book by Zhu Hsi, the qualities of an ideal child include filial piety, duty, loyalty, and honesty (Chang, 2021). These emphases are, in fact, consistent with the recent proposal of Positive Psychology that character strengths and virtues are important developmental goals.

14.2.6 Enhance the Psychosocial Well-Being of Adolescents

The sixth response is that there is a wealth of empirical evidence showing the importance of non-cognitive skills and psychosocial competencies in shaping positive developmental outcomes. With specific reference to positive youth development (PYD) attributes, Shek et al. (2023a) emphasized that focusing on non-cognitive competence empowers young people to embrace the idea that "Everyone is Number One." Cultivating non-cognitive skills and abilities redefines the meaning of "achievement," which can enhance the well-being of adolescents. Shek et al. (2019b) highlighted that SEL programs could promote the students' quality of life. Zhou et al. (2021) confirmed that qualities of moral character are positively related to adolescents' responsible behavior and life satisfaction, and responsible behavior is positively related to life satisfaction. Additionally, the research showed that moral character has a positive impact on adolescents' well-being, which supported the value of the PYD approach.

Shek (2013) showed that courses with PYD elements are positively related to adolescents' psychosocial competencies and mental well-being. In terms of adolescents' behavioral problems, Zhu and Shek (2020) conducted a longitudinal study and proposed that PYD attributes mediated concurrent and future delinquency behaviors of adolescents. Moreover, the quality of self-identity and general PYD attributes were negatively related to delinquency, while life satisfaction acted as a mediating factor. Cognitive-behavioral competence was also positively related to adolescents' delinquency. The study confirmed that PYD attributes have a predictive impact on participants' life satisfaction and delinquency. More importantly, the study emphasized the importance of PYD attributes and proposed that cultivating PYD qualities is a practical approach to reducing adolescents' delinquency. Shek and Israelashvili (2023) concluded that PYD programs can reduce risk behaviors among adolescents, such as substance abuse, violence, consumption of tobacco, alcohol, and video gaming problems. Additionally, PYD programs such as the P.A.T.H.S. project can cultivate adolescents' developmental assets, such as "moral competence," "positive identity," and "general PYD attributes." The programs enable adolescents to develop psychosocial skills, which facilitate them to react to various psychosocial challenges, stressors, and changes in their daily lives.

14.2.7 The Effectiveness of Leadership and Service-Learning Subjects

The final response is that there is strong support for leadership and SL subjects in our case. For Tomorrow's Leaders, plenty of studies have been conducted to show its effectiveness. Firstly, objective outcome evaluation studies showed that students experienced positive changes after taking this subject. Besides, quasi-experimental studies showed that this subject is effective in cultivating cognitive-behavioral competence. In a review regarding its effectiveness, Shek (2019) concluded that the subject is impactful in enhancing the psychological well-being of students. Secondly, regular subjective outcome evaluation studies revealed that students generally evaluated the subject, teachers, and benefits positively. In particular, they agreed that their competencies in different areas (such as emotional competence and resilience), as well as their holistic development, were enhanced after taking this subject. Third, qualitative findings such as focus groups and reflection exercises also pointed to the value of the subject. Students remarked that the subject is very relevant to their needs, and they learned many skills, such as being empathetic and having effective communication with others. In the past decade, many students have asked why they must study leadership. Our direct answer is to invite them to look at the evaluation findings, particularly the positive views of the students.

For Service Leadership, we similarly argue that the positive evaluation findings speak for the value of this subject. Many studies analyzed pretest and posttest data and confirmed that students benefit from the subject positively, and such positive changes also occurred during the COVID-19 pandemic. For instance, students showed positive changes in different developmental outcomes, including "PYD attributes" and "Service Leadership qualities (values, attitudes, and skills)." In these studies, we also showed that changes in Service Leadership attributes were related to changes in students' mental health. Besides, quasi-experimental studies revealed that students in the experimental group developed better than students in the control group. We also conducted subjective outcome evaluations regularly using a validated student feedback questionnaire. Results consistently revealed that the students evaluated the subject (such as the design and class atmosphere) and the instructors (such as their professionalism and concern for the students) positively, and they viewed that there were many benefits of taking this subject (such as promotion of holistic development and specific psychosocial skills). Finally, qualitative evaluation using focus groups and qualitative reflection exercises highlighted students' positive learning experience as well as their gains from the subjects.

In the "Promotion of Children and Adolescent Development" subject, we have implemented it in Hong Kong and offshore. Different evaluation studies showed that the subject was effective in cultivating the holistic development of the students as well as the service recipients. Shek et al. (2022) found that the subject has a positive impact on both teachers and students in terms of their competence, care, and social responsibility. Teachers were empowered to act as youth resource mobilizers to help students explore their potential and develop social responsibility. At the same time, the students are willing to make active contributions to enhance the well-being of society. Lin and Shek (2021) employed the "Chinese Positive Youth Development Scale" in their research and found that this subject has a positive impact on students' PYD competencies, service leadership qualities, and life satisfaction. Similarly, in the subject "Service Leadership through Serving Children and Families with Special Needs," research showed that students benefited a lot in terms of holistic development. In the study conducted by Leung et al. (2021), both objective and subjective outcome evaluation findings supported the conclusion that the project benefited the students and the service recipients in terms of PYD attributes and service leadership. Ma et al.

(2019) applied qualitative and quantitative methods in their study and found that both students and service recipients evaluated the subjects positively. We also found that the impact of this SL subject was very good during the COVID-19 pandemic.

14.3 Lessons Learned and Issues to Be Addressed

14.3.1 Using Good Conceptual Frameworks to Guide the Development of the Subjects

There are several lessons we have learned from our experience gained in the past 12 years. The first lesson is to use good conceptual frameworks to guide the development of evidence-based leadership and SL credit-bearing subjects. For Tomorrow's Leaders, we developed the curriculum based on the PYD framework. Actually, before we designed and implemented the leadership program, we had been working on a PYD program entitled Project P.A.T.H.S. in the high school context, which has been shown to promote the holistic development of the program participants. Hence, we always regard "Tomorrow's Leaders" as a university version of Project P.A.T.H.S. in Hong Kong, which aims to cultivate the PYD attributes of university students. As we have mentioned, research studies have underscored the value of PYD attributes and PYD programs.

For Service Leadership, we have utilized the Service Leadership Theory proposed by Po Chung, which highlights the importance of competence, character, and care in leadership. The theory adopts an ecological model and emphasizes the importance of Chinese values in leadership, such as the "dark side" of leadership in light of Confucian thoughts. Finally, we used experiential learning theory (e.g., focus on learning by doing and reflection) and civic engagement model (e.g., understanding the needs of the community and attempting to solve them) to develop the pedagogy of SL.

Several issues need to be resolved in the future. The first issue is to further align the needs of university students (e.g., emergent adults) with models of leadership and SL models. For example, with law abidance as a growing challenge in Hong Kong, the topic of law abidance leadership has been incorporated in Tomorrow's Leaders. Second, it would be exciting to examine the possible integration of Western models on leadership and SL into indigenous Chinese concepts and philosophies. For example, with reference to the Chinese Confucian virtues, Po Chung formulated the "dark side" of service leadership. For SL, it would be conceptually stimulating to integrate the Chinese concepts of care and humanity.

14.3.2 Utilization of Innovative Pedagogies

The second lesson learned is that innovative pedagogies play an essential role in effective leadership and SL subjects. In traditional pedagogy, which is commonly used by Chinese teachers, a one-way didactic teaching mode is adopted with passive involvement and loose student engagement in the teaching and learning process. In contrast, we adopted interactive pedagogies through active student involvement to promote learning effectiveness in these subjects. For the leadership subjects, we used many interactive approaches, including group reflection, role-play, group presentation, and games, to engage the students and promote student reflection (Shek et al., 2020). For the SL subjects, asking students to write SL proposals can empower them to investigate the needs of their service targets and develop a sense of empathy, which eventually promotes their sense of civic-mindedness and civic engagement.

There are several issues surrounding the pedagogies of the leadership and SL subjects. First, it would be helpful to develop curriculum manuals for the leadership subjects. There are two advantages to doing so. The first advantage is that it can standardize the teaching through a manualized approach, particularly when a group of teachers is involved. Secondly, teaching manuals would help new teachers to understand the subjects. For Service Leadership, we have already developed a blended learning curriculum program, which was used during the COVID-19 pandemic. Another issue is the constant updating and revision of the curriculum in view of the changing needs of the students and societal circumstances. For example, with the need to strengthen law abidance in university students, we have included curriculum materials on law abidance and the Hong Kong National Security Law in Tomorrow's Leaders. Besides, to increase the flexibility of teaching under COVID-19, we have developed 24 videos (15 animated videos and 9 case-based videos) to facilitate teaching and learning in the subject. Third, technological advances (AR, VR, and the metaverse) provide many opportunities for the further development of pedagogies.

14.3.3 Teachers Need to Embrace Positive Teaching Philosophy

The third lesson is that the teachers have to "buy-in," including understanding and trying to identify with the teaching philosophy of the subjects developed. This lesson is crucial. Without identification with the teaching philosophy (e.g., believing that students have the potential to be leaders), it would not be easy to reinforce this belief in class. Besides, teachers have to reflect on their teaching methods, such as using interactive teaching methods to promote student engagement and motivation to learn. The practice is not easy because teachers are generally not trained to teach using experiential learning strategies. Hence, regular meetings with the teachers and support networks are essential to promote teacher engagement and empowerment.

There are two issues related to teaching engagement and empowerment. The first issue is teacher training. Besides regular team meetings, there is a need to provide adequate training for colleagues. For example, when we were forced to change from face-to-face teaching to online teaching during the COVID-19 Pandemic in 2020, we organized workshops for teachers to familiarize themselves with online learning platforms (Blackboard) and conducted mock teaching using online teaching. Another example is the teaching of law abidance leadership. When we decided to include National Security Law education under leadership education, colleagues were very anxious and stressed because of two reasons. Firstly, they did not know the reactions of the students. Moreover, they were worried that students would have negative responses to National Security Law education. The second issue is how to empower teachers and promote teacher well-being in their teaching. Using National Security Law education as an example again, we have strived to empower teachers to teach and re-iterate our position of not brainwashing the students. We have strived to respect the views of the students. At the same time, we upheld our role as educators to encourage and admonish them to be law-abiding citizens as well as to discuss issues related to NSL education.

14.3.4 Appreciate the Importance of Evaluation

The fourth lesson is to appreciate the importance of evaluation in assessing the quality of the subjects and the impact of teaching and learning on the students. For teachers, it may be a self-fulfilling prophecy to "feel" that one is teaching well. However, one essential indicator of whether one teaches well is the learning outcomes of the students. Hence, systematic evaluation is an important consideration. In these four subjects, we employ several evaluation strategies to understand how teaching influences students and what their changes are. Firstly, objective outcome evaluation is applied by collecting self-report behaviors of the students. Through the collection of pretest and posttest data, we can have an idea of the changes in the students. Besides, with the addition of a comparison group, we can also rule out some of the threats to internal validity, such as the natural maturation of the students. The second strategy is subjective outcome evaluation, which is widely applied in universities. Through the use of standardized and validated scales, we can understand how students evaluated the program, teacher, and benefits. In our four subjects, besides the routine Student Feedback Questionnaire data collected by the University, we also collected data via a more validated subjective outcome evaluation tool (Yu et al., 2022). The third strategy is qualitative evaluation, which attempts to capture the students' subjective experiences and personal journeys. Through individual interviews, focus group interviews, reflection exercises (e.g., metaphors and descriptors for the subjects), and personal journals, we have collected qualitative data to evaluate students' learning and personal experiences. Obviously, these evaluation mechanisms can serve as prototypes and pointers for colleagues who wish to evaluate their subjects in the future.

There are several issues for consideration here. First, we need different evaluation mechanisms for different subjects. For example, in SL subjects, we need to evaluate how SL subjects influence the service recipients as well as the community. Besides, looking at the personal journals of the students in SL subjects is helpful. For the Leadership subjects, we have to look at how the subjects nurture different leadership qualities in the students. It would also be helpful to examine the class dynamics as well. Second, teachers should be sensitive to the changes in the ecology and examine how such changes would affect student learning. For example, under COVID-19, it is a challenge to change the face-to-face learning to online and hybrid modes. The challenge is evident for online SL. In the same vein, one should ask whether leadership and SL subjects work well for different types of students (e.g., students from mainland China and international students).

The third issue is the evaluation methodologies involved. If human resources and financial resources permit, we should include a control group for comparison. However, this may not be easy for SL subjects where comparable control activities may not be easily arranged. Besides, for qualitative evaluation, it would be helpful if we could invite the different stakeholders to document their experiences throughout the learning process. Of course, many resources are needed for this kind of research, and it is not helpful for the junior staff, who usually need "quick" publications for tenure and appraisal exercises. Furthermore, besides collecting data from the students, we should also collect data from teachers, who can also be regarded as the primary stakeholders. The final issue is the long-term impact of these subjects. The fundamental questions are "What happens after graduation?" and "Have these subjects nurtured them to be better people?"

14.3.5 Disseminate the Experience and Findings

The fifth lesson is that it is essential to disseminate the teaching experience and evaluation findings (e.g., scholarship of Teaching and Learning). According to Boyer (1990), there are different types of scholarship (Almeida, 2010). As he remarked, "Scholarship means engaging in original research. However, the work of the scholar also means stepping back from one's investigation, looking for connections, building bridges between theory and practice, and communicating one's knowledge effectively to students. Specifically, we conclude that the work of the professoriate might be thought of as having four separate yet overlapping functions." These include "the scholarship of discovery; the scholarship of integration; the scholarship of application; and the scholarship of teaching" (p. 17). Specifically, scholarship of discovery (basic research) refers to "not just the outcomes, but the process, and especially the passion, give meaning to the effort" (p. 17); scholarship of integration (interdisciplinary research) means "doing research at the boundaries, where fields converge" (p. 19); scholarship of application (applied research) where "new intellectual understandings can arise out of the very act of application… theory and practice vitally interact, and one renews the other" (p. 23). Besides, scholarship of teaching (teaching research) is essential because "while well-prepared lectures surely have a place, teaching, at its best, means not only transmitting knowledge but transforming and extending it as well" (p. 24).

According to Darling (2003), "Scholarship of Teaching and Learning is work that encourages an empirical examination of teaching in relation to student learning. It is distinct from scholarly teaching in that it goes beyond teaching well, even superbly, to participating in a focused inquiry process and reflective practice about one's own teaching" (p. 47). McKinney (2004) similarly pointed out that "The scholarship of teaching and learning goes beyond scholarly teaching and involves the systematic study of teaching and/or learning and the public sharing and review of such work through presentations or publications. Clearly, there is a focus here on the product or outcome" (p. 8). Furthermore, Hutchings and Shulman (1999) highlighted that "Scholarship of teaching is not synonymous with excellent teaching. It requires a kind of 'going meta,' in which faculty frame and systematically investigate questions related to student learning" (p. 13).

In their discussion of the scholarship of teaching, Trigwell et al. (2000) pointed out that it seeks "to understand teaching by consulting and using the literature on teaching and learning, by investigating their own teaching, by reflecting on their teaching from the perspective of their intention in teaching while seeing it from the students' position, and by formally communicating their ideas and practice to their peers" (p. 164). Shulman (2002) argued that scholarship of teaching and learning inquires "into the consequences of one's work with students … an obligation that devolves on individual faculty members, on programs, on institutions, and even on disciplinary communities" (p. vii). Moreover, "Scholars of teaching and learning (SoTL) are prepared to mess with the world even more boldly than their colleagues who are satisfied to teach well and leave it at that. They mess with their students' minds and hearts as they instruct, and then they mess again as they examine the quality of those practices and ask how they could have been even more effective. SoTL are prepared to confront the ethical as well as the intellectual and pedagogical challenges of their work. They are not prepared to be drive-by educators. They insist on stopping at the scene to see what more they can do" (p. viii).

Shulman (2002) pointed out several reasons for SoTL. The first reason is professionalism, and professionals and educators have the responsibility to discover, connect, apply, teach, and pass on professional wisdom. The second reason is pragmatism, where SoTL supports improvement in teaching and promotes transparency. The third reason is policy. Through SoTL, teachers can demonstrate the extent to which the educational goals are achieved. SoTL also serves as an educational audit, strengthening accountability and assessment. Regarding the benefits of SoTL projects, Haigh (2010) highlighted several benefits, including enhanced learning, a vehicle to channel their views on teaching and learning, learning about research methods, understanding the learning of other students, engagement in reflection, engagement in inquiry and serve as co-inquirers, enhanced understanding of teaching professionals and teaching scholarship, know more about academic life, and appreciation of student-centered teaching.

14.3.6 Plan for the Sustainability of the Subjects

The sixth lesson is that we should have made forward planning, particularly with reference to the sustainability of the subjects. Using a SWOT analysis, we can have several observations. For strengths, we have four quality leadership and SL subjects, which are award-winning. We also have experienced teachers. We also regularly conduct evaluations of these subjects. However, there are two weaknesses. The first one is staff turnover, which means that we have to increase training. The second weakness is that there is a need to groom leaders for this teaching team who can take up responsibilities in a more proactive manner. Regarding opportunities, with growing importance attached to student holistic development and social responsibility, there are growing opportunities for offshore SL and leadership subjects. Concerning threats, because the income is based on student numbers, colleagues have to work hard to attract students for the SL subjects. Besides, as SL subjects operate on a competitive basis, sharpening the competitive advantage is an issue that needs to be considered. Furthermore, in view of the tight teaching space, whether the three credits of leadership development will be used for other purposes should be carefully addressed. Additionally, pending the retirement of Daniel Shek, the conductor and forerunner of these subjects, the question of how to succeed is a problem to be considered. In short, we need planning, nurturance of leadership, and marketing of the four subjects for the long-term sustainability of the subjects.

Besides SWOT analyses, colleagues should also highlight several arguments to "defend" the importance of these subjects. First, we should always be mindful of the importance of university students' development issues. The fundamental question is how we can help to reduce such problems and promote the positive development of the students. Second, the theoretical support for leadership and SL subjects, particularly from theories embracing the concepts of developmental assets and PYD, should be highlighted. Third, empirical support for the positive relationship between leadership and SL development and positive developmental outcomes in university students should be reinforced. Fourth, the empirical support shown by the evaluation findings should be emphasized. The most substantial support for the subjects should be the multifaceted evidence showing that they are making an impact and saving lives. Fifth, it highlights international recognition of the value of the subjects. Obviously, we do not develop and teach these subjects for the sake of getting teaching awards. The awards are consequences of our modest work.

14.3.7 Consolidate and Deepen Leadership and SL Education

The final lesson is that there is a need to consolidate and deepen leadership and SL education for university students. Our experience in the past decade is that different stakeholders, particularly the students, find the leadership and SL subjects to be beneficial for them. With reference to the challenges of the 21st-century and the service economy, we believe that leadership and SL education are fundamental to adolescents' holistic youth development.

Consistent with this belief, we have carried out several initiatives in the past decade. First, we have held two international conferences on Service Leadership. The first one was entitled "Service Leadership Education for University Students: Experience in Hong Kong," which included presentations on the Service Leadership development initiatives in the eight public universities under the Fung Service Leadership Initiative. With the support of the Victor and William Fung Foundation, the Fung Service Leadership Initiative (SLI) is a collaborative project of the Victor and William Fung Foundation, HKI-SLAM, and the eight UGC-funded universities in Hong Kong from 2012 to 2015. This collaboration constitutes a unique platform for curriculum development and related research for the participating universities. Each participating university can develop and design its curriculum materials to be aligned with the Service Leadership framework and the unique characteristics of the university concerned. Based on this symposium, we published a book entitled "Promoting Service Leadership Qualities in University Students: The Case of Hong Kong" (Shek & Chung, 2015). The second symposium, entitled "Service Leadership Education in Service Economies," was held in 2016 and concluded the efforts made by various universities over the past three years. We also published a special issue based on the presentations at the symposium (Shek et al., 2018).

Besides the two international conferences, we also conducted two symposiums to introduce leadership subjects to colleagues in the field. The first symposium, entitled "How to Promote Leadership Qualities in University Students via a Credit-bearing Subject?" was held in November 2020. In view of the transition of the manufacturing economy to a global service economy, we argue that it is necessary to promote 21st-century skills as well as intrapersonal and interpersonal competencies in university students. Besides, student mental health and adjustment problems are growing in higher education. To address these issues, we have developed and implemented a credit-bearing subject entitled "Tomorrow's Leaders" to nurture psychosocial competencies and ethical leadership in university students using a leadership framework. The whole-day workshop introduced a series of e-learning modules to teachers and allied professionals who were interested in implementing leadership subjects/programs in higher education institutions in Hong Kong. The second symposium, "Promoting Leadership Qualities of University Students in the Service Economy," was held in February 2021. As the service sector is the core of the economy of Hong Kong and contributes to over 93% of the GDP of Hong Kong, we urge educators to ask two fundamental questions: (a) "What are the attributes of effective leadership under the service economy, particularly with respect to 21st-Century skills, non-cognitive skills, social-emotional learning, and character development?" (b) "Do universities in Hong Kong nurture undergraduate students to be effective leaders via credit-bearing subjects and/or non-credit-bearing programs?" Through these two symposiums, colleagues can further understand the leadership subjects that we have developed and the associated vision and beliefs.

Finally, to promote Service Leadership to universities in mainland China, we have organized two international conferences on Service Leadership in May 2019 and September 2022, respectively. Besides, we have provided training to colleagues and students at the Southwestern University of Finance and Economics to conduct SL through teaching Service Leadership to the students (Zhou et al., 2022).

Acknowledgements The preparation of this chapter is financially supported by The Hong Kong Polytechnic University (ZZ4U and ZZUE), Li and Fung Endowed Professorship in Service Leadership Education, Wofoo Foundation, and the Matching Fund of Research Grants Council (ZECL and ZH4Q).

References

Almeida, P. A. (2010). Scholarship of teaching and learning: An overview. *Journal of the World Universities Forum, 3*(2), 143–154. https://doi.org/10.18848/1835-2030/CGP/v03i02/56669

American College Health Association. (2022). National college health assessment III: Undergraduate student reference group data report. *American College Health Association.* https://portal.acha.org/documents/ncha/NCHA-III_SPRING_2022_UNDERGRAD_REFERENCE_GROUP_DATA_REPORT.pdf

American Foundation for Suicide Prevention. (n.d.). *University and college campus suicide prevention.* American Foundation for Suicide Prevention. https://afsp.org/university-and-college-campus-suicide-prevention/

Berg, J., Diffenderffer, A., & Osher, D. (2022). School climate assessments: Measuring the conditions that support students' social and emotional competencies. In S. H. R. Jeremy Burrus, & M. W. Brenneman (Eds.), *Assessing competencies for social and emotional learning* (pp. 210–226). Routledge.

Boyer, E. L. (1990). *Scholarship reconsidered: Priorities of the professoriate.* ERIC. https://files.eric.ed.gov/fulltext/ED326149.pdf

Breet, E., Matooane, M., Tomlinson, M., & Bantjes, J. (2021). Systematic review and narrative synthesis of suicide prevention in high-schools and universities: A research agenda for evidence-based practice. *BMC Public Health, 21*(1), 1116. https://doi.org/10.1186/s12889-021-11124-w

Chang, H.-K. (2021). Zhu Zi's elementary learning-a Confucian outline of fundamental education. *Tsing Hua Journal of Educational Research, 38*(1), 1–41. https://doi.org/10.6869/THJER.202106_38(1).0001

Chong, W. H., & Lee, B. O. (2015). Social-emotional learning: Promotion of youth wellbeing in Singapore schools. In K. Wright, & J. McLeod (Eds.), *Rethinking youth wellbeing: Critical perspectives* (pp. 161–177). Springer. https://doi.org/10.1007/978-981-287-188-6_10

Collie, R. J., Martin, A. J., & Frydenberg, E. (2017). Social and emotional learning: A brief overview and issues relevant to Australia and the Asia-Pacific. In E. Frydenberg, A. Martin, & R. Collie (Eds.), *Social and emotional learning in Australia and the Asia-Pacific*, (pp. 1–13). Springer. https://doi.org/10.1007/978-981-10-3394-0_1

Conley, C. S. (2015). SEL in higher education. *Handbook of Social and Emotional Learning: Research and Practice*, 197–212. https://ecommons.luc.edu/cgi/viewcontent.cgi?article=1035&context=psychology_facpubs

Corcoran, R. P., Cheung, A. C., Kim, E., & Xie, C. (2018). Effective universal school-based social and emotional learning programs for improving academic achievement: A systematic review and meta-analysis of 50 years of research. *Educational Research Review, 25*, 56–72. https://doi.org/10.1016/j.edurev.2017.12.001

Darling, A. L. (2003). Scholarship of teaching and learning in communication: New connections, new directions, new possibilities. *Communication Education, 52*(1), 47–49. https://doi.org/10.1080/03634520302458

Haigh, N. (2010). *The scholarship of teaching & learning: A practical introduction and critique*. Auckland University of Technology. https://www.researchgate.net/profile/Neil-Haigh/publication/276922073_The_scholarship_of_teaching_and_learning_-_A_practical_introduction_and_critique/links/555c142208ae6aea0817313b/The-scholarship-of-teaching-and-learning-A-practical-introduction-and-critique.pdf

Hutchings, P., & Shulman, L. S. (1999). The scholarship of teaching: New elaborations, new developments. *Change: The Magazine of Higher Learning, 31*(5), 10–15. https://doi.org/10.1080/00091389909604218

Lee, S. K., & Bong, M. (2017). Social and emotional learning as a solution for adolescent problems in Korea. In E. Frydenberg, A. Martin, & R. Collie (Eds.), *Social and emotional learning in Australia and the Asia-Pacific*. Springer. https://doi.org/10.1007/978-981-10-3394-0_13

Leung, H., Shek, D. T. L., & Dou, D. Y. (2021). Evaluation of service-learning in project WeCan under COVID-19 in a Chinese context. *International Journal of Environmental Research and Public Health, 18*(7), Article 3596. https://doi.org/10.3390/ijerph18073596

Li, X., Shek, D. T. L., & Shek, E. Y. W. (2021). Offline victimization, psychological morbidity, and problematic online behavior among Chinese secondary school students. *International Journal of Environmental Research and Public Health, 18*(18), 9462. https://doi.org/10.3390/ijerph18189462

Liem, G. A. D., Chua, B. L., Seng, Y. B., Kamarolzaman, K., & Cai, E. Y. L. (2017). Social and emotional learning in Singapore's schools: Framework, practice, research, and future directions. In E. Frydenberg, A. Martin, & R. Collie (Eds.), *Social and emotional learning in Australia and the Asia-Pacific: Perspectives, programs and approaches* (pp. 187–203). https://doi.org/10.1007/978-981-10-3394-0_10

Lin, L., & Shek, D. T. L. (2021). Serving children and adolescents in need during the COVID-19 pandemic: Evaluation of service-learning subjects with and without face-to-face interaction. *International Journal of Environmental Research and Public Health, 18*(4), 2114. https://doi.org/10.3390/ijerph18042114

Lipson, S. K., Zhou, S., Abelson, S., Heinze, J., Jirsa, M., Morigney, J., Patterson, A., Singh, M., & Eisenberg, D. (2022). Trends in college student mental health and help-seeking by race/ethnicity: Findings from the national healthy minds study, 2013–2021. *Journal of Affective Disorders, 306*, 138–147. https://doi.org/10.1016/j.jad.2022.03.038

Ma, C. M. S., Shek, D. T. L., & Li, P. P. K. (2019). Service leadership through serving socially deprived students: Experience gained from corporate-community-university partnership (project WeCan). In D. T. L. Shek, G. Ngai, & S. Chan (Eds.), *Service-learning for youth leadership* (pp. 83–112). Springer Nature Singapore. https://doi.org/10.1007/978-981-13-0448-4_6

McKinney, K. (2004). The scholarship of teaching and learning: Past lessons, current challenges, and future visions. In C. Wehlburg & S. Chadwick-Blossey (Eds.), *To improve the academy* (Vol. 22, pp. 3–19). Anker Pub. Co. https://doi.org/10.1002/j.2334-4822.2004.tb00399.x

NCSSLE. (2017). *Campus drug prevention*. National Center on Safe Supportive Learning Environments. https://safesupportivelearning.ed.gov/resources/campus-drug-prevention

Peterson, C., & Seligman, M. E. P. (2004). *Character strengths and virtues: A handbook and classification*. Oxford University Press.

Rith-Najarian, L. R., Boustani, M. M., & Chorpita, B. F. (2019). A systematic review of prevention programs targeting depression, anxiety, and stress in university students. *Journal of Affective Disorders, 257*, 568–584. https://doi.org/10.1016/j.jad.2019.06.035

Shek, D. T. L. (2013). Promotion of holistic development in university students. *Best Practices in Mental Health, 9*(1), 47–61. https://www.ingentaconnect.com/content/follmer/bpmh/2013/00000009/00000001/art00005

Shek, D. T. L. (2019). Leadership qualities as a foundation of service learning: The Hong Kong experience. *International Journal of Child and Adolescent Health, 12*(1), 9–18.

Shek, D. T. L. (2024). Do student mental health problems disappear over night in the postpandemic Era? *The Journal of Adolescent Health, 74*(6), 1066–1067. https://doi.org/10.1016/j.jadohealth.2024.01.037

Shek, D. T. L., Chau, C. C., Zhou, K. J., Chu, C. K. M., Chu, K., & Li, A. T. (2023a). Nurturing holistic development of university students: The role of non-cognitive skills. *International Journal of Child and Adolescent Health, 16*(2), 111–122.

Shek, D. T. L., & Cheung, B. P. (2013). Developmental issues of university students in Hong Kong. *International Journal of Adolescent Medicine and Health, 25*(4), 345–351. https://doi.org/10.1515/ijamh-2013-0032

Shek, D. T. L., & Chung, P. (Eds.). (2015). *Promoting service leadership qualities in university students: The case of Hong Kong*. Springer. https://doi.org/10.1007/978-981-287-515-0

Shek, D. T. L., Chung, P. P., Lin, L., & Merrick, J. (2018). Service leadership education for university students [Special issue]. *International Journal on Disability and Human Development, 17*(1), 3–158.

Shek, D. T. L., Dou, D. Y., & Cheng, M. N. S. (2019a). Transition from adolescence to emerging adulthood. In D. T. L. Shek, & J. T. Y. Leung (Eds.), *The encyclopedia of child and adolescent development. (Volume 7: History, Theory, and Culture in Adolescence)*, (pp. 3145–3154). Wiley. https://doi.org/10.1002/9781119171492.wecad325

Shek, D. T. L., Dou, D. Y., Zhu, X. Q., & Chai, W. Y. (2019b). Positive youth development: Current perspectives. *Adolescent Health, Medicine and Therapeutics, 10*, 131–141. https://doi.org/10.2147/AHMT.S179946

Shek, D. T. L., & Israelashvili, M. (2023). The transition to secondary school: A definition and conceptualization of adjustment during adolescence. In M. Israelashvili (Ed.), *Prevention of maladjustment to life course transitions* (pp. 247–288). Springer. https://doi.org/10.1007/978-3-031-26700-0_10

Shek, D. T. L., Keung Ma, H., & Sun, R. C. F. (2011). A brief overview of adolescent developmental problems in Hong Kong. *The Scientific World Journal, 11*, 2243–2256. https://doi.org/10.1100/2011/896835

Shek, D. T. L., & Law, M. Y. M. (2019). "Di Zi Gui" (Standards for being a good student and child): Implications for children and youth development and parenting. *International Journal of Child & Adolescent Health, 12*(4), 403–418.

Shek, D. T. L., Li, X., Chak, Y. L. Y., & Lin, L. (2022). Service-learning in the context of business-community-university partnership: The project WeCan in Hong Kong. In G. Ngai & D. T. L. Shek (Eds.), *Service-learning capacity enhancement in Hong Kong higher education* (pp. 181–201). Springer. https://doi.org/10.1007/978-981-19-2437-8_10

Shek, D. T. L., Lin, L., Siu, A. M. H., & Lee, B. M. (2019c). Materialism in Chinese adolescents in Hong Kong: Profiles and socio-demographic correlates. *International Journal of Child Health and Human Development, 12*(3), 259–268.

Shek, D. T. L., & Siu, A. M. H. (2019). "UNHAPPY" environment for adolescent development in Hong Kong. *Journal of Adolescent Health, 64*(6), S1–S4. https://doi.org/10.1016/j.jadohealth.2019.01.007

Shek, D. T. L., & Wong, K. K. (2011). Do adolescent developmental issues disappear overnight? Reflections about holistic development in university students. *The Scientific World Journal, 11*, 353–361. https://doi.org/10.1100/tsw.2011.5

Shek, D. T. L., Zhao, L., Dou, D. Y., Zhu, X. Q., & Xiao, C. H. (2021). The impact of positive youth development attributes on posttraumatic stress disorder symptoms among Chinese adolescents under COVID-19. *Journal of Adolescent Health, 68*(4), 676–682. https://doi.org/10.1016/j.jadohealth.2021.01.011

Shek, D. T. L., Zhu, X. Q., & Dou, D. Y. (2023b). A mental health survey and the promotion of psychological well-being in university students under COVID-19. *Journal of Alternative Medicine Research, 15*(1), 9–173.

Shek, D. T. L., Zhu, X. Q., Dou, D. Y., Law, Y. M., Yu, L., Ma, M. S., & Lin, L. (2020). Nurturing holistic development in university students through leadership courses: The Hong Kong experience. In G. Tonon (Ed.), *Teaching quality of life in different domains. Social indicators research series* (pp. 61–80). Springer. https://doi.org/10.1007/978-3-030-21551-4_4

Shulman, L. (2002). Forward. In P. Hutchings (Ed.), *Ethics of inquiry: Issues in the scholarship of teaching and learning* (pp. v–viii). The Carnegie Foundation for the Advancement of Teaching.

Trigwell, K., Martin, E., Benjamin, J., & Prosser, M. (2000). Scholarship of teaching: A model. *Higher Education Research & Development, 19*(2), 155–168. https://doi.org/10.1080/072943600445628

UNESCO. (2013). *Transversal skills.* International Centre for Technical and Vocational Education and Training. Retrieved March 10, 2024, from https://unevoc.unesco.org/home/TVETipedia+Glossary/lang=en/show=term/term=transversal+skills#top

Yu, K., & Jiang, Z. (2017). Social and emotional learning in China: Theory, research, and practice. In E. Frydenberg, A. J. Martin, & R. J. Collie (Eds.), *Social and emotional learning in Australia and the Asia-Pacific: Perspectives, programs and approaches* (pp. 205–217). Springer. https://doi.org/10.1007/978-981-10-3394-0_11

Yu, L., Lin, L., Shek, D. T. L., & Chai, W. Y. (2022). Students' perceived attributes and benefits of a leadership course: Subjective outcome evaluation. *Research on Social Work Practice, 32*(2), 199–214. https://doi.org/10.1177/10497315211042823

Zhou, Z., Mu, L. P., Qi, S. J., & Shek, D. T. L. (2022). Service leadership through serving minority adolescents in rural China using a rural version of a positive youth development program. *Applied Research in Quality of Life, 19*, 3057–3079.https://doi.org/10.1007/s11482-022-10098-0

Zhou, Z., Shek, D. T. L., Zhu, X. Q., & Lin, L. (2021). The influence of moral character attributes on adolescent life satisfaction: The mediating role of responsible behavior. *Child Indicators Research, 14*(3), 1293–1313. https://doi.org/10.1007/s12187-020-09797-7

Zhu, X. Q., & Shek, D. T. L. (2020). Predictive effect of positive youth development attributes on delinquency among adolescents in mainland China. *Frontiers in Psychology, 11*, 615900. https://doi.org/10.3389/fpsyg.2020.615900

MIX
Papier aus verantwortungsvollen Quellen
Paper from responsible sources
FSC® C105338

If you have any concerns about our products,
you can contact us on
ProductSafety@springernature.com

In case Publisher is established outside the EU,
the EU authorized representative is:
Springer Nature Customer Service Center GmbH
Europaplatz 3, 69115 Heidelberg, Germany

Printed by Libri Plureos GmbH
in Hamburg, Germany